To George,

From Jeff Shula
1996

ADVANCES IN

Obstetrics and Gynecology

VOLUME 1

ADVANCES IN

Obstetrics and Gynecology

VOLUME 1

Editor-in-Chief
John A. Rock, M.D.
Chairman, Department of Gynecology and Obstetrics, Emory University School of Medicine, Atlanta, Georgia

Associate Editors
Sebastian Faro, M.D., Ph.D.
Chairman, Department of Obstetrics and Gynecology, University of Kansas, Kansas City, Kansas

Norman F. Gant, Jr., M.D.
Executive Director, American Board of Obstetrics and Gynecology; Professor, Department of Obstetrics and Gynecology, University of Texas, Southwestern Medical School, Dallas, Texas

Ira R. Horowitz, M.D.
Associate Professor, Department of Gynecology and Obstetrics; Director of Gynecologic Oncology, Emory University School of Medicine, Atlanta, Georgia

Ana A. Murphy, M.D.
Associate Professor, Department of Gynecology and Obstetrics, Emory University School of Medicine, Atlanta, Georgia

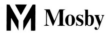 Mosby

St. Louis Baltimore Boston Chicago London Madrid Philadelphia Sydney Toronto

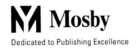

Mosby
Dedicated to Publishing Excellence

Vice President, Continuity Publishing: Kenneth H. Killion
Sponsoring Editor: Donna Steinhagen
Project Manager: Denise Dungey
Project Supervisor: Maria Nevinger
Proofroom Manager: Barbara M. Kelly

Printed in the United States of America
Composition by The Clarinda Company
Printing/binding by The Maple-Vail Book Manufacturing Group

Mosby-Year Book, Inc.
11830 Westline Industrial Drive
St. Louis, Missouri 63146

Editorial Office:
Mosby–Year Book, Inc.
200 North LaSalle Street
Chicago, IL 60601

International Standard Serial Number: 1070-5392
International Standard Book Number: 0-8151-7356-3

Contributors

Mark D. Adelson, M.D.
Clinical Associate Professor, Department of Obstetrics and Gynecology, State University of New York, Health Science Center at Syracuse College of Medicine, Crouse-Irving Memorial Hospital, Syracuse, New York

N. Scott Adzick, M.D.
Fetal Treatment Center and Division of Pediatric Surgery, University of California, San Francisco, School of Medicine, San Francisco, California

Kevin Ault, M.D.
Fellow in Infectious Diseases, Department of Gynecology and Obstetrics, University of Kansas School of Medicine, University of Kansas Medical Center, Kansas City, Kansas

Kathleen R. Cho, M.D.
Assistant Professor, Departments of Pathology, Oncology, and Gynecology and Obstetrics, The Johns Hopkins University School of Medicine, The Johns Hopkins Hospital, Baltimore, Maryland

Stephen H. Cruikshank, M.D.
Professor and Vice-Chairman, Obstetrics and Gynecology, University of Minnesota Medical School; Chief, Department of Obstetrics and Gynecology, Hennepin County Medical Center, Minneapolis, Minnesota

Randall C. Dunn, M.D.
Assistant Professor, Department of Obstetrics and Gynecology, Division of Reproductive Endocrinology, Baylor College of Medicine; Active Staff, Assistant Professor, St. Luke's Episcopal Hospital, The Methodist Hospital, Ben Taub General Hospital, Woman's Hospital of Texas, Houston, Texas

Gregory F. Erickson, Ph.D.
Department of Reproductive Medicine, University of California, San Diego, School of Medicine, La Jolla, California

Mark I. Evans, M.D.
Professor and Vice-Chief of Obstetrics and Gynecology, Professor of Molecular Biology and Genetics, Professor of Pathology, Director, Division of Reproductive Genetics, Director, Center for Fetal Diagnosis and Therapy, Wayne State University School of Medicine, Hutzel Hospital, Detroit, Michigan

Sebastian Faro, M.D., Ph.D.
Professor and Chairman, Department of Gynecology and Obstetrics, University of Kansas School of Medicine, University of Kansas Medical Center, Kansas City, Kansas

Andrew Friedman, M.D.
Associate Professor, Obstetrics, Gynecology, and Reproductive Biology, Harvard Medical School; Department of Obstetrics and Gynecology, Brigham and Women's Hospital, Boston, Massachusetts

Joseph W. Goldzieher, M.D.
Professor and Director of Endocrine Research (retired), Department of Obstetrics and Gynecology, Baylor College of Medicine, Houston, Texas

R. Ian Hardy, M.D., Ph.D.
Clinical Fellow, Obstetrics, Gynecology, and Reproductive Biology, Harvard Medical School; Department of Obstetrics and Gynecology, Brigham and Women's Hospital, Boston, Massachusetts

Michael R. Harrison, M.D.
Fetal Treatment Center and Division of Pediatric Surgery, University of California, San Francisco, School of Medicine, San Francisco, California

Lora Hedrick, M.D.
Instructor, Departments of Pathology, Oncology, and Gynecology and Obstetrics, The Johns Hopkins University School of Medicine, The Johns Hopkins Hospital, Baltimore, Maryland

Thomas J. Herzog, M.D.
Clinical Instructor, Fellow, Department of Obstetrics and Gynecology, Division of Gynecologic Oncology, Washington University School of Medicine, Barnes Hospital, St. Louis, Missouri

John Hesla, M.D.
Assistant Professor, Division of Reproductive Endocrinology, Director of In Vitro Fertilization, The Johns Hopkins University School of Medicine, Baltimore, Maryland

Mark P. Johnson, M.D.
Associate Director, Division of Reproductive Genetics, Center for Fetal Diagnosis and Therapy, Assistant Professor, Departments of Obstetrics/ Gynecology, Molecular Biology and Genetics, and Pathology, Wayne State University School of Medicine, Hutzel Hospital, Detroit, Michigan

L. Michael Kettel, M.D.
Assistant Professor of Reproductive Medicine, University of California, San Diego, School of Medicine, San Diego, California

Frank W. Ling, M.D.
Associate Professor, Division of Gynecology, Director, Residency Training Program, Department of Obstetrics and Gynecology, University of Tennessee, Memphis, College of Medicine, Memphis, Tennessee

Susan S. Martier, MSSA, BA
Research Assistant, Wayne State University School of Medicine; Associate Director, Fetal Alcohol Research Center, Hutzel Hospital, Detroit, Michigan

Bruce Patsner, M.D.
Professor, Clinical Obstetrics and Gynecology, University of Medicine and Dentistry of New Jersey; New Jersey Gynecologic Oncology, River View Medical Center, Newark, New Jersey

Janet S. Rader, M.D.
Assistant Professor, Department of Obstetrics and Gynecology, Washington University School of Medicine, St. Louis, Missouri

Harry Reich, M.D.

Director of Gynecologic Surgery, Department of Gynecology, Graduate Hospital, Philadelphia, Pennsylvania

Avihai Reichler, M.D.

Center for Fetal Diagnosis and Therapy, Departments of Obstetrics/Gynecology, Molecular Biology and Genetics, Wayne State University School of Medicine, Hutzel Hospital, Detroit, Michigan

Ramada S. Smith, M.D.

Fellow, Clinical Instructor, Wayne State University School of Medicine, Hutzel Hospital, Detroit, Michigan

Thomas E. Snyder, M.D.

Associate Professor, Department of Gynecology and Obstetrics, University of Kansas School of Medicine, University of Kansas Medical Center, Kansas City, Kansas

Robert J. Sokol, M.D.

Dean, Professor of Obstetrics and Gynecology, Wayne State University School of Medicine; Chairman of the Medical Board and Senior Vice President for Medical Affairs, Detroit Medical Center, Hutzel Hospital, Detroit, Michigan

David E. Soper, M.D.

Associate Professor, Departments of Obstetrics and Gynecology, and Medicine, Division of Infectious Diseases, Medical College of Virginia, Virginia Commonwealth University Medical College of Virginia, Richmond, Virginia

Thomas G. Stovall, M.D.

Associate Professor and Head, Section on Gynecology, Department of Obstetrics and Gynecology, Bowman Gray School of Medicine of Wake Forest University, Winston-Salem, North Carolina

Scott A. Washburn, M.D.

Assistant Professor, Section on Gynecology, Bowman Gray School of Medicine of Wake Forest University, North Carolina Baptist Hospital, Winston-Salem, North Carolina

Preface

Obstetrics and gynecology are perhaps the oldest forms of medical practice, founded on intuition and existing since the birth of humankind itself. Religious beliefs were intimately bound up in the birthing practices of different cultures—in some instances furthering an understanding of anatomy and the development of simple surgical tools and techniques but in many instances inhibiting any kind of progress. A few towering geniuses light the path from these ancient times to the beginnings of the modern eras—Galen, Soranus, Leonardo da Vinci, Fallopio, William Harvey—but their knowledge was not widely disseminated, nor could it be effectively implemented: the patient usually died. It was not until the mid-1800s that the concept of antisepsis was introduced and the late 1800s when ether anesthesia was discovered, thus making possible the beginnings of modern surgery. Now, almost exactly a century later, new technological developments in physics, material sciences, molecular and genetic biology, computer science, and communications have once again brought the field of obstetrics and gynecology to the brink of a new age.

In addressing the Johns Hopkins Historical Club in January 1901, the Canadian physician Sir William Osler eulogized the old century in the following words:

> In the fullness of time, long expected, long delayed, at last Science emptied upon /mankind/ . . . blessings which have made the century forever memorable; and which have followed each other with a rapidity so bewildering that we know not what next to expect. . . . Measure as we may the progress of the world . . . there is no one measure which can compare with the decrease of physical suffering in man, woman, and child when stricken by disease or accident. . . . This is the Promethean gift of the century to man.

As appropriate as these words were to the 19th century, they are equally descriptive of the 20th century and are prophetic of the unimaginable spiraling outward and upward that will take place in the field of medicine in the century that lies before us.

The Mosby series *Advances in Obstetrics and Gynecology* will chronicle what will undoubtedly be an exponential rate of development in this new age. This series will present practical information, current practices and techniques, and significant developments in procedures and clinical research. Volume 1 covers four major topics: gynecology, reproductive endocrinology, obstetrics, and gynecologic oncology; it is intended to serve as a baseline of information upon which future volumes can build to highlight advances in these various areas. Each future volume in the series will be devoted to a few broad topics selected from areas of significant advancement and areas of vital discussion.

I wish especially to thank our editors who have brought into focus the significant advances in obstetrics and gynecology that are represented in this volume. Professor and Department Chairman Sebastian Faro, M.D., Kansas University Medical Center; Professor Norman F. Gant, M.D., University of Texas Southwestern School of Medicine; and Associate Professors Ira R. Horowitz, M.D., and Ana A. Murphy, M.D., Emory University School of Medicine. The editors wish to thank not only the individual authors who contributed chapters to this volume but also Donna Steinhagen, assistant managing editor for this series, and Nancy G. Puckett, managing editor, for their help in the preparation of this volume.

It is with great pride that we present to you this 1994 inaugural volume of *Advances in Obstetrics and Gynecology*.

John A. Rock, M.D.
Editor-in-Chief

Contents

Contributors   *v*

Preface   *ix*

PART I.   General Gynecology

Hysteroscopy.
By Randall C. Dunn   3

   Historical Perspective   3

   Indications and Contraindications   3

   Complications of Hysteroscopy   6

   Technique   6

   Media for Hysteroscopy   8

   Therapeutic Hysteroscopy Considerations   10

Complications of Endoscopy.
By Scott A. Washburn and Thomas G. Stovall   13

   Surveys   13

   Descriptive and Cohort Studies   16

   Specific Complications   18

      Anesthesia-Related Complications   18

      Complications of Pneumoperitoneum   19

      Analgesic Complications   20

      Incision and Infectious Complications   20

      Bowel Injuries   21

      Urologic Injuries   21

      Vascular Injuries   22

      Veress Needle and Trocar Injuries   22

      Miscellaneous Complications   23

   Summary   23

The Role of Laparoscopy in Hysterectomy.
By Harry Reich   29

   Definitions   30

   Indications   31

   Contraindications   32

   Equipment   33

      Preoperative Preparation   34

      Positioning of the Patient   34

Total Laparoscopic Hysterectomy Technique 35
  Incisions 35
  Vaginal Preparation 43
  Exploration 43
  Ureteral Dissection 43
  Bladder Mobilization 43
  Upper Uterine Blood Supply 44
  Uterine Vessel Ligation 44
  Circumferential Culdotomy (Division of Cervicovaginal
    Attachments) 44
  Laparoscopic Vaginal Vault Closure and Suspension With
    McCall Culdoplasty 44
  Underwater Examination 45

Postoperative Considerations 45

Complications 45

Special Problems Related to Laparoscopic Hysterectomy ... 46
  Very Large Fibroid Uterus (16 Weeks' Size or Above) ... 46
  Stage IV Endometriosis 47
  Laparoscopic Uterosacral-Vaginal Suspension 50
  Laparoscopic Rectocele Repair 50

Scoring System 50

Conclusions 52

Update on the Diagnosis and Management of Ectopic
Pregnancy.
By Frank W. Ling and Thomas G. Stovall 55

Diagnosis 55
  History 57
  Physical Examination 58
  Laboratory Evaluation 60
  Sonography 64
  Invasive Testing 66
  Algorithms for Nonsurgical Diagnosis 68

Management 69
  Ruptured Vs. Unruptured Ectopic Pregnancy 69
  Surgical Approaches 71
  Nonsurgical Treatment 72
  Nontubal Ectopic Pregnancy 75

Summary 76

Pelvic Inflammatory Disease.
By David E. Soper 85

Epidemiology 85
Microbiology and Pathogenesis 85
  Fitz-Hugh−Curtis Syndrome 87
  Atypical Pelvic Inflammatory Disease ("Silent Salpingitis") ... 88

Diagnosis   88
   Endometrial Biopsy   91
   Ultrasound   91
   Laparoscopy   91
   Tubo-ovarian Abscess   92

Treatment   92
   Medical Treatment   93
   Surgical Treatment   96

Long-Term Sequelae   96

Prevention   96

Summary   97

Urinary Incontinence—Untying the Gordian Knot.
By Thomas E. Snyder   103

Scope of the Problem   103

Anatomy   106

Contemporary Concepts   107

Pathophysiology   111

Evaluation   117

Nonsurgical Management   124

Surgical Therapy   127

Summary   132

Vaginal Vault Prolapse—Prevention and Surgical Management.
By Stephen H. Cruikshank   141

Anatomy   141

Preventing Vaginal Prolapse at the Time of Hysterectomy   142

Preventing Enterocele   144

Adjunct Support to the Vaginal Cuff   148

Vaginal Vault Prolapse   153

Summary   155

PART II. Reproductive Endocrinology

Menopause—A Deficiency Disease.
By Joseph W. Goldzieher   159

Replacement Therapy   160
   Androgens   160
   Estrogens and Progestins   161
Osteoporosis   165
   Laboratory Workup   166
   Therapeutic Intervention   167
Summary   172

The Role of Gonadotropin-Releasing Hormone Agonists in Gynecology.
By R. Ian Hardy and Andrew J. Friedman   179

   Biochemistry, Pharmacology, and Drug Information   179
      Structure and Activity   179
      Mechanism of Action   180
      Bioavailability and Delivery Systems   182
      Initiation and Monitoring of Therapy   183
      Side Effects   184
   GnRH Agonist Therapy for Uterine Leiomyomas   187
      Mechanism of Action   188
      Preoperative GnRH Agonist Therapy   188
   GnRH Agonist Therapy for Endometriosis   189
      Mechanism of Action   190
      GnRH vs. Danazol   190
      Effects of Infertility in Patients With Endometriosis   190
      CA-125 Levels and Endometriosis   191
      Endometriomas   191
   GnRH Agonist Therapy for Ovulation Induction   191
      Ovulation Induction in the Patient With Polycystic Ovaries 191
      Use of GnRH Agonists in In Vitro Fertilization-Embryo
        Transfer   192
      Effect on Oocyte Quality and Granulosa Cell Function   194
      Prognostic Value of GnRH Agonist Response in In Vitro
        Fertilization-Embryo Transfer Cycles   194
      Effects of GnRH Agonists on Endometrial Receptivity   194
      Use of GnRH Agonists in Intrauterine Insemination Cycles   195
      Use of GnRH Agonists for Triggering Ovulation   195
   GnRH Agonists and Estrogen-Progestin Replacement Therapy   196
      Progestin Replacement Therapy   196
      Estrogen Replacement Therapy   197
   Emerging Applications With GnRH Agonists   198
      Premenstrual Syndrome   198
      Hirsutism   198
      Use of GnRH Agonists Before Endometrial Ablation   199
      Use of GnRH Agonists in Fibrocystic Breast Disease and
        Mastalgia   199
      Use of GnRH Agonists in Ovarian, Breast, and Endometrial
        Cancers   200
   Summary   201

Basic and Clinical Concepts in Ovulation Induction.
By L. Michael Kettel and Gregory F. Erickson   211

   Basic Advances in Ovulation Induction   211
      The Structure of the Follicle Compartment   213
      The Two-Gonadotropin/Two-Cell Concept   214

The Growth Factor Concept   215
The Ovarian Insulin-Like Growth Factor System Example   217
Clinical Advances in Ovulation Induction   219
Human Menopausal Gonadotropins   219
Superovulation   219
Human Menopausal Gonadotropin Cotreatment With
Growth Hormone   220
Pulsatile Gonadotropin-Releasing Hormone   221
Premature Ovarian Failure   222
Ovarian Ablation in Polycystic Ovary Disease   223
Summary   223

Current Concepts in Assisted Reproductive Technology.
By John S. Hesla

                                                              231
Controlled Ovarian Hyperstimulation for In Vitro Fertilization 231
Treatment Schedules   231
Progesterone Monitoring   237
The Luteal Phase   238
Micromanipulation of Embryos and Gametes   238
Preimplantation Diagnosis   239
Gamete Micromanipulation as Therapy for Male Infertility   242
Assisted Hatching   243
Cryopreservation   243
Donor Oocyte In Vitro Fertilization   246
Coculture of Embryos   248
Tubal Transfer Procedures   249
Summary   251

PART III. Oncology

Diagnosis and Contemporary Management of Cervical Intraepithelial Neoplasia.
By Bruce Patsner

                                                              261
Epidemiology and Screening of Cervical Dysplasia   261
How Often Should Patients Be Screened, and Who Should
Be Screened?   263
Improvements in Papanicolaou Smear Collection   264
The Bethesda System   265
What Are the Merits of the Bethesda System?   266
What Are the Problems With the Bethesda System as It Is
Presently Formulated?   267
How Are We to Resolve All of These Issues?   268
Management of the "Atypical" Papanicolaou Smear and
Cervical Intraepithelial Neoplasia I   269
Which Patients With "Atypical" Papanicolaou Smears
Should Undergo Colposcopic Evaluation?   269

Treatment of Cervical Intraepithelial Neoplasia: Excisional Vs. Destructive Methods   270
    What Are the Therapeutic Options, and What New Treatments Are Available?   271
Loop Excision Procedures: The "Newest" Development   274
    How Valid Are the Reasons for Choosing One Technique Over Another?   276
Summary   278

The Role of Laparoscopy in the Gynecologic Oncology Patient.

By Mark D. Adelson   283
    Preoperative Preparation   286
    Positioning   286
    Anesthesia   288
    Procedure   288
    Closed Laparoscopy   288
    Hysterectomy   292
    Laparoscopy With Hysterectomy   293
    Laparoscopic-Assisted Vaginal Hysterectomy   293
    Laparoscopic Abdominal Hysterectomy   293
    Lymphadenectomy   299
    Diagnosis and Treatment of Adnexal Masses   301
    Appendicitis   305
    Second-Look Laparoscopy   309
    Future Advances   309
        Radical Hysterectomy   309
        Bowel Resection   310
        Cytoreduction   316
        Splenectomy   317
    Summary   321

The Ultrasonic Surgical Aspirator in the Gynecologic Oncology Patient.

By Thomas J. Herzog and Janet S. Rader   325
    Historical Background   325
    Physics of the Ultrasonic Surgical Aspirator   327
    The Ultrasonic Surgical Aspirator Unit   331
    Ultrasonic Surgical Aspirator in Gynecologic Oncology   333
        Ovary and Fallopian Tube   334
        Uterus and Cervix   337
        Vulva   338
        Vagina   340

Wound healing   341
Pathologic Analysis of Ultrasonic Aspirates   341

Molecular Biology of Gynecological Tumors.
By Kathleen R. Cho and Lora Hedrick   347

Background   347
Gynecologic Tumors   349
Cervical Cancer   350
Vulvar Cancer   354
Endometrial Cancer   355
Ovarian Cancer   356
Summary   360

PART IV. Obstetrics

Substance Abuse in Pregnant Women.
By Ramada S. Smith, Susan S. Martier, and Robert J. Sokol   369

Alcohol   370
  Pathophysiology   370
  Fetal Alcohol Syndrome   370
  Alcohol-Related Birth Defects   371
  Screening for Exposure   372
  Comments   374
Cocaine   374
  Pathophysiology   375
  Maternal and Fetal Complications   375
  Comments   376
Marijuana   377
Opioids   377
  Maternal and Fetal Complications   377
  Comments   378
Summary   379

HIV and AIDS in the Obstetrical and Gynecological Patient: A Review of the Literature With Guidelines for Care and Screening.
By Kevin A. Ault and Sebastian Faro   383

Heterosexual Transmission   385
Gynecologic Diseases and HIV Infection   386
Interaction of HIV and Other Sexually Transmitted Diseases   389
Pregnancy and HIV Infection   391
Summary   395

Fetal Surgical and Medical Interventions.
By Mark I. Evans, Michael R. Harrison, N. Scott Adzick, Avihai Reichler, and Mark P. Johnson   401

Percutaneous Fetal Surgery   402
Fetal Ventriculomegaly   402
Obstructive Uropathy in the Fetus   404
Shunt Procedures   409
Open Fetal Surgery   413
Medical Fetal Therapy   414
Fetal Cardiac Therapy   415
Neural Tube Defects   417
Summary   420

Fetal Gene Therapy.
By Mark Paul Johnson, Michael R. Harrison, N. Scott Adzick, Avihai Reichler, and Mark I. Evans   423

Approaches to Gene Therapy   423
Modification   423
Removal   424
Addition   424
Somatic Cell Gene Therapy   425
Techniques for Gene Insertion   426
Current Status   427
Germ Line Gene Therapy   429
Enhancement of Genetic Engineering   430
Ethical Issues   431
Summary   432

Index   435

General Gynecology

Hysteroscopy

RANDALL C. DUNN, M.D.

HISTORICAL PERSPECTIVE

Hysteroscopy, like other forms of endoscopy, had its origin in technology developed in the first half of the 19th century. Hysteroscopes developed at that time used reflected light.[1] Hysteroscopy could not continue at the pace set by cystocopy because of the limited distension of the uterus as compared with the bladder. Modified cystoscopic equipment that had inflow-outflow channels or contact hysteroscopy were the only options in the early 1900s. Difficulty in maintaining uterine distension was what primarily hampered the early hysteroscopists, although the use of water and CO_2 were discussed in the 1910s and 1920s by Heineberg and Rubin, respectively.[1] Advances in hysterosalpingography in the 1920s and 1930s resulted in a decline in further development and interest in hysteroscopy.

The lack of a suitable medium to distend the uterine cavity, which had hampered early hysteroscopic development, was positively affected by the introduction of three different media, and instrumentation for performing hysteroscopy began to improve in the early 1970s. Initially, Edstrom and Fernstrom[2] used high–molecular-weight dextran, which allowed improved intrauterine visualization and intrauterine surgery because of the nonmiscibility of dextran with blood and cervical mucus. Five percent dextrose in water delivered under pressure was introduced by Quinones-Guerrero et al.[3] Carbon dioxide (CO_2) insufflation with specially designed CO_2 regulators was most recently introduced by Lindemann.[4]

INDICATIONS AND CONTRAINDICATIONS

The indications for hysteroscopy have continued to grow in number as physicians have gained experience in interpreting hysteroscopic findings. The more common indications are evaluation of abnormal uterine bleeding, whether premenopausal or postmenopausal, without a hormonal etiology; evaluation of the uterine cavity in infertility patients; confirmation of abnormal hysterograms; directed removal of intrauterine devices; diagnosis and treatment of müllerian fusion defects; diagnosis and treatment of intrauterine adhesions; diagnosis and treatment of submucous leiomyomas; evaluation of the uterine cavity and cervical canal in women with repeated abortions; evaluation of possible uterine wall defects following surgical procedures such as caesarean section, hysterotomy, or myomectomy; directed removal of intrauterine or intracervical polyps; management of patients undergoing first-trimester pregnancy termination from whom products of conception have not been obtained; and uterine ablation for menometrorrhagia. Additional specialized uses for hysteroscopy have been more recently reported. They include (1) evaluation of the extent of carcinoma of the endometrium; (2) sterilization by electrosurgical, mechanical, or chemical tubal occlusion; (3) embryo transfer under direct control; (4) gamete or zygote intrafallopian transfer; and (5) proximal tubal recanalization.[1, 5, 6]

Although all of the aforementioned are indications for hysteroscopy, the most common reasons for diagnostic hysteroscopy are the first three mentioned in the first list given in the previous paragraph. The first of these, the evaluation of abnormal uterine bleeding, has been one of the leading indications for hysteroscopy since its inception as a clinical tool. Many early investigators reported their findings in the evaluation of premenopausal and postmenopausal abnormal uterine bleeding (Table 1). All of the authors in this table reported significant hysteroscopic abnormalities in patients with abnormal bleeding. A more recent (1988) study evaluating women with persistent abnormal bleeding who had failed prior dilatation and curettage within 1 year of their hysteroscopy found that most had significant intrauterine pathology such as leiomyoma.[14] This has led many investigators to recommend hysteroscopy to patients who have persistent abnormal bleeding despite recent dilatation and curettage. The principal advantage of hysteroscopy over other gynecologic diagnostic methods is that it permits observation of the entire uterine cavity. This increases the diagnostic accuracy of suspected intrauterine pathology up

TABLE 1.

Hysteroscopic Evaluation of Women With Abnormal Uterine Bleeding

Author	Year	No. of Patients	Comments
Norment[7]	1956	100	50% with endometrial hyperplasia; 43% with other lesions
Englund[8]	1957	165	44 with pathology inadequately diagnosed by prior dilatation and curettage
Burnett[9]	1964	59	55.5% with abnormalities
Valle[10]	1977	172	131 premenopausal women, 70% with abnormalities; 41 postmenopausal women, 63.4% with abnormalities
Mohr[11]	1978	60	60% with abnormalities in postmenopausal women
Parent[12]	1978	120	85% with abnormalities (with contact hysteroscopy)
Sugimoto[13]	1978	1,824	60.1% with abnormalities (including cervical lesions and trophoblastic tumors)

to 70%, depending on the criteria used (Table 2). When hysteroscopy biopsy specimens of uterine lesions were compared with curettage specimens in patients with focal pathologic lesions, hysteroscopic detection and biopsy were far more accurate than was random curettage; only in extensive lesions did curettage adequately reveal the pathology.[10] In this study of 553 patients, 66.1% of 419 premenopausal patients and 55.9% of 134 postmenopausal patients had intrauterine abnormalities that could explain their abnormal bleeding.[10]

Hysteroscopy in the evaluation of infertility patients has revealed uterine abnormalities at reported rates that vary from 19% to 62%.[1] The clinical significance of these findings remains to be completely evaluated, but relevant intrauterine conditions and their impact on fertility are known. Recently, similar findings and their influence on the success of couples undergoing in vitro fertilization–embryo transfer (IVF-ET) have been reviewed.[19, 20] Most studies emphasize that a significant number of infertility and IVF-ET patients will have intrauterine or intracervical abnormalities that can sometimes be missed if hysterosalpingography is the sole diagnostic tool used.

Evaluation of suspected intrauterine pathology determined by hysteroscopy rather than by hysterography has been advocated because of the improved diagnostic accuracy of hysteroscopy. Several investigators have shown that up to one third of hysterograms may have false positive findings[21] and that 25% of the cases reported as normal by hysterography demonstrated a uterine lesion by hysteroscopy.[22] The relative sensitivity and specificity of hysterosalpingography and hysteroscopy depend, however, on both the pathology involved and the size of the abnormality. Submucous fibroids and polyps are better diagnosed hysteroscopically.[17] The pressure of injection or the amount of contrast media during hysterosalpingography can obliterate polyps or leiomyomas and lead to a false negative result.[23]

Contraindications to hysteroscopy are primarily those that are also contraindications to hysterosalpingography.[1, 6, 24] A recent or existing uterine infection can result in salpingitis or peritonitis after hysterosalpinography with any type of distending media. Vaginal infections should also be cleared before hysteroscopy to avoid spreading a lower genital tract infection by direct extension. Pregnant women should generally not undergo hysteroscopy unless they are aware of the risks of abortion, in-

TABLE 2.
Intrauterine Abnormalities Revealed or Confirmed by Hysteroscopy

Author	No. of Patients	Abnormalities, %
Hepp[15]	211	35.0
Lindemann[16]	1,100	28.9
Quinones-Guerrero[17]	60	43.3
Siegler[18]	257	48.0
Valle[10]	350	71.0

fection, and bleeding. In selected cases the value of the information obtained by hysteroscopy may outweigh the risk. For instance, an intrauterine device may be removed in a patient who conceives and desires to continue the pregnancy. Excessive uterine bleeding may need to be suppressed before hysteroscopy so that the cavity can be adequately inspected and intravasation of the distending medium will be less likely to occur. Cervical malignancy is a contraindication to hysteroscopy because of the concern that disease spread may occur.

COMPLICATIONS OF HYSTEROSCOPY

Many of the complications of hysteroscopy are similar to those associated with dilatation and curettage. Uterine perforation may occur during uterine sounding or cervical dilatation. Hysteroscopy should commence as soon as the hysteroscope is introduced into the cervical canal without advancing the instrument until visualization is achieved. Application of force without adequate visualization can result in perforation, and the intestines quickly come into endoscopic view. In complicated hysteroscopic procedures such as resection of large uterine septa, concomitant laparoscopy is recommended to avoid perforations and injury to adjacent organs. Infection is a rare complication of hysteroscopy. In one series, 7 mild infections occurred in 4,000 hysteroscopies,[1] and in another series, no infections occurred in over 1,000 hysteroscopies.[24] Bleeding after hysteroscopic examination has not been reported except in patients with intrauterine dissections. Postoperative bleeding has been reported after resection of submucous myomas, but this can usually be controlled by intrauterine tamponade with an intrauterine balloon such as a Foley bulb. Many patients have minimal spotting for the first 24 hours after hysteroscopic procedures. Electrosurgical injuries have been reported after hysteroscopic procedures involving electrocoagulation. Any patient with increasing abdominal pain should be examined for signs of peritonitis and the need for initiation of appropriate surgical intervention. Media-related complications are dependent primarily on the type of media used for distension. Excessive rates of flow of CO_2 or excessive quantities of liquid media can be hazardous. Fatal and nonfatal accidents have been reported with CO_2 for distension in therapeutic hysteroscopy, and the Food and Drug Administration (FDA) does not allow concurrent use of CO_2 with hysteroscopic lasers. The insufflator equipment used to create a pneumoperitoneum during laparoscopy must never be used for hysteroscopy since flow rates are invariably greater than or equal to 1 L/min. Rare anaphylactic reactions have been reported with dextran.[25] Pulmonary edema and prolongation of bleeding times have both been reported with various liquid media, especially with dextran.[26, 27] Prolonged hysteroscopic procedures require the use of large amounts of liquid media, and accurate inflow and outflow must be measured.

TECHNIQUE

A complete pelvic examination, including a recent Papanicolaou cervical smear, is performed before hysteroscopy. Cultures of the vagina and cervix are performed when appropriate. The procedure and its attendant risks and possible complications must be discussed with the patient to ensure informed consent. Diagnostic hysteroscopy performed within the first week after the cessation of menses will provide optimal visualization and minimize the chance for bleeding because the endometrium is in its thinnest state.[16] An office setting for diagnostic hysteroscopy is safe, economical, and practical. Hospitalization is required for therapeutic procedures, especially when significant intrauterine abnormalities are suspected by prior studies. The patient should empty her bladder (or it should be emptied if the patient is under general anesthesia), and the table should elevate the buttocks or rotate the patient into the dorsolithotomy position before the procedure. The cervix should be cleaned with antiseptic solution in the office setting or with routine preparation for vaginal procedures in the hospital setting. Generally, hysteroscopy requires some cervical dilatation, especially when operating hysteroscopes are used. Therefore, some type of anesthesia is usually required. Paracervical blockade, approximately 10 mL of 1% lidocaine, is often used in the office setting, especially when dilation is required. One milliliter of 1% lidocaine injected under the anterior cervical mucosa may also be useful to blunt the effect of a tenaculum. When office anesthetics are used, it is necessary to maintain agents, equipment (e.g., "crash cart"), and personnel training that may be necessary to treat an allergic response. General anesthesia is used for operative hysteroscopy or when laparoscopy is also a planned procedure, although regional anesthesia may be an option in selected cases. Many parous patients will tolerate the procedure without paracervical blockade or do well if systemic analgesia is used concomitantly.

The endocervical canal and uterine cavity are generally sounded and the canal dilated as necessary for entry of the particular hysteroscope. When hysteroscopes that have an obturator are used, the sheath with the obturator in place is placed to the level of the internal cervical os. The obturator is then removed and the telescope with its separable bridge introduced and fixed in the encasing sheath. Modern hysteroscopes are 25 cm in length. Visualization of the uterine cavity begins at the level of the internal os. Most hysteroscopes have a fore-oblique view, which may require a rotational motion to visualize the entire cavity unless a contact hysteroscope is used.

The two primary methods of hysteroscopy are "contact" and "panoramic." The focal length of each hysteroscope's optics determines the field of vision. In the former, the lens is placed directly in contact with the area to be examined; in the latter the tissue is viewed from a distance. A recent application made possible by a combination of both types of optics is called microhysteroscopy.[28]

The contact hysteroscopy technique was introduced in the early 1900s and has the advantage of being self-contained. The uterine cavity does not have to be distended, so expensive adjunctive equipment or media for this purpose are not required. The uterine cavity must be examined systematically since only the small area in direct contact with the lens of the hysteroscope, usually about 7 mm, is visualized. Illumination is obtained from ambient light that enters the scope through a translucent proximal light collector and is transmitted down to the distal rod lens.[29-31] Since the field of view is limited, it may be difficult to do a complete examination of the uterine cavity. Additionally, with the technology available today for panoramic hysteroscopy, this technique is less used.

Panoramic hysteroscopy is the most common type of hysteroscopy performed. Most current residency and postgraduate instrumentation training courses use this technique for hysteroscopy. Panoramic hysteroscopic instrumentation requires an external illumination source and media for distension. At a distance of 3 cm the hysteroscope has unit magnification. Increasing the magnification, by coming closer to the uterine wall or structure in question, decreases the resolution and depth of focus. The actual hysteroscope has a telescope (usually 4 to 6 mm); a fore-oblique lens or 0-degree lens; an outer sheath with a separate channel for the media or similar function via a nonseparable bridge; fiber-optic bundle; and additional ancillary instrumentation such as forceps, scissors, electrodes, cutting loops, laser fibers, suction cannulas, or catheters. One feature that most hysteroscopes have is that the inflow and outflow channels communicate at the proximal end and therefore fluid does not necessarily produce a "washing" effect within the cavity. This often requires a longer initial distension time within the cavity before clear visualization is achieved. Additional instrumentation that is helpful, particularly in the teaching situation, is the use of video cameras so that the student has the same view as the operator. This also allows for permanent documentation via videotapes, video image printers, or photography. More recently, flexible and steerable hysteroscopes have been developed and will, no doubt, continue to become smaller with improved visualization as optical and illumination problems are solved. These will advance the routine practice of office hysteroscopy, in particular.

MEDIA FOR HYSTEROSCOPY

The principle media used for hysteroscopy are CO_2 gas, high-viscosity dextran 70, and low-viscosity 5% dextrose. Each medium has certain characteristics that offer unique advantages and disadvantages.

Carbon dioxide gas is the only gas medium in use today. (Nitrous oxide should never be used because it can increase the partial pressure of CO_2 and lead to profound bradycardia and cardiac arrest). Carbon dioxide is colorless and innocuous, does not conduct electrical current, does not support combustion, and is not flammable. Advantages also include a long history of safety, rapid absorption, excellent visualization, and immiscibility with blood. These qualities have made it the most commonly used distension medium for office hysteroscopy. One of the disadvantages of CO_2 for distension is the initial expense of the insufflator because of the sophisticated nature of this instrumentation. Easy intravasation of CO_2 into venous sinuses of the uterus requires the CO_2 to be closely monitored. This type of problem has led to reports of possible acidosis secondary to hypercarbia, cardiac arrhythmias, and risk of pulmonary embolus. Therefore, proper instrumentation and pressure settings are extremely important with the use of CO_2. Again, it should be emphasized that only instrumentation specifically designed for hysteroscopy provides appropriate control of CO_2 for its safe use. The insufflator should limit the maximum flow rate to 100 mL/min, and the maximum intrauterine pressure should not exceed 200 mm Hg. These two readings act as checks for each other, and the flow rate is automatically reduced as intrauterine pressure increases. A flow rate of 40 to 60 mL/min of CO_2 and, in women with patent tubes, an average uterine pressure of 50 to 70 mm Hg usually give excellent results for visualization. A test taking approximately 5 minutes will use about 250 mL of CO_2. Often patients will report shoulder pain after the use of CO_2 because of diaphragmatic nerve irritation similar to that reported after laparoscopy, but of a lesser degree. Carbon dioxide is the primary distension medium used for office hysteroscopy.

Dextran 70 is the only high-viscosity liquid in use at this time. It is a 32% concentration of dextran 70 (glucose molecules linked by glycosidic bonds with minimal branching) with 10% dextrose and has a molecular weight of 70,000.[32] It is colorless, optically clear with a high refractory index, and immiscible with blood; does not require an expensive insufflator; and is electrolyte free and nonconductive. However, disadvantages include its requirement for greater care of the instrumentation because of its high viscosity (220 centistoke at room temperature). Careful cleansing with hot water and rinsing is necessary to prevent hardening and crystallization of the material around and within the instrument after the procedure. Valves in hysteroscopes or accessory instruments may be bent or broken by excessive use of force to open it if an incomplete cleansing has left residual dextran 70. Although an excellent media for diagnostic purposes, dextran's viscosity makes it a more difficult medium to work with for prolonged cases. Another problem is that allergic and anaphylactic reactions have been reported with the use of dextran 70.[33] Finally, pulmonary edema resulting from plasma volume expansion and coagulopathies (usually prolonged bleeding time) have been reported with use of dextran 70.[26, 34]

Dextrose 5% is the most frequently used low-viscosity liquid. (Glycine and Ringer's lactate are also used and have essentially similar advantages and disadvantages.) The primary advantages are the inexpensive cost, physiologic absorption, and intrauterine cooling effect when an intrauterine laser or electrical instruments are used. The primary disadvantage relates to its low viscosity and therefore relatively easy retrograde passage out of patent tubes resulting in potential fluid overload. It is also more difficult to maintain a clear visual field, so more volume is needed to clear the field to continue the diagnostic or therapeutic procedure. Because of their conductivity, mixtures that contain saline should never be used when electrosurgical procedures are performed. The external pressure of approximately 100 mm Hg that must be applied to this distending medium can be achieved by applying a blood pressure cuff to small bags or large urologic pressure cuffs to large bags. Recently, automatic systems to control pressure have become commercially available. Because of the potential for fluid overload, the final input and output should be within 1 L of each other. If they are not, careful postoperative monitoring is essential, and potential electrolyte abnormalities should be checked. Frequently, operative uses of low-viscosity media require large volumes, often several liters. Fluid overload can usually be simply controlled by the use of furosemide (20 to 80 mg intravenously). Direct intravascular fluid overload is rare except where extensive uterine wall vessels are exposed. This can be minimized by chilling the media preoperatively, which will constrict blood vessels in the uterus in cases where this is a significant preoperative concern.

THERAPEUTIC HYSTEROSCOPY CONSIDERATIONS

Hysteroscopic intrauterine procedures require experience in the interpretation of the topography of the uterus and great skill in manipulation of the instruments required. These procedures should not be attempted until significant experience has been gained in diagnostic hysteroscopy and qualified assistants are available to assist the procedure; credentialing is an important consideration. The indications for hysteroscopy previously mentioned demonstrate that with appropriate training, almost all uterine abnormalities can be or have been treated hysteroscopically. The value to the patient in decreased morbidity, decreased convalescence time, and decreased expense affords this modality an increased role in routine gynecology and reproductive surgery.

One procedure that has recently gained increased acceptance is ablation of the endometrium in women with menorrhagia or metrorrhagia with or without other intrauterine pathology. This has opened a new frontier for the treatment of irregular bleeding in premenopausal and postmenopausal women. Many methods have been used to destroy the endometrial lining, but only laser ablation and electrocoagulation are being regularly used to ablate the endometrium. Laser ablation of the endometrium was introduced in 1981.[35] The Nd:YAG laser delivered hysteroscopically to ablate the endometrium is the most common intrauterine laser used. Two basic techniques are used: touch (dragging) and nontouch (blanching). Laser settings of 55 and 70 W, respectively, are used for these two techniques.[36, 37] Ablation of the endometrium by electrocoagulation has been performed with a resectoscopic wire loop, borrowed and adapted from urologists, or a resectoscopic ball-end electrode.[38, 39] Both methods require adequate uterine distension, usually with non–electrolyte-containing low-viscosity media. There have been serious complications associated with these techniques, and they should not be attempted by novice hysteroscopists.[40] The ball-end electrode has the advantage of expediting the procedure—it is usually performed in 15 to 30 minutes—and of being much less expensive than laser ablation because of the high cost of the Nd:YAG laser. It also provides better control by the operator and is easy to teach. In short, the ball-end electrode is superior to the laser in simplicity and safety.

REFERENCES

1. Valle RF, Sciarra JJ: Current status of hysteroscopy in gynecologic practice. *Fertil Steril* 1979; 32:619.
2. Edstrom K, Fernstrom I: The diagnostic possibilities of a modified hysteroscopic technique. *Acta Obstet Gynecol Scand* 1970; 49:327.

3. Quinones-Guerrero R, Alvarado-Duran A, Agnar-Ramos R: Tubal catheriza-
tion: Applications of a new technique. *Am J Obstet Gynecol* 1971; 114:674.
4. Lindemann HJ: Eine neue Untersuchingsmethode fur die Hysteroskopie. *Endoscopy* 1971; 4:194.
5. Shamma FN, DeCherney AH: The role of hysteroscopy in in vitro fertilization–embryo transfer. *Assist Reprod Rev* 1992; 2:132.
6. Siegler AM: Gynecologic endoscopy in infertility. *Obstet Gynecol Clin North Am* 1987; 14:1015.
7. Norment WB: The hysteroscope. *Am J Obstet Gynecol* 1956; 71:426.
8. Englund SE, Ingelman-Sundberg A, Westin B: Hysteroscopy in diagnosis and treatment of uterine bleeding. *Gynaecologia* 1957; 143:217.
9. Burnett JE: Hysteroscopy-controlled curettage for endometrial polyps. *Obstet Gynecol* 1964; 24:621.
10. Valle RF: Hysteroscopic evaluation of patients with abnormal uterine bleeding. *Surg Gynecol Obstet* 1981; 153:521.
11. Mohr JW: Hysteroscopy as a diagnostic tool in postmenopausal bleeding, in Phillips JM (ed): *Endoscopy in Gynecology.* Downey, Calif, American Association of Gynecologic Laparoscopists, 1978, p 347.
12. Parent B, Doerler B, Barbot J, et al: Metrorragies postmenopausiques: Diagnostic par 1-hysteroscope de contact. *Acta Endosc* 1978; 8:13.
13. Sugimoto O: *Diagnostic and Therapeutic Hysterocopy.* New York, Igaku-Shoin, 1978.
14. Brooks PS, Serden SP: Hysteroscopic findings after unsuccessful dilatation and curettage for abnormal uterine bleeding. *Am J Obstet Gynecol* 1988; 158:1354.
15. Hepp H, Roll H: Die Hysteroskopie. *Gynaekologie* 1974; 7:166.
16. Lindemann HL, Mohr JM: CO_2 hysteroscopy: Diagnosis and treatment, in Phillips JM, Keith L (eds): *Gynecologic Laparoscopy: Principles and Techniques.* New York, Stratton, 1974.
17. Edstrom K, Fernstrom I: The diagnostic possibilities of a modified hysteroscopic technique. *Acta Obstet Gynecol Scand* 1970; 49:327.
18. Siegler AM, Kemmann E, Gentile GP: Hysteroscopic procedures in 257 patients. *Fertil Steril* 1976; 27:1267.
19. Frydman R, Eibshictz I, Fernandez H, et al: Uterine evaluation by microhysteroscopy in IVF candidates. *Hum Reprod* 1987; 2:481.
20. Seinera R, Maccario S, Visentin L, et al: Hysteroscopy in an IVF-ET program. Clinical experience with 360 infertile patients. *Acta Obstet Gynecol Scand* 1988; 67:135.
21. La-Sala GB, Dessanti L, Sacchetti F: Hysteroscopy and female sterility: Analysis of the results from 213 patients. *Acta Eur Fertil* 1985; 16:47.
22. La-Sala GB, Sachetti F, Deglincerti-Tocci, et al: Complementary use of hysterosalpingography, hysteroscopy, and laparoscopy in 100 infertile patients: Results and comparison of their diagnostic accuracy. *Acta Eur Fertil* 1987; 18:369.
23. Taylor PJ, Lewinthal D, Leader A, et al: A comparison of dextran 70 with carbon dioxide as the distension medium for hysteroscopy in patients with infertility or requesting reversal of a prior tubal sterilization. *Fertil Steril* 1987; 47:861.
24. Salet-Baroux J, Hamon J, Maillard G, et al: Complications from microhysteroscopy, in Siegler AM, Lindemann HM (eds): *Hysteroscopy: Principle and Practice.* Philadelphia, JB Lippincott, 1984, p 112.
25. Maddi VI, Wyso EM, Zinner EN: Dextran anaphylaxis. *Angiology* 1969; 20:243.
26. Leake JF, Murphy AA, Zacur HA: Noncardiogenic pulmonary edema: A complication of operative hysteroscopy. *Fertil Steril* 1987; 48:497.

27. Zbella EA, Moise J, Carson SA: Noncardiogenic pulmonary edema secondary to intrauterine instillation of 32% dextran 70. *Fertil Steril* 1985; 43:479.
28. Hamou J: Microhysteroscopy, a new procedure and its original application. *J Reprod Med* 1981; 26:375.
29. Marleschki V: Del moderne zerviscopie und hysteroskopie. *Zentralbl Gynakol* 1966; 88:637.
30. Barbot JI: *Hysteroscope de Contact* (thesis). University of Paris, 1975.
31. Baggish MS, Barbot J: Contact hysteroscopy. *Clin Obstet Gynecol* 1983; 26:219.
32. Diamond MP, Lavy G, Shapiro BS, et al: A new device to facilitate intrauterine instillation of dextran 70 for hysteroscopy. *Obstet Gynecol* 1987; 70:955.
33. Borten M, Seibert CP, Taymor ML: Recurrent anaphylactic reaction to intraperitoneal dextran 75 used for the prevention of postsurgical adhesions. *Obstet Gynecol* 1983; 61:755.
34. Zbella EA, Moise J, Carson SA: Noncardiogenic pulmonary edema secondary to intrauterine instillation of 32% dextran 70. *Fertil Steril* 1985; 43:479.
35. Goldrath MH, Fuller TA, Segal S: Laser photovaporization of the endometrium for the treatment of menorrhagia. *Am J Obstet Gynecol* 1981; 140:14.
36. Goldrath MH: Hysteroscopic laser surgery, in Baggish MS (ed): *Basic and Advanced Laser Surgery in Gynecology*. East Norwalk, Conn, Appleton-Century-Crofts, 1985, p 357.
37. Loffer FD: Hysteroscopic endometrial ablation with the Nd:YAG laser using a nontouch technique. *Obstet Gynecol* 1987; 69:679.
38. DeCherney AH, Diamond MP, Lavy G, et al: Endometrial ablation for intractable uterine bleeding: Hysteroscopic resection. *Obstet Gynecol* 1987; 70:668.
39. Vancaillie TG: Electrocoagulation of the endometrium with the ball-end resectoscope. *Obstet Gynecol* 1989; 74:425.
40. Baggish MS, Daniell JF: Death caused by air embolism associated with neodymium-yttrium-aluminum-garnet laser surgery and artificial sapphire tips. *Am J Obstet Gynecol* 1989; 161:877.

Editor's Comment

Dr. Dunn has presented an erudite discussion on the indications and applications of hysteroscopy. The discussion on the contraindications to hysteroscopy are precisely stated, leaving the reader with clear recommendations. Although hysteroscopy allows for visual examination of the uterine cavity, its therapeutic applications are limited. The present discussion describes the benefits to be derived from, as well as the limitations and potential complications of, this technique.

Sebastian Faro, M.D., Ph.D.

Complications of Endoscopy

SCOTT A. WASHBURN, M.D.

THOMAS G. STOVALL, M.D.

T he laparoscope is an essential diagnostic and treatment tool in gynecologic practice. Kelling[1] described the first diagnostic laparoscopy in humans in 1902. Anderson[2] introduced laparoscopic tubal sterilization in 1937. However, laparoscopic surgery did not gain widespread acceptance until the late 1960s when fiber-optic lighting and controlled insufflation pumps became widely available. During the last 30 years laparoscopic technology has experienced a sustained and rapid increase in advances that shows no signs of weakening. Today, state-of-the-art laparoscopy allows virtually all gynecologic laparoscopic procedures to be conducted in the outpatient setting, and patients tolerate these procedures well and perceive laparoscopic procedures to be relatively safe. The discussion of laparoscopy presented below is a review of some of the potential hazards and complications that have been reported in the literature over the past 30 years.

SURVEYS

The American Association of Gynecologic Laparoscopists (AAGL), established in 1972, has conducted extensive surveys of its membership. Although these surveys rely on self-report instead of medical records, much useful information may be derived from them because of the diversity of experience and expertise of the membership and the many years spanned by the information. Unfortunately, direct comparisons between years cannot be made because questionnaire end points did not overlap and definitions of what constituted complications varied over the years. Perhaps the most important contribution of the AAGL surveys was the observation that the highest frequency of complications occurred in the group of surgeons who had relatively little experience.

Table 1 summarizes the results of the AAGL surveys.[3-9] The surveys were designed to ascertain the number of cases that physicians performed each year as well as the number of deaths and major complications that occurred during the survey period. The death rate reported in the survey declined during the first several years and then stabilized between 1.5 and 2.8 deaths per 100,000 cases. The major complication rate declined steadily over the survey period.

The cumulative German experience in laparoscopy[10] from 1949 to 1988 revealed many similarities to the AAGL experience and is summarized in Table 2. Unfortunately, this extensive experience also relied on

Advances in Obstetrics and Gynecology, vol 1
© 1994, Mosby–Year Book, Inc.

TABLE 1.
American Association of Gynecologic Laparoscopists Surveys of Laparoscopic Experience

Year	No. of MDs/ Total Forms	Total Cases*	No. of Deaths	Death Rate/ 100,000 Cases	No. of Complications Reported†	No. of Complications/ 1,000 Cases
1974[3]	872/1,030	236,253	8	3.4	743	3.14
1975[4]	966/1,300	113,253	4	3.5	674	5.95
1976[5]	964/2,800	108,759	3	2.8	376	3.46
1977[6]	837/3,300	87,275	N/A	N/A	N/A	N/A
1979[7]	1,452/3,827	144,190	2	1.4	309	2.14
1982[8]‡	1,024/4,737	125,560	N/A	N/A	181	1.44
1988[9]	816/4,832	71,640	2	2.79	192	2.68

*Represents the combined number of diagnostic and sterilization procedures reported.
†Generally represents those complications requiring laparotomy but may also include anesthetic-related complications.
‡Indicates survey of sterilization procedures only.

TABLE 2.
German Surveys of Laparoscopic Experience

Years	No. of Forms Reported	No. of Cases Reported*	No. of Deaths Reported	Deaths/100,000 Cases	No. of Complications†	No. of Complications/ 1,000 Cases
1949–77	682	265,900	24	9.0	949	3.56
1978–82	438	292,462	15	5.1	563	1.93
1983–85	464	253,109	6	2.4	496	1.96
1986–88	530	260,206	2	0.8	615	2.36

*Represents the total number of diagnostic, operative, and sterilization laparoscopies reported.
†Generally represents those complications requiring laparotomy and not anesthetic complications. A trend toward handling complications without laparotomy was noted in the teaching institutions that participated in the survey; a similar trend was not found in the private sector.

data from surveys, but it is remarkable for its parallelism to the AAGL data. Both the AAGL and German surveys reveal essentially stable complication and decreasing mortality rates despite a shift from diagnostic and sterilization procedures to the more technically complicated operative laparoscopic procedures.

Both the German and the AAGL surveys report the number of cases, deaths, and complication rates. The German survey also separated out academic and private practice experience. Death rates in the German survey declined continuously across the years reported. The complication rate, however, seemed to stabilize in the "modern era" of laparoscopy. The German and the AAGL surveys report similar trends toward greater use of operative laparoscopy and away from exclusive use of the laparoscope for sterilization and diagnostic procedures.

Both surveys provide valuable clues about the prevailing use and complications of laparoscopic surgery during the survey periods. The reports are remarkably similar in death and complication rates and report similar trends in use of the laparoscope. However, neither report can be used to draw conclusions regarding the efficacy and safety of any particular technique relative to any other.

DESCRIPTIVE AND COHORT STUDIES

Several authors have reported series of laparoscopic experience. These contributions are invaluable for their descriptions of the actual experience of laparoscopy at a particular institution or by a particular individual. The series we examined[11-21] appeared in the literature between 1973 and 1989 and encompass both the gynecologic and gastrointestinal disciplines. The series results are compiled in Table 3.

These descriptive and cohort studies represent a wide range of experiences. Soderstrom and Butler's[11] series highlights the absolute necessity of adequate training and supervision of the laparoscopist. The institution of a rigorous training and supervision program for beginning laparoscopists in two Seattle, Washington, hospitals resulted in 9.5-fold reduction in the major complication rate.[11] The mean for the major complication rate of the series we examined is approximately 6- to 8-fold higher than the complication rate reported in the survey conducted by the AAGL and the German laparoscopists. However, the mean complication rate of the descriptive and cohort studies declines to approximately 3.5- to 4.5-fold higher than the AAGL and German surveys when the "pre-education" data, which include complication rates of inadequately trained physicians, are excluded from the calculation. In addition, the complication rate of the gastroenterologists approximates that of the gynecologists when one excludes the "pre-educational" data of Soderstrom from the calculation. It is important to remember that both the AAGL and German data were collected by using a mail-in survey instrument. It is possible that minor complications were sometimes not reported and that even major complications were occasionally forgotten.

Perhaps the most remarkable series is the one reported by Mehta[21] in which he details his personal experience with over 250,000 laparoscopic tubal occlusion sterilizations. Not only is his death rate much lower than

TABLE 3.
Descriptive and Cohort Studies of Laparoscopic Complications

Author	Years	No. of Cases	No. of Deaths	Deaths/ 100,000 Cases	No. of Complications*	No. of Complications/ 1,000 Cases
Soderstrom[11]	1970–71	199	0	0	19	95.4
Soderstrom[11]	1971–72	294	0	0	3	10.2
Rawlings[12]	1967–71	417	0	0	20	48.0
Uribe-Ramirez[13]	1974–75	2,000	0	0	18	9.0
Cunanan[14]	1970–78	5,018	0	0	43	8.6
Frenkel[15]	1965–79	2,757	0	0	6	2.2
Kane[16]	1976–83	603	3	166	20	33.2
Henning[17]	1954–80	36,207	24	66	66	1.8
Patel[18]	pre–1985	8,600	0	0	13	1.5
Franks[19]	1978–82	5,027	0	0	51	10.1
Orlando[20]	pre–1987	1,845	0	0	10	5.4
Mehta[21]	1979–88	250,136	12	4.8	118	0.5

*Generally refers to those complications requiring laparotomy; failure to accomplish the procedure. Anesthetic-related complications were also included when reported.

that of the survey, his complication rate is also extremely low. In addition, all of the laparoscopies were done in "sterilization camps" in India, with tents as operating rooms and benches as operating tables. Only intramuscular sedation and local anesthetic were used for the entire procedure, and Silastic bands were used to accomplish the tubal occlusion. These data further support the importance of operator experience as a factor in the incidence of laparoscopic complications.

The cohort study of Franks et al.[19] details relative risk factors for unintended laparotomy at laparoscopic tubal ligation. They determined that the relative risk of unintended laparotomy was 10.2 (95% confidence interval [CI], 5.3 to 19.7) in patients who had undergone previous abdominal surgery as compared with controls. History of an intrauterine device or known history of pelvic inflammatory disease was not a statistically significant risk factor unless they were combined with each other or with a history of previous pelvic surgery. The relative risk of unintended laparotomy was 5.5 (95% CI, 2.5 to 12.1) when compared with controls when the combination of these risk factors was considered.

The most common complication of laparoscopy found in both the surveys and the series is bleeding. However, bowel perforation and bowel burns are also very common. The remainder of this discussion will detail most of the reported complications of laparoscopy. Fortunately, death is an extremely rare complication of laparoscopy and will not be elaborated on further.

SPECIFIC COMPLICATIONS

ANESTHESIA-RELATED COMPLICATIONS

Postoperative nausea and vomiting with subsequent aspiration are well-known complications of general anesthesia. Hovorka et al.[22] conducted a prospective cohort study of the effects of nitrous oxide on the incidence of postoperative nausea and vomiting and found no differences between groups. Beattie et al.[23] also conducted a retrospective cohort analysis and determined that postoperative nausea and vomiting occurred at a much higher frequency (51.6 vs. 21.6, $P < .001$) in women during the first 8 days of the follicular phase than during the remainder of the menstrual cycle.

The practice of routinely intubating patients to avoid aspiration is controversial. The Royal College of Obstetricians and Gynecologists' review of laparoscopy[24] revealed that of the 38 "anesthetic" complications, only 1 occurred in the group of 4,750 managed with spontaneous ventilation and a face mask. In addition, no clinical evidence of aspiration in any of the 50,247 cases was noted. However, the importance of preoperative gastric prophylaxis was emphasized by the prospective cohort analysis of Duffy.[25] Two of 93 patients (2.2%) were found to have evidence of gastric regurgitation into the pharynx despite overnight fasts in all of the patients in the study. Local anesthesia for laparoscopic procedures reduces the number of patients requiring intubation, thus reducing the risk of aspiration resulting from postoperative nausea and vomiting.

COMPLICATIONS OF PNEUMOPERITONEUM

The circulatory effects of pneumoperitoneum have been assessed by several investigators. Hodgson et al.[26] noted that carbon dioxide (CO_2) pneumoperitoneum significantly increased arterial P_{CO_2} in both spontaneously ventilated and intubated patients. The increase in minute ventilation in the spontaneously ventilating group allowed better compensation for the increased P_{CO_2} than in the intubated group in which minute ventilation remained constant. Marshall et al.[27, 28] further clarified the effects of both CO_2 and nitrous oxide on the circulation. They determined that pneumoperitoneum obtained with either agent resulted in increased mean arterial pressure, heart rate, and central venous pressure. Carbon dioxide pneumoperitoneum did not affect cardiac output in Marshall and colleagues' study, but Hodgson et al.[26] and Smith et al.[29] demonstrated increases in cardiac output with CO_2 pneumoperitoneum. Nitrous oxide decreased cardiac output in Marshall and associates' study.[28] Intra-abdominal pressure irrespective of the pneumoperitoneum agent was found to dictate the effects on cardiac output in the trial of Ivankovich et al.[30] in dogs. They demonstrated an increase in cardiac output with an increase in intra-abdominal pressure until the intra-abdominal pressure exceeded inferior vena cava pressure. In fact, they documented a 60% decrease in cardiac output and inferior vena cava flow with intra-abdominal pressures of 40 mm Hg.

Two studies have addressed the effects of CO_2 pneumoperitoneum on arterial blood gases.[31, 32] Drury et al.[31] reported no change in Pa_{CO_2} during assisted ventilation with CO_2 pneumoperitoneum pressures of 30 to 50 cm water. However, Diamant et al.[32] reported a significant increase in Pa_{CO_2} during laparoscopic tubal sterilization performed with local anesthesia and intravenous sedation. They reported no significant increases in heart rate, PaO_2, blood pressure, or electrocardiogram.

Cardiac arrhythmias are relatively common during laparoscopy. Myles[33] reported a 30% incidence of bradyarrhythmias during a short prospective series of laparoscopic sterilization. The highest frequency of bradyarrhythmias occurred during introduction of the CO_2 pneumoperitoneum and during traction on the pelvic organs. Both peritoneal distension, which compresses the inferior vena cava and triggers a vagal response, and traction on the pelvic visceral structures have resulted in asystolic cardiac arrest or severe hypotension.[34, 35] The incidence of asystole has been reported as 1 in 2,500 cases.[14] Carbon dioxide embolism is also a reported complication of pneumoperitoneum. Gas embolism is rare and not often fatal, but it is certainly a dramatic complication. Although direct injection of CO_2 into the venous circulation has been reported,[36] several other case reports[37–41] postulate that increased intraperitoneal partial pressures of CO_2 lead to venous embolization of CO_2. One study of gas embolization in dogs[42] revealed that air has a fivefold lower lethal embolization dose than CO_2 does. It was interesting to note that two of the case reports of CO_2 embolism were associated with laparoscopy immediately after evacuation of pregnant uteri.[39, 41] Management of CO_2 embolism is supportive and relies on prompt correction of any cardiac dysrhythmias and aggressive hyperventilation to facilitate expulsion of the intravascular CO_2.

Additional complications of pneumoperitoneum include subcutaneous emphysema, pneumothorax, pneumomediastinum, and pneumopericardium.[43-49] Whereas subcutaneous emphysema is usually trivial and self-limiting, pneumothorax, pneumomediastinum, and pneumopericardium can require intervention and decompression. The mechanism of pneumothorax, pneumomediastinum, and pneumopericardium is escape of gas into the chest cavity through weak points or defects in the diaphragm. All of the case reports of pneumomediastinum and pneumothorax reviewed here documented the appearance of subcutaneous emphysema in the neck before the diagnosis of the pneumothorax and pneumomediastinum.

Shoulder-hand syndrome has also been reported as a complication of pneumoperitoneum at laparoscopic tubal ligation.[50] This rare complication resulted in permanent disability of arm movement on the affected side. The most dramatic complication of the pneumoperitoneum is intraperitoneal explosion and subsequent patient death during nitrous oxide pneumoperitoneum laparoscopy, an occurrence that has been reported on two occasions.[51] Although Vickers[52] trivialized the potential hazards of nitrous oxide explosion, the actual occurrence of the complication makes nitrous oxide a poor choice for insufflation of the pneumoperitoneum. The inability of CO_2 to support a fire or explosion makes CO_2 pneumoperitoneum insufflation preferable.

ANALGESIC COMPLICATIONS

Several studies have addressed the issue of pain morbidity associated with laparoscopy. Harvey[53] examined the effect of outpatient status on the incidence of morbidity. Despite a significantly greater incidence of emesis and pain in the recovery room, outpatients reported less vomiting 24 hours postoperatively, but the outpatients continued to report more nausea but less drowsiness than the inpatients through 48 hours postoperatively. Dobbs et al.[54] reported that Falope rings for tubal ligation were associated with significantly more pain than were Hulka clips, and Lipscomb et al.[55] have recently shown that the use of local analgesia with Falope ring tubal occlusion markedly reduces tubal pain when compared with tubal electrocoagulation. The Dobbs group also found that the intraoperative posture, lithotomy or supine, made no difference in postoperative pain. Rosenblum et al.[56] demonstrated that postoperative ibuprofen provides longer-lasting postoperative analgesia than does intraoperative fentanyl. Narchi et al.[57] have provided preliminary data supporting intraperitoneal local anesthetic as an effective agent in reducing postoperative shoulder pain.

INCISION AND INFECTIOUS COMPLICATIONS

Several cases of herniation of either the omentum or small bowel through the umbilical laparoscopic incision have been reported.[58-61] These hernias often result in intestinal obstruction and must be surgically reduced and repaired. Computed tomography may be a useful diagnostic tool if the incisional site does not readily reveal itself as the point of obstruction.[62]

Bacterial peritonitis following laparoscopic tubal ligation and diagnostic laparoscopy has been reported. Goodnough et al.[63] reported a case of culture-positive gonococcal peritonitis following laparoscopic sterilization in a previously asymptomatic patient, and House[64] reported a case of pelvic actinomycosis following diagnostic laparoscopy in a patient with an intrauterine device. Iwamura et al.[65] reported that 5 (4.4%) of 113 patients undergoing laparoscopy for liver disease had positive blood cultures during the procedure. Peritonitis did not develop in any of these 5 patients. Pyper et al.[66] demonstrated a 90% culture-positive rate of bacteria in peritoneal fluid at chromopertubation in previously sterile peritoneum tissue. All of the bacterial counts were less than 10^5 organisms per milliliter, and clinically evident salpingitis or peritonitis did not develop in any patient. A more serious postlaparoscopic infectious complication is detailed in the report by Sotrel et al.[67] of the development of necrotizing fasciitis in a diabetic patient after diagnostic laparoscopy. The laparoscopic instruments had been steam sterilized, and the laparoscope was soaked in 2% activated glutaraldehyde. Huezo et al.[68] reviewed the Collaborative Review of Laparoscopic Sterilization (CREST) data and determined that soaking instruments in 2% activated glutaraldehyde was not associated with an increased risk of either pelvic or skin infections as compared with ethylene oxide sterilization.

BOWEL INJURIES

It is evident in both the surveys and the cohort and descriptive studies of laparoscopic complications that next to bleeding, burns are the second most common complication of laparoscopy. Improvement in the quality of cautery generators and instruments has markedly reduced the number of inadvertent burn injuries. Operator error still allows burn injuries to occur, however; unfortunately, as detailed in the AAGL data, most of the burn injuries occur during the initial experience of the laparoscopic surgeon.

In addition to burn injuries of the bowel, several investigators have reported perforation injuries to the stomach and the small and large bowel.[69-75] All cases of Veress needle perforations were managed conservatively, and no patients had subsequent adverse outcomes. In contrast, the vast majority of the trocar puncture and burn injuries had to be managed by laparotomy and repair. Farooqui et al.[76] reported the incidence of radiographically evident free peritoneal air 24 hours postlaparoscopy. Of the 26 patients examined, 38.5% had more than 2 cm^2 of free air despite a complete lack of clinical evidence of bowel perforation.

UROLOGIC INJURIES

Several cases of bladder injury during laparoscopy have been reported.[77-82] Most of these cases occurred by trocar perforation of the bladder as a result of inadequate preoperative bladder drainage. Thermal injury to the bladder has also been reported.[79] Despite the fact that many of the perforations went unrecognized until the patients were investigated for urinary ascites, the perforations spontaneously healed during continuous bladder drainage. Patients with urinary ascites have intense abdominal pain and distension, fever and chills, nausea and vomiting, and oliguria. They appear to have diffuse peritonitis. They usually have leukocytosis as well. Abdominal films and ultrasound will reveal intraperitoneal fluid. The test that distinguishes urinary ascites from bacterial peritonitis is serum blood urea nitrogen (BUN) and creatinine concentrations. Patients with urinary ascites will respond to aggressive hydration and continuous bladder drainage. Antibiotics are usually not indicated. Physicians faced with a patient with urinary ascites should not attempt to drain the ascites because the frequent result is circulatory collapse from inadequate intravascular volume. Bladder injuries can generally be prevented by complete drainage of the bladder immediately before insertion of the suprapubic trocar.

Laparoscopic ureteral injury is a relatively rare but serious complication, and at least 14 cases have been reported in the literature.[83, 84] Grainger et al.[83] reviewed 13 of these injuries and determined that 12 of the 13 injuries occurred as a result of thermal injury. Five of the 13 injuries occurred at the level of the uterosacral ligament, and 3 of the 13 patients lost renal function on the affected side. Unlike the bladder injuries, all of the ureteral injuries required laparotomy and ureteral reconstruction and reanastomosis.

In addition to trocar and thermal injury of the ureter, two cases of ureteral injury have been reported during laparoscopic-assisted vaginal hysterectomy (LAVH).[85] The possibility of ureteral injury at hysterectomy by LAVH may be increased if scrupulous care in identification of the ureter is not exercised. There are presently no series that might allow estimation of the incidence of LAVH-related ureteral injury and the factors that increase the risk of ureteral injury.

VASCULAR INJURIES

Bleeding is the most common complication of laparoscopy. Although most bleeding results from injuries to the inferior epigastric and mesosalpingeal vessels, perforation of the great vessels in the pelvis is a well-known, dramatic, and life-threatening event. Baadsgard et al.[86] reviewed 16 reported cases of great-vessel injury. Two of the 16 patients died as a result of the injuries, and the other 14 required immediate surgical repair to halt rapid retroperitoneal hemorrhage. Fourteen of the 16 injuries resulted from Veress needle injury. Injury to the inferior epigastric vessels can also occur during operative laparoscopy. Repair of these vessels can be effected by a transabdominal horizontal mattress suture placed under direct laparoscopic visualization. Attempts at cauterization of the vessels are generally ineffectual.

VERESS NEEDLE AND TROCAR INJURIES

Many laparoscopic complications occur during insertion of the Veress needle or trocar; several series have examined the relative safety of different methods of trocar introduction. Yuzpe[87] reported that 25% of Canadian obstetricians and gynecologists who responded to a survey about laparoscopic practices reported experiencing at least one complication resulting from sharp trocar or needle injury. Penfield[88] reported 19 wound infections and 6 bowel lacerations in 10,840 cases of open laparoscopy. Cohen and Scoccia[89] proposed a "double insertion technique" that allowed peritoneal insufflation through a supraumbilical site in cases of previous midline and umbilical surgery. The large trocar could then be placed under direct visualization. Bhidwandiwala et al.[90] reviewed 1,400 cases of open and "conventional" laparoscopic insertion technique and found no differences in surgical difficulty or complication rates between techniques. Nezhat et al.[91] performed a randomized trial of direct insertion of a "disposable trocar" vs. "conventional" technique using peritoneal insufflation with the Veress needle before trocar insertion. Although there were no major complications in the study, the "conventional" insertion group had a significantly higher incidence of subcutaneous and omental emphysema than did the group with direct insertion of a "disposable" trocar.

MISCELLANEOUS COMPLICATIONS

The common but relatively innocuous complication of uterine perforation has a reported incidence of between 1.8 and 30 per 1,000 cases.[92, 93] The major risk factors identified for uterine perforation are delivery within the past year, age older than 34 years, parity greater than 4, and body weight more than 20% above ideal. None of the cases reported in the literature required operative intervention.

The use of operative laparoscopy for the management of adnexal masses is controversial. Virtually no data exist on the outcome of patients undergoing ovarian cystectomy or oophorectomy with subsequent discovery of a malignancy in the specimen. Therefore, no recommendations are possible regarding either the safety or efficacy of laparoscopic treatment of malignant adnexal masses until the appropriate studies have been conducted to adequately examine the issue. Three cases of skin metastasis of malignant ovarian neoplasms following diagnostic laparoscopy in women with pelvic masses appear in the literature.[94, 95] This complication underlines the necessity of scrupulous preoperative testing, especially in perimenopausal and postmenopausal women with pelvic masses, to rule out intraperitoneal carcinoma before proceeding to laparoscopy.

Reports of rare laparoscopic complications include splenic rupture,[96] femoral neuropathy,[97] appendicitis secondary to erosion of a Filshie clip into the lumen of the appendix,[98] intestinal obstruction following herniation of the small bowel into a defect in the broad ligament peritoneum,[98] and cutaneous endometriosis following laparoscopic tubal ligation.[98]

SUMMARY

Laparoscopic surgery is a relatively safe and minimally invasive technique for the diagnosis and treatment of many intraperitoneal disease entities. However, the procedure is not innocuous, and extreme diligence on the part of the operator during the procedure itself, adequate training, and close supervision of laparoscopic novices are essential in minimizing the rate and seriousness of complications.

No data exist on the amount or type of training necessary to become a proficient laparoscopic surgeon. Nor is there any nationally accepted standard that can be used to gauge when a gynecologic surgeon should be capable of progressing from less complicated procedures (diagnostic laparoscopy or tubal sterilization) to the more complicated procedures (severe endometriosis or laparoscopic hysterectomy). Our experience is that the process of skills acquisition is a continuum and that it is impractical and ill-advised to progress too rapidly from experience with laparoscopic tubal sterilization to the more complicated surgical procedures. There is little question that didactic and laboratory experience as well as observational preceptorships aid in learning surgical skills. However, these should precede and cannot replace skill-building experiences in the operating room and progression from less complicated to more complicated surgical procedures.

REFERENCES

1. Kelling G: Über Oesophagoskopie, Gastroskopie, und Zölioskopie. *Munch Med Wochenscher* 1902; 49:21–24.
2. Anderson ET: Peritoneoscopy. *Am J Surg* 1937; 35:36–39.
3. Phillips J, Keith D, Keith L, et al: Survey of gynecologic laparoscopy for 1974. *J Reprod Med* 1975;15:45–50.
4. Phillips J, Keith D, Hulka J, et al: Gynecologic laparoscopy in 1975. *J Reprod Med* 1976; 16:105–117.
5. Phillips J, Hulka J, Hulka B, et al: American Association of Gynecologic Laparoscopists' 1976 membership survey. *J Reprod Med* 1978; 21:3–6.
6. Phillips J, Hulka J, Hulka B, et al: American Associate of Gynecologic Laparoscopists' 1977 membership survey. *J Reprod Med* 1979; 23:61–64.
7. Phillips JM, Hulka JF, Hulka B, et al: 1979 AAGL membership survey. *J Reprod Med* 1981; 26:529–533.
8. Phillips JM, Hulka JF, Peterson HB: American Association of Gynecologic Laparoscopists' 1982 membership survey. *J Reprod Med* 1984; 29:592–594.
9. Hulka JF, Peterson HB, Phillips JM: American Association of Gynecologic Laparoscopists' 1988 membership survey on laparoscopic sterilization. *J Reprod Med* 1990; 35:584–586.
10. Lehmann-Willenbrock E, Riedel H-H, Mecke H, et al: Pelviscopy/laparoscopy and its complications in Germany, 1949–1988. *J Reprod Med* 1992; 37:671–677.
11. Soderstrom RM, Butler JC: A critical evaluation of complications in laparoscopy. *J Reprod Med* 1973; 10:245–248.
12. Rawlings EE, Balgobin B: Complications of laparoscopy. *BMJ* 1975; 1:727–728.
13. Uribe-Ramirez LC, Camerena R, Hernandez F, et al: Outpatient laparoscopic sterilization: A review of complications in 2,000 cases. *J Reprod Med* 1977; 18:103–108.
14. Cunanan RG Jr, Courey NG, Lippes J: Complications of laparoscopic tubal sterilization. *Obstet Gynecol* 1980; 55:501–506.
15. Frenkel Y, Oelsner G, Ben-Baruch G, et al: Major surgical complications of laparoscopy. *Eur J Obstet Gynecol Reprod Biol* 1981; 12:107–111.
16. Kane MG, Krejs GJ: Complications of diagnostic laparoscopy in Dallas: A 7-year prospective study. *Gastrointest Endosc* 1984; 30:237–240.

17. Henning H: The Dallas report on laparoscopic complications. *Gastrointest Endosc* 1985; 31:104–105.

18. Patel DN, Parikh M, Nanavati MS, et al: Complications of laparoscopy. *Asia Oceania J Obstet Gynaecol* 1985; 11:87–91.

19. Franks AL, Kendrick JS, Peterson HB: Unintended laparotomy associated with laparoscopic tubal sterilization. *Am J Obstet Gynecol* 1987; 157:1102–1105.

20. Orlando R, Lirussi F, Nassuato G, et al: Complications of laparoscopy in the elderly: A report on 345 consecutive cases and comparison with a younger population. *Endoscopy* 1987; 19:146–146.

21. Mehta PV: A total of 250, 136 laparoscopic sterilizations by a single operator. *Br J Obstet Gynaecol* 1989; 96:1024–1034.

22. Hovorka J, Korttila K, Erkola O: Nitrous oxide does not increase nausea and vomiting following gynaecological laparoscopy. *Can J Anaesth* 1989; 36:145–148.

23. Beattie WS, Lindblad T, Buckley DN, et al: The incidence of post-operative nausea and vomiting in women undergoing laparoscopy is influenced by the day of menstrual cycle. *Can J Anaesth* 1991; 38:298–302.

24. Scott DB: Gynaecological laparoscopy. *BMJ* 1978; 2:1695.

25. Duffy BL: Regurgitation during pelvic laparoscopy. *Br J Anaesth* 1979; 51:1089.

26. Hodgson C, McClelland RMA, Newton JR: Some effects of the peritoneal insufflation of carbon dioxide at laparoscopy. *Anaesthesia* 1970; 25:382–390.

27. Marshall RL, Jebson PJR, Davie IT, et al: Circulatory effects of carbon dioxide insufflation of the peritoneal cavity for laparoscopy. *Br J Anaesth* 1972; 44:680–684.

28. Marshall RL, Jebson PJR, Davie IT, et al: Circulatory effects of peritoneal insufflation with nitrous oxide. *Br J Anaesth* 1972; 44:1183–1187.

29. Smith I, Benzie RJ, Gordon MLM, et al: Cardiovascular effects of peritoneal insufflation of carbon dioxide for laparoscopy. *BMJ* 1971; 3:410–411.

30. Ivankovich AD, Miletich DJ, Albrecht RF, et al: Cardiovascular effects of intraperitoneal insufflation with carbon dioxide and nitrous oxide in the dog. *Anesthesiology* 1975; 42:281–287.

31. Drury WL, LaVallee DA, Vacanti CJ: Effects of laparoscopic tubal ligation on arterial blood gases. *Anesth Analg* 1971; 50:349–354.

32. Diamant M, Benumof JL, Saidman LJ, et al: Laparoscopic sterilization with local anesthesia: Complications and blood-gas changes. *Anesth Analg* 1977; 56:335–337.

33. Myles PS: Bradyarrhythmias and laparoscopy: A prospective study of heart rate changes with laparoscopy. *Aust N Z J Obstet Gynaecol* 1991; 31:171–173.

34. Shifren JL, Adlestein L, Finkler NJ: Asystolic cardiac arrest: A rare complicaton of laparoscopy. *Obstet Gynecol* 1992; 79:840–841.

35. Lee CM: Acute hypotension during laparoscopy: A case report. *Anesth Analg* 1975; 54:142–143.

36. Parewijck W, Thiery M, Timperman J: Serious complications of laparoscopy. *Med Sci Law* 1979; 19:199–201.

37. DePlater RMH, Jones ISC: Non-fatal carbon dioxide embolism during laparoscopy. *Anaesth Intensive Care* 1989; 17:359–361.

38. Wadhwa RK, McKenzie R, Wadhwa SR, et al: Gas embolism during laparoscopy. *Anesthesiology* 1978; 48:74–76.

39. Östman PL, Pantle-Fisher FH, Faure EA: Circulatory collapse during laparoscopy. *J Clin Anesth* 1990; 2:129–132.

40. Bradfield ST: Gas embolism during laparoscopy. *Anaesth Intensive Care* 1991; 19:474.

41. Yacoub OF, Cardona I, Coveler LA, et al: Carbon dioxide embolism during laparoscopy. *Anesthesiology* 1982; 57:533–535.

42. Graff TD, Arbegast NR, Phillips OC, et al: Gas embolism: A comparative study of air and carbon dioxide as embolic agents in the systemic venous system. *Am J Obstet Gynecol* 1959; 78:259–265.

43. Pascual JB, Baranda MM, Tarrero MT, et al: Subcutaneous emphysema, pneumomediastinum, bilateral pneumothorax and pneumopericardium after laparoscopy. *Endoscopy* 1990; 22:59.

44. Bard PA, Chen L: Subcutaneous emphysema associated with laparoscopy. *Anesth Analg* 1990; 71:100–106.

45. Kent RB III: Subcutaneous emphysema and hypercarbia following laparoscopic cholecystectomy. *Arch Surg* 1991; 126:1154–1156.

46. Kalhan SB, Reaney JA, Collins RL: Pneumomediastinum and subcutaneous emphysema during laparoscopy. *Cleve Clin J Med* 1990; 57:639–642.

47. Berman ND: Pneumopericardium following laparoscopy. *Chest* 1980; 77:811.

48. Herrerias JM, Ariza A, Garrido M: An unusual complication of laparoscopy: Pneumopericardium. *Endoscopy* 1980; 12:254–255.

49. Doctor NH, Hussain Z: Bilateral pneumothorax associated with laparoscopy. *Anesthesiology* 1973; 28:57–81.

50. Low LCK, McCruden DC, Ramsay LE: Shoulder-hand syndrome after laparoscopic sterilisation. *BMJ* 1978; 14:1060–1061.

51. Robinson JS, Thompson JM, Wood AW: Fire and explosion hazards in operating theatres: A reply and new evidence. *Br J Anaesth* 1978; 51:908.

52. Vickers MD: Fire and explosion hazards in operating theatres. *Br J Anaesth* 1978; 50:659–664.

53. Harvey DO, Charlton AJ, Findley IL: Comparison of morbidity between inpatients and outpatients following gynaecological laparoscopy. *Ann R Coll Surg Engl* 1985; 67:103–104.

54. Dobbs EF, Kumar V, Alexander JI, et al: Pain after laparoscopy related to posture and ring versus clip sterilization. *Br J Obstet Gynaecol* 1987; 94:262–266.

55. Lipscomb GH, Stovall TG, Ramanathan JA, et al: Comparison of Silastic rings and electrocoagulation for laparoscopic tubal ligation under local anesthesia. *Obstet Gynecol* 1992; 80:645.

56. Rosenblum M, Weller RS, Conard PL, et al: Ibuprofen provides longer lasting analgesia than fentanyl after laparoscopic surgery. *Anesth Analg* 1991; 73:255–259.

57. Narchi P, Benhamou D, Hernandez H: Intraperitoneal local anaesthetic for shoulder pain after day-case laparoscopy. *Lancet* 1991; 338:1569–1570.

58. Hiilholma P, Mäkinen J: Incarcerated Richter's hernia after laparoscopy: A case report. *Eur J Obstet Gynecol Reprod Biol* 1988; 28:75–77.

59. Bourke JB: Small-intestinal obstruction from a Richter's hernia at the site of insertion of a laparoscope. *BMJ* 1977; 2:1393–1394.

60. Bishop HL, Halpin TF: Dehiscence following laparoscopy: Report of an unusual complication. *Am J Obstet Gynecol* 1973; 116:585–586.

61. Sauer M, Jarrett JC II: Small bowel obstruction following diagnostic laparoscopy. *Fertil Steril* 1984; 42:653–654.

62. Maio A, Ruchman RB: Case report: CT diagnosis of postlaparoscopic hernia. *J Comput Assist Tomogr* 1991; 15:1054–1055.

63. Goodnough JE, O'Shaughnessy R, Shoff D: Gonococcal peritonitis following uterine manipulation at laparoscopy. *Am J Obstet Gynecol* 1981; 139:218–219.

64. House MJ: Abdominal actinomycosis complication of laparoscopy? *Br J Obstet Gynaecol* 1981; 88:459–460.

65. Iwamura K, Ueno F, Itakura M, et al: Evaluation of blood cultures following laparoscopy. *Tokai J Exp Clin Med* 1980; 5:323–327.
66. Pyper RJD, Ahmet Z, Houang ET: Bacteriological contamination during laparoscopy with dye injection. *Br J Obstet Gynaecol* 1988; 95:367–371.
67. Sotrel G, Hirsch E, Edelin KC: Necrotizing fasciitis following diagnostic laparoscopy. *Obstet Gynecol* 1983; 62(suppl):67–69.
68. Huezo CM, DeStefano F, Rubin GL, et al: Risk of wound and pelvic infection after laparoscopic tubal sterilization: Instrument disinfection versus sterilization. *Obstet Gynecol* 1983; 61:598–602.
69. Roopnarinesingh S, Raj-Kumar G, Woo J: Laparoscopic trocar point perforation of the small bowel. *Int Surg* 1976; 62:76.
70. Milliken RA, Milliken GM: Gastric perforation: Rare complication of laparoscopy. *N Y State J Med* 1975; 75:77–79.
71. Endler GC, Moghissi KS: Gastric perforation during pelvic laparoscopy. *Obstet Gynecol* 1976; 47(suppl):40–42.
72. Esposito JM: Hematoma of the sigmoid colon as a complication of laparoscopy. *Am J Obstet Gynecol* 1973; 117:581–582.
73. Birns MT: Inadvertent instrumental perforation of the colon during laparoscopy: Nonsurgical repair. *Gastrointest Endosc* 1989; 35:54–56.
74. Thompson BH, Wheeless CR Jr: Gastrointestinal complications of laparoscopy sterilization. *Obstet Gynecol* 1973; 41:669–676.
75. Shell JH Jr, Myers RC: Small bowel injury after laparoscopic sterilization. *Am J Obstet Gynecol* 1973; 115:285.
76. Farooqui MO, Bazzoli JM: Significance of radiologic evidence of free air following laparoscopy. *J Reprod Med* 1976; 16:119–125.
77. Georgy FM, Fetterman HH, Chefetz MD: Complication of laparoscopy: Two cases of perforated urinary bladder. *Obstet Gynecol* 1974; 120:1121–1122.
78. Homburg R, Segal T: Perforation of the urinary bladder by laparoscope. *Am J Obstet Gynecol* 1978; 130:597.
79. Deshmukh AS: Laparoscopic bladder injury. *Urology* 1982; 19:306–307.
80. Sherer DM: Inadvertent transvaginal cystotomy during laparoscopy. *Int J Gynaecol Obstet* 1990; 32:77–79.
81. Yong EL, Prabhakaran K, Lee YS, et al: Peritonitis following diagnostic laparoscopy due to injury to a vesicourachal diverticulum: Case report. *Br J Obstet Gynaecol* 1989; 96:365–368.
82. Schapira M, Dizerens H, Essinger A, et al: Urinary ascites after gynaecological laparoscopy. *Lancet* 1978; 1:871–872.
83. Grainger DA, Soderstrom RM, Schiff SF, et al: Ureteral injuries at laparoscopy: Insights into diagnosis, management, and prevention. *Obstet Gynecol* 1990; 75:839–843.
84. Gomel V, James C: Intraoperative management of ureteral injury during operative laparoscopy. *Fertil Steril* 1991; 55:416–418.
85. Woodland MB: Ureter injury during laparoscopic-assisted vaginal hysterectomy. *Am J Obstet Gynecol* 1992; 167:757–757.
86. Baadsgaard SE, Bille S, Egeblad K: Major vascular injury during gynecologic laparoscopy. *Acta Obstet Gynecol Scand* 1989; 68:283–285.
87. Yuzpe AA: Pneumoperitoneum needle and trocar injuries in laparoscopy: A survey of possible contributing factors and prevention. *J Reprod Med* 1990; 35:489–490.
88. Penfield AJ: How to prevent complications of open laparoscopy. *J Reprod Med* 1985; 30:660–663.
89. Cohen MR, Scoccia B: Double laparoscopy: An alterative two-stage procedure to minimize bowel and blood vessel injury. *J Gynecol Surg* 1991; 7:203–206.
90. Bhiwandiwala PP, Memford SD, Kennedy KI: Comparison of the safety of

open and conventional laparoscopic sterilization. *Obstet Gynecol* 1985; 66:391–394.

91. Nezhat FR, Silfen SL, Evans D, et al: Comparison of direct insertion of disposable and standard reusable laparoscopic trocars and previous pneumoperitoneum with Veress needle. *Obstet Gynecol* 1991; 78:148–150.
92. White MK, Ory HW, Goldenberg LA: A case-control study of uterine perforations documented at laparoscopy. *Am J Obstet Gynecol* 1977; 129:623.
93. Chi I-C, Feldblum P: Uterine performation during sterilization by laparoscopy and minilaparotomy. *Am J Obstet Gynecol* 1981; 139:735–736.
94. Hsiu JG, Given FR Jr, Kemp GM: Tumor implantation after diagnostic laparoscopic biopsy of serous ovarian tumors of low malignant potential. *Obstet Gynecol* 1986; 68(suppl):90–93.
95. Miralles RM, Petit J, Gine L, et al: Metastatic cancer spread at the laparoscopic puncture site. Report of a case in a patient with carcinoma of the ovary. *Eur J Gynaecol Oncol* 1989; 10:442–444.
96. Dancygier H, Jacob RA: Splenic rupture during laparoscopy. *Gastrointest Endosc* 1983; 29:63.
97. Hershlag A, Loy RA, Lavy G, et al: Femoral neuropathy after laparoscopy: A case report. *J Reprod Med* 1990; 35:575–576.
98. Denton GWL, Schofield JB, Gallagher P: Uncommon complications of laparoscopic sterilisation. *Ann R Coll Surg Engl* 1990; 72:210–211.

Editor's Comment

The author stresses that endoscopy has the potential for complications especially when performed by improperly trained individuals. The most common complications are bleeding, bowel perforations, and burns. The section on complications of pneumoperitoneum is timely and important, because it explicitly details the effects of instilling CO_2 into the peritoneal cavity. The shoulder pain that is associated with laparoscopy typically has been considered to be the only significant complication. Most surgeons do not consider the other complications associated with the CO_2 instilled within the peritoneal cavity.

An interesting complication of laparoscopy is herniation of the small bowel or omentum through the umbilical incision. This is a significant complication because of intestinal obstruction. Recognizing that a spectrum of infections has been reported associated with laparoscopy, including necrotizing infections is important. The small nature of the incision tends to conceal the infection and allow it to go undetected until it is far advanced.

The authors have provided an excellent and comprehensive discussion of the complications of laparoscopy. This chapter should be read by all gynecologists and residents in training, and by all practicing gynecologic surgeons.

Sebastian Faro, M.D., Ph.D.

The Role of Laparoscopy in Hysterectomy

HARRY REICH, M.D.

O f the 600,000 hysterectomies performed each year, over 60% are presently accomplished by using an abdominal incision.[1] Abdominal hysterectomy will probably become a rarely used procedure, however, because laparoscopy, properly applied, can be effectively used to accomplish a less invasive vaginal hysterectomy. Laparoscopic-assisted vaginal hysterectomy (LAVH) may encourage surgeons to become skilled in vaginal surgery.

Laparoscopic hysterectomy (LH), defined as laparoscopic ligation of the uterine vessels, is an alternative to abdominal hysterectomy that allows precise attention to ureteral identification.[2–4] First performed in January 1988,[5] LH has stimulated general interest in the laparoscopic approach to hysterectomy that has reached its zenith in LAVH. Laparoscopically assisted vaginal hysterectomy has become an expensive procedure, and skilled vaginal surgeons will not often see sufficient indication for its use. Laparoscopic hysterectomy remains a reasonable substitute for abdominal hysterectomy.

Most hysterectomies presently requiring an abdominal approach may be performed by laparoscopic dissection of part or all of the abdominal portion followed by vaginal removal. There are many surgical advantages to laparoscopy, particularly magnification of anatomy and pathology, easy access to the vagina and rectum, and the ability to achieve complete hemostasis and clot evacuation during underwater examination. Patient advantages are many. They include avoidance of a painful abdominal incision, reduced duration of hospitalization and recuperation, and an extremely low rate of infection and ileus. When compared with abdominal surgery, vaginal surgery by competent surgeons reduces blood loss and respiratory problems and does not require exposure of the bowel.

The goal of vaginal hysterectomy, LAVH or LH, is to safely avoid an abdominal wall incision. The surgeon must remember that if vaginal hysterectomy is possible after ligating the utero-ovarian ligaments, it should be done. Laparoscopic inspection at the end will still allow the surgeon to control any bleeding and evacuate clots. Unnecessary operations should not be done because of the surgeon's preoccupation with the development of new surgical skills. Laparoscopic hysterectomy is not indicated when vaginal hysterectomy is possible.

Advances in Obstetrics and Gynecology, vol 1
© 1994, Mosby–Year Book, Inc.

DEFINITIONS

There is a variety of procedures for which the laparoscope is useful as an aid to hysterectomy (Table 1). It is important that these different procedures be clearly delineated.

Diagnostic laparoscopy with vaginal hysterectomy is use of the laparoscope for *diagnostic* purposes, when indications for a vaginal approach are equivocal, to determine whether *vaginal hysterectomy* is possible.[6] It also ensures that vaginal cuff and pedicle hemostasis is complete and allows clot evacuation.

Laparoscopic-assisted vaginal hysterectomy is a vaginal hysterectomy after laparoscopic adhesiolysis, endometriosis excision, or oophorectomy.[7–9] Unfortunately, this term is also used to refer to staple ligation of the upper uterine blood supply of a relatively normal uterus. It must be emphasized that in most cases the easy part of both abdominal and vaginal hysterectomy is upper pedicle ligation.

Laparoscopic hysterectomy denotes laparoscopic ligation of the uterine arteries either by electrosurgical desiccation, suture ligature, or staples. All maneuvers after uterine vessel ligation can be done vaginally or laparoscopically, including anterior and posterior vaginal entry, cardinal and uterosacral ligament division, uterine removal intact or by morcellation, and vaginal closure vertically or transversely. Laparoscopic ligation of the uterine vessels is the sine qua non for LH. Ureteral isolation has always been advised.

Total laparoscopic hysterectomy (TLH) is a laparoscopically assisted abdominal hysterectomy. Laparoscopic dissection continues until the uterus lies free of all attachments in the peritoneal cavity. The uterus is removed through the vagina with morcellation if necessary. The vagina is closed with laparoscopically placed sutures.

Laparoscopic supracervical hysterectomy (LSH) has recently regained advocates after suggestions that total hysterectomy results in a decrease in libido.[10] The uterus is removed by morcellation from above or below.

Kurt Semm's version of supracervical hysterectomy, called the CASH procedure (classic abdominal Semm hysterectomy), leaves the cardinal

TABLE 1.
Laparoscopic Hysterectomy Classification

Diagnostic laparoscopy with vaginal hysterectomy
Laparoscopic-assisted vaginal hysterectomy (LAVH)
Laparoscopic hysterectomy (LH)
Total laparoscopic hysterectomy (TLH)
Laparoscopic supracervical hysterectomy (LSH), including classic
  abdominal Semm hysterectomy (CASH)
Vaginal hysterectomy with laparoscopic vault suspension (LVS) or
  laparoscopic pelvic reconstruction (LPR)
Laparoscopic hysterectomy with lymphadenectomy
Laparoscopic hysterectomy with lymphadenectomy and omentectomy
Laparoscopic radical hysterectomy with lymphadenectomy

ligaments intact while eliminating the columnar cells of the endocervical canal. After perforating the uterine fundus with a long sound-dilator, a calibrated uterine resection tool (CURT) that fits around this instrument is used to core out the endocervical canal. Thereafter, at laparoscopy, suture techniques are used to ligate the utero-ovarian ligaments. An Endoloop is placed around the uterine fundus to the level of the internal os of the cervix and tied. The uterus is divided at its junction with the cervix and removed by laparoscopic morcellation.

Laparoscopic pelvic reconstruction (LPR) with vaginal hysterectomy is useful when vaginal hysterectomy alone cannot accomplish appropriate repair for prolapse. Ureteral dissection and suture placement before the vaginal hysterectomy aid in high uterosacral ligament identification and plication near the sacrum. Levator muscle plication from below or above is often necessary. Retropubic colposuspension can also be done laparoscopically.

INDICATIONS

Indications for LH include benign pathology such as endometriosis, fibroids, adhesions, and adnexal masses usually requiring the selection of an abdominal approach to hysterectomy. It is also appropriate when vaginal hysterectomy is contraindicated because of a narrow pubic arch, a narrow vagina with no prolapse, or severe arthritis that prohibits placement of the patient in a sufficient lithotomy position for vaginal exposure. Laparoscopic procedures in obese women allow the surgeon to make an incision above the panniculus and operate below it. Laparoscopic hysterectomy may also be considered for stage I endometrial, ovarian, and cervical cancer.[11-13] Pelvic reconstruction procedures including cuff suspension, retropubic colposuspension, and rectocele repair may be accomplished through the laparoscope.

The most common indication for LH is a symptomatic fibroid uterus. Morcellation is often necessary. Fibroids fixed in the pelvis or abdomen without descent are easier to mobilize laparoscopically. Uterine size and weight measurements are important to document the appropriateness of LH since most small uteri can be removed vaginally. The normal uterus weighs 70 to 125 g. A 12-week gestational age uterus weighs 280 to 320 g, a 24-week uterus weighs 580 to 620 g, and a term uterus weighs 1,000 to 1,100 g.

Hysterectomy should not be done for stage IV endometriosis with extensive cul-de-sac involvement unless the surgeon has the capability and the time to resect all deep fibrotic endometriosis from the posterior of the vagina, uterosacral ligaments, and anterior of the rectum. Excision of the uterus with an intrafascial technique leaves the deep fibrotic endometriosis behind to cause future problems. It is much more difficult to remove deep fibrotic endometriosis when there is no uterus between the anterior of the rectum and the bladder; after hysterectomy, the endometriosis left in the anterior of the rectum and vaginal cuff frequently becomes densely adherent or invades into the bladder and one or both ureters. In many cases of stage IV endometriosis with extensive cul-de-sac obliteration, it is better to preserve the uterus to prevent future vaginal cuff, bladder, and ureteral problems.[14] Obviously, this approach will not be effective when uterine adenomyosis is present. In these cases, after excision of cul-de-sac endometriosis, persistent pain will lead ultimately to hysterectomy. Oophorectomy is not always necessary at hysterectomy; if the endometriosis is carefully removed, it is less likely to recur. Bilateral oophorectomy is rarely indicated in women under the age of 40 years who are undergoing hysterectomy for endometriosis.

Hysterectomy is performed for abnormal uterine bleeding in women of reproductive age. Abnormal uterine bleeding is defined as excessive uterine bleeding or irregular uterine bleeding for more than 8 days during more than a single cycle or as profuse bleeding requiring additional protection (large clots, gushes, or limitations on activity). There should be no history of a bleeding diathesis or use of medication that may cause bleeding. A negative effect on quality of life should be documented. Physical examination, laboratory data, ultrasound, and hysteroscopy findings are frequently negative. Hormone treatment is attempted before hysterectomy, and its failure, contraindication, or refusal is documented. The presence of anemia is recorded and correction attempted. If hysterectomy is chosen, a vaginal approach is usually appropriate. Laparoscopic hysterectomy is done when vaginal hysterectomy is not possible, including a history of previous surgery, lack of prolapse (nulliparous or multiparous), or inexperience of the operator with the vaginal approach. Recognition of vaginal surgery inexperience is important; in many countries vaginal hysterectomy is not done.

CONTRAINDICATIONS

Laparoscopic hysterectomy is not advised for the diagnosis and treatment of a pelvic mass that is too large to fit intact into an impermeable sack. The largest available sack for removal of intraperitoneal masses is the Lap-Sac (Cook Ob/Gyn, Spencer, Ind), which measures 8 × 5 in. Although cyst aspiration is advocated by some investigators,[15] this author feels that postmenopausal cystic ovaries should not be subjected to fluid aspiration before oophorectomy because the inevitable spillage changes the diagnosis from a stage IA ovarian cancer to a stage IA with spill. Its effect on survival is unknown, but it may be detrimental. It must be emphasized that small-gauge needles, placement through thickened portions of the ovary, and cyst aspiration devices with surrounding suction and Endoloop placement (Cook) do not prevent spillage. Ovaries should be removed intact through a culdotomy incision.[16]

The medical status of the patient may prohibit surgery. Anemia, diabetes, lung disorders, cardiac disease, and bleeding diathesis must be evaluated before surgery. Age should rarely be a deterrent.

Cesarean hysterectomy is an absolute contraindication. Placenta accreta, uterine atony, unspecified uterine bleeding, and uterine rupture are relative contraindications for peripartum hysterectomy at present. Laparoscopic hysterectomy may be considered for patients needing a postpartum hysterectomy.

Another contraindication is stage III ovarian cancer that requires a large abdominal incision. Finally, inexperience of the surgeon is a contraindication to the laparoscopic approach.

EQUIPMENT

High-flow CO_2 insufflation up to 10 to 15 L/min is necessary to compensate for the rapid loss of CO_2 during suctioning. The ability to maintain a relatively constant intra-abdominal pressure between 10 and 15 mm Hg during laparoscopic hysterectomy is essential. Gasless laparoscopy with abdominal wall retractors is used to minimize abdominal wall subcutaneous emphysema during retroperitoneal surgery since peritoneal defects resulting in free subcutaneous communication may compromise peritoneal cavity operating space. A useful technique is to insert a Laparolift anterior abdominal wall retractor (Origin Medsystems, Menlo Park, Calif) once the vagina is opened to maintain working space.

Operating room tables capable of a 30-degree Trendelenburg position are extremely valuable for LH. Unfortunately these tables are rare, and this author has much difficulty operating when only a limited degree of body tilt can be attained. For the past 16 years a steep Trendelenburg position (20 to 40 degrees) with shoulder braces and the arms at the patient's sides has been used without adverse effects.

A Valtchev uterine mobilizer (Conkin Surgical Instruments, Toronto) is the best available single instrument to antevert the uterus and delineate the posterior of the vagina.[17] The uterus can be anteverted to about 120 degrees and moved in an arc about 45 degrees to the left or right by turning the mobilizer around its longitudinal axis. Either the 100-mm-long and 10-mm-thick or the 80-mm-long and 8-mm-thick obturator may be used for uterine manipulation during hysterectomy.

If a Valtchev uterine mobilizer is not available, a sponge on a ring forceps is inserted into the posterior vaginal fornix, and an 81 F rectal probe (Reznik Instruments, Skokie, Ill) is placed in the rectum to define the rectum and posterior of the vagina and excise endometriosis or to open the posterior of the vagina (culdotomy). In addition, a no. 3 or 4 Sims curette is placed in the endometrial cavity to antevert the uterus markedly and stretch out the cul-de-sac. The rectal probe and intraoperative rectovaginal examinations remain important techniques even when the Valtchev mobilizer is available. Whenever rectal location is in doubt, it is identified by placing a probe.

Trocar sleeves are available in many sizes and shapes. For most cases, 5.5-mm cannulas are adequate. Newer electrosurgical electrodes that eliminate capacitance and insulation failures (Electroshield from Electroscope, Boulder, Colo) require 7/8 mm sleeves. Laparoscopic stapling is performed through 12/13 mm Surgiports (U.S. Surgical Corp., Norwalk, Conn). However, disposable stapling instruments (U.S. Surgical) are rarely used for large-vessel hemostasis during LH.

Short trapless 5-mm trocar sleeves with a retention screw grid around the external surface (Richard Wolf Medical Instruments, Vernon Hills, Ill; Apple Medical, Bolton, Mass) are used to facilitate efficient instrument exchanges and evacuation of tissue while allowing unlimited freedom during extracorporeal suture tying.[18] With practice, a good laparoscopic surgical team will be able to make instrument exchanges so fast that little pneumoperitoneum will be lost.

Bipolar forceps use a high-frequency low-voltage cutting current (20 to 50 W) to coagulate vessels as large as the ovarian and uterine arteries. The Kleppinger bipolar forceps (Richard Wolf) are excellent for large-vessel hemostasis. Specially insulated bipolar forceps are available that allow current to pass through their tips for precise hemostasis. Microbipolar forceps contain a channel for irrigation and a fixed distance between the electrodes. They are used to irrigate bleeding sites for vessel identification before coagulation and to prevent sticking of the electrode to the eschar that is created. Irrigation is used during underwater examination to identify the bleeding vessel before coagulation by removing surrounding blood products.

Disposable stapling instruments (U.S. Surgical) are rarely used during laparoscopic hysterectomy because of their expense. Suture and/or bipolar desiccation work better.

PREOPERATIVE PREPARATION

The preoperative use of gonadotropin-releasing hormone (GnRH) analogues for at least 2 months before hysterectomy for large myomas is encouraged. Such analogues may reduce the total uterine and leiomyoma volumes and make laparoscopic or vaginal hysterectomy easier.[19, 20] During treatment with leuprolide (Lupron Depot) at a dose of 3.75 mg intramuscularly once per month for 3 to 6 months, anemia secondary to hypermenorrhea will resolve, and autologous blood donation can be considered before LH. Packed red blood cells have a shelf life of 35 days if stored at 1 to 6° C. In addition, Lupron Depot is often administered after ovulation in the cycle preceding surgery to avoid operating on ovaries containing a corpus luteum.

Patients are encouraged to drink and eat lightly for 24 hours before admission on the day of surgery. When extensive cul-de-sac involvement with endometriosis is suspected, mechanical bowel preparation is ordered (polyethylene glycol–based isosmotic solution: GoLYTELY or Colyte). Lower abdominal, pubic, and perineal hair is *not* shaved. A Foley catheter is inserted during surgery and removed the next morning. Antibiotics (usually cefoxitin) are administered at the 2-hour mark in all surgeries lasting over 2 hours.

POSITIONING OF THE PATIENT

All laparoscopic surgical procedures are done under general anesthesia with endotracheal intubation and an orogastric tube. The routine use of an orogastric tube is recommended to diminish the possibility of a trocar injury to the stomach and to reduce small bowel distension. The patient is flat (0 degrees) until the umbilical trocar sleeve has been inserted and then is placed in the steep Trendelenburg position (20 to 30 degrees). The lithotomy position with the hip extended (thigh parallel to the abdomen) is obtained with Allan stirrups (Edgewater Medical Systems, Mayfield Heights, Ohio) or knee braces that are adjusted to each individual patient before anesthesia. Self-retaining lateral vaginal wall retractors or Vienna retractors (Brisky-Navatril) are used when quick vaginal uterine extraction is anticipated. With large fibroids, the stirrups are replaced with candy-cane stirrups for the vaginal part in order to obtain better hip flexion so that vaginal sidewall retractors can be used. Examination under anesthesia is always performed before preparing the patient.

Laparoscopy was never thought to be a sterile procedure before the incorporation of video because the surgeon operated with his head in the surgical field, looking through the laparoscopic optic. It is not possible to sterilize skin. Since 1983, this author has maintained a policy of not sterilizing or draping the camera or laser arm. Infection has been rare: less than 1 per 200 cases. The umbilical incision is closed with a single 4-0 polyglactin 910 (Vicryl) suture opposing deep fascia and skin dermis, with the knot buried beneath the fascia to prevent the suture from acting like a wick to transmit bacteria into the soft tissue or peritoneal cavity. The lower quadrant incisions are loosely approximated with a Javid vascular clamp (V. Mueller, McGaw Park, Ill) and covered with Collodion (AMEND, Irvington, NJ) to allow drainage of excess Ringer's lactate solution.

TOTAL LAPAROSCOPIC HYSTERECTOMY TECHNIQUE

The technique for total laparoscopic hysterectomy is depicted in Figures 1 through 14.

INCISIONS

Three laparoscopic puncture sites including the umbilicus are used: 10 or 12 mm umbilical, 5 mm right, and 5 mm left lower quadrant. The left

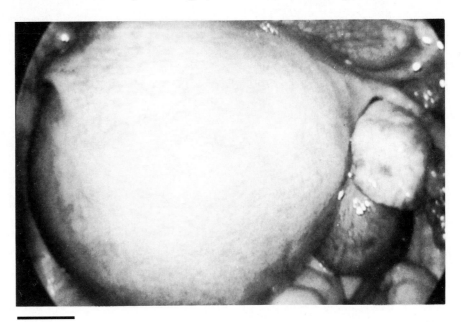

FIGURE 1.
A large fibroid uterus fills the lower part of the abdomen.

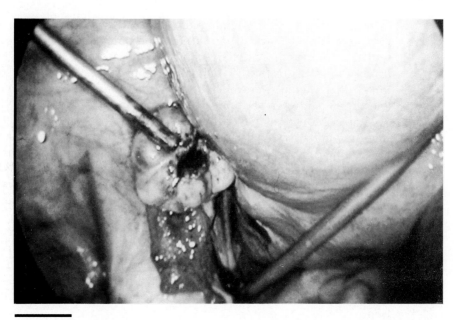

FIGURE 2.
Left ovary mobilized, left ovarian endometrioma excised, and the left ureter grasped and pulled medially.

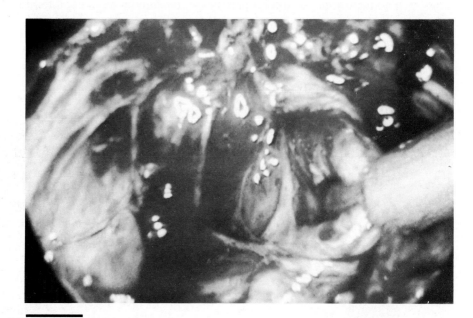

FIGURE 3.
Close-up of the left ureter in grasping forceps after the overlying peritoneum has been divided.

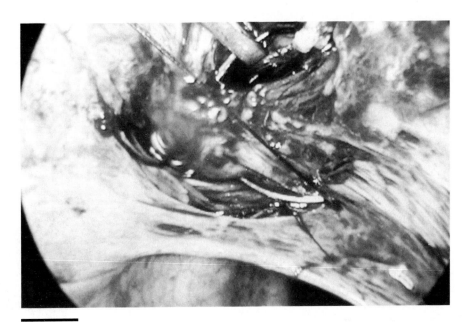

FIGURE 4.
CT-1 needle around the left uterine vessels.

lower quadrant puncture is the major portal for operative manipulation. The right trocar sleeve is used for retraction with atraumatic grasping forceps. When the Multi-Fire Endo GIA 30 was used, it was inserted through the umbilical incision, and the procedure was viewed through a 5-mm laparoscope in one of the 5-mm lower quadrant sites. This is no longer used.

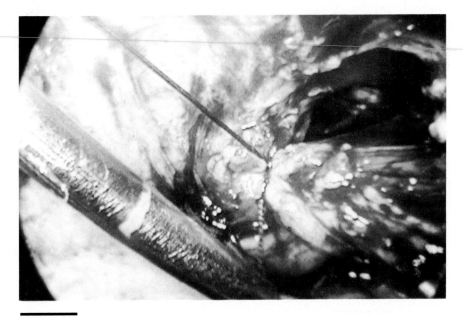

FIGURE 5.
Suture ligature tightened on the left uterine vessels with a Clarke knot pusher.

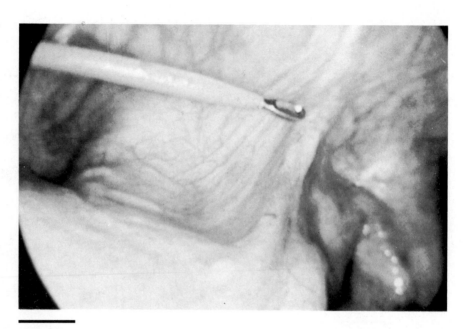

FIGURE 6.
A spoon electrode at 150-W cutting current is used to divide round ligaments and the vesicouterine peritoneal fold.

In most cases, a vertical midline incision on the inferior wall of the umbilical fossa extending to and just beyond its lowest point is used. Veress needle insufflation is continued until a pressure of 20 to 25 mm Hg is obtained, usually after 4 to 6 L. It is not necessary to lift the anterior abdominal wall during trocar insertion after establishment of a 4- to

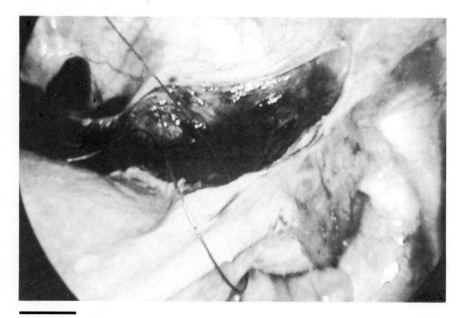

FIGURE 7.
Suture ligature around the right utero-ovarian ligament.

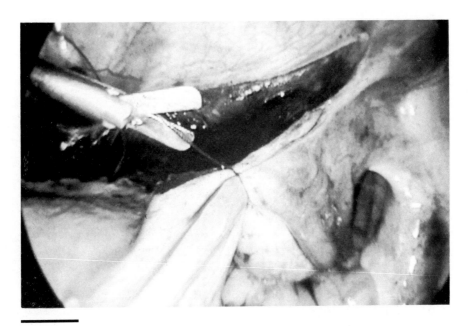

FIGURE 8.
Ligature tightened around the right utero-ovarian ligament and the suture divided.

6-L pneumoperitoneum at 20 to 25 mm Hg because the parietal peritoneum and skin move as one. The palmed Apple trocar is positioned with
moderate pressure in the incision to the peritoneum at a 90-degree angle
and is upturned to approximately 30 degrees in one continuous thrusting motion with the wrist rotating nearly 90 degrees. The result is a parietal peritoneal puncture directly beneath the umbilicus. The high-

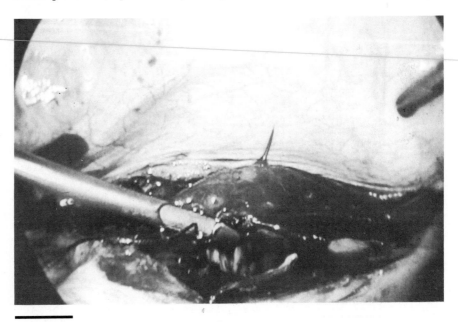

FIGURE 9.
Right uterine vessels suture ligated after exposure of the right ureter.

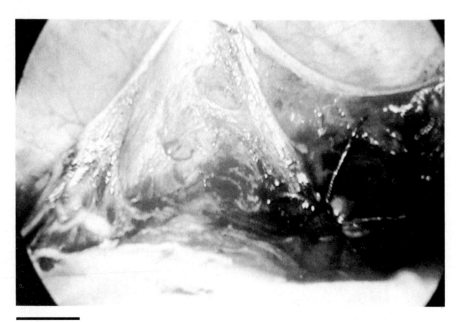

FIGURE 10.
Vesicouterine peritoneal fold reflection completed to the upper anterior portion
of the vagina.

pressure settings used during initial insertion of the trocar are lowered
thereafter to diminish the development of vena caval compression and
subcutaneous emphysema. A relatively constant 10- to 15-mm Hg intra-
abdominal pressure is maintained during long laparoscopic procedures.

Special entry techniques are necessary in patients who have under-

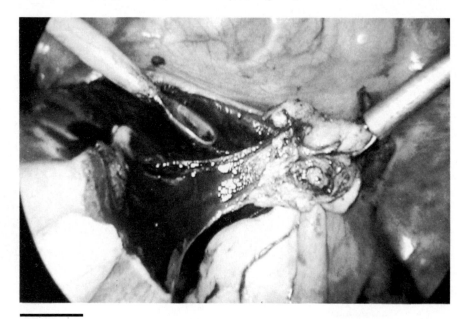

FIGURE 11.
A spoon electrode at 150-W cutting current is used to divide the right utero-
ovarian ligament and right cardinal ligament.

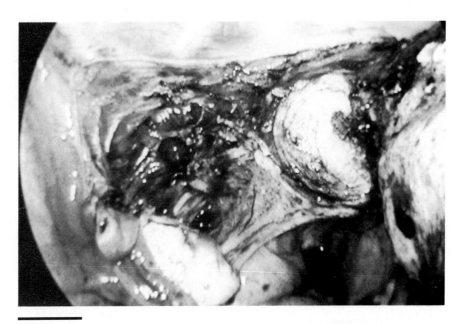

FIGURE 12.
On the left side, the left cardinal ligament has been divided and the left vaginal fornix exposed (white sponge in it).

gone multiple laparotomies, who have lower abdominal incisions travers-ing the umbilicus, or who have extensive adhesions either clinically or from a previous surgery. Open laparoscopy or microlaparotomy carries the same risk for bowel laceration if the bowel is fused to the umbilical undersurface. In these cases, Veress needle puncture is done in the left

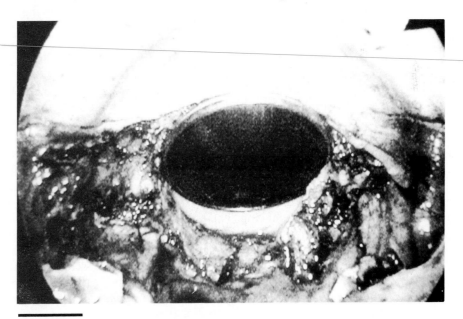

FIGURE 13.
An operating sigmoidoscope (Wolf) is used to maintain pneumoperitoneum dur-ing circumferential culdotomy.

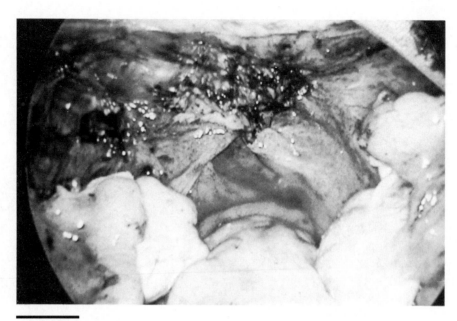

FIGURE 14.
Vertical midline closure of the vaginal cuff completed, with the uterosacral ligaments adjoined in the midline.

ninth intercostal space, anterior axillary line. Adhesions are rare in this area, and the peritoneum is tethered to the undersurface of the ribs, which makes subcutaneous insufflation unusual. A disposable Veress needle is grasped near its tip like a dart, between the thumb and forefinger. The needle tip is then inserted at right angles to the skin, but at a 45-degree angle to the horizontal anterior abdominal wall between the ninth and tenth ribs. A single pop is felt on penetration of the peritoneum. Pneumoperitoneum to a pressure of 20 to 25 mm Hg is obtained. A 5- or 10-mm trocar is then inserted at the left costal margin in the midclavicular line to give a panoramic view of the entire peritoneal cavity.

Placement of the lower quadrant trocar sleeves under direct laparoscopic vision just above the pubic hairline and lateral to the rectus abdominis muscles (and thus, the deep epigastric vessels) is preferred. These vessels, an artery flanked by two veins (venae comitantes), are located lateral to the umbilical ligaments (obliterated umbilical artery). These can be identified by direct laparoscopic inspection of the anterior abdominal wall. The deep epigastric vessels arise near the junction of the external iliac vessels with the femoral vessels and make up the medial border of the internal inguinal ring. The round ligament curls around these vessels to enter the inguinal canal. When the anterior abdominal wall parietal peritoneum is thickened from previous surgery or obesity, the position of these vessels is judged by palpating and depressing the anterior abdominal wall with the back of the scalpel; the wall will appear thicker where rectus muscle is enclosed, and the incision site is made lateral to this area near the anterior superior iliac spine.

VAGINAL PREPARATION

The endocervical canal is dilated to Pratt no. 25, and the Valtchev uterine mobilizer (Conkin Surgical Instruments) is inserted to antevert the uterus and delineate the posterior of the vagina. When the uterus is in the anteverted position, the cervix sits on a wide pedestal, thus making the vagina readily visible between the uterosacral ligaments when the cul-de-sac is viewed laparoscopically. Hysteroscopy with CO_2 may be done during insufflation of pneumoperitoneum to identify the location of the fibroids.

EXPLORATION

The upper part of the abdomen is inspected and the appendix identified. If appendiceal pathology is present, i.e., dilatation, adhesions, or endometriosis, appendectomy is performed after ureteral isolation by mobilizing the appendix, desiccating its blood supply, and placing three Endoloops (Endoloop [chromic gut ligature], Ethicon, Somerville, NJ) at the appendiceal-cecal junction after desiccating the appendix just above this juncture. The appendix is left attached to the cecum; its stump is divided later in the procedure, after opening the cul-de-sac, so that removal from the peritoneal cavity is accomplished immediately after separation.

URETERAL DISSECTION

Immediately after exploration of the upper part of the abdomen and pelvis, each ureter is isolated deep in the pelvis, if possible. This is done early in the operation, before the pelvic sidewall peritoneum becomes edematous and/or opaque from irritation by the CO_2 pneumoperitoneum or aquadissection and before ureteral peristalsis is inhibited by surgical stress, pressure, or the Trendelenburg position. The ureter and its overlying peritoneum are grasped deep in the pelvis on the left below the lateral rectosigmoid attachments at the pelvic brim. An atraumatic grasping forceps is used from a right-sided cannula to grab the ureter and its overlying peritoneum on the left pelvic sidewall below and caudad to the left ovary, lateral to the left uterosacral ligament. Scissors are used to divide the peritoneum overlying the ureter and are inserted into the defect created and spread. Thereafter one blade of the scissors is placed on top of the ureter, the buried scissors blade is visualized through the peritoneum, and the peritoneum is divided. This is continued deep into the pelvis where the uterine vessels cross the ureter, lateral to the cardinal ligament insertion into the cervix. Connective tissue between the ureter and the vessels is separated with scissors. Bleeding is controlled with microbipolar forceps. Often, the uterine vessel ligation procedure below is accomplished at this time to diminish backbleeding from the upper pedicles.

BLADDER MOBILIZATION

The round ligaments are divided at their midportion with a spoon electrode (Electroscope) at 150-W cutting current with minimal bleeding. Persistent bleeding is controlled with monopolar fulguration at 80-W coagulation current or bipolar desiccation at 30-W cutting current (fulguration is the noncontact application of high-voltage coagulation current). Thereafter scissors or the same electrode is used to divide the vesicouterine peritoneal fold, starting at the left side and continuing across the midline to the right round ligament. The bladder is mobilized off the uterus and upper portion of the vagina by using scissors or the same spoon electrode until the anterior of the vagina is identified by elevating it from below with ring forceps.

UPPER UTERINE BLOOD SUPPLY

When ovarian preservation is desired, the utero-ovarian ligament and fallopian tube pedicle are suture-ligated adjacent to the uterus with O-Vicryl. When ovarian preservation is not desired, the infundibulo-pelvic ligaments and broad ligaments are coagulated until desiccated with bipolar forceps at 25- to 35-W cutting current and then divided.

UTERINE VESSEL LIGATION

The broad ligament on each side is skeletonized down to the uterine vessels. Each uterine vessel pedicle is suture-ligated with O-Vicryl (27 in.) on a CT-1 needle. The needles are introduced into the peritoneal cavity by pulling them through a 5-mm incision.[21] The curved needle is inserted on top of the unroofed ureter where it turns medially toward the previously mobilized bladder. A short rotary movement of the Cook oblique curved needle holder brings the needle around the uterine vessel pedicle. Sutures are tied extracorporeally with a Clarke knot pusher.[22] A single suture placed in this manner on each side serves as a "sentinel stitch" to identify and watch over the ureter for the rest of the procedure.

CIRCUMFERENTIAL CULDOTOMY (DIVISION OF CERVICOVAGINAL ATTACHMENTS)

The cardinal ligaments on each side are divided with the CO_2 laser at high power (80 W) or with the spoon electrode at 150-W cutting current. Often, bipolar forceps are necessary to control bleeding. The vagina is entered posteriorly over the Valtchev retractor near the junction of the cervix and vagina. A ring forceps inserted into the anterior of the vagina above the tenaculum on the anterior cervical lip identifies the anterior cervicovaginal junction, which is entered by using the laser. Following insertion of the ring forceps or the Aquapurator tip and using them as backstops, the lateral vaginal fornices are divided. The uterus is morcellated if necessary and pulled out of the vagina. Alternately, a 4-cm-diameter operative colonoscope (Richard Wolf) is used to circumferentially outline the cervicovaginal junction; it also serves as a backstop for laser work.

LAPAROSCOPIC VAGINAL VAULT CLOSURE AND SUSPENSION WITH McCALL CULDOPLASTY

Vaginal repair is accomplished after packing the vagina and placing a Laparomed (Irvine, Calif) port saver retraction device at the cuff apex (12 o'clock). The left uterosacral ligament and posterolateral aspect of the vagina are first elevated. A suture is placed through this uterosacral ligament into the vagina, exits the vagina including posterior vaginal tissue near the midline on the left, and reenters just adjacent to this spot on the right. Finally, an opposite-sided oblique Cook needle holder is used to fix the right posterolateral portion of the vagina to the right uterosacral ligament. This suture is tied extracorporeally and gives excellent support to the vaginal cuff apex while elevating it superiorly and posteriorly toward the hollow of the sacrum. The rest of the vagina and the overlying pubocervical fascia are closed vertically with a figure-of-8 suture. In most cases the peritoneum is not closed.

UNDERWATER EXAMINATION

At the close of each operation, an underwater examination is used to detect bleeding from vessels and viscera tamponaded during the procedure by the increased intraperitoneal pressure of the CO_2 pneumoperitoneum. The CO_2 pneumopertioneum is displaced with 2 to 5 L of Ringer's lactate solution, and the peritoneal cavity is vigorously irrigated and suctioned until the effluent is clear of blood products. Any further bleeding is controlled underwater by using microbipolar forceps to coagulate through the electrolyte solution, and at least 2 L of lactated Ringer's solution is left in the peritoneal cavity.

POSTOPERATIVE CONSIDERATIONS

Postoperatively, the vaginal cuff is checked for granulation tissue between 6 and 12 weeks since sutures are usually absorbed by then. Patients usually experience some fatigue and discomfort for approximately 6 weeks after the operation but may perform gentle exercise such as walking and return to routine activities between 2 and 6 weeks. Sexual activity may be resumed when the vaginal incision has healed, usually after 6 weeks.

COMPLICATIONS

Complications of LH are those of hysterectomy and laparoscopy in general: anesthetic accidents; respiratory compromise; thromboembolic phenomena; urinary retention; injury to vessels, ureters, bladder, and bowel; and infections, especially of the vaginal cuff.[23] Complications unique to laparoscopy include large-vessel injury and subcutaneous emphysema. Since the introduction of prophylactic antibiotics, vaginal cuff abscess, pelvic thrombophlebitis, septicemia, pelvic cellulitis, and adnexal abscesses are rare. Abdominal wound infection is rare, but the incidence of incisional hernias after operative laparoscopy is greatly increased if 10-mm or larger trocars are placed at extraumbilical sites. These sites should be closed. If the incision is lateral to the rectus muscle, the deep fascia is elevated with skin hooks and suture-repaired. If the incision is through the rectus muscle, the peritoneal defect is closed with a laparoscopically placed suture.

Febrile morbidity with a vaginal approach is about half that of abdominal hysterectomy. Laparoscopic treatment with evacuation of all blood clots and the sealing of all blood vessels after the uterus is out should reduce the infection rate further. Morcellation during laparoscopic or vaginal hysterectomy results in a slightly increased risk of fever, especially if prophylactic antibiotics are not used.

SPECIAL PROBLEMS RELATED TO LAPAROSCOPIC HYSTERECTOMY

VERY LARGE FIBROID UTERUS (16 WEEKS' SIZE OR ABOVE)

The laparoscope is maneuvered into the deep cul-de-sac, and its tip may be used as a lever or retractor to lift the uterus. The ureters are identified and isolated if possible; if this is not possible, the surgeon should go below early in the procedure. If endometriosis or rectal tenting are present, the peritoneum is opened and the rectum is reflected off the posterior of the vagina to the loose areolar tissue of the rectovaginal space. The vagina is incised between the uterosacral ligaments with a CO_2 laser through the operating laparoscope or with a spatula electrode, and this incision is tamponaded with a sponge or balloon to avoid battling to maintain pneumoperitoneum for the rest of the procedure.

The ovaries are examined. In most cases involving a very large fibroid uterus, it is better to preserve the ovaries at the start of surgery to avoid problems with the pelvic sidewall. The ovaries should be reexamined after the uterus is out and excised if indicated. In cases where an ovary has been pulled away from its sidewall by interligamentous fibroid growth, early oophorectomy may be necessary for better exposure.

With a large fibroid uterus, the utero-ovarian ligament/round ligament/fallopian tube pedicle is markedly elongated. It is suture ligated twice to prevent backbleeding as the procedure continues. In many cases, bipolar desiccation is used.

The vesicouterine peritoneal fold is divided with scissors, electrode, or CO_2 laser. This part of the procedure is done after ligation of the utero-ovarian ligament/round ligament/fallopian tube pedicle in cases where a very large fibroid is present because the bladder is far down in the pelvis and the vesicouterine peritoneal fold is stretched out. The round ligament is divided with cutting-current electrosurgery through a spoon electrode.

At this juncture, it is usually possible to incise both the anterior and posterior of the vagina laparoscopically and then proceed vaginally. Allan stirrups are switched to candy-cane stirrups, and the surgeon sits between the patient's legs. Vaginal clamps are applied; the uterosacral ligaments, cardinal ligaments, and uterine vessels are clamped, divided, and suture-ligated. The uterus is then removed after extensive morcellation.

When very large fibroids are located high above the level of the internal os of the cervix, it is often possible to manipulate the laparoscope above or beneath the large fibroid into deep areas of the pelvis. The ureters on each side are identified by using atraumatic forceps and are then separated from the uterine vessels, which are suture ligated as previously described with curved needle techniques. The vagina is entered anteriorly and posteriorly and the cardinal ligaments are divided between these two incisions. The free uterus is removed from below after extensive morcellation.

After securing the ovarian arteries from above and the uterine arteries from above or below, a no. 10 blade on a long knife handle is used to make a circumferential incision into the fundus of the uterus, with the cervix used as a fulcrum. The myometrium is incised circumferentially parallel to the axis of the uterine cavity and the serosa of the uterus. The incision is continued around the full circumference of the myometrium in a symmetrical fashion beneath the uterine serosa. Traction is maintained on the cervix, and the avascular myometrium is cut so that the endometrial cavity with a surrounding thick layer of myometrium is delivered with the cervix to bring the outside of the uterus closer to the operator for further excision by wedge morcellation.[24, 25]

Wedge morcellation is done by removing wedges of myometrium from the anterior and posterior uterine wall, usually in the midline, to reduce the bulk of the myometrium. After excision of a large core, the fundus is morcellated with multiple wedge resection around either a tenaculum or an 11-mm corkscrew (WISAP, Sauerlach, Germany, or Tomball, Tex). The remaining fundus, if still too large for removal, can be bivalved for easier removal from the peritoneal cavity.

At the end of the procedure, a look with a laparoscope should be considered even if a large myomatous uterus is removed by using solely vaginal techniques. Bleeding from the vaginal cuff or from the stretched-out pedicles is common and can be readily coagulated laparoscopically, and blood clot seeded with vaginal organisms can be aspirated laparoscopically. Adding laparoscopy to vaginal hysterectomy should reduce the morbidity of vaginal hysterectomy.

STAGE IV ENDOMETRIOSIS

In cases of severe endometriosis with cul-de-sac obliteration, the surgeon must first free the ovaries, then the ureters, and finally the rectum from the posterior of the vagina to the rectovaginal septum (Figs 15 through

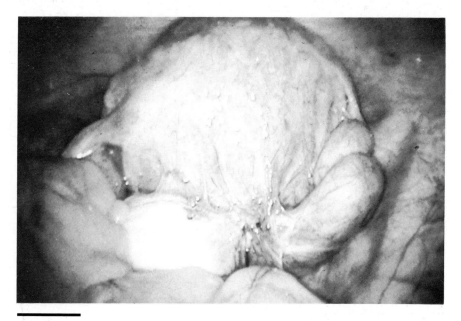

FIGURE 15.
Stage IV endometriosis with complete cul-de-sac obliteration (laparoscopic view).

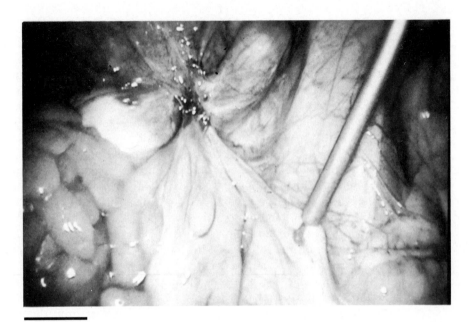

FIGURE 16.
Right ureter grasped. The right ureter is attached to the right side of the uterus.

19). Deep fibrotic nodular endometriosis involving the cul-de-sac requires excision of nodular fibrotic tissue from the uterosacral ligaments, posterior of the cervix, posterior of the vagina, and the rectum. Attention is first directed to complete dissection of the anterior of the rectum throughout its area of involvement until loose areolar tissue of the rectovaginal space is reached. In all cases, a rectal probe (Reznik Instruments, Skokie,

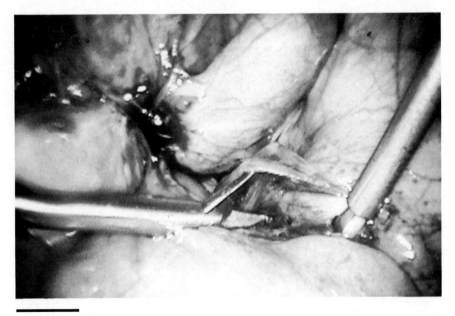

FIGURE 17.
Right ureter unroofed and freed from attachments to the right side of the ureter.

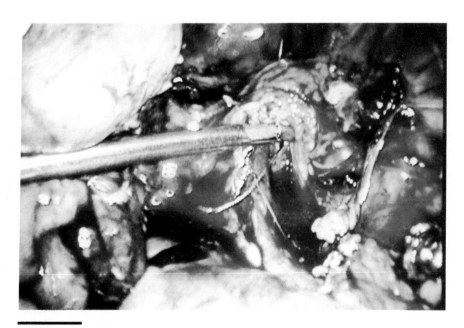

FIGURE 18.
Right uterine vessels suture ligated with the Cook oblique curved needle holder.
The right ureter is well visualized during this ligation and lies beneath the vessel
pedicle.

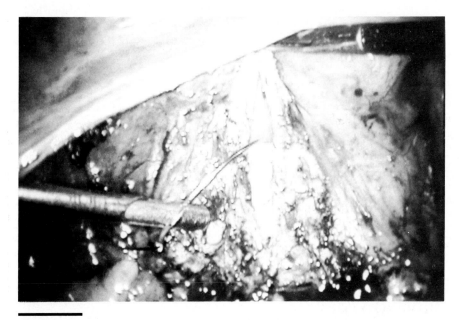

FIGURE 19.
At close of the procedure, the vaginal cuff is repaired by using a modified McCall
culdoplasty stitch followed by a figure-of-8 suture through the endopelvic fascia
and vaginal wall in the midline.

Ill) is placed in the rectum. With the rectal probe used as a guide, the rectal interface with the cul-de-sac lesion is identified and opened at this junction with a CO_2 laser or scissors. Careful blunt dissection then ensues using the aquadissector for aquadissection and suction-traction. Laser or scissors are used for sharp dissection until the rectum, with or without fibrotic endometriosis, is separated from the posterior of the uterus and upper portion of the vagina and is identifiable below the lesion. Loose areolar tissue of the rectovaginal space should be reached. Only after the rectum is mobilized should excision of the fibrotic endometriosis be attempted from the posterior of the vagina, uterosacral ligaments, and rectum. Full-thickness excision of the vaginal nodular areas usually results in relief of the patient's pain and/or bleeding.[14]

LAPAROSCOPIC UTEROSACRAL-VAGINAL SUSPENSION

It is possible to suspend the vagina after hysterectomy by using laparoscopic surgical techniques. In cases where hysterectomy is done for vaginal and uterine prolapse, the ureters are dissected laparoscopically before vaginal hysterectomy to better identify the uterosacral ligaments close to the sacrum in a very high position. Sutures are applied to these firm ligaments adjacent to the sacrum and upper part of the rectum. The suture material is left long in the peritoneal cavity for later fixation.

After vaginal removal of the uterus, the previously applied sutures are grasped with the surgeon's index finger high in the pelvis and are brought into the vagina. These sutures are then applied to the vaginal cuff by free curved needles and are tied after completion of the vaginal closure repair to bring the vagina into a higher position than is obtained with conventional vaginal surgery.

LAPAROSCOPIC RECTOCELE REPAIR

Enteroceles and rectoceles are amenable to a laparoscopic approach. Laparoscopic plication of the levator ani muscles from the sphincter results in excellent vaginal and rectal support. To do this procedure, the rectovaginal space is opened with aquadissection or retroperitoneal space expanders (Preperitoneal Distention Balloon, Origin Medsystems). Separation of the rectum laterally results in identification of the levator ani muscles. These are opposed across the midline with O-Vicryl or Ethibond in an interrupted fashion. Thereafter, the vaginal vault is suspended to the uterosacral ligaments overlying the levator plate and sacrum, as previously described, by using a combined laparoscopic and vaginal approach.[26, 27]

SCORING SYSTEM

The degree of difficulty of LH is most dependent on the number of previous laparotomies. The severity of endometriosis surrounding the cervix and the degree of entrapment of the ovaries are also important. Fibroid size is rarely related to increased difficulty because its blood supply is usually easy to identify and is separate from that of the ureter; these procedures can be time consuming, however, because of the degree of morcellation necessary. Unfortunately for the occasional surgeon, the degree of anticipated difficulty is directly related to the severity of symptoms, which makes indicated procedures demanding in both time and technical expertise required.

A laparoscopic scoring system for determining the operative approach has been developed by Kovac, Reich, and Cruikshank (Table 2).

Uterine and adnexal mobility are first assessed by pelvic examination and by the use of a tenaculum placed in the cervix to move the uterus. The stretched length of the infundibulopelvic ligament is evaluated laparoscopically by placing a probe (marked in centimeters) at the junction of the ovary's distal pole with the infundibulopelvic ligament.

Uterine and adnexal size and mobility and the presence and degree of adhesions and endometriosis, including the cul-de-sac, are evaluated and recorded. Each parameter is assigned a point count. The total cumulative points provide the surgeon with a basis for deciding the operative approach.

TABLE 2.

Laparoscopic Scoring System for Determining the Operative Approach

Parameter	Points
Uterine size	
Grade I: 8 wk or less	1
Grade II: 8–12 wk	3
Grade III: 12–16 wk	5
Grade IV: >16 wk	8
Mobility of the adnexa as judged by the stretched length of the infundibulopelvic ligament	
Good: >5 cm	1
Moderate: 2–5 cm	3
Poor: <2 cm	5
Adhesion of adnexa (Rock's criteria)	
None/mild: no significant paratubal or periovarian adhesions	1
Moderate: periovarian and/or paratubal adhesions without fixation and minimal cul-de-sac adhesions	3
Severe: dense pelvic or adnexal adhesions with fixation of the ovary and tube to either the broad ligament, pelvic wall, omentum, and/or bowel; severe cul-de-sac adhesions	5
Status of the cul-de-sac	
Accessible	0
Obliterated	5
Rectal nodule	8
Endometriosis (American Fertility Society classification)	
Stage I	1
Stage II	2
Stage III	3
Stage IV	4

In this scoring system, the maximum total points in any given case is 30. Patients with scores less than 10 have a successful surgical outcome with traditional vaginal hysterectomy. Conversely, total scores in excess of 10 suggest that LH or abdominal hysterectomy may be preferred. It should be noted that vaginal surgery may still be considered (laparoscopically and vaginally) by an experienced surgeon in the presence of the following relative contraindications: a very large uterus, severe endometriosis where the rectum is adherent to the back of the uterus, and extensive adhesions. An abdominal incisional approach (total abdominal hysterectomy) with bilateral salpingo-oophorectomy should be performed, however, on most ovarian masses over 10 cm if malignancy cannot be ruled out.

CONCLUSIONS

The place of LH in the future will be determined by the skill of surgeons with the vaginal approach. This skill will increase as surgeons are stimulated to do the difficult part of an LAVH vaginally. This author suspects that over 50% of indicated hysterectomies can be performed via the vaginal route without laparoscopy. The laparoscope will be used in the remaining 50%. Vaginal hysterectomy after diagnostic laparoscopy will be possible in half of those with some relative contraindication to the vaginal approach. In these cases, the laparoscope will be used for diagnosis, but no laparoscopic surgery will be done. Half of the remaining indicated hysterectomies will require laparoscopic oophorectomy or adhesiolysis, i.e., LAVH. Of the remaining 12.5% of the total, skilled laparoscopic surgeons will consider LH in all but 1%.

REFERENCES

1. Bachmann GA: Hysterectomy: A critical review. *J Reprod Med* 1990; 35:839–862.
2. Reich H: Laparoscopic hysterectomy. *Surg Laparosc Endosc* 1992; 2:85–88.
3. Liu CY: Laparoscopic hysterectomy: A review of 72 cases. *J Reprod Med* 1992; 37:351–354.
4. Liu CY: Laparoscopic hysterectomy. Report of 215 cases. *Gynaecol Endosc* 1992; 1:73–77.
5. Reich H, DeCaprio J, McGlynn F: Laparoscopic hysterectomy. *J Gynecol Surg* 1989; 5:213–216.
6. Kovac SR, Cruikshank SH, Retto HF: Laparoscopy-assisted vaginal hysterectomy. *J Gynecol Surg* 1990; 6:185–189.
7. Summit RL, Stovall TG, Lipscomb GH, et al: Randomized comparison of laparoscopy-assisted vaginal hysterectomy with standard vaginal hysterectomy in an outpatient setting. *Obstet Gynecol* 1992; 80:895–901.
8. Minelli L, Angiolillo M, Caione C, et al: Laparoscopically-assisted vaginal hysterectomy. *Endoscopy* 1991; 23:64–66.
9. Maher PJ, Wood EC, Hill DJ, et al: Laparoscopically assisted hysterectomy. *Med J Aust* 1992; 156:316–318.
10. Lyons TL: Laparoscopic supracervical hysterectomy, in Hunt RB, Martin DC (eds): *Endoscopy in Gynecology. Proceedings of the World Congress of Gynecologic Endoscopy. AAGL 20th Annual Meeting, Las Vegas Nevada.* Baltimore, Port City Press, 1993, pp 129–131.

11. Reich H: Laparoscopic extrafascial hysterectomy with bilateral salpingo-oophorectomy using stapling techniques for endometrial adenocarcinoma. Presented at the AAGL 19th Annual Meeting, Orlando Fla, Nov 14–18, 1990.
12. Reich H, McGlynn F, Wilkie W. Laparoscopic management of stage I ovarian cancer. *J Reprod Med* 1990; 35:601–605.
13. Canis M, Mage G, Wattiez A, et al: Does endoscopic surgery have a role in radical surgery of cancer of the cervix uteri? *J Gynecol Obstet Biol Reprod* 1990; 19:921.
14. Reich H, McGlynn F, Salvat J: Laparoscopic treatment of cul-de-sac obliteration secondary to retrocervical deep fibrotic endometriosis. *J Reprod Med* 1991; 36:516–522.
15. Parker WH, Berek JS: Management of selected cystic adnexal masses in postmenopausal women by operative laparoscopy: A pilot study. *Am J Obstet Gynecol* 1990; 163:1574–1577.
16. Mann WJ, Reich H: Laparoscopic adnexectomy in postmenopausal women. *J Reprod Med* 1992; 37:254–256.
17. Valtchev KL, Papsin FR: A new uterine mobilizer for laparoscopy: Its use in 518 patients. *Am J Obstet Gynecol* 1977; 127:738–740.
18. Reich H, McGlynn F: Short self-retaining trocar sleeves. *Am J Obstet Gynecol* 1990; 162:453–454.
19. Stovall TG, Ling FW, Henry LC, et al: A randomized trial evaluating leuprolide acetate before hysterectomy as treatment for leiomyomas. *Am J Obstet Gynecol* 1991; 164:1420–1425.
20. Schlaff WD, Zerhouni EA, Huth JA, et al: A placebo-controlled trial of a depot gonadotropin-releasing hormone analogue (leuprolide) in the treatment of uterine leiomyomata. *Obstet Gynecol* 1989; 74:856–862.
21. Reich H, Clarke HC, Sekel L: A simple method for ligating in operative laparoscopy with straight and curved needles. *Obstet Gynecol* 1992; 79:143–147.
22. Clarke HC: Laparaoscopy—New instruments for suturing and ligation. *Fertil Steril* 1972; 23:274–277.
23. Woodland MB: Ureter injury during laparoscopy-assisted vaginal hysterectomy with the endoscopic linear stapler. *Am J Obstet Gynecol* 1992; 167:756–757.
24. Lash AF: A method for reducing the size of the uterus in vaginal hysterectomy. *Am J Obstet Gynecol* 1941; 42:452–459.
25. Kovac SR: Intramyometrial coring as an adjunct to vaginal hysterectomy. *Obstet Gynecol* 1986; 57:131–136.
26. Zacharin RF: Pulsion enterocele: Review of functional anatomy of the pelvic floor. *Obstet Gynecol* 1980; 55:135–140.
27. Zacharin RF, Hamilton NT: Pulsion enterocele: Long-term results of an abdominoperineal technique. *Obstet Gynecol* 1980; 55:141–148.

Editor's Comment

To say that laparoscopic hysterectomy in its various forms is controversial is probably a major understatement. These operations have engendered much discomfort among physicians because this operation is so basic to all obstetricians and gynecologists. Part of the problem is that the proper indications for these endoscopic hysterectomies are still being explored. Unfortunately, most laparoscopically assisted vaginal hysterectomies (LAVHs) are not converting abdominal hysterectomies into vaginal ones. In a landmark article, Summit et al. (*Obstet Gynecol* 1992; 80:895) showed that LAVH and vaginal hysterectomy were comparable when performed on an outpatient basis. The problem is also compounded by the patient who is anxious for "new, less invasive" ways of accomplishing these operations. The "experimental" nature of these operations is not understood by the general public. Dr. Reich, who reported the first laparoscopic hysterectomy, has written an excellent article that defines the different endoscopic hysterectomies, offers indications/contraindications for each, describes these procedures, and offers a scoring system for determining the appropriate approach.

Ana Murphy, M.D.

Update on the Diagnosis and Management of Ectopic Pregnancy

FRANK W. LING, M.D.

THOMAS G. STOVALL, M.D.

T he number and rate of ectopic pregnancies in the United States have increased to epidemic proportions. The Centers for Disease Control reported that the number of ectopic pregnancies (Table 1) has more than quadrupled from 17,800 in 1970 to 88,000 in 1987.[1] During this time, the rate per 1,000 pregnancies also increased from 4.5 to 16.8. Although many explanations for this increase have been offered, the increased incidence of pelvic inflammatory disease, the use of intrauterine devices, and prior tubal surgery appear to have contributed significantly to this clinical problem. In addition to the changing epidemiology, improved diagnostic methods have made the identification of ectopic pregnancy possible at an earlier time in gestation. Because the cases are identified at an earlier stage, the incidence of unruptured ectopic pregnancy at the time of diagnosis is increasing. As a result, a greater number of surgical or nonsurgical alternatives are now available to the clinician. With the advent of earlier diagnosis and less invasive therapy, the long-term implications for reduced morbidity and mortality for patients have become apparent. Although the absolute number and incidence of ectopic pregnancy have been rising, the number of deaths and the mortality rate have steadily declined since 1970 (Table 2). Given the technology that is now available for earlier diagnosis, this discussion will focus on those techniques used to identify cases of ectopic pregnancy at an earlier period in gestation, thus allowing for implementation of the newer therapeutic management alternatives that will follow.

DIAGNOSIS

The clinical manifestations of an ectopic pregnancy are highly variable. On one hand, a woman may have no signs or symptoms, with the result that the diagnosis is made in the course of what has been presumed to be a routine early pregnancy. On the other hand, a woman may have an acute abdomen or be in hemorrhagic shock. The natural course of ectopic preg-

TABLE 1.
Numbers and Rates of Ectopic Pregnancies Reported in the United States, 1970–1987*

Year	Number†	Rate‡
1970	17,800	4.5
1971	19,300	4.8
1972	24,500	6.3
1973	25,600	6.8
1974	26,400	6.7
1975	30,500	7.6
1976	34,600	8.3
1977	40,700	9.2
1978	42,400	9.4
1979	49,900	10.4
1980	52,200	10.5
1981	68,000	13.6
1982	61,800	12.3
1983	69,600	14.0
1984	75,400	14.9
1985	78,400	15.2
1986	73,700	14.3
1987	88,000	16.8
Total	877,400§	10.7

*From Centers for Disease Control: *MMWR* 1990; 39:11.
†Rounded to the nearest hundred.
‡Rate per 1,000 pregnancies (live births, legally induced abortions, and ectopic pregnancies).
§Because of rounding, the total differs from the sum of the numbers.

TABLE 2.
Numbers of Deaths Due to Ectopic Pregnancy and Case-Fatality Rates for the United States, 1970–1987*

Year	Number	Rate†
1970	63	35.5
1971	61	31.7
1972	48	19.6
1973	46	18.0
1974	51	19.4
1975	50	16.4
1976	39	11.3
1977	44	10.8
1978	37	8.7
1979	45	9.0
1980	46	8.8
1981	34	5.0
1982	43	7.0
1983	37	5.3
1984	39	5.2
1985	33	4.2
1986	36	4.9
1987	30	3.4
Total	782	8.9

*From Centers for Disease Control: *MMWR* 1990; 39:14.
†Deaths from ectopic pregnancy per 10,000 ectopic pregnancies.

nancy is similarly unpredictable. At one extreme, the pregnancy may progress to tubal rupture with intra-abdominal hemorrhage; at the other extreme, the ectopic gestation may be resorbed spontaneously without medical or surgical intervention. Because the traditional approach to ectopic pregnancy has been to remove the products of conception in order to prevent further clinical deterioration, little is known about the true natural course of these pregnancies. Therefore, the goals remain to diagnose the condition as early as possible, to minimize anatomic distortion, to stop the progression of the condition, and to prevent long-term morbidity while maximizing the options available for therapy. Diagnostic modalities that will aid in the early identification of ectopic pregnancy are therefore preferred by astute clinicians.

HISTORY

Risk Factors

Over half of patients with an ectopic pregnancy have one or more identifiable risk factors. Table 3 lists those factors associated with an increased incidence of ectopic pregnancy. Delayed ovum transport is likely a primary cause of ectopic pregnancy. Risk factors associated with delayed implantation are nonmechanical (factors that change the affinity of the timing of the fallopian tubes for the embryo) and mechanical (obstructive) factors. Four conditions that have a strong causal relationship with ectopic pregnancy are current intrauterine device use (relative risk, 13.7), prior fallopian tube surgery (relative risk, 4.5), history of pelvic infection (relative risk, 3.3), and history of infertility (relative risk, 2.6).[2] In taking a thorough history, identification of risk factors does not, however, make the diagnosis firm, just as absence of factors does not exclude the presence of an ectopic pregnancy. The clinician should therefore use appropriate diagnostic modalities to identify the location of a pregnancy when a pregnancy test is positive.

Common Symptoms

Common symptoms associated with ectopic pregnancy are listed in Table 4. Symptoms are usually present for approximately 10 days before diagnosis. Pain, amenorrhea, and vaginal bleeding are the classic triad of symptoms, but the clinician should be vigilant to variations. Pain initially

---

TABLE 3.

Risk Factors for Ectopic Pregnancy

Nonmechanical factors
  Endometriosis
  Fallopian tube disorders
    Diverticuli
    Motility disorders
  Progestin-only contraceptives
  Postcoital estrogens
  Diethylstilbestrol exposure
  Prior history of infertility
  Use of fertility-inducing agents
  History of prior ectopic pregnancy
Mechanical factors
  Previous history of pelvic inflammatory disease
    Gonococcal
    Chlamydial
    Tuberculous
    Other
  Intrauterine contraceptive device use
  Bilateral tubal ligation
  Previous abdominal surgery

TABLE 4.

Symptoms of Ectopic Pregnancy

Symptom	Prevalence, %
Abdominal pain	95–100
Generalized	50
Unilateral	35
Shoulder	20
Back	5–10
Abnormal uterine bleeding	65–85
Amenorrhea	75–95
<2 wk	45
<6 wk	35
Syncope	10–18
Dizziness	20–35
Pregnancy symptoms	10–20
Nausea	15
Urge to defecate	5–15

is described as dull or cramping in the lower quadrants and is associated with bleeding that is characterized as spotting. The woman usually seeks medical attention because of an acute change in the nature and intensity of pain. This sudden change likely occurs around the time of rupture and is often associated with shoulder pain resulting from peritoneal and diaphragmatic irritation from blood. Syncopal episodes often occur at this time. The location of abdominal pain is of little help in diagnosing the site of the ectopic pregnancy. In fact, one fourth of women localize abdominal pain from a tubal pregnancy to the contralateral side; ipsilateral pain occurs in only about half of the cases.

The amount or character of abnormal vaginal bleeding is not helpful in identifying the etiology. Approximately 15% of women report bleeding heavy enough to resemble that seen with a spontaneous abortion. Up to 45% of women with an ectopic pregnancy have no vaginal bleeding. When bleeding does occur, it may precede the onset of pain in half of the women, whereas pain and bleeding may occur within 4 hours of each other in about one third of patients.[5–8]

Common symptoms of normal pregnancy may also occur in women with ectopic pregnancies. These include symptoms such as breast tenderness, nausea, and vomiting. Syncope is relatively uncommon during normal pregnancy and is found three times more frequently in women who are subsequently found to have an ectopic pregnancy.[9]

PHYSICAL EXAMINATION

Women with ectopic pregnancies, when seen very early in their clinical course and before rupture of the ectopic pregnancy, may be totally asymptomatic. Conversely, they may be initially seen after the ectopic pregnancy has ruptured and may be in a hemodynamically unstable condition. Because of the clinical spectrum that is possible, the incidence of physical findings will to a great extent reflect the sophistication and timeliness with which the diagnosis is made. Listed in Table 5 is a summary of examination findings derived from several series of patients before the development and implementation of aggressive surveillance techniques that now allow physicians to diagnose ectopic pregnancy before rupture.

Vital Signs

Shock as an initial symptom has decreased from as high as 50% in 1967 to less than 15%.[6, 10] Because the amount and the rate of bleeding vary from patient to patient, the clinician should know that a woman may have minimal and extremely subtle orthostatic changes in pulse and pressure. Subtle early changes include a narrowing of pulse pressure and an elevation of the diastolic blood pressure. Additionally, it is not uncommon for hypovolemia to presage frank hypotension. Therefore, progressive orthostatic vital signs (supine as well as upright pulse and pressure) and urine output may help in earlier identification of an ectopic pregnancy. Even with significant hemorrhage, a young, healthy woman may be able to compensate well for quite extensive blood loss and have minimal changes in vital signs. Pain may itself cause a slightly increased blood pressure and pulse.

Temperature elevation is uncommon in ectopic pregnancy. Most often, a woman's temperature is normal or even below normal if acute hemorrhage occurs. High fevers rarely occur with a hemoperitoneum, and a temperature greater than 38.5° C is extremely uncommon in patients with ectopic pregnancy.[11]

TABLE 5.
Physical Examination in Ectopic Pregnancy

Finding	Prevalence, %
Abdominal tenderness	80–95
Peritoneal signs	
Ruptured	50
Unruptured	5
Adnexal tenderness	75–90
Unilateral	40–75
Bilateral	50–75
Cervical motion tenderness	50–75
Adnexal mass	30–50
Contralateral	20
Uterus	
Normal size	70
Enlarged	15–30
Orthostatic changes	10–15
Temperature >37° C	5–10
Vomiting	15

Abdominal Tenderness

Abdominal tenderness remains the most common positive physical examination finding in patients with ectopic pregnancy. Findings suggestive of peritoneal irritation, e.g., rebound tenderness, guarding, abdominal distension, and absence of bowel sounds, are present in fewer than one third of patients.[6, 10] If, however, tubal rupture or retrograde bleeding from the implantation site has occurred, the chances for generalized abdominal tenderness and evidence of peritoneal irritation increase. The commonly cited but rarely seen Cullen sign is a bluish discoloration of the periumbilical skin resulting from extensive intra-abdominal hemorrhage. The absence of Cullen sign does not exclude extensive intraabdominal bleeding.

Pelvic Examination

As expected, pelvic examination findings also vary, ranging from normal to exquisite tenderness with the presence of a large pelvic mass. Vaginal inspection may reveal blood and tissue being passed through the cervix. The tissue may be a decidual cast that may be mistaken for menstrual flow or the products of conception. The uterus is typically not markedly enlarged; in fact, it may be slightly smaller than expected for gestational age. Approximately three fourths of patients have a normal-sized uterus. Women with an interstitial pregnancy have larger uteri.[12] An adnexal mass is palpable in no more than one half of ectopic pregnancies and may consist not only of the products of conception but also of blood, omentum, and other adherent intra-abdominal structures. A mass palpated on the contralateral side to the ectopic site may be a corpus luteum cyst. Tenderness in the adnexal region is found in over three fourths of patients, and tenderness is therefore of little clinical usefulness in localizing the ectopia. A mass may also be palpable in the cul-de-sac. This may be due either to tubal rupture or to intermittent retrograde flow through the fallopian tubes and may result in an accumulation of blood in the lower portion of the pelvis.

Despite a clinician's careful consideration of the possibility of an ectopic pregnancy, the standard history and physical examination remain insensitive methods for detecting this condition. Information presented in a recent report helped reinforce the concept that history and physical examination alone are insufficiently sensitive in detecting an unruptured ectopic pregnancy.[11] Only 89 of 161 ectopic pregnancies (55.3%) were detected on initial examination. Of these 89, 53 (60%) were ruptured at the time of surgery to treat the condition. The 72 patients with undetected ectopic pregnancies were discharged from the emergency department only to return later.[11] There were no significant differences in the initial symptoms of patients with unruptured ectopic pregnancies when compared with normal intrauterine pregnancies. After careful follow-up evaluation and questioning, only 91 of the 161 patients with ectopic pregnancies acknowledged having one or more of the risk factors.

LABORATORY EVALUATION

The physician should keep in mind at all times the premise that any woman of childbearing age who has abdominal pain and/or menstrual complaints must have ectopic pregnancy ruled out as a primary consideration. Because some of the available tests are no more sensitive than are the history or the physical examination, it is critical that the appropriate tests be ordered and that they be interpreted in light of their inherent limitations.

Blood Count

A decrease in hemoglobin and hematocrit may reflect hemorrhage if there has been a significant amount and duration of bleeding. A repeat evaluation may be helpful when the diagnosis is in doubt.[8] Similarly, the leukocyte count is variable in women with ectopic pregnancy. White blood cell counts are typically normal, but values have been reported up to 30,000/mL. This is an important consideration for physicians who are trying to differentiate pelvic inflammatory disease from ectopic pregnancy; a significant leukocytosis should not be assumed to exclude an ectopic pregnancy. The erythrocyte sedimentation rate (ESR) also may be elevated in 10% to 15% of patients. It should therefore not be used to exclude or confirm the diagnosis of an ectopic pregnancy.

Human Chorionic Gonadotropin Assays

Improved sensitivity and specificity of urinary test kits for human chorionic gonadotropin (hCG) have greatly improved the ability to diagnose an ectopic pregnancy. Formerly, urine pregnancy tests were latex agglutination inhibition assays that detected hCG in the 500 to 800-mIU/mL range. These were sensitive enough to detect up to only 50% to 60% of ectopic pregnancies. Hemagglutination inhibition assays are sensitive for hCG in the 150- to 250-mIU/ML range and are positive in up to 85% of cases. Although these assays are more sensitive, negative results cannot exclude a pregnancy and therefore do not rule out an ectopic pregnancy.[13] Enzyme-linked immunosorbent assays (ELISAs) are sensitive down to 50 mIU/mL, and the ELISA tests are therefore the present standard for urinary screening for ectopic pregnancy. At 50 mIU/mL, these tests can detect hCG as early as 14 days after conception and have been found to be positive in over 90% of cases of ectopic pregnancy. No special expertise is required on the part of laboratory personnel, no specialized equipment is necessary, and the test can be performed rapidly.[14, 15] Although serum hCG assays can detect hCG down to 5 mIU/mL and are positive as early as 5 days after conception, they are not useful in emergencies or for screening in a general setting because they require a considerable amount of time to perform.

There are two reference standards of the β-subunit of hCG gonadotropin measurement. In 1964, the Second International Standard (SIS) was established for bioassays. This material had varying amounts of both α- and β-subunits of hCG in addition to the intact hormone. The International Reference Preparation (IRP) was introduced 10 years later. It contains highly purified β-hCG distributed by the National Institutes of Health. One nanogram of purified β-hCG is approximately equivalent to 5.5 mIU (SIS) or 9.3 mIU (IRP).[16] Interpretation of the literature should take into account the standard used (Table 6).

Levels of β-hCG increase by approximately two thirds every 48 hours in a normal intrauterine pregnancy, with a doubling time of approxi-

TABLE 6.

Two Reference Standards Used for Measuring Human Chorionic
Gonadotropin

Reference Standard	Measures	Amount of Reference Standard Equivalent to 1 ng of Purified β-hCG*
Second International Standard (SIS)	α and β fragments and intact hCG	5.5 mIU
International Reference Preparation (IRP)	β-hCG	9.3 mIU

*hCG = human chorionic gonadotropin.

mately 2 days.[17, 18] A distinction between normal or abnormal pregnancy
is not always possible with serial hCG measurements, however, since up
to 15% of normal pregnancies may have an abnormal hCG rise.

Similarly, there is no single hCG value that can be used in isolation
to make a diagnosis of or exclude an ectopic pregnancy. Only when an
hCG assay is negative should it be used by itself to exclude the diagnosis
of ectopic pregnancy with reasonable certainty. Otherwise, the use of a
single positive value of hCG is extremely limited. Either serial determinations of hCG should be used to determine whether or not hCG levels
are doubling appropriately for a normal pregnancy, or a single value of
hCG should be used in conjunction with other diagnostic methods such
as ultrasound.

In summary, a normal hCG doubling time does not exclude an ectopic pregnancy, nor does an abnormal hCG doubling time establish the
diagnosis of an ectopic pregnancy. These measurements do, however,
greatly increase the suspicion that there is an abnormal pregnancy, either uterine or extrauterine.

Serum Progesterone

The measurement of serum progesterone may be used as an adjunct
screening tool for ectopic pregnancy. Progesterone is primarily secreted
from the corpus luteum until the luteal-placental shift occurs at approximately 6 to 8 weeks of gestation. In 1977, Milwidsky et al. observed no
correlation between progesterone and hCG in patients with ectopic pregnancy; however, the mean serum progesterone level was noted to be lower
in women with ectopic pregnancies when compared with normal intrauterine pregnancies.[19] In 1986, Matthews and colleagues[20] reported that
women who were subsequently found to have a normal pregnancy had a
serum progesterone content exceeding 20 ng/mL, whereas patients with
ectopic pregnancies had progesterone levels less than 15 ng/mL. Yeko et
al.[21] reported in a retrospective study that a progesterone level of less than

15 ng/mL was found in 28 of 28 ectopic pregnancies whereas in all 24 normal pregnancies evaluated, the serum progesterone concentration exceeded 15 ng/mL.

The use of a single serum progesterone measurement has been compared with two serial hCG measurements in screening for an abnormal pregnancy. With the use of receiver operating characteristic (ROC) curves, serum progesterone was found to be significantly more sensitive.[22] Use of a serum progesterone level for early screening for ectopic pregnancy has also reduced the incidence of ectopic pregnancy rupture at one institution from 79.2% to 38%.[23] Unfortunately, the use of a screening serum progesterone value to detect an ectopic pregnancy has resulted in no single "magic" cutoff value above which an ectopic pregnancy can be excluded. In an effort to determine the lowest serum progesterone value with which a viable intrauterine pregnancy could be found, a retrospective review was done in 1,028 consecutive first-trimester pregnancies.[24] After identifying a progesterone level below which no pregnancy was found to progress to viability, the level was tested in a prospective fashion in an additional 630 patients. It was found that no viable pregnancies were associated with a serum progesterone value less than 5.0 ng/mL. Subsequently, 2 patients whose cases have not yet been reported had pregnancies progress to viability with a serum progesterone concentration of 3.9 ng/mL. Therefore, not even a serum progesterone value of 5.0 ng/mL is 100% predictive of a nonviable pregnancy.

Serum progesterone can be used effectively to aid in screening for ectopic pregnancy. On the high end, using 25 ng/mL as an upper-level marker, the clinician can feel confident that only approximately 2.5% of abnormal pregnancies will have serum progesterone above this level. On the low end, a serum progesterone concentration of less than 5 ng/mL, although not 100% accurate, is nonetheless highly predictive of an abnormal pregnancy, either uterine or extrauterine. Whether or not a serum progesterone determination is necessary when quantitative hCG titers and transvaginal ultrasound are readily available remains to be established.

Other Serum Markers

Estradiol has been investigated as a possible marker for pregnancy outcome since it is produced by the β-hCG−dependent corpus luteum. Although a threshold has not been established, estradiol levels have been found to be lower in ectopic pregnancies than in viable pregnancies.[25−28] Schwangerschafts protein 1 (SP1) is a glycoprotein secreted by syncytiotrophoblasts that appears in the maternal circulation shortly after implantation. Its usefulness as a marker for ectopic pregnancy has also been investigated. Because it will not cross-react with hCG at low levels, it may be useful for women treated with hCG for ovulation induction. It does not differentiate, however, between viable and nonviable pregnancies.[28] Its primary utility would be in the diagnosis of conception in patients who have already received hCG. Schwangerschafts protein 1 may also serve as a prognostic indicator of pregnancy, although a single value has not been shown to have any prognostic value.[29]

Relaxin has been found to be significantly lower both in resorbing ectopic pregnancies and spontaneous abortions than in normal pregnancies.[28, 30] Because relaxin levels sometimes take several days to determine, their clinical utility has been limited. A rapid ELISA has been developed recently that will allow relaxin levels to be measured more quickly. It is hoped that such measurements will prove to be clinically useful in determining the status of early pregnancies.

Renin has also been looked at as a possible ectopic pregnancy marker. It, along with hCG, progesterone, and prorenin, has been found to be lower in ectopic pregnancy.[31] The use of CA-125, the tumor-associated glycoprotein, has also been investigated in ectopic pregnancy with mixed results.[28, 32] α-Fetoprotein (AFP) levels have been reported to be markedly elevated in five ectopic pregnancies, but its role as a screening marker for ectopic pregnancy has not been evaluated.[33, 34] Pregnancy-associated plasma protein A (PAPP-A) is a protein synthesized by syncytiotrophoblasts. Low levels of PAPP-A have been found to be associated with poor pregnancy outcome.[35–37] It could be detected in fewer than half the patients with proven ectopic pregnancy. C-reactive protein levels increase significantly in patients who have infection, trauma, or infarction. Levels were lower in patients with ectopic pregnancy than in those with acute infectious processes. Its role in differentiating an ectopic pregnancy from an intrauterine gestation, however, has not been studied.[38] Pregnancy-specific β_1-glycoprotein (PSBG) is also secreted by trophoblasts. Its concentrations, however, are lower than that of β-hCG, making it a currently unusable test.[39]

The potential clinical utility of using a host of serum proteins for the diagnosis of an ectopic pregnancy remains unclear. Until further studies are performed, the role of laboratory testing in identifying an ectopic pregnancy remains limited to blood count, quantitative β-hCG, and in some circumstances, serum progesterone.

SONOGRAPHY

Transabdominal Sonography

The importance of pelvic ultrasound in the diagnosis of a suspected ectopic pregnancy has undergone significant evolution. At one time, ultrasound was used primarily only to exclude patients with an intrauterine pregnancy because of the unlikely coexistence of an intrauterine and extrauterine pregnancy.[40–42] Ultrasound is now relied upon to demonstrate the ectopic mass itself, to characterize its size, and even to guide or follow the course of nonsurgical therapy.[43–46] Although the experience of the sonographer and the sophistication of the equipment are important variables, cardiac activity can normally be recognized between 6 and 7 weeks' gestation by transabdominal sonography. In general, if ultrasound evidence exists for an early intrauterine pregnancy, it is felt that an ectopic pregnancy is essentially excluded. If, however, no definite sonographic signs of intrauterine pregnancy exist (empty uterus sign), the following are possible conclusions: (1) a normal intrauterine pregnancy exists, but it is too small to be seen at this early stage; (2) there is/was an abnormal intrauterine pregnancy; (3) there is an ectopic pregnancy; and (4) the patient is not pregnant.

Because of the wide range of possibilities, both transabdominal and transvaginal ultrasound should be used together with other laboratory measurements. Totally normal pelvic ultrasound findings do not exclude an ectopic pregnancy, and further follow-up must be initiated if warranted by clinical circumstances. Identification of an adnexal gestational sac with embryo and cardiac activity confirms an ectopic pregnancy. When there are adnexal masses that do not fit classic ectopic gestational sac descriptions, the certainty of an ectopic pregnancy is far less. For abdominal ultrasound, a quantitative hCG level of 6,500 mIU/mL (IRP) has been used as a standard cutoff for identification of intrauterine pregnancies. Patients with an hCG level above this and no evidence of intrauterine gestation should be managed as though they had ectopic pregnancies.[47, 48]

Visualization of a strong double decidual ring is important to diagnose an intrauterine pregnancy. A pseudogestational sac may be identified in up to 20% of women with an ectopic gestation. It is therefore important for fetal cardiac activity to be identified within the gestational sac in order for a definitive diagnosis of intrauterine pregnancy to be established.

Transvaginal Ultrasound
The transvaginal approach to pelvic ultrasound is now widely accepted as superior to the transabdominal approach in the diagnosis of an ectopic pregnancy. Some of the advantages of vaginal over abdominal ultrasound are listed in Table 7. Not only can transvaginal ultrasound diagnose an intrauterine pregnancy 1 week earlier, but by using this more sensitive technique an empty uterus can be identified with greater confidence. Adnexal structures are better visualized with this approach, which therefore increases the ability to detect adnexal evidence of an ectopic gestation.

Just as Kadar[18] established an hCG level of 6,500 mIU/mL (IRP) above which a normal intrauterine pregnancy should be seen with transabdominal ultrasound and established 6,000 mIU/mL as a level below which evidence of a normal intrauterine pregnancy would not be expected, so

TABLE 7.

Transvaginal and Transabdominal Ultrasound in the Diagnosis of Ectopic Pregnancy

	Transvaginal	Transabdominal
Bladder preparation	Empty	Full
Distance from target organ (cm)	0.5–4	5–10
Anatomic distortion from urinary bladder	No	Yes
Earliest identification of IUP* (wk)	4	5
Able to displace organs with transducer pressure	Yes	No

*IUP = intrauterine pregnancy.

also have discriminatory levels of hCG corresponding to transvaginal ultrasound been published. As sonographic resolution has improved, the discriminatory zone for hCG has progressively fallen. With transvaginal sonography, the discriminatory zone has been reported to be as low as 100 mIU/mL.[49] Levels between 1,000 and 1,500 mIU/mL are more realistic, however. By knowing the hCG level and using a discriminatory zone, an experienced sonographer should know when to expect (high levels) and when not to expect (low levels) evidence of an intrauterine gestational sac. If levels are high and there is no evidence of a sac, suspicion of an ectopic pregnancy should be high.

INVASIVE TESTING

With the development of sensitive assays for β-hCG, both qualitative and quantitative, the need for invasive tests such as endometrial curettage and culdocentesis has decreased dramatically. These tests have not been rendered totally useless, however, and a need for them still exists.

Culdocentesis

Culdocentesis is a method by which the presence of intraperitoneal blood can be rapidly identified. Culdocentesis is based upon the principle that blood in the peritoneal cavity will undergo clotting and subsequent fibrinolysis, after which it will not clot again. It is performed by using a single-toothed tenaculum to grasp the cervix and elevate it anteriorly. The pouch of Douglas is then entered with a 20-gauge spinal needle attached to a syringe to aspirate whatever material is present. If blood is aspirated and subsequently clots, it is assumed to be from a vascular structure, whereas nonclotting blood, particularly if the hematocrit exceeds 15%, is felt to be compatible with the diagnosis of a hemoperitoneum. Aspiration of serous fluid is considered negative (no hemoperitoneum), whereas failure to aspirate any fluid is considered nondiagnostic (dry tap). It should be remembered, however, that should there be brisk bleeding, the aspirated blood may not have had time to clot and the test would thereby yield a false negative result if interpreted as above. Patients with such active bleeding, however, typically demonstrate evidence of hypovolemia. Culdocentesis may also be compromised because of pelvic scarring in women with chronic pelvic inflammatory or other disease. In such instances, the cul-de-sac may be partially obliterated. With the availability of more sensitive noninvasive and similarly rapid tests, the role of culdocentesis has diminished significantly. In the past, culdocentesis as a diagnostic tool had a positive predictive value of up to 95%.[50] When used in conjunction with a positive pregnancy test, a positive culdocentesis is associated with an ectopic pregnancy in up to 99% of cases.[51] It should be noted, however, that false positive taps occurred in up to 17% of cases; at laparotomy or laparoscopy, a benign adnexal process was detected rather than an ectopic pregnancy.[52, 53] Vermesh et al.[54] reported that only 50% of patients who had a positive culdocentesis actually had a ruptured ectopic pregnancy when surgery was performed.[54] These authors also reported that a negative culdocentesis was predictive of an unruptured ectopic pregnancy in only 58% of cases.

In summary, culdocentesis cannot be used to predict the status of the fallopian tube in patients who have an ectopic pregnancy. Therefore, the clinician cannot depend on the results of this test to determine the best surgical operation, if any, to pursue for a patient suspected of having an ectopic pregnancy. Although its advantages include speed and simplicity, culdocentesis is very uncomfortable for the patient (even with topical anesthesia used for the needle insertion), has significant false positive and false negative results, and can only identify the presence or absence of blood in the peritoneal cavity, not its source. A very limited role for this procedure may be for the few patients who are hemodynamically unstable but who require a rapid confirmation of the need for emergency surgery.

Endometrial Sampling by Dilation and Curettage

The primary role of endometrial sampling is to document the absence of products of conception within the uterine cavity and thereby increase the likelihood that a pregnancy is ectopic in location. The likelihood of a heterotopic, i.e., coexistent intrauterine and extrauterine, pregnancy has been estimated at 1 in 4,000 in the general population,[55] but other estimates put the number as low as 1 in 30,000[66] and as high as 3 in 100,[57] a number drawn from patients undergoing ovarian hyperstimulation and assisted reproductive techniques. Any instrumentation of the uterine cavity should clearly be reserved only for those circumstances in which a viable, intrauterine pregnancy has been excluded. If chorionic villi are obtained from the uterine cavity, the presence of a concurrent ectopic gestation along with the documented intrauterine pregnancy is highly unlikely. Removing tissue from the uterine cavity for this purpose has been used both for viable, but undesired pregnancies and for nonviable intrauterine pregnancies that would proceed to spontaneous abortion if allowed to continue their clinical course.[58–60]

Formerly, the optimal technique for obtaining the endometrial tissue was at the time of dilation and curettage in an operating room setting. The technique is commonly performed now in an office or emergency department setting under local, i.e. paracervical, anesthesia. Often, minimal cervical dilation is required as the patient is actively bleeding, a clinical presentation not unlike that seen in a patient with an incomplete abortion. Sampling with biopsy instruments such as the endometrial Pipelle or the Novak curette has not yet been proven to be the equal of uterine evacuation techniques, and should therfore not be recommended at the present time. The tissue obtained through uterine evacuation should be evaluated for chorionic villi, either by floating in saline to identify the lacy fronds characteristic of their gross appearance, or by means of frozen or histologic preparations. The Arias-Stella reaction is a nonspecific finding, compatible with not only ectopic pregnancy, but also with ongoing intrauterine pregnancy, as well as failed intrauterine pregnancy.[61]

The clinical decision to proceed with uterine evacuation/sampling in the investigation of ectopic pregnancy must always take into consideration the possible unintentional interruption of a desired early intrauterine pregnancy. Endometrial curettage should be used only in conjunction with documented abnormal hCG progression, an abnormally low serum progesterone value, and/or ultrasound documentation of loss of pregnancy integrity. When used appropriately, uterine curettage can be both therapeutic and diagnostic. For those patients who are subsequently followed via hCG levels, it also can provide a baseline point at which hormonally active trophoblastic tissue is known to have been removed.

Diagnostic Laparoscopy

In contemporary gynecologic practice, laparoscopy remains the standard for the diagnosis of an ectopic pregnancy. It is the best invasive procedure because it misses the diagnosis of an ectopic pregnancy in fewer than 3% of cases and then typically only in extremely early gestations. This approach also allows for therapy to be incorporated at one operative setting. The likelihood of an ectopic pregnancy being missed increases as the diagnosis of pregnancy is made at increasingly earlier gestational ages. For patients who are hemodynamically stable, diagnostic laparoscopy is the single best operation for both diagnosis and therapy.

As diagnostic capabilities improve, attempts are being made to move away from laparoscopy for diagnosis, thus leaving it as a treatment modality only. If the need for diagnosis with laparoscopy is eliminated, the risks, complications, and morbidity of medical therapy as an alternative to surgery become more appealing. False negative laparoscopy results can be avoided when hormonal markers and ultrasound are used in conjunction with the diagnostic procedure. In addition, false positive laparoscopy findings, i.e., tubal discoloration or dilation, can be misinterpreted as ectopic gestations. These are factors that will have to be considered as the role of laparoscopy in the diagnosis of ectopic pregnancy is further defined in the future.

Laparotomy

Although to a great extent replaced by laparoscopy with its reduced morbidity, laparotomy remains a diagnostic modality in selected patients. For patients who are hemodynamically unstable or in cases in which laparoscopic instrumentation is not available, patients with suspected ectopic gestations are best served by this surgical approach. Like laparoscopy, it allows for both diagnosis and therapy.

ALGORITHMS FOR NONSURGICAL DIAGNOSIS

Diagnostic algorithms for ectopic pregnancy that allow the diagnosis of ectopic pregnancy to be confirmed without the use of laparoscopy have been developed. Our currently employed algorithm, which uses quantitative β-hCG, serum progesterone, transvaginal ultrasound, and endometrial curettage, was tested in a randomized, controlled fashion.[62] In this series, all patients who were randomized to have laparoscopic confirmation of the diagnosis of ectopic pregnancy did have an ectopic gestation, and they all were subsequently successfully treated medically. Those who did not undergo laparoscopic confirmation were also successfully treated medically with methotrexate. The algorithms in Figures 1 and 2 rely on dependable laboratory methodology for the measurement of both quantitative hCG and serum progesterone.[62] For these algorithms to work, access to an accomplished transvaginal ultrasonographer is also essential. By strict adherence to these algorithms, inadvertent instrumentation of

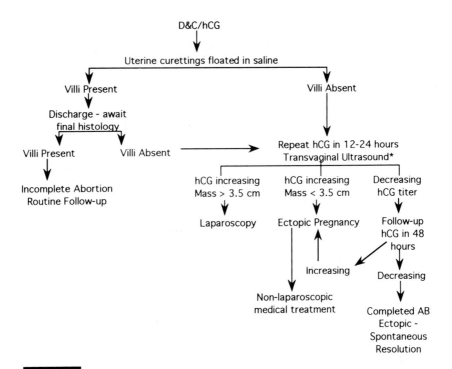

FIGURE 1.

Management of patients following dilatation and curettage (D&C) for an abnormal pregnancy (hCG = human chorionic gonadotropin; AB = abortion).* Repeat transvaginal ultrasound if performed more than 48 hours previously.

an intact intrauterine pregnancy may be avoided, and women are not exposed to unnecessary surgical or medical therapy.

MANAGEMENT

RUPTURED VS. UNRUPTURED ECTOPIC PREGNANCY

A ruptured ectopic gestation is not, in and of itself, an indication for laparotomy. A laparoscopic approach may be considered if the woman is not in hypovolemic shock. The choice of laparoscopic surgery vs. laparotomy should be based on clinician experience, equipment availability, and the patient's physical status. The surgeon should also feel comfortable that there will be relatively free access to the pelvic structures with adequate mobilization of the diseased tube. Obesity, multiple previous abdominal procedures, diaphragmatic hernia, and a patient history of bleeding diathesis should be considered negative factors when laparoscopic surgery is considered. Because reproductive outcome has not been found to be significantly different between patients undergoing laparoscopy and laparotomy,[63] the surgeon should consider both intraoperative and postoperative factors in selecting a surgical approach. The laparoscopic approach has been associated with reduced morbidity and hospital costs, less attendant postoperative pain, improved cosmetic outcome, shorter hospitalization and recuperation time, earlier return to work, and overall reduced costs.[64] Assuming adequate surgical expertise and assuming that

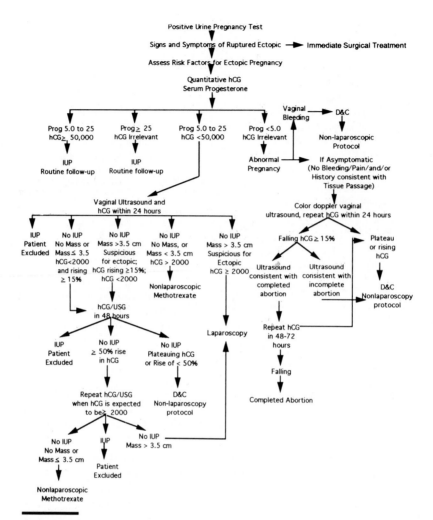

FIGURE 2.

Nonsurgical diagnostic and treatment algorithm for ectopic pregnancy diagnosis. Units for progesterone are nanograms per milliliter and those for human chorionic gonadotropin (hCG) are milli-International units per milliliter. Note: (1) If cardiac activity in adnexa and mass < 3.5 cm, treat with methotrexate; if mass > 3.5 cm in largest dimension, surgery is indicated. (2) If hCG level is falling (>15% decline between two consecutive levels), follow hCG. Consider completed abortion or spontaneously resolving ectopic pregnancy. (3) Any time the patient develops significant symptoms, or ultrasound reveals a ruptured ectopic pregnancy, laparoscopy should be performed. (Prog = progesterone; D&C = dilatation and curettage; IUP = intrauterine pregnancy; USG = ultrasonogram).

the laparoscopic approach does not significantly extend exposure to the anesthetic agents, a hemodynamically stable patient is likely to be better served with laparoscopy than with laparotomy.

Nonsurgical therapy for a ruptured ectopic pregnancy cannot be advocated at the present time because the diagnosis of ruptured ectopic gestation would necessarily be made at the time of laparoscopy or laparotomy. It would not be clinically prudent to identify a ruptured ectopic pregnancy and not initiate appropriate surgical treatment unless the specific circumstances required no surgery. Nonsurgical alternatives have typically been reserved for those patients in whom the pregnancy has not yet ruptured.

In women desiring future fertility, conservative management of a ruptured tubal pregnancy has been recommended. Although salpingectomy may be necessary to control hemostasis, segmental resection may also be accomplished. In the past, recommendations were promulgated that included ipsilateral oophorectomy and cornual resection at the time of surgery for ruptured ectopic pregnancy. Today, neither is considered appropriate surgical management.[65]

SURGICAL APPROACHES

Virtually all surgical procedures that have been described for ectopic gestation by laparotomy can also be performed laparoscopically. Preoperatively, the physician should be prepared for both conservative as well as extirpative surgery. If the woman desires to maintain the potential for future childbearing, conservative management should be the primary consideration. In women who have completed their childbearing, extirpative surgery should be anticipated. If there is significant concern about avoiding the subsequent risk of another ectopic pregnancy, a nonconservative approach may be considered, even to include the possibility of a contralateral ligation of the fallopian tube. This latter consideration should be considered very carefully because there is a significant risk of subsequent patient regret if a decision for permanent sterilization is made under stress.

Salpingostomy

Linear salpingostomy is the most conservative procedure available for treating an ectopic pregnancy. With or without infiltration of a dilute solution of vasopressin (10 units in 100 mL of normal saline), an incision is made on the antimesenteric border of the tube over the bulge of the ectopic gestation. The products of conception are then removed, hemostasis is achieved at the incision site as well as the ectopic pregnancy bed, and the tube is allowed to heal by secondary intention. Salpingotomy with closure of the incision site by fine interrupted sutures such as 7-0 interrupted polyglactin 910 (Vicryl) has also been used. There are no differences in subsequent pregnancy rates, adhesion formation, or fistula formation with or without closure of the incision site. Presently, closure is reserved for instances requiring hemostasis.[66, 67]

A significant concern after salpingostomy is the potential risk of residual placental tissue. Because hCG levels may normally persist for up to 12 days,[68] a continued rise in hCG levels is suggestive of a persistent ectopic pregnancy, whereas plateauing or slowly decreasing levels of hCG probably reflect incomplete (partial) removal of trophoblastic tissue. Sequential hCG determinations are needed to exclude the possibility of persistent trophoblastic function.

In segmental resection, the ectopic pregnancy and the affected portion of the fallopian tube are resected, with proximal and distal stumps left. If the contralateral tube is patent, the distal segment that remains is a potential site for a recurrent ectopic pregnancy. Typically, this procedure is used when there is an isthmic gestation or when hemostasis cannot be achieved without removal of a portion of the tube. Reanastomosis can be achieved at the same time or in a later operation. Both immediate and delayed reanastomosis procedures have had reported success rates of up to 85%.[69]

Fimbrial Expression

Fimbrial expression consists of "milking" the ectopic pregnancy out of the distal end of the tube. The technique has been associated with a higher incidence of persistent trophoblastic tissue, a higher incidence of postoperative bleeding, and a higher rate of subsequent ectopic pregnancy.[70] Sherman and associates[71] reported that 25 of 27 patients (93%) conceived after fimbrial expression, with no repeat ectopic pregnancies. This too-optimistic conclusion may have resulted from case selection in which many of these patients had incomplete tubal abortions.

Salpingectomy

Salpingectomy is the procedure of choice when a woman expresses a desire for no more pregnancies. This procedure may also be necessary if hemostasis cannot be obtained in the process of performing conservative surgery or if the tube cannot be salvaged. If a woman expresses a desire for future fertility, salpingectomy should be considered only as a last resort. Surgery for an interstitial pregnancy has typically been managed via laparotomy with cornual resection; however, successful resection of cornual ectopic pregnancies with the laparoscope has been reported.[72]

Persistent Ectopic Pregnancy

As more conservative laparoscopic management of ectopic pregnancy is pursued, there is an increasing chance for incomplete evacuation of trophoblastic tissue. Persistent ectopic pregnancy after laparotomy has been reported in up to 5% of cases,[73] whereas the incidence following laparoscopic linear salpingostomy has been reported to be as high as 20%. The final choice of management depends on the patient's status and symptomatology. Laparoscopic diagnosis and surgical management may be appropriate. Medical therapy may also be appropriate. Both laparoscopic salpingectomy and salpingostomy have been used for persistent ectopic pregnancy.[73]

NONSURGICAL TREATMENT

Because ectopic pregnancy is being diagnosed earlier, treatment priorities have shifted from the emergency surgical management of a ruptured ectopic pregnancy toward interventions with the least detrimental effect on the woman's reproductive potential. By using the diagnostic algorithms shown in Figures 1 and 2, an ectopic pregnancy may be confidently diagnosed without surgical intervention. These women are ideal patients for a nonsurgical treatment modality, and all surgical risk may be avoided. At the present time, methotrexate is the primary medical therapy available, although the use of other agents such as actinomycin D, potassium chloride, hyperosmolar glucose, prostaglandins, and RU 486 has been reported.

Methotrexate is a folic acid analogue that inhibits dehydrofolate reductase and thereby prevents DNA synthesis. This agent has been shown to inhibit normal trophoblasts in vitro.[74] Side effects such as thrombocytopenia, leukopenia, ulcerative stomatitis, diarrhea, and hemorrhagic enteritis can be reduced by the use of citrovorum factor.[75, 76] The first reported use of methotrexate for an unruptured ectopic pregnancy was by Tanaka et al.[77] in 1982, who treated an interstitial pregnancy with a 15-day course of intramuscular methotrexate. Before this time, methotrexate had been used to treat persistent trophoblastic tissue following abdominal pregnancy.[78–80] The initial successful treatment was followed by a series of case reports and small clinical series using varying doses of methotrexate and citrovorum.[81–84] A prospective trial using intramuscular methotrexate (1 mg/kg/day) followed by citrovorum factor (0.1 mg/kg/day) on alternate days was reported in which all patients were treated as outpatients and the methotrexate/citrovorum factor was given only until the hCG titer began to decrease.[85, 86] The protocol for this multidose regimen is listed in Table 8. In this protocol, the methotrexate/citrovorum factor was administered until a 15% decline between two consecutive hCG titers was noted. Citrovorum factor may always be given on the day following the methotrexate dose, even when another methotrexate dose was not anticipated. Once medication is discontinued, hCG titers are followed weekly until negative. A second course of methotrexate/citrovorum factor is begun only if the hCG titer begins to plateau or rise. With a 96% success rate, we concluded that methotrexate/citrovorum factor could be used successfully on an outpatient basis, that a significant portion (17%) of patients could be treated with only a single dose, that side effects were minimal, and that cardiac activity seen in the ectopic pregnancy by ultrasound represented a relative contraindication to methotrexate therapy (20% failure rate).

TABLE 8.

Ectopic Pregnancy Protocol for Outpatient Multidose Administration of Methotrexate

Day	Time	Therapy*
1	Variable	CBC, SGOT, MTX, hCG, blood type + Rh, BUN, creatinine
2	8:00 A.M.	CF, hCG
3	8:00 A.M.	MTX, hCG
4	8:00 A.M.	CF, hCG
5	8:00 A.M.	MTX, hCG
6	8:00 A.M.	CF, hCG
7	8:00 A.M.	MTX, hCG
8	8:00 A.M.	CF, hCG

*CBC = complete blood count with differential and platelet count; SGOT = serum glutamic oxaloacetic transaminase, units/L; MTX = intramuscular methotrexate, 1.0 mg/kg; hCG = quantitative β-human chorionic gonadotropin, mIU/mL; BUN = blood urea nitrogen; CF = intramuscular citrovorum, 0.1 mg/kg.

Based on this successful experience and the consideration that weekly intramuscular methotrexate without citrovorum factor had been reported for the treatment of nonmetastatic trophoblastic disease,[87] a single-dose methotrexate protocol for ectopic pregnancy was implemented. The initial single-dose methotrexate protocol resulted in a 96.7% success rate with no methotrexate-related side effects. This protocol is summarized in Table 9.[88] When compared with the multidose protocol, single-dose methotrexate costs less, requires less hormonal monitoring during treatment, has fewer side effects, and has similar clinical results and reproductive potential.

Methotrexate also has been given via the oral route. Several investigators have documented the safety and efficacy of oral methotrexate in the treatment of persistent ectopic pregnancy following initial conservative surgical therapy.[84, 88, 89] The optimal dosage regimen has not been identified. The optimal oral methotrexate regimen for treating primary ectopic pregnancy has also not been established.

Direct injection of various agents into ectopic gestations has also been described in the primary treatment of ectopic pregnancy. Injection of methotrexate under ultrasound guidance is associated with an approximately 80% success rate. Its primary advantage is the avoidance of potential systemic complications of methotrexate. This theoretical advantage is minimized, however, when the low rate of side effects of systemic methotrexate therapy is considered. Injection of methotrexate by ultrasound also has the advantage of avoiding laparoscopy. Because of the limited number of cases reported and because reproductive function following this type of treatment has not been described, this treatment as yet has not been widely used.[91, 92] Methotrexate, prostaglandin E_2 (PGE_2), and hyperosmolar glucose have also been reported as agents injected di-

---

TABLE 9.

Single-Dose Methotrexate Protocol for Ectopic Pregnancy Treatment

Day	Therapy*
0†	hCG, D&C, CBC, SGOT, BUN, creatinine, blood type + Rh
1	MTX, hCG
4	hCG
7‡	hCG

*hCG = quantitative β-human chorionic gonadotropin, mIU/mL; D&C = dilation and curettage; CBC = complete blood count; SGOT = serum glutamic oxaloacetic transaminase, units/L; BUN = blood urea nitrogen; MTX = intramuscular methotrexate, 50 mg/m^2.
†In those patients not requiring D&C before MTX initiation (hCG < 2,000 mIU/mL and no gestational sac on transvaginal ultrasound), day 0 and day 1 are combined.
‡If < 15% decline in hCG titer between days 4 and 7, give a second dose of methotrexate, 50 mg/m^2 on day 7. If ≥ 15% decline in hCG titer between days 4 and 7, follow weekly until hCG < 10 mIU/mL.

rectly into ectopic gestations at the time of laparoscopy. The clinical dilemma associated with these cases is that surgery and its inherent risks have already been undertaken and the addition or substitution of medical treatment instead of definitive surgery may be adding risk beyond that of the accepted surgical procedures.[93-99] Injection of KC1 with methotrexate has also been reported.[99, 100] There is a single case report in which intravenous actinomycin D was administered in four 0.5-mg doses. As an alternative to methotrexate, actinomycin D has minimal data upon which to judge its potential. RU 486 is an antiprogesterone that has been used extensively as an abortifacient. A single case report describes RU 486 given as a single oral dose and then followed 1 week later with a course of methotrexate.[101]

Because the natural course of any given ectopic pregnancy is unknown, the role of expectant management remains unclear. Without surgical or medical intervention, some ectopic pregnancies can proceed to spontaneous tubal abortion and minimal bleeding or total resorption with or without resulting tubal patency. Unfortunately, identification of those pregnancies that will resolve spontaneously without intervention is not presently possible. Women whose serial quantitative β-hCG levels are decreasing would be considered the most appropriate for this management approach. Because the failure rate for expectant management using only β-hCG levels as a measurement can be significant, a better predictor of spontaneous resolution is needed.[102-107] Until a reliable marker is identified, expectant management of ectopic pregnancy will have limited use. Methotrexate as a medical alternative offers clinical efficacy, minimal side effects, minimal time off work, 95% success rates, and reproductive outcomes similar to those obtained with surgery.

NONTUBAL ECTOPIC PREGNANCY

Because of improved diagnostic capabilities and because of a greater vigilance on the part of physicians seeing women of reproductive age, the prognosis for nontubal ectopic pregnancy has improved greatly. Fewer patients are diagnosed only at the time of hypovolemic shock and resulting exploratory surgery, and reproductive organs are more commonly preserved.

Cervical Pregnancy

Because cervical pregnancies are prone to massive hemorrhage, hysterectomy has often been the only treatment choice. Although cervical pregnancies are uncommon (from 1 in 2,400 to 1 in 50,000 pregnancies),[5, 108] early ultrasound diagnosis has resulted in a greater range of choices being made available to both the woman and her physician. Some patients with a cervical pregnancy may be treated with methotrexate, either intra-amniotically or systemically.[109-111] Oral etoposide as well as combination chemotherapy have also been reported as successful therapies for cervical pregnancy.[112, 113] Surgical alternatives less radical than hysterectomy can also be successful. A variety of hemostatic techniques have been used in an attempt to arrest the profuse bleeding that is commonly encountered in these cases. The techniques include uterine packing, use of an intracervical Foley catheter balloon, deep lateral cervical stitches, or cerclage with either the MacDonald or Shirodkar techniques.[114-120]

Abdominal Pregnancy

With frequency reported to be from 1 in 372 live births to as rare as 1 in 9,174 live births,[121, 122] abdominal pregnancy may originate from the early rupture of a tubal gestation and subsequent intra-abdominal reimplantation. Maternal mortality rates have been reported to be 2% to 18%.[123, 124] No maternal deaths are reported in the more recent studies.[125, 126] Blood loss can be massive when the placenta is removed at the primary operation, but significant postoperative morbidity is also encountered if the placenta is left in place. These complications include further bleeding, abscess formation, septicemia, bowel obstruction, and gastrointestinal fistula formation. Even with the use of ultrasound, only about 50% of cases are diagnosed preoperatively.[122] Because the clinical manifestation is so variable, the diagnosis is not easily made. When this condition is encountered, it is recommended that the placenta be removed only if the vascular supply can be identified and controlled because partial placental removal may result in massive bleeding. If left in place, the placenta may remain functional for up to 50 days.[127] Methotrexate has been used to hasten the resorption of functional trophoblastic tissue, but not all results using methotrexate have been satisfactory. When massive bleeding is encountered, abdominal packs can be used to control bleeding and left in place with removal at a second procedure. Arterial embolization has also been used successfully.[128, 129]

Ovarian Pregnancy

Of the nontubal ectopic pregnancies, ovarian pregnancy is the most common and carries the least morbidity. The classically described Spiegelberg criteria include the following four conditions that must be met to make the diagnosis of ovarian pregnancy: (1) the tube on the affected side must be intact, (2) the fetal sac must occupy the normal position of the ovary, (3) the ovary must be connected to the uterus by the ovarian ligament, and (4) ovarian tissue must be found in the sac wall.[130] The incidence has been estimated to range from 1 in 7,000 to 1 in 40,000 deliveries.[131, 132] The clinical symptoms are typically the same as in a tubal gestation. Because ovarian pregnancy tends to rupture early, the standard of care in the past has been oophorectomy. Ovarian cystectomy, however, has now become a standard practice.[133–135] Like other operations for ectopic pregnancy, this procedure has also been accomplished successfully through the laparoscope.[136, 137]

SUMMARY

In order to minimize both short- and long-term morbidity, ectopic pregnancies must be diagnosed as early as possible in their clinical course. It is critical that the clinician consider the possibility of an ectopic gestation in all patients of reproductive age who have pain and/or vaginal bleeding. Patients with risk factors should have early ultrasound and hormonal screening to exclude the possibility of an ectopic pregnancy. With a timely diagnosis, an increased proportion of patients will be candidates for conservative treatment modalities such as nonextirpative surgery and/or medical treatment. With increased vigilance and continued applications of the newest technology, morbidity and mortality from ectopic pregnancies will continue to be reduced.

REFERENCES

1. Centers for Disease Control: Ectopic pregnancy surveillance in the United States, 1970–1987. *MMWR* 1990; 39:11.
2. Marchbanks PA, Annegers JF, Coulam CB, et al: Risk factors for ectopic pregnancy. A population-based study. *JAMA* 1988; 259:1823.
3. Papano R: Ectopic pregnancy—a seven year survey. *Med J Aust* 1981; 2:586.
4. Patrick JD: Ectopic pregnancy—a brief review. *Ann Emerg Med* 1982; 11:576.
5. Breen JL: A 21 year old survey of 659 ectopic pregnancies. *Am J Obstet Gynecol* 1970; 106:1004.
6. Helvacioglu A, Long EM, Yang SL: Ectopic pregnancy: An eight year review. *J Reprod Med* 1979; 22:87.
7. Weeks AR, Hutchins CJ: Ectopic pregnancy: A five year review. *Br J Clin Pract* 1976; 30:104.
8. Brenner PF, Roy S, Mishell DR: Ectopic pregnancy: A study of 300 consecutive surgically treated cases. *JAMA* 1980; 243:673.
9. Halpin TF: Ectopic pregnancy—the problem of diagnosis. *Am J Obstet Gynecol* 1970; 106:227.
10. Powers DN: Ectopic pregnancy: A five year experience. *South Med J* 1980; 73:1012.
11. Stovall TG, Kellerman AL, Ling FW, et al: Emergency department diagnosis of ectopic pregnancies. *Ann Emerg Med* 1990; 19:1098.
12. Stabile I, Grudzinskas JG: Ectopic pregnancy: A review of incidence, etiology and diagnostic aspects. *Obstet Gynecol Surv* 1990; 45:335.
13. Derman R, Edelman DA, Berger GS: Current status of immunologic pregnancy tests. *Int J Gynaecol Obstet* 1979; 17:190.
14. Rasor JL, Braunstein GD: A rapid modification of the beta-hCG radioimmunoassay. Use as an aid in the diagnosis of ectopic pregnancy. *Obstet Gynecol* 1977; 50:553.
15. Vaitukaitis JL, Braunstein GD: Radioimmunoassay which specifically measured human chorionic gonadotropin in the presence of luteinizing hormone. *Am J Obstet Gynecol* 1972; 113:751.
16. Storring PL, Gaine-Des RE, Bangham DR: International Reference Preparation of human chorionic gonadotropin for immunoassay; potency estimates in various bioassay and protein binding assay systems; and International Reference Preparations of the alpha and beta subunits of human chorionic gonadotropin for immunoassay. *J Endocrinol* 1980; 84:295.
17. Kadar N, Caldwell BV, Romero R: A method for screening for ectopic pregnancy. *Obstet Gynecol* 1981; 58:162.
18. Kadar N, DeVore G, Romero R: The discriminatory hCG zone: Its use in the sonographic evaluation of ectopic pregnancy. *Obstet Gynecol* 1981; 58:156.
19. Milwidsky A, Adoni A, Segal S, et al: Chorionic gonadotropin and progesterone levels in ectopic pregnancy. *Obstet Gynecol* 1977; 50:145.
20. Matthews CP, Coulson PB, Wild RA: Serum progesterone levels as an aid in the diagnosis of ectopic pregnancy. *Obstet Gynecol* 1986; 68:390.
21. Yeko TR, Rodi IA, Gorrill MJ, et al: Timely diagnosis of early ectopic pregnancy using a single blood progesterone measurement. *Fertil Steril* 1987; 48:1048.
22. Stovall TG, Ling FW, Andersen RN, et al: Improved sensitivity and specificity of a single measurement of serum progesterone over serial quantita-

tive beta-human chorionic gonadotropin in screening for ectopic pregnancy. *Hum Reprod* 1992; 7:723.

23. Stovall TG, Ling FW, Cope BJ, et al: Preventing ruptured ectopic prgnancy with a single serum progesterone. *Am J Obstet Gynecol* 1989; 160:1425.

24. Stovall TG, Ling FW, Carson SA, et al: Serum progesterone and uterine curettage in differential diagnosis of ectopic pregnancy. *Fertil Steril* 1992; 57:456.

25. Barnea ER, Oelsner G, Benvenisto R, et al: Progesterone, estradiol and β-human chorionic gonadotropin secretion in patients with ectopic pregnancy. *J Clin Endocrinol Metab* 1986; 62:529.

26. Guillaume J, Benjamin F, Sicuranza BJ, et al: Maternal serum levels of estradiol, progesterone, and human chorionic gonadotropin in ectopic pregnancy and their correlation with endometrial histologic findings. *Surg Gynecol Obstet* 1978; 165:9.

27. Guillaume J, Benjamin F, Sicuranza BJ, et al: Serum estradiol as an aid in the diagnosis of ectopic pregnancy. *Obstet Gynecol* 1990; 76:1126.

28. Witt BR, Wolf GC, Wainwright CJ, et al: Relaxin, CA-125, progesterone, estradiol, Schwangerschafts protein, and human chorionic gonadotropin as predictors of outcome in threatened and nonthreatened pregnancies. *Fertil Steril* 1990; 53:1029.

29. Ho PC, Chan SYW, Tang GWK: Diagnosis of early pregnancy by enzyme immunoassay of Schwangerschafts-protein 1. *Fertil Steril* 1988; 49:76.

30. Garcia A, Skurnick JH, Goldsmith LT, et al: Human chorionic gonadotropin and relaxin concentrations in early ectopic and normal pregnancies. *Obstet Gynecol* 1990; 75:77.

31. Meunier K, Mignot T, Maria B, et al: Predictive value of the active renin assay for the diagnosis of ectopic pregnancy. *Fertil Steril* 1991; 55:432.

32. Sauer MV, Vasilev SA, Campeau J, et al: Serum cancer antigen 125 in ectopic pregnancy. *Gynecol Obstet Invest* 1989; 27:164.

33. Stabile I, Olajide F, Chard T, et al: Maternal serum alpha-fetoprotein levels in ectopic pregnancy. Circulating alpha-fetoprotein levels in women with ectopic pregnancy. *Hum Reprod* 1989; 4:835.

34. Cederquest LL, Killackey MA, Abdel-Latif N, et al: Alpha-fetoprotein and ectopic pregnancy. *BMJ* 1983; 286:1247.

35. Coddington CC, Sinosich MJ, Boston EG, et al: Pregnancy-associated protein-A does not improve predictability of pregnancy success or failure over human chorionic gonadotropins levels in early normal and abnormal pregnancy. *Fertil Steril* 1989; 52:854.

36. Poulsen HK, Westergaard JG, Teisner B, et al: Measurements of hCG and PAPP-A in uncommon types of ectopic gestation. *Eur J Obstet Gynecol Reprod Biol* 1987; 26:33.

37. Sauer MV, Sinosich J, Yeko TR, et al: Predictive value of a single pregnancy-associated plasma protein-A or progesterone in the diagnosis of abnormal pregnancy. *Hum Reprod* 1989; 4:331.

38. Theron GB, Sheperd EGS, Strachan AE: C-reactive protein levels in ectopic pregnancy, pelvic infection and carcinoma of the cervix. *S Afr Med J* 1986; 69:661.

39. Seppälä M, Venesmaa P, Rutann E-M: Pregnancy-specific beta-1 glycoprotein in ectopic pregnancy. *Am J Obstet Gynecol* 1980; 136:189.

40. Lawson TL: Ectopic pregnancy: Criteria and accuracy of ultrasonic diagnosis. *AJR Am J Roentgenol* 1978; 131:153–156.

41. Pelosi MA: The value of pelvic ultrasound in the diagnosis of ectopic pregnancy. *Diagn Gynecol Obstet* 1981; 3:337–346.

42. Bradley WG, Fiske CE, Filly RA: The double sac sign of early intrauterine

pregnancy: Use in exclusion of ectopic pregnancy. *Radiology* 1982; 143:223–226.

43. Cacciatore B: Can the status of tubal pregnancy be predicted with transvaginal sonography? A prospective comparison of sonographic, surgical, and serum hCG findings. *Radiology* 1990; 177:481–484.

44. Stovall TG, Ling FW, Buster JE: Outpatient chemotherapy of unruptured ectopic pregnancy. *Fertil Steril* 1989; 51:435–438.

45. Menard A, Crequat J, Mandelbrot L, et al: Treatment of unruptured tubal pregnancy by local injection of methotrexate under transvaginal sonographic control. *Fertil Steril* 1990; 54:47–50.

46. Brown DL, Felker RE, Stovall TG, et al: Serial endovaginal sonography of ectopic pregnancies treated with methotrexate. *Obstet Gynecol* 1991; 77:406–409.

47. Romero R, Kadar N, Castro D, et al: Diagnosis of ectopic pregnancy: Value of the discriminatory human chorionic gonadotropin zone. *Obstet Gynecol* 1985; 66:357.

48. Kadar N, DeVore G, Romero R: Discriminatory hCG zone: Its use in the sonographic evaluation for ectopic pregnancy. *Obstet Gynecol* 1981; 58:156–161.

49. Bree RL, Edwards M, Bohm VM, et al: Transvaginal sonography in the evaluation of normal early pregnancy: Correlation with hCG level. *AJR Am J Roentgenol* 1989; 153:75–79.

50. Weckstein LN: Current perspective on ectopic pregnancy. *Obstet Gynecol Surv* 1985; 40:259–272.

51. Romero R, Copel JA, Kadar N, et al: Value of culdocentesis in the diagnosis of ectopic pregnancy. *Obstet Gynecol* 1985; 65:519–522.

52. Tancer ML, Delke I, Veridiano NP: A fifteen year experience with ectopic pregnancy. *Surg Gynecol Obstet* 1981; 152:179.

53. Sandvei R: Diagnosis of ectopic pregnancy. *Diagn Gynecol Obstet* 1981; 3:15–21.

54. Vermesh M, Graczykowski JW, Sauer MV: Reevaluation of the role of culdocentesis in the management of ectopic pregnancy. *Am J Obstet Gynecol* 1990; 162:411–413.

55. Bello GV, Schonholz D, Moshirpur J, et al: Combined pregnancy: The Mount Sinai experience. *Obstet Gynecol Surv* 1986; 41:603–613.

56. DeVoe R, Pratt J: Simultaneous intrauterine and extrauterine pregnancy. *Am J Obstet Gynecol* 1948; 56:1119.

57. Cartwright PS: Diagnosis of ectopic pregnancy. *Obstet Gynecol Clin North Am* 1991; 18:19–37.

58. Sauer MV, Rodi IA: Utility of an algorithm to diagnose ectopic pregnancy. *Int J Gynaecol Obstet* 1990; 31:29–34.

59. Kim DS, Chung SR, Park MI, et al: Comparative review of diagnostic accuracy in tubal pregnancy: A 14-year survey of 1040 cases. *Obstet Gynecol* 1987; 70:547–554.

60. Stovall TG, Ling FW, Carson SA, et al: Nonsurgical diagnosis and treatment of tubal pregnancy. *Fertil Steril* 1990; 54:537–538.

61. Mackles A, Wolfe S, Pozner S: Cellular atypia in endometrial glands (Arias-Stella reaction) as an aid in the diagnosis of ectopic pregnancy. *Am J Obstet Gynecol* 1961; 81:1209.

62. Stovall TG, Ling FW: Ectopic pregnancy: Diagnostic and therapeutic algorithms minimizing surgical intervention. *J Reprod Med*, in press.

63. Vermesh M, Presser SC: Reproductive outcome after linear salpingostomy for ectopic gestation. A prospective 3-4 year follow-up. *Fertil Steril* 1992; 57:682.

64. Brumsted J, Kessler C, Gibson C, et al: A comparison of laparoscopy and

laparotomy for the treatment of ectopic pregnancy. *Obstet Gynecol* 1988; 71:889.

65. Kalchman GG, Meltzer RM: Interstitial pregnancy following homolateral salpingectomy: Report of two cases and a review of the literature. *Am J Obstet Gynecol* 1966; 96:1139.

66. Nelson LM, Margara RA, Winston RML: Primary and secondary closure of ampullary salpingostomy compared in the rabbit. *Fertil Steril* 1986; 45:292.

67. DeCherney AH, Jones EE: Ectopic pregnancy. *Clin Obstet Gynecol* 1985; 28:365.

68. Kamrava MM, Taymor ML, Berger MJ, et al: Disappearance of human chorionic gonadotropin following removal of ectopic pregnancy. *Obstet Gynecol* 1983; 62:486.

69. Smith HO, Toledo AA, Thompson JD: Conservative surgical management of isthmic ectopic pregnancies. *Am J Obstet Gynecol* 1987; 157:604.

70. Bell OR, Awadalla SG, Mattox H: Persistent ectopic syndrome: A case report and literature review. *Obstet Gynecol* 1987; 69:521.

71. Sherman D, Langer R, Herman A, et al: Reproductive outcome after fimbrial evacuation of tubal pregnancy. *Fertil Steril* 1987; 47:420.

72. Pasic R, Wolfe WM: Laparoscopic diagnosis and treatment of interstitial ectopic pregnancy: A case report. *Am J Obstet Gynecol* 1990; 163:587.

73. Seifer DB, Gutmann JN, Doyle MB, et al: Persistent ectopic pregnancy following laparoscopic linear salpingostomy. *Obstet Gynecol* 1990; 76:1121.

74. Sand PK, Stubblefield PA, Ory SJ: Methotrexate inhibition of normal trophoblasts in vitro. *Am J Obstet Gynecol* 1986; 155:324.

75. Bleyer WA: The clinical pharmacology of methotrexate: New applications of an old drug. *Cancer* 1978; 41:36.

76. Berkowitz RS, Goldstein DP, Jones MA, et al: Methotrexate with citrovorum factor rescue: Reduced chemotherapy toxicity in the management of gestational trophoblastic neoplasms. *Cancer* 1980; 45:423.

77. Tanaka T, Hayaski H, Kutsuzawa T, et al: Treatment of interstitial ectopic pregnancy with methotrexate: Report of a successful case. *Fertil Steril* 1982; 37:851.

78. Hreshchyshyn MM, Naples JD Jr, Randall CL: Amethopterin in abdominal pregnancy. *Am J Obstet Gynecol* 1965; 93:286.

79. Lathrop JC, Bowles GE: Methotrexate in abdominal pregnancy. Report of case. *Obstet Gynecol* 1968; 32:81.

80. St. Clair JT, Whealer DA: Methotrexate in abdominal pregnancy. *JAMA* 1969; 21:529.

81. Ory SJ, Villanueva AL, Sand PK, et al: Conservative treatment of ectopic pregnancy with methotrexate. *Am J Obstet Gynecol* 1986; 154:1299.

82. Ichinoe K, Wake N, Shinkai N, et al: Nonsurgical therapy to preserve oviduct function in patient with tubal pregnancies. *Am J Obstet Gynecol* 1987; 156:484.

83. Sauer MV, Gorrill MJ, Rodi IA, et al: Nonsurgical management of unruptured ectopic pregnancy: An extended clinical trial. *Fertil Steril* 1987; 48:754.

84. Patsner B, Kenigsberg D: Successful treatment of persistent ectopic pregnancy with oral methotrexate therapy. *Fertil Steril* 1988; 50:982.

85. Stovall TG, Ling FW, Buster JE: Outpatient chemotherapy of unruptured ectopic pregnancy. *Fertil Steril* 1989; 51:435.

86. Stovall TG, Ling FW, Gray LA, et al: Methotrexate treatment of unruptured ectopic pregnancy: A report of 100 cases. *Obstet Gynecol* 1991; 77:749.

87. Homesly HD, Blessing JA, Rettenmaier M, et al: Weekly intramuscular methotrexate for non-metastatic gestational trophoblastic disease. *Obstet Gynecol* 1988; 72:413.

88. Fernandez H, Deziegler D, Bourget P, et al: The place of methotrexate in the management of interstitial pregnancy. *Hum Reprod* 1991; 6:302.

89. Higgins KA, Schwartz MB: Treatment of persistent trophoblastic tissue after salpingostomy with methotrexate. *Fertil Steril* 1986; 45:427.

90. Bengtsson G, Bryman I, Thorburn J, et al: Low dose oral methotrexate as second line therapy for persistent trophoblast after conservative treatment of ectopic pregnancy. *Obstet Gynecol* 1991; 79:589.

91. Vermesh M: Conservative management of ectopic gestation. *Fertil Steril* 1989; 51:550.

92. Tulandi T, Atri M, Bret P, et al: Transvaginal intratubal methotrexate treatment of ectopic pregnancy. *Fertil Steril* 1992; 58:98.

93. Robertson DE, Moye MA, Hansen JH, et al: Reduction of ectopic pregnancy by injection under ultrasound control. *Lancet* 1987; 1:974.

94. Tulandi T, Bret PM, Atri M, et al: Treatment of ectopic pregnancy by transvaginal intratubal methotrexate administration. *Obstet Gynecol* 1991; 77:627.

95. Clark LC, Raymond S, Stranger J, et al: Treatment of ectopic pregnancy with intraamniotic methotrexate: A case report. *Aust N Z J Obstet Gynaecol* 1989; 29:84.

96. Porreco RP: Percutaneous, ultrasound-directed ablation of ectopic pregnancy with methotrexate: A report of three cases. *J Reprod Med* 1992; 37:363.

97. Timor-Trisch I, Baxi L, Peisner DB: Transvaginal salpingocentesis: A new technique for treating ectopic pregnancy. *Am J Obstet Gynecol* 1989; 160:459.

98. Timor-Trisch IE, Montequdo A, Matera C, et al: Sonographic evolution of cornual pregnancies treated without surgery. *Obstet Gynecol* 1992; 79:1044.

99. Guingis RR: Simultaneous intrauterine and ectopic pregnancies following in-vitro fertilization and gamete intra-fallopian transfer: A review of nine cases. *Hum Reprod* 1990; 5:484.

100. Abolghar MA, Mansour RT, Serour GI: Transvaginal injection of potassium chloride and methotrexate for the treatment of tubal pregnancy with a live fetus. *Hum Reprod* 1990; 5:887.

101. Kenigsberg D, Porte J, Hull M, et al: Medical treatment of residual ectopic pregnancy: RU486 and methotrexate. *Fertil Steril* 1987; 47:702.

102. Lund SS: Early ectopic pregnancy treated nonsurgically. *J Obstet Gynaecol Br Emp* 1955; 62:70.

103. Mäkinen JI, Kivijarvi AK, Irjala KMA: Success of non-surgical management of ectopic pregnancy. *Lancet* 1990; 335:1099.

104. Fernandez H, Rainhorn J, Papiernik E, et al: Spontaneous resolution of ectopic pregnancy. *Obstet Gynecol* 1988; 71:171.

105. Carp HJA, Oelsner G, Serr DM, et al: Fertility after nonsurgical treatment of ectopic pregnancy. *J Reprod Med* 1986; 31:119.

106. Carson SA, Stovall TG, Ling FW, et al: Low human chorionic somatomammotropin fails to predict spontaneous resolution of unruputed ectopic pregnancies. *Fertil Steril* 1980; 55:629.

107. Ylöstalo P, Cacciatore B, Koskimies A, et al: Conservative treatment of ectopic pregnancy. *Ann N Y Acad Sci* 1991; 626:516.

108. Parente JT, Ou CS, Levy J, et al: Cervical pregnancy analysis: A review and report of five cases. *Obstet Gynecol* 1983; 62:79.

109. Farabow WS, Fulton JW, Fletcher V, et al: Cervical pregnancy treated with methotrexate. *N C Med J* 1983; 44:91.

110. Stovall TG, Ling FW, Smith WC, et al: Successful nonsurgical treatment of cervical pregnancy with methotrexate. *Fertil Steril* 1988; 50:672.

111. Oyer R, Tarakjian D, Lev-Toaff A, et al: Treatment of cervical pregnancy with methotrexate. *Obstet Gynecol* 1988; 71:469.

112. Segna RA, Mitchell Dr, Misas JE: Successful treatment of cervical pregnancy with oral etoposide. *Obstet Gynecol* 1990; 76:945.

113. Baakri YN, Badawi A: Case report: Cervical pregnancy successfully treated with chemotherapy. *Acta Obstet Gynecol Scand* 1990; 69:655.

114. Sheldon RS, Aaro LA, Welch JS: Conservative management of cervical pregnancy. *Am J Obstet Gynecol* 1963; 87:504.

115. Ratten GJ: Cervical pregnancy treated by ligation of the descending branch of the uterine arteries. Case report. *Br J Obstet Gynaecol* 1983; 90:367.

116. Bernstein D, Holzinger M, Ovadia J, et al: Conservative treatment of cervical pregnancy. *Obstet Gynecol* 1981; 58:741.

117. Wharton KR, Gore B: Cervical pregnancy managed by placement of a Shirodkar cerclage before evacuation: A case report. *J Reprod Med* 1988; 33:227.

118. Nolan TE, Chandler PE, Hess LW, et al: Cervical pregnancy managed without hysterectomy: A case report. *J Reprod Med* 1989; 34:241.

119. Reginald PW, Reid JE, Paintin DB: Control of bleeding in cervical pregnancy: Two case reports. *Br J Obstet Gynaecol* 1985; 92:1199.

120. Patchell D: Cervical pregnancy managed by balloon tamponade (letter). *Am J Obstet Gynecol* 1983; 149:107.

121. Beecham WD, Hernquist WC, Beacham DW, et al: Abdominal pregnancy at Charity Hospital in New Orleans. *Am J Obstet Gynecol* 1962; 84:1257.

122. Atrash HK, Friede A, Hogue CJR: Abdominal pregnancy in the United States: Fequency and maternal mortality. *Obstet Gynecol* 1987; 69:333.

123. Hreshchyshyn MM, Bogen B, Loughran CH: What is the actual present-day management of the placenta in late abdominal pregnancy? *Am J Obstet Gynecol* 1961; 81:302.

124. Ware HH: Observations on 13 cases of late extrauterine pregnancy. *Am J Obstet Gynecol* 1948; 55:561.

125. Martin JN Jr, Sessums JK, Martin RW, et al: Abdominal pregnancy: Current concepts of management. *Obstet Gynecol* 1988; 71:549.

126. Delke I, Veridiano NP, Tancer ML: Abdominal pregnancy: Review of current management and addition of 10 cases. *Obstet Gynecol* 1982; 60:200.

127. Siegler AH, Zeichner S, Rubenstein I, et al: Endocrine studies in two instances of term abdominal pregnancy. *Am J Obstet Gynecol* 1987; 76:542.

128. Martin JN Jr, Ridgway LE III, Connors JJ, et al: Angiographic arterial embolization and computed tomography–directed drainage for the management of hemorrhage and infection with abdominal pregnancy. *Obstet Gynecol* 1990; 76:941.

129. Kivikoske AI, Martin C, Weyman P, et al: Angiographic arterial embolization to control hemorrhage in abdominal pregnancy: A case report. *Obstet Gynecol* 1988; 71:456.

130. Spiegelberg O: Casusistik der Ovarialschwangerschaft. *Arch Gynaekol* 1878: 13:73.

131. Lehfeldt H, Tietze C, Gorstein F: Ovarian pregnancy and the intrauterine device. *Am J Obstet Gynecol* 1970; 108:1005.

132. Vasilev SA, Sauer MV: Diagnosis and modern surgical management of ovarian pregnancy. *Surg Gynecol Obstet* 1990; 170:395.

133. Hallatt JG: Primary ovarian pregnancy: A report of twenty-five cases. *Am J Obstet Gynecol* 1982; 143:55.

134. DeVrier K, Atad J, Arodi J, et al: Primary ovarian pregnancy: A conservative surgical approach by wedge resection. *Int J Fertil* 1981; 26:293.

135. Dougherty RE, Diddle AW: Intrafollicular ovarian pregnancy: Management with ovarian conservation. *Obstet Gynecol* 1969; 33:20.

136. Russell JB, Cutler LR: Transvaginal ultrasonographic detection of primary ovarian pregnancy with laparoscopic removal: A case report. *Fertil Steril* 1989; 51:1055.

137. Van Coevering RJ, Fisher JE: Laparoscopic management of ovarian pregnancy: A case report. *J Reprod Med* 1988; 33:774.

Editor's Comment

This update provided by Drs. Ling and Stovall is a concise summary of their series of brilliant clinical and laboratory studies of ectopic pregnancy. Through their investigative work and publications, these physicians have simplified the diagnosis and management of this extremely deadly complication of pregnancy.

Any clinician reading this update will be able to diagnose an ectopic pregnancy at a much earlier time in its clinical course. Moreover, once the diagnosis is made, the clinician will have the choice of operative or medical therapy to treat the condition. In any event, this will result in less danger to the woman and will more likely help preserve her future childbearing capacity.

In summary, hundreds of women today, and likely hundreds yet unborn, will one day owe their lives, and perhaps the lives of their children, to these two obstetrician/gynecologists.

Norman F. Gant, Jr., M.D.

Pelvic Inflammatory Disease

DAVID E. SOPER, M.D.

EPIDEMIOLOGY

Pelvic inflammatory disease (PID) remains a common complication of cervicovaginal sexually transmitted diseases (STDs). In 1988, over 10% of American women in the reproductive age group reported that they had received treatment for PID.[1] This is probably an underestimate of the true magnitude of PID because of the poor reliability of the diagnosis and the realization that many women with PID will have atypical symptoms or no symptoms at all.[2] Direct costs for PID and its associated sequelae of ectopic pregnancy and infertility approach 3 billion dollars annually. These costs are projected to approach 10 billion dollars annually by the year 2000, with an increasing proportion being covered by public payment sources.[3] Although there has been a decreased incidence of hospitalization for acute PID since 1983, the average annual numbers of women visiting private physicians' offices for this disorder has increased, thus suggesting a higher proportion of women with clinically mild disease associated with *Chlamydia trachomatis*,[4] which remains the most common bacterial STD in America. Rates of *Neisseria gonorrhoeae* infection have been decreasing since the 1970s.[5]

Population differences will have a significant effect on the clinical manifestations and microbiology of PID. Women evaluated in an urban emergency room will generally have the more classic signs and symptoms of PID including fever and the "chandelier sign" associated with gonococcal PID, whereas women selected from an STD clinic or college population may have the more benign clinical symptoms associated with chlamydial PID.[6–8] However, universal risk assessment for the development of PID and its sequelae depends primarily on the identification of variables associated with the acquisition of an STD. Risk markers include young age, lower socioeconomic status, substance abuse, and certain contraceptive practices. Risk factors associated with ascending infection include poor health-care–seeking behavior (allowing more prolonged STD infection), intrauterine device (IUD) use, and douching.[9]

MICROBIOLOGY AND PATHOGENESIS

The microbial etiology of PID can be divided into three categories: sexually transmitted microorganisms, respiratory pathogens, and endogenous vaginal and/or bowel microorganisms (Table 1). In North America the microbial etiology of PID has been defined by endocervical cultures for the STD microorganisms. Studies that use culdocentesis specimens from hos-

Advances in Obstetrics and Gynecology, vol 1
© 1994, Mosby–Year Book, Inc.

TABLE 1.
Microbial Pathogenesis of Pelvic
Inflammatory Disease

Sexually transmitted microorganisms
  Neisseria gonorrhoeae
  Chlamydia trachomatis
Respiratory pathogens
  Haemophilus influenzae
  Streptococcus pyogenes
  Streptococcus pneumoniae
Endogenous microorganisms
  "Bacterial vaginosis microorganisms"
    Bacteroides sp.
    Peptostreptococcus sp.
    Mycoplasma hominis
  Bowel microorganisms
    Bacteroides fragilis
    Escherichia coli

pitalized patients with the clinical diagnosis of PID suggest that as many as 80% of cases are associated with mixed infections of both aerobic and anaerobic microorganisms.[10–13] However, it has become apparent that culdocentesis is an unreliable method for defining the microbiology of the upper genital tract and may, in fact, even contaminate the cul-de-sac and yield false positive cultures.[14, 15] Subsequent reports in which only laparoscopically obtained isolates were used and culdocentesis was restricted have confirmed a polymicrobial etiology in only 30% to 40% of cases.[6, 7, 16, 17] *Neisseria gonorrhoeae* remains the single most frequent pathogen recovered. *Chlamydia trachomatis* can be detected in up to 40% of women with PID in some populations. Studies done in Scandinavian countries reflect a different bacterial pathogenesis in that *C. trachomatis* is the most frequently recovered pathogen; anaerobic bacteria are conspicuously absent.[18]

Respiratory pathogens are isolated from the fallopian tube in approximately 5% of cases of acute salpingitis.[17] *Haemophilus influenzae* is the most commonly isolated microorganism in this category and is commonly associated with pyosalpinx formation.[19] *Streptococcus pyogenes*, *Neisseria meningitidis*, and *Streptococcus pneumoniae* have also been isolated from the upper genital tract of women with PID. That respiratory pathogens can initiate PID should come as no surprise since there is substantial similarity between the histology of the respiratory and upper genital tracts.[20]

Endogenous bacteria isolated from the upper genital tract of women with PID have generally been "bacterial vaginosis (BV) microorganisms." These are predominantly anaerobic bacteria such as *Bacteroides* sp. and *Peptostreptococcus* sp. commonly found in high concentrations in the vagina of women with BV. An increased concentration of *Mycoplasma hominis*, a genital mycoplasma, is also found in women with BV. Bacterial vaginosis has been associated with adnexal tenderness and, therefore, presumptive PID.[21] Moreover, the recovery of BV microorganisms has been shown to be associated with histologic endometritis in women with clinical signs of PID.[22] Microorganisms found in the gut may also translocate across the bowel wall in cases involving significant bowel inflammation such as patients with tubo-ovarian abscesses (TOAs). Uncommonly, PID may be secondary to direct extension of an inflammatory process resulting from appendicitis or Crohn's disease. Rarely, PID caused by *Actinomyces israelii* develops in women using an intrauterine contraceptive device.

The pathogenesis of PID involves the ascending spread of pathogens found in the endocervix. Cervical mucus, by virtue of its gel structure and cell composition, is a mechanical barrier to ascending infection. Cervical mucus proteins such as lactoferrin possess antibacterial activity that inhibits bacterial penetration into the endometrium. Secretions of endometrial and oviductal fluids, aided by myometrial and ciliary activity, help to wash out cellular debris and possibly bacteria from the upper genital tract. These secretions also possess lactoferrin and lysosomal enzymes with antibacterial activity.[23, 24] By mechanisms that are poorly understood, bacterial pathogens are able to gain entrance into the endometrium and fallopian tube mucosa of women with PID. It has been suggested that both passive transport and vectors such as spermatozoa and trichomonads assist in establishing this ascending infection.[25] In addition, it is well known that tubal regurgitation of menstrual blood is common, and this may also transport microorganisms into the fallopian tube. Intrauterine instrumentation and intrauterine contraceptive device insertion are obvious mechanisms by which the endometrium can be inoculated with potentially pathogenic bacteria. Once present in the upper genital tract in sufficient numbers and with sufficient virulence, these bacteria initiate an inflammatory reaction (endometritis-salpingitis-peritonitis) that results in the symptoms and signs of PID.

The mildest form of salpingitis can be visualized as (1) fallopian tube hyperemia, (2) edema of the tubal wall, and (3) a sticky exudate on the tubal surface and from the fimbriated ends. If left untreated, more advanced inflammatory changes of the pelvic organs occur. The tubes become involved with inflammatory adhesions, and tubal paraphimosis with fimbrial agglutination occurs.[26, 27] The pelvic organs may then become adherent to one another, and a pyosalpinx or tubo-ovarian complex may develop. Tubo-ovarian abscess formation, the most severe consequence of PID, complicates approximately 15% of cases. Presumably through an ovulation site, microorganisms gain entry to the ovarian stroma.[28] This can lead to destruction of the ovary and the formation of an abscess cavity. Loculations of pus can occur between pelvic structures (tube, ovary, uterus), and in many cases bowel becomes involved. These loculations act as abscess cavities and result in persistent inflammation and destruction of the adjacent organs.

FITZ-HUGH–CURTIS SYNDROME

The Fitz-Hugh–Curtis syndrome (FHCS), an extrapelvic manifestation of PID,[29] is composed of two phases, acute and chronic. In the acute phase, a perihepatitis and a focal peritonitis result from the transport of inflammatory peritoneal fluid either directly or by lymphatics to the subphrenic and subdiaphragmatic space. Both N. gonorrohoeae and C. trachomatis have been isolated from the liver surface of women with FHCS. Microscopic examination of the liver parenchyma reveals acute inflammation of the capsule without parenchymal involvement. Liver function test results are normal in women with FHCS. The chronic phase is characterized by "violin-string" adhesions between the anterior surface of the liver and the anterior abdominal wall.

ATYPICAL PELVIC INFLAMMATORY DISEASE ("SILENT SALPINGITIS")

Although more than half of women with tubal factor infertility (TFI) give no history of PID, antibodies to C. trachomatis and/or N. gonorrhoeae are noted in the majority of these patients, thus suggesting that prior infection has occurred.[30, 31] Moreover, both gross and microscopic examinations of the fallopian tubes of women with TFI fail to differentiate between those patients with or without a history of PID.[32] These data indirectly suggest that salpingitis and subsequent tubal damage may develop without the typical clinical symptoms, primarily lower abdominal pain and fever, associated with the traditional diagnosis of PID. Many of these patients may have abdominal or pelvic discomfort (dysmenorrhea or dyspareunia), but not to such a degree that it alerts the clinician to the diagnosis of PID. Other women may have symptoms associated with PID (metrorrhagia, vaginal discharge), but in the absence of abdominal pain many clinicians will not relate these symptoms to a sexually transmitted genital infection.[33] The absence of significant abdominal pain in these patients is most likely related to the lack of an associated peritonitis.[34]

Women with mucopurulent endocervicitis often have histologic evidence of endometritis.[27] This is direct evidence that upper genital tract inflammation may be present in the absence of signs and symptoms suggesting PID. In addition, almost half of women with chlamydial endocervical infections may have concurrent endometrial infections without evidence of endometritis or salpingitis on physical examination.[35] Many women with infertility and positive chlamydial serology will also have silent but active chlamydial infections of the endometrium.[36]

DIAGNOSIS

The clinical criteria for the diagnosis of PID have never been validated in large prospective studies (Table 2). Two similar sets of guidelines for the diagnosis are in current use.

Jacobson and Westrom[37] were the first to evaluate the accuracy of conventional signs and symptoms of PID as assessed by the visual confirmation of acute salpingitis. Diagnostic accuracy was improved by increasing the number of positive parameters. Westrom suggested that the basis for the diagnosis of PID should be a minimum of three criteria, with supportive signs, laboratory tests, or both, to improve the specificity of the diagnosis. Of particular importance is Westrom's uniform finding of a marked increase in the number of inflammatory cells (leukorrhea) in the wet smear of the vaginal secretions of women with PID.[38] It appears that

TABLE 2.
Clinical Criteria for the Diagnosis of Pelvic Inflammatory Disease*

Westrom and Mardh	Hager	Suggested
Major criteria (all must be present)		
Symptoms		
Abdominal pain	None required	None required
Signs		
Adnexal tenderness	Abdominal tenderness	Pelvic organ tenderness
Signs of an LGTI†	Cervical motion tenderness	Leukorrhea and/or MPC†
	Adnexal tenderness	
Minor criteria (additional criteria increase the specificity of the diagnosis)		
Palpable adnexal mass	Gram's stain of endocervix is positive for GND†	Endometrial biopsy showing endometritis
ESR† ≥15 mm/hr	Temperature >38°C	Elevated CRP† or ESR
Temperature >38°C	Leukocytosis (>10,000/mm³)	Temperature >38°C
	Purulent material by culdocentesis	Leukocytosis
	Pelvic complex by examination or sonography	Positive test for chlamydia or GC†

*Adapted from Soper DE: Am J Obstet Gynecol 1991; 164:1370–1376.
†LGTI = lower genital tract infection; MPC = mucopurulent endocervicitis; ESR = erythrocyte sedimentation rate; GND = gram-negative diplococci; CRP = C-reactive protein; GC = Neisseria gonorrhoeae.

this simple test can be used to exclude the possibility of PID in women with abdominal pain. In other words, women with PID almost always have leukorrhea, but women with leukorrhea do not necessarily have PID. In a separate analysis of Westrom's data, purulent vaginal discharge, an elevated erythrocyte sedimentation rate, positive culture for N. gonorrhoeae, adnexal swelling on bimanual examination, and a temperature greater than 38°C were good predictors of laparoscopically confirmed salpingitis.[39]

Hager et al.[40] published similar guidelines suggesting that clinicians rely on three major clinical signs and at least one of five supportive parameters. Their guidelines eliminate the necessity for a chief complaint of abdominal pain, an important improvement if we accept the possibility that many patients with atypical PID may not have abdominal pain. However, they diminish the importance of assessing the patient's vaginal secretions, although a Gram stain of the endocervix revealing gram-negative diplococci is an adjunctive criterion. As Hager et al. point out, it is important to use criteria that will not exclude patients with mild disease. Recently, a comprehensive analysis of symptoms, physical signs, laboratory data, and combinations of these indicators failed to reveal an algorithm that would reliably predict PID.[41] In light of these findings, adnexal tenderness or cervical motion tenderness was felt to be sufficient to allow a diagnosis of mild PID. For women with a more serious degree of clinical illness, additional evaluation including invasive tests such as endometrial biopsy and laparoscopy was recommended.

The goal for the diagnosis of PID is to establish diagnostic guidelines sufficiently sensitive to avoid missing mild cases but sufficiently specific to avoid antibiotic therapy in women with no infection. Since symptoms are what bring the patient to the physician, the first step is to define symptoms that are potential indicators of upper genital tract infection. As has already been mentioned, any number of genital tract symptoms may be indicators of PID, and none have sufficient specificity to warrant a diagnosis of PID on historical grounds alone. However, the diagnosis of PID should be considered for all patients with any genitourinary symptoms. These symptoms include but are not limited to lower abdominal pain, excessive vaginal discharge, menorrhagia, metrorrhagia, fever/chills, and urinary symptoms. In addition, if the physical findings suggested in Table 2 are noted, a diagnosis of PID may be made even in an asymptomatic woman.

The next crucial step is an evaluation of the lower genital tract secretions, both vaginal and endocervical. The vaginal secretions should be evaluated for the presence of increased numbers of polymorphonuclear leukocytes (leukorrhea) and for the composite clinical criteria (including clue cells) contributing to a diagnosis of BV. The endocervix should be evaluated for the presence of mucopurulent endocervicitis (MPC). Endocervicitis is characterized by a mucopurulent (green or yellow) endocervical discharge and an endocervix that is erythematous, edematous, and friable. Tests from the endocervix for the detection of N. gonorrhoeae and C. trachomatis should be conducted. A bimanual pelvic examination should then be performed and any uterine, adnexal, or cervical motion tenderness noted. Management of the patient can then be based on findings of the above evaluation.

Women without pelvic organ tenderness and no evidence of MPC or BV need not be treated with antibiotics unless the history suggests the need for epidemiologic therapy (exposure to a known gonorrhea or chlamydia carrier). Women with pelvic organ tenderness and no evidence of MPC or BV should have other diagnoses considered such as a ruptured ovarian cyst, mittelschmerz, or other lower abdominal disorders. These women should not require antibiotic treatment. Women with pelvic organ tenderness, no evidence of lower genital tract inflammation (i.e., no leukorrhea or MPC), and evidence of BV should be treated systemically for BV (metronidazole, 500 mg orally twice daily for 7 days). Women with pelvic organ tenderness and evidence of MPC should be started on antibiotic therapy for a presumed diagnosis of PID. Blood for a complete blood count and C-reactive protein should be drawn, but the results need only be used retrospectively to support the presumptive diagnosis. Positive tests for gonorrhea and/or chlamydia will reveal which women with no evidence of lower genital tract inflammation, who therefore were not started on antimicrobial therapy for gonorrhea or chlamydia, should be treated for these endocervical infections.

These recommendations are an attempt to provide a rationale for instituting antimicrobial therapy in women with or at risk for PID. These guidelines provide a "low threshold for diagnosis" of PID but do not allow indiscriminate use of antibiotic treatment for any woman with lower abdominal pain or pelvic organ tenderness. Note that women without evidence of lower genital tract inflammation (leukorrhea or MPC) are not considered to have PID. However, because of the association of BV microorganisms with PID, systemic treatment with metronidazole is indicated in women with BV and pelvic organ tenderness.[21]

ENDOMETRIAL BIOPSY

Endometritis is commonly associated with salpingitis.[42-44] Endometrial biopsy and subsequent histologic confirmation of acute or chronic endometritis confirms the diagnosis of PID. The procedure is technically uncomplicated and can be performed by all primary care physicians. Although not imperative in the evaluation of a woman with suspected PID, biopsy allows the clinician to objectively evaluate the upper genital tract for inflammation but stops short of requiring general anesthesia and laparoscopy. When performed with the Pipelle endometrial suction curette, only minor discomfort is experienced by the patient.

ULTRASOUND

Endovaginal sonography has been shown to correlate well with laparoscopic findings of patients with severe PID. Sonographic findings will be only minimal, however, in women with mild salpingitis,[45] thus limiting its usefulness in evaluating women with atypical or mild symptoms. For the most part, sonographic findings in women with PID are not specific enough to add to the overall diagnosis of a patient with suspected PID. There may be some utility in the use of ultrasound for the evaluation of women with TOA formation. Sonographic evaluation can objectively measure abscess diameters and can therefore be used to monitor the decreasing size of TOAs during the course of antimicrobial therapy. In addition, in women too tender to allow adequate assessment of the adnexa during bimanual pelvic examination, ultrasound may allow detection of adnexal complexes suggestive of TOAs.

LAPAROSCOPY

Laparoscopy remains the gold standard for the diagnosis and grading of acute salpingitis. The minimum criteria for the visual confirmation of acute salpingitis include (1) pronounced hyperemia of the tubal surface, (2) edema of the tubal wall, and (3) a sticky exudate on the tubal surface and from the fimbriated ends when patent.[37] In some cases erythema and edema can be overinterpreted because of observer bias.[46] Because visual confirmation of salpingitis without the presence of exudate may be erroneous (false positive), evaluation of the peritoneal exudate to document the presence of inflammatory cells is suggested. Peritoneal fluid in normal patients and in those with endometriosis will contain predominantly macrophages. Peritoneal fluid cytologic examinations in patients with acute salpingitis will inevitably reveal a predominance of neutrophils. The value of histologic evaluation of minute fimbrial biopsy specimens to pathologically confirm the visual diagnosis of salpingitis has yet to be defined. However, Sellors et al.[46] have demonstrated the importance of minute fimbrial biopsy as an additional objective parameter in preventing both a false positive and false negative laparoscopic diagnosis of salpingitis. Most important, patients who do not meet the minimum criteria for visual confirmation of salpingitis may actually have subclinical disease, possibly because of an endosalpingitis. Minute fimbrial biopsy may play a role in defining this subset of women with visually mild salpingitis. Moreover, it is imperative to perform an endometrial biopsy during the performance of diagnostic laparoscopy to add objective evidence of upper genital tract inflammation.

The severity of clinical disease is unrelated to laparoscopic findings.[7, 47] Women with indolent symptoms who therefore delay seeking health care tend to have more severe tubal abnormalities noted at laparoscopy than their benign clinical symptoms would suggest.[8] Interestingly, at the Medical College of Virginia, patients admitted with four-quadrant rebound and significant temperature elevation are more likely to have a laparoscopically mild salpingitis than a ruptured TOA.

TUBO-OVARIAN ABSCESS

The diagnosis of TOA is made when bimanual pelvic examination reveals a palpable adnexal mass in a patient with the clinical diagnosis of PID. Further characterization of this mass can be undertaken with endovaginal sonography. In addition, some patients are too tender to allow adequate evaluation of the adnexa when admitted to the hospital. Sonography can help determine the presence of inflammatory complexes in these patients.

TREATMENT

Treatment of patients with PID encompasses more than just prescribing the appropriate antimicrobial regimen. Patient education, management of sexual partners, determining the need for hospitalization, and exercising careful follow-up are key treatment issues.

Before choosing an antibiotic regimen, a decision as to the advisability of hospitalization is required. It is unknown whether parenteral regimens are superior to oral regimens for the treatment of PID. However, the high cost of in-hospital treatment prevents routine hospitalization of all patients with the diagnosis of PID. A particular patient's need for hospitalization can be based on the severity of clinical illness, likelihood of compliance with an outpatient regimen, suspected anaerobic infection, and certainty of the diagnosis (Table 3).

Bed rest and avoidance of sexual intercourse during therapy are an integral part of the treatment of PID. Bed rest in the semi-Fowler position allows purulent material to pool in the cul-de-sac and promotes patient comfort. Sexual abstinence should continue until all signs and symptoms of PID have resolved and until male sexual partners have completed treatment.

The male sexual partners of women with PID should be tested for *N. gonorrhoeae* and *C. trachomatis* and treated empirically with ceftriaxone,

TABLE 3.

Indications for Hospitalization in Pelvic Inflammatory Disease*

Compliance with outpatient regimen
  Addicts
  Adolescents
  Nausea/vomiting precludes oral therapy
Severe clinical disease
  Temperature >101° F
  White blood cell count >15,000/mm^3
  Upper peritoneal signs
  Septic shock
Suspected anaerobic infection
  History of intrauterine instrumentation
  IUD use
  Suspected pelvic or tubo-ovarian abscess
Uncertain diagnosis
  Failure to respond to outpatient treatment
  Pregnancy and PID (rule out ectopic pregnancy)
  Rule out appendicitis

*From Soper DE: Treatment, in Berger GS, Westrom L (eds): *Pelvic Inflammatory Disease.* New York, Raven Press, 1992. Used by permission.

250 mg intramuscularly, and doxycycline, 100 mg orally every 12 hours for 7 days. Over half of male sexual partners of women with gonococcal PID will have cultures positive for N. *gonorrhoeae* even though many are asymptomatic.[58, 59] Chlamydial infection has also been found in approximately one third of male sexual partners of women with PID.[60] In women with PID in whom neither N. *gonorrhoeae* or C. *trachomatis* is cultured, testing the male sexual partner may disclose a sexually transmitted cause for the episode of acute salpingitis.

MEDICAL TREATMENT

Patients with severe clinical disease require hospitalization to monitor early response to therapy and to rule out the possibility of a rupturing TOA. These patients generally have high white blood cell counts (>15,000/mm^3), significant fever (>101°F), and/or upper peritoneal signs. Patients with significant nausea and vomiting that precludes oral therapy will also require admission for parenteral antimicrobial therapy. Concerns about compliance with oral antibiotic regimens may make the hospitalization of adolescents and addicts appropriate.[48] Patients with a history of intrauterine surgery or IUD use or patients who have a pelvic mass during bimanual pelvic examination should be admitted for treatment with inpatient antimicrobial regimens that more effectively cover anaerobic bacteria. Patients with an uncertain diagnosis may also warrant admission for observation and possible diagnostic laparoscopy. Laparoscopy is particularly recommended for women with a history of recurrent outpatient-treated PID; their symptoms may have an alternative etiology such as endometriosis. An alternative etiology is also the rule for most women failing to respond to outpatient antibiotic treatment. Patients with a positive pregnancy test and a diagnosis of PID should undergo laparoscopy to rule out the possibility of ectopic pregnancy.

Treatment is based on a consensus that PID is polymicrobial in cause, and the two currently recommended antimicrobial inpatient regimens are broad spectrum in coverage (Table 4).[49, 50] Treatment must usually be initiated before the microbial cause is established, and treatment is usually empirical. The first regimen is a combination of cefoxitin and doxycycline. Cefoxitin was selected for coverage of N. gonorrhoeae, the Enterobacteriaceae, and anaerobes. Doxycycline was chosen primarily to cover C. trachomatis. The second regimen is a combination of clindamycin and gentamicin. Clindamycin was selected to cover anaerobes and gram-

---

TABLE 4.
Centers for Disease Control Guidelines for Treatment of Pelvic Inflammatory Disease*

Outpatient treatment
    Cefoxitin, 2 g IM, plus probenedid, 1 g orally concurrently, or
        ceftriaxone, 250 mg IM, or equivalent cephalosporin
plus
    Doxycycline, 100 mg orally 2 times daily for 10–14 days
or
    Tetracycline, 500 mg orally 4 times daily for 10–14 days
    (The alternative for patients not tolerating doxycycline is
        erythromycin, 500 mg orally 4 times daily for 10–14 days)

Inpatient treatment†
    Regimen A
        Cefoxitin, 2 g IV every 6 hr
or
        Cefotetan,‡ 2 g IV every 12 hr
plus
        Doxycycline, 100 mg every 12 hr orally or IV§
    Regimen B
        Clindamycin, 900 mg IV every 8 hr
plus
        Gentamicin loading dose, IV or IM (2 mg/kg), followed by a
            maintenance dose (1.5 mg/kg) every 8 hr

---

*From Centers for Disease Control: MMWR 1991; 40:1–25.
†One of the regimens is given for at least 48 hours after the patient clinically improves.
‡Other cephalosporins such as ceftizoxime, cefotaxime, and ceftriaxone, which provide adequate gonococcal, other facultative gram-negative aerobic, and anaerobic coverage, may be used in appropriate doses.
§After discharge from the hospital, continue doxycyline, 100 mg two times daily to a total of 10 to 14 days.

positive aerobes. Gentamicin was chosen to cover gram-negative aerobes, including N. gonorrhoeae. This second regimen is thought to be potentially more useful than the first for patients with pelvic abscesses but provides less coverage for C. trachomatis.

The two recommended inpatient regimens have been studied extensively (over 1,000 patients studied), and these studies strongly suggest that both regimens are clinically effective. A recent study suggests that extended-spectrum antibiotic regimens, including single-agent broad-spectrum antibiotics such as cefoxitin in conjunction with doxycycline, have efficacy that is equivalent to that of clindamycin-containing regimens for the treatment of TOA.[51] In addition, more than 75% of patients with TOAs will respond to antibiotic treatment alone and will not require surgical intervention.

Data regarding the treatment of PID in an outpatient setting are limited, and the microbial etiology of PID seen in this setting is not well established. It is assumed that the etiology mirrors the bacterial pathogenesis seen in the clinically severe cases of PID that require hospitalization. The regimen of a β-lactam antibiotic with doxycycline has been used extensively in the treatment of outpatient PID since its recommendation in 1984. A recent study revealed rather poor coverage by doxycycline of facultative bacteria and anaerobic microorganisms isolated from women with PID.[55] In addition, a single dose of a β-lactam antibiotic should not be sufficient to treat a significant anaerobic soft tissue infection. Despite this, clinical efficacy varies from 81% to 94%.[49, 56, 57] Limited study of the quinolone ofloxacin suggests that this agent may be useful in the treatment of women with PID in an outpatient setting.[52]

A number of regimens other than the two discussed appear to have promise for the treatment of PID. Penicillins with β-lactamase inhibitors (ampicillin-sulbactam, ticarcillin-clavulanate, amoxicillin-clavulanate) appear to be effective in the treatment of PID, but use of these agents in treating those infections attributable to C. trachomatis remains in question. Quinolones such as ofloxacin have in vitro activity against some facultative gram-positive cocci, gram-negative organisms including N. gonorrhoeae, and C. trachomatis. They have limited anaerobic activity, however. Quinolones appear to be effective in the treatment of salpingitis not complicated by TOA.[7, 52]

Antibiotic therapy should be continued to complete a 10- to 14-day course. Patients should be followed for criteria indicative of a therapeutic response, including lysis of fever, normalization of the white blood cell count, total disappearance of rebound tenderness, and marked amelioration of pelvic organ tenderness. Although a prompt response is common in women with even severe clinical manifestations of PID, patients with laparoscopically severe disease and/or TOAs tend to require a longer duration of hospitalization. Patients failing to show a response to antimicrobial treatment within 96 hours should be reevaluated with respect to both the accuracy of diagnosis and the possibility of the presence of a TOA that may require surgical intervention. In some cases, percutaneous drainage of TOAs can be effected under computed tomographic (CT) scan or sonographic guidance, thus obviating the need for surgical intervention.[53]

SURGICAL TREATMENT

The initial surgical approach usually involves laparoscopy to confirm the diagnosis and establish disease severity. Laparoscopy is particularly helpful in ruling out the possibility of acute appendicitis. Patients with severe disease may benefit from operative endoscopy to lyse adhesions, aspirate pyosalpinx, dissect and drain loculations of pus, and irrigate the pelvic and abdominal cavities.[54] Laparotomy is recommended in cases of generalized peritonitis associated with signs of sepsis from a suspected ruptured TOA or in case of severe PID refractory to medical therapy. A great deal of judgment must be used to determine the extent of extirpative surgery necessary to cure the patient. In patients who want to preserve fertility, unilateral adnexectomy may be elected if the disease is predominantly one-sided. In some cases, bilateral salpingectomy or bilateral salpingo-oophorectomy may be necessary. Patients without adnexa may still be able to conceive with the help of in vitro fertilization and ovum donation as long as the uterus remains. Total abdominal hysterectomy with bilateral salpingo-oophorectomy continues to be the procedure of choice for severe PID refractory to medical therapy in women not desiring to become pregnant.

LONG-TERM SEQUELAE

It is well known that the reproductive sequelae of TFI and ectopic pregnancy are common consequences of PID. Tubal factor infertility was shown to be related to the severity of salpingitis and to the number of episodes of PID in a longitudinal study of over 1,800 women.[61] For patients with only one episode of PID, the incidence of proven TFI increases significantly with the severity of the infection as visually judged at the time of the index laparoscopy. The rate of TFI was 0.6% after a case of mild salpingitis, 6.2% after a case of moderate salpingitis, and 21.4% after severe salpingitis. Each repeated episode of PID roughly doubled the rate of TFI. Overall, after one, two, and three or more episodes, the rates were 8.0%, 19.5%, and 40.0%, respectively.

Damage to the fallopian tubes after PID is a well-documented etiologic risk for tubal pregnancy. Westrom et al.[61] confirmed this in his earlier population study and noted that when compared with controls, the rate of ectopic pregnancy was increased by almost a factor of 4 in women with a visually documented case of salpingitis. Such an increased risk applied even after an eventual intrauterine pregnancy.[62]

In a retrospective study, Safrin et al.[63] noted that 24% of women with PID had pelvic pain for 6 months or more after hospitalization. This confirms earlier work by Westrom[64] in which he reported an 18% incidence of chronic pelvic pain following an episode of PID. Patients may also complain of longer and more painful menstruation and pain during sexual intercourse.[65]

PREVENTION

Prevention options for PID can be identified for the individual, the health care provider, and the community and can be categorized as primary, secondary, or tertiary prevention.[66] Primary prevention focuses on avoiding either exposure to STDs or acquisition of infection following exposure. Secondary prevention involves keeping the lower genital tract infection from ascending and limiting further sexual transmission. Tertiary prevention attempts to minimize sequelae such as tubal damage once ascending infection occurs.

Prevention strategies for individuals involve healthy sexual behavior. Healthy sexual behavior can be characterized as postponing one's sexual debut, choosing uninfected sex partners, and limiting the number of sex partners. Mechanical and chemical barriers can be used for personal prophylaxis against acquiring an STD and therefore PID. Oral contraceptive use apparently protects women from acquiring symptomatic PID and is also associated with laparoscopically milder disease in those women in whom PID develops.[61, 67, 68] Increasing symptom awareness in women may lead to prompt detection and early treatment of chlamydial and gonococcal infection for themselves and their partners.

Prevention strategies for health care providers include increasing the amount of clinical training in STD. This will lead to appropriate screening of high-risk individuals as well as improved recognition and treatment of clinically recognizable infections. Aggressive identification and treatment of women infected with N. gonorrhoeae and/or C. trachomatis and/or BV should greatly reduce the risk for development of PID. Counseling to reduce future STD risk is an important adjunct when treating any STD.

Communities also bear a responsibility in the fight to control STDs and consequent PID. Health promotion and education are an integral part of STD intervention activities, and patients need to be guaranteed access to medical care. The final common pathway for preventing both lower and upper genital tract infections is through effective clinical STD services, including laboratory support.

Most of these prevention options are primary. However, prompt identification and appropriate treatment of women with STDs can prevent PID.[69] In addition, prompt treatment of women with PID seems to arrest what visible evidence of tubal damage is present at the time the diagnosis is laparoscopically confirmed.[7]

SUMMARY

Pelvic inflammatory disease continues to be a cause of significant morbidity in reproductive age group women. The microbial pathogenesis of this disease is predominately related to the sexually transmitted bacteria Neisseria gonorrhoeae and Chlamydia trachomatis. Bacterial vaginosis and "BV microorganisms" are also involved in the pathogenesis of PID. Less commonly, respiratory pathogens such as Haemophilus influenzae cause PID. The diagnosis is based upon the recognition of clinical signs of genital tract inflammation in women with any genitourinary complaint, not necessarily including pelvic pain. Outpatient antimicrobial therapy is acceptable therapy for women with mild clinical disease, while more severely ill patients require admission and parenteral antibiotics. Adjunctive measures include the contact tracing of sexual partners and patient education regarding to the sexually transmitted nature of this infection. Aggressive screening and treatment of uncomplicated lower genital tract gonococcal and/or chlamydial infection can decrease the development of PID.

REFERENCES

1. Aral SO, Mosher WD, Cates W: Self-reported pelvic inflammatory disease in the United States, 1988. *JAMA* 1991; 266:2570–2573.
2. Wolner-Hanssen PW, Kiviat NB, Holmes KK: Atypical pelvic inflammatory disease: Subacute, chronic, or subclinical upper genital tract infection in women, in Holmes KK, Mardh P-A, Sparling PF, et al (eds): *Sexually Transmitted Diseases*, ed 2. New York, McGraw-Hill, 1990, pp 615–620.
3. Washington AE, Katz P: Cost of and payment source for pelvic inflammatory disease. Trends and projections, 1983 through 2000. *JAMA* 1991; 266:2565–2569.
4. Rolfs RT, Galaid EI, Zaidi AA: Pelvic inflammatory disease: Trends in hospitalizations and office visits, 1979 through 1988. *Am J Obstet Gynecol* 1992; 166:983–990.
5. Centers for Disease Control: Summary of notifiable diseases, United States 1991. *MMWR* 1991; 40:24.
6. Wasserheit JN, Bell TA, Kiviat NB, et al: Microbial causes of proven pelvic inflammatory disease and efficacy of clindamycin and tobramycin. *Ann Intern Med* 1986; 104:187–193.
7. Soper DE, Brockwell NJ, Dalton HP: Microbial etiology of urban emergency department acute salpingitis: Treatment with ofloxacin. *Am J Obstet Gynecol* 1992; 167:653–660.
8. Svennson L, Westrom L, Ripa KT, et al: Differences in some clinical and laboratory parameters in acute salpingitis related to culture and serologic findings. *Am J Obstet Gynecol* 1980; 138:1017–1021.
9. Washington AE, Aral SO, Wolner-Hanssen P, et al: Assessing risk for pelvic inflammatory disease and its sequelae. *JAMA* 1991; 266:2581–2586.
10. Eschenbach DA, Buchanan TM, Pollock HM, et al: Polymicrobial etiology of acute pelvic inflammatory disease. *N Engl J Med* 1975; 293:166–171.
11. Cunningham FG, Hauth JC, Gilstrap LC, et al: The bacterial pathogenesis of acute pelvic inflammatory disease. *Obstet Gynecol* 1978; 52:161–164.
12. Chow WC, Malkasian KL, Marshall JR, et al: The bacteriology of acute pelvic inflammatory disease: Value of cul-de-sac cultures and relative importance of gonococci and other aerobic and anaerobic bacteria. *Am J Obstet Gynecol* 1975; 122:876–879.
13. Monif GRG, Welkos SL, Baer H, et al: Cul-de-sac isolates from patients with endometritis-salpingitis-peritonitis and gonococcal endocervicitis. *Am J Obstet Gynecol* 1976; 126:158–161.
14. Sweet RL, Draper DL, Schachter J, et al: Microbiology and pathogenesis of acute salpingitis as determined by laparoscopy: What is the appropriate site to sample? *Am J Obstet Gynecol* 1980; 138:985–989.
15. Soper DE, Brockwell NJ, Dalton HP: False-positive cultures of the cul-de-sac associated with culdocentesis in patients undergoing elective laparoscopy. *Obstet Gynecol* 1991; 77:134–138.
16. Sweet RL, Draper DL, Hadley WK: Etiology of acute salpingitis: Influence of episode number and duration of symptoms. *Obstet Gynecol* 1981; 58:62–68.
17. Brunham RC, Binns B, Guijon F, et al: Etiology and outcome of acute pelvic inflammatory disease. *J Infect Dis* 1988; 158:510–517.

18. Mardh P-A, Moller BR, Paavonen J: Chlamydial infection of the female genital tract with emphasis on pelvic inflammatory disease: A review of Scandinavian studies. *Sex Transm Dis* 1981; 8:140–155.

19. Teisala K, Heinonen PK, Punnonen R: Laparoscopic diagnosis and treatment of acute pyosalpinx. *J Reprod Med* 1990; 35:19–21.

20. McGee ZA, Pavia AT: Is the concept, "agents of sexually transmitted disease" still valid (editorial)? *Sex Transm Dis* 1991; 18:69–71.

21. Eschenbach DA, Hillier S, Critchlow C, et al: Diagnosis and clinical manifestations of bacterial vaginosis. *Am J Obstet Gynecol* 1988; 158:819–828.

22. Hillier SL, Kiviat NB, Critchlow C, et al: Bacterial vaginosis (BV)-associated bacteria as etiologic agents of pelvic inflammatory disease (abstract). Presented at the Annual Meeting of the Infectious Disease Society for Obstetrics and Gyecology, San Diego, 1992.

23. Chow AW, Carlson C, Sorrell TC: Host defenses in acute pelvic inflammatory disease. I. Bacterial clearance in the murine uterus and oviduct. *Am J Obstet Gynecol* 1980; 138:1003.

24. Ogra PL, Yamanaka T, Losonsky GA: Local immunologic defenses in the genital tract, in Barber HK (ed): *Reproductive Immunology*. New York, Alan R Liss, 1981, pp 381–394.

25. Keith LG, Berger GS, Edelman DA, et al: On the causation of pelvic inflammatory disease. *Am J Obstet Gynecol* 1984; 149:215–224.

26. Soper DE: Diagnosis and laparoscopic grading of acute salpingitis. *Am J Obstet Gynecol* 1991; 164:1370–1376.

27. Paavonen J, Kiviat NG, Brunham RC, et al: Prevalence and manifestations of endometritis among women with cervicitis. *Am J Obstet Gynecol* 1985; 152:280–286.

28. Landers DV, Sweet RL: Current trends in the diagnosis and treatment of tuboovarian abscess. *Am J Obstet Gynecol* 1985; 151:1098.

29. Lopez-Zeno JA, Keith LG, Berger GS: The Fitz-Hugh–Curtis syndrome revisited. Changing perspectives after half a century. *J Reprod Med* 1985; 30:567–582.

30. Sellors JW, Mahony JB, Chernesky MA, et al: Tubal factor infertility: An association with prior chlamydial infection and asymptomatic salpingitis. *Fertil Steril* 1988; 49:451–457.

31. Tjiam KH, Zeilmaker GH, Alberda AT, et al: Prevalence of antibodies to *Chlamydia trachomatis*, *Neisseria gonorrhoeae*, and *Mycoplasma hominis* in infertile women. *Genitourin Med* 1985; 61:175–178.

32. Patton DL, Moore DE, Spadoni LR, et al: A comparison of the fallopian tube's response to overt and silent salpingitis. *Obstet Gynecol* 1989; 73:622–630.

33. Curran JW, Rendtorff RC, Chandler RW, et al: Female gonorrhea: Its relation to abnormal uterine bleeding, urinary tract symptoms, and cervicitis. *Obstet Gynecol* 1975; 45:195–198.

34. Wolner-Hanssen P, Kiviat NB, Holmes KK: Atypical pelvic inflammatory disease: Subacute, chronic, or subclinical upper genital tract infection in women, in Holmes KK, et al (eds): *Sexually Transmitted Diseases*. New York, McGraw-Hill, 1990.

35. Jones RB, Mammel JB, Shepard MK, et al: Recovery of *Chlamydia trachomatis* from the endometrium of women at risk for chlamydial infection. *Am J Obstet Gynecol* 1986; 155:35–39.

36. Cleary RE, Jones RB: Recovery of *Chlamydia trachomatis* from the endometrium in infertile women with serum antichlamydial antibodies. *Fertil Steril* 1985; 44:233–235.

37. Jacobson L, Westrom L: Objectivized diagnosis of acute pelvic inflammatory disease: Diagnostic and prognostic value of routine laparoscopy. *Am J Obstet Gynecol* 1969; 105:1088–1098.

38. Westrom L: Diagnosis and treatment of salpingitis. *J Reprod Med* 1983; 28:703–708.

39. Hadgu AH, Westrom L, Brooks CA, et al: Predicting acute pelvic inflammatory disease: A multivariate analysis. *Am J Obstet Gynecol* 1986; 155:954–960.

40. Hager WD, Eschenbach DA, Spence MR, et al: Criteria for the diagnosis and grading of salpingitis. *Obstet Gynecol* 1983; 72:7–12.

41. Kahn JG, Walker CG, Washington AE, et al: Diagnosing pelvic inflammatory disease. A comprehensive analysis and considerations for developing a model. *JAMA* 1991; 266:2594–2604.

42. Paavonen J, Aine R, Teisala K, et al: Comparison of endometrial biopsy and peritoneal fluid cytologic testing with laparoscopy in the diagnosis of acute pelvic inflammatory disease. *Am J Obstet Gynecol* 1985; 151:645–650.

43. Kiviat NB, Wolner-Hanssen P, Eschenbach DA, et al: Endometrial histopathology in patients with culture-proved upper genital tract infection and laparoscopically diagnosed acute salpingitis. *Am J Surg Pathol* 1990; 14:167–175.

44. Sellors J, Mahony J, Goldsmith C, et al: Accuracy of clinical findings and laparoscopy for pelvic inflammatory disease. *Am J Obstet Gynecol* 1991; 164:113–120.

45. Patten RM, Vincent LM, Wolner-Hanssen P, et al: Pelvic inflammatory disease. Endovaginal sonography with laparoscopic correlation. *J Ultrasound Med* 1990; 9:681–689.

46. Sellors J, Mahony J, Goldsmith C, et al: The accuracy of clinical findings and laparoscopy for pelvic inflammatory disease. *Am J Obstet Gynecol* 1991; 164:113–120.

47. Livengood CH, Hill GB, Addison WA: Pelvic inflammatory disease: Findings during inpatient treatment of clinically severe, laparoscopy-documented disease. *Am J Obstet Gynecol* 1992; 166:519–524.

48. Katz BP, Zwickl BW, Caine VA, et al: Compliance with antibiotic therapy for *Chlamydia trachomatis* and *Neisseria gonorrhoeae*. *Sex Transm Dis* 1992; 19:351–354.

49. Peterson HB, Walker CK, Kahn JG, et al: Pelvic inflammatory disease. Key treatment issues and options. *JAMA* 1991; 266:2605–2611.

50. Centers for Disease Control: Pelvic inflammatory disease: Guidelines for prevention and management. *MMWR* 1991; 40:1–25.

51. Reed SD, Landers DV, Sweet RL: Antibiotic treatment of tuboovarian abscess: Comparison of broad-spectrum β-lactam agents versus clindamycin-containing regimens. *Am J Obstet Gynecol* 1991; 164:1556–1562.

52. Wendel GC, Cox SM, Bawdon RE, et al: A randomized trial of ofloxacin versus cefoxitin and doxycycline in the outpatient treatment of acute salpingitis. *Am J Obstet Gynecol* 1991; 164:1390–1396.

53. Casola G, vanSonnenberg E, D'Agostino HB, et al: Percutaneous drainage of tubo-ovarian abscesses. *Radiology* 1992; 182:399–402.

54. Reich H: Laparoscopic treatment of tuboovarian and pelvic abscess. *J Reprod Med* 1987; 32:747.

55. Hasselquist MB, Hillier S: Susceptibility of upper genital tract isolates from women with pelvic inflammatory disease to ampicillin, cefotaxime, metronidazole, and doxycycline. *Sex Transm Dis* 1991; 18:146–149.

56. Brunham RC: Therapy for acute pelvic inflammatory disease: A critique of recent treatment trials. *Am J Obstet Gynecol* 1984; 148:235–240.

57. Soper DE: Treatment, in Berger GS, Westrom L (eds): *Pelvic Inflammatory Disease*. New York, Raven Press, 1992.

58. Gilstrap LC, Herbert WNP, Cunningham FG, et al: Gonorrhea screening in the male consorts of women with pelvic infection. *JAMA* 1977; 238:965–966.

59. Potterat JJ, Phillips L, Rothenberg RB, et al: Gonococcal pelvic inflamma-

tory disease: Case-finding observations. *Am J Obstet Gynecol* 1980; 138: 1101–1104.

60. Moss TR, Hawkswell J: Evidence of infection with *Chlamydia trachomatis* in patients with pelvic inflammatory disease: Value of partner investigation. *Fertil Steril* 1986; 45:429–430.

61. Westrom L, Joesoef R, Reynolds B, et al: Pelvic inflammatory disease and fertility. A cohort study of 1,844 women with laparoscopically verified disease and 657 control women with normal laparoscopic results. *Sex Transm Dis* 1992; 19:185–192.

62. Joesoef R, Reynolds G, Westrom L, et al: Recurrence of ectopic pregnancy: The role of salpingitis. *Am J Obstet Gynecol* 1991; 165:46–50.

63. Safrin S, Schachter J, Dahrouge D, et al: Long-term sequelae of acute pelvic inflammatory disease. A retrospective cohort study. *Am J Obstet Gynecol* 1992; 166:1300–1305.

64. Westrom L: Pelvic inflammatory disease: Bacteriology and sequelae. *Contraception* 1987; 36:111–128.

65. Adlet MW, Belsey EH, O'Connor BH: Morbidity associated with pelvic inflammatory disease. *Br J Vener Dis* 1982; 58:151–157.

66. Washington AE, Cates W, Wasserheit JN: Preventing pelvic inflammatory disease. *JAMA* 1991; 266:2574–2580.

67. Svensson L, Westrom L, Mardh P-A: Contraceptives and acute salpingitis. *JAMA* 1984; 251:2553–2555.

68. Wolner-Hanssen P: Oral contraceptive use modifies the manifestations of pelvic inflammatory disease. *Br J Obstet Gynaecol* 1986; 93:619–624.

69. Stamm WE, Guinan ME, Johnson C, et al: Effect of treatment regimens for *Neisseria gonorrhoeae* on simultaneous infection with *Chlamydia trachomatis*. *N Engl J Med* 1984; 310:545–551.

Editor's Comment

Dr. Soper provides a current description of the significance of pelvic inflammatory disease. The discussion on the microbiology of PID is presented in a logical manner and positions the bacteria properly with regard to frequency of involvement. However, the discussion of the association between bacterial vaginosis and pelvic inflammatory disease might lead the reader to conclude there is a cause and effect. The reader should be reminded that bacterial vaginosis has not been shown to be a cause of PID.

An excellent point is made in the discussion of the significance of obtaining an endometrial biopsy. Since there is good correlation between endometritis and PID, the endometrial biopsy provides an easy method to diagnose PID. This is more valid than a culdocentesis and is less invasive, as well as less costly, than laparoscopy. However, the latter provides the physician and patient with information on tubal damage, and perhaps a prognosis.

Dr. Soper relates that PID and its sequelae results in costs that will soon exceed 3 billion dollars. This is due to the fact that early signs of PID are unrecognized because cervicitis is usually asymptomatic. Signs of cervicitis are endocervical hypertrophy, bleeding that occurs when the endocervix is gently touched with a cotton-tipped applicator, or bleeding following sexual intercourse. Recognition of cervicitis, appropriate treatment, follow-up, and education can have a significant impact on the incidence of PID. Specifically, early recognition and appropriate treatment can result in a reduction of PID and its sequelae.

Sebastian Faro, M.D., Ph.D.

Urinary Incontinence—
Untying the Gordian Knot

THOMAS E. SNYDER, M.D.

U rinary incontinence is one of the great paradoxes of modern gynecology, especially stress urinary incontinence. Why should a problem so superficially simple as loss of urine with coughing or sneezing
generate such an inordinate volume of contradictory, confusing, and un-
intelligible literature?

The material regarding incontinence epitomizes the axiom that "the
less understood, the more written." Few subjects in our specialty have
been addressed for so long and have resulted in so much contradictory
information, so little agreement on issues such as anatomy, and so many
surgical approaches, all claiming to be highly successful. The result is
substantial confusion regarding the basic facts of anatomy, physiology,
and surgery.

A recent survey of board-eligible and board-certified gynecologists
currently performing incontinence surgery revealed that few could even
accurately describe genuine stress incontinence as defined by the International Continence Society or by appropriate preoperative studies in the
current literature.[1] Even more significant, few could accurately describe
the rationale for choosing one methodology of repair over another or the
pitfalls of the approach they were using for their patients.

As with the Gordian knot of mythology, the key to understanding is
to slice through the confusing literature with a sword like Alexander's
and to deal in a straightforward fashion with the basic anatomic and
physiologic facts. It is the goal of this chapter to present a comprehen-
sible summary of the current literature regarding our collective understanding of the basic anatomy, physiology, and surgical correction of female incontinence. The current approach used at this institution, derived
from experience of greater than 5,000 cases, will be presented.[2] Decision
making, correct surgical technique, and avoidance of common pitfalls often encountered during attempted repairs will be emphasized.

SCOPE OF THE PROBLEM

Urinary incontinence is defined by the International Continence Society[3]
to be "a condition in which involuntary loss of urine is a social or hy-
gienic problem and is objectively demonstrable." Despite this simple definition, it remains one of the most underrecognized and undertreated of
gynecologic conditions. A National Institutes of Health National Consen-

Advances in Obstetrics and Gynecology, vol 1
© 1994, Mosby–Year Book, Inc.

sus Development Conference was convened in 1988 to address the major issues regarding urinary incontinence. A minimum of 10 million adults in this country are affected. These numbers include 15% to 30% of the community-dwelling elderly, 20% to 25% of whom are severe cases, and greater than 50% of nursing home patients.

Numerous studies are available regarding elderly patients and this problem. Ouslander et al.[4] studied 842 elderly patients in seven nursing homes and found that 72% had at least one episode of incontinence during the day. Fecal incontinence was often associated with urinary incontinence, perhaps secondary to overlap in pathophysiologic mechanics. Decreased mental status, lack of mobility, and a variety of drugs including diuretics, psychotropics, and autonomic agents adversely affect continence. As a result, these patients are treated with catheters, which may cause a variety of complications. Others, including Campbell et al.[5] and Tobin et al.,[6] have recently reviewed the prevalence of incontinence in elderly institutionalized patients and have reported similar findings.

It is difficult to obtain accurate estimates of the prevalence of urinary incontinence in the general population. Only 50% of affected persons outside nursing homes have consulted their physicians. Diokno and colleagues[7] surveyed almost 2,000 community-dwelling older persons in Michigan and found a 37% incidence of incontinence. Brink et al.[8] interviewed 200 women from age 55 to 90. Sixty-nine percent registered severe wetting on a daily basis; many (56%) of these women had experienced the problem for greater than 5 years. Sixty-two percent of those interviewed used protective padding consisting of homemade pads (20%) and commercial menstrual pads (63%).

Incontinence is not limited to the elderly. Holst and Wilson[9] interviewed 851 women 18 years or older in Dunedin, New Zealand. Of this population, 31% admitted to some degree of incontinence, 17% regularly and 5% with some degree of social distress. Fifty-two percent of the sample experienced stress incontinence, 25% urge incontinence, and 22% combined stress/urge ("complex") incontinence. Incontinence was associated with parity and was found to be uncommon in nulliparous women; however, incontinence did not increase with increasing parity in this study. It is a matter of current debate whether increasing parity or pregnancy per se rather than labor[10, 11] or injury to pelvic floor innervation plays a role in incontinence.[12]

Yarnell et al.[13] interviewed 1,000 females aged 18 or older in South Wales. Forty-five percent admitted to incontinence within the last year. Approximately 22% experienced historical stress incontinence, 10% urge incontinence, and 14% complex incontinence. Greater than 3% stated that urinary incontinence interfered with their social or domestic life, but only half had sought medical care (Fig 1).

A staggering estimate of $10.3 billion annually is spent in care products for these individuals. Although knowledge of the problem has increased among professional and laypersons, the consensus conference concluded that therapy remains inadequate because of several factors.

First, incontinence is embarrassing and is often considered a part of aging or the natural consequence of childbirth. Resnick[14] has estimated that fewer than 20% of females will volunteer information regarding in-

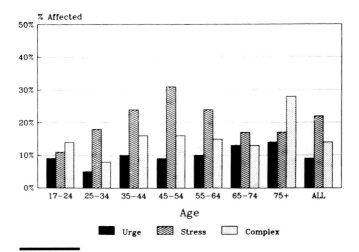

FIGURE 1.

Prevalence of urinary incontinence by type and age. (Adapted from Yarnell JWG, Voyle GJ, Richards CJ, et al: *J Epidemiol Community Health* 1981; 35:71–74.)

continence and that only one third are properly evaluated when they do. In Holst and Wilson's study,[9] reasons given for not seeking help included nonperception as an abnormality, low expectation of benefit, and lack of knowledge of treatment programs (Table 1).

The clinical, psychological, and social impact of urinary incontinence is significant. Wyman et al.[15] interviewed 69 community-dwelling women greater than 55 years old and found that self-perception and daily activities were affected more than social interactions. Activities such as shopping, entertainment, long distance travel, physical recreation, and vacations were most affected, secondary not only to incontinence but also to urgency and frequency. Walters et al.[16] analyzed a group of patients with detrusor instability by using the Minnesota Multiphasic Personality Inventory (MMPI). They found patients with incontinence to be more anxious and depressed than controls. Other studies report that patients with urinary frequency, urgency, and urge incontinence describe somatization, hysteria, depression, anxiety, and abnormal levels of situational life

TABLE 1.

Reasons for Not Obtaining Medical Advice About Incontinence*

Reason	Percentage
Not abnormal	82
No benefit of treatment	10
Self-help exercise	3
Unaware of treatment	2
Incontinence related to other conditions	2
Can't afford M.D.	1

*Adapted from Holst K, Wilson PD: *N Z Med J* 1988; 101:756–758.

stresses.[17, 18] Thiede[19] reviewed multiple problems that may be experienced by those with incontinence (Table 2).

The socioeconomic impact of urinary incontinence is now and will remain directly proportional to the growing number of elderly persons in the population. Based on 1987 dollars, a conservative estimate of the direct costs of incontinence was $7 billion in the community and $3.3 billion in nursing homes.[20] Brazda[21] reported the cost of undergarments for females in institutions alone to be $8 billion. Marked variation in the cost of providing appropriate care was noted by Hu et al.,[22] including the minimum use of basic tests such as urinalysis. In addition, they estimate that greater than $20 million per year could be saved by applying the standard guidelines for treatment of stress and urge incontinence developed by the Agency for Health Care Policy and Research (AHCPR).[23]

ANATOMY

Just as detailed knowledge of intrapelvic anatomy is key to performance of pelvic surgery, knowledge of the anatomy of the space of Retzius, the urethra, bladder, and anterior of the vagina are critical to the performance of incontinence surgery. One might presume that anatomy would be a point of mutual agreement among authors; however, it continues to be an area of great controversy. Is there an intrinsic urethral sphincter? How does it function if it exists? Where is it located? How does it interact with the other anatomic elements to maintain continence? A complete review of the anatomy and physiology of all types of incontinence is beyond the intent of this chapter. Therefore, attention will be directed to the anatomy and physiology pertinent to surgically correctable incontinence, or "genuine stress incontinence."

The earliest anatomic treatises concerning the musculature of the urethra and vaginal wall were by Galen,[24] who described the musculature of the bladder as composed of longitudinal, transverse, and oblique fibers

---

TABLE 2.
Problems of Patients With
Incontinence*

Emotional
Disruption of sexual life
Odor
Interference with household chores
Interference with employment
Inability to perform physical exercise
Increased costs
Dietary restrictions
Limitation of social activities
Discomfort

---

*Adapted from Thiede HA: *Obstet Gynecol
Clin North Am* 1989; 16:709–716.

with a sphincter in the region of the urethal meatus. Spiegel[25] first used the term "detrusor" to refer to the longitudinal muscle of the bladder. As might be expected, many misconceptions were stated as fact; i.e., Cowper[26] believed the bladder to be merely a dilatation of the ureters. Galen first described the concept of a sphincter in the bladder neck; however, Vicary[27] identified the vesical neck as having the ability to retain or release urine. Vasalius[28] first identified the sphincter as a separate muscle, later termed the "sphincter-vesicae internus" by Bell.[29]

Kennedy[30] (1946) described a smooth muscle sphincter of the urethra located in the middle and inner thirds that was associated with the longitudinal smooth muscle coursing the length of the urethra. Von Ludinghausen[31] (1931) described the smooth muscle sphincter of the bladder as two opposing horseshoe arrangements that were able to relax at the same time while the remainder of the bladder contracted. Bonney[32] (1923) stated that the bladder trigone rested on a sheet of smooth muscle and named this layer the "pubocervical sheet," now often termed "pubocervical fascia." However, as Krantz[33] has demonstrated, there is no demonstrable fascial layer in this area.

Descriptions of historical anatomic treatises regarding the urethra and vagina were detailed by Krantz[34] and later reiterated by Ullery.[35]

CONTEMPORARY CONCEPTS

The magnum opus of urethral and anterior vaginal wall anatomy that is still consistent with current physiologic concepts is that of Krantz,[33] and it is the basis for the following descriptions (Fig 2).

The urethra of the adult female varies from 2.5 to 8.0 cm, averaging 3.5 cm, and assumes an angle of 16 degrees from the external to internal meatus measured against the anterior vaginal wall. The external two thirds of the urethra is inseparable from the anterior vaginal wall, and fibers of the vaginal musculature may be easily seen encircling it. However, these fibers are not present in the inner third. The epithelial lining of the lower third is squamous and changes to columnar in the middle and transitional segments like that of the bladder in the upper third.

The arterial supply of the upper third of the urethra is from the bladder by anastomosis. The middle and lower thirds receive blood supply from the interior vesical artery, as do the corresponding portions of the vagina. Venous drainage is via the inferior, middle, and superior vesical veins. The nerve supply is from the hypogastric plexus, which courses with the arterial supply. Lymphatics course to the vestibular plexus, then anteriorly to the inguinal nodes, and posteriorly to (1) the anterior bladder wall and external iliac chain from the anterior superior portion; (2) the lateral bladder wall and subsequently the internal iliacs, hypogastrics, or obturator chain; or (3) posteriorly with the bladder and uterine channels. The musculature of the urethra occupies the most interest in discussion of the anatomy of urinary stress incontinence. The lower two thirds of the urethra and vagina cannot be separated, and one cannot distinguish two separate layers in the upper third—a fact that is readily discovered when attempting anterior vaginal dissection during performance of anterior repair. The so-called "sphincter vaginae" consists of the de-

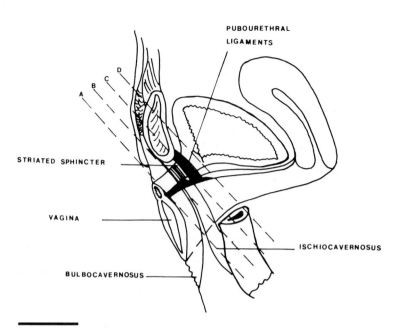

FIGURE 2.

Sagittal view of the relationship of the urethra, bladder, and vagina. Note the lack of a plane of separation between the vagina and lower two thirds of the urethra. The fibers of the striated sphincter are formed by decussating fibers of the bulbo-cavernosus/urethrocavernosus. The pubourethral ligaments arise at the junction of the middle and inner thirds of the urethra.

cussating fibers of the bulbocavernosus as they course over the lower third of the urethra. The main body of the bulbocavernosus lies along the lateral sides of the urethra in the region of the external meatus. The ischio-cavernosus lies more medially and superiorly, with fibers coursing over the urethra in the midline, and is inseparable from the fibers of the bul-bocavernosus. The levator ani lies lateral to the urethra. Its thick fascia prevents muscular decussation from the urethra to its surface (Fig 3).

The urethra of the female is analogous to the prostatic portion of the male urethra. At the junction of the middle and upper thirds of the ure-thra are heavy fibrous bands of tissue from the anterior vaginal wall to the pubic ramus, variously called the puboprostatic (from the analogous structure in the male) or pubourethral ligaments. Zacharin[36] demon-strated that these ligaments are continuous with the suspensory ligament of the clitoris. These structures were recently studied by light electron microscopy and neurohistochemistry in both continent and incontinent females.[37] They were found to consist of dense connective tissue enclos-ing smooth muscle bundles with associated cholinergic autonomic nerve endings. Although there were no observable morphologic differences noted in incontinent and continent subjects, the authors concluded that the pubourethral ligaments play a role in stabilizing the proximal por-tion of the urethra. Similar conclusions were reached in a study by Mil-ley and Nichols.[38]

The mucosa of the urethra is squamous varying to columnar and tran-sitional epithelium as it approaches the bladder and forms many longi-tudinal folds. The periurethral glands dispersed in the longitudinal

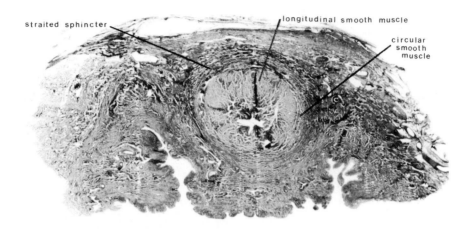

FIGURE 3.

Diagram of a section through B, Figure 2, taken at the junction of the lower and middle thirds of the urethra. Note the inner longitudinal and outer circular smooth muscle and the presence of striated sphincter externally formed by decussation of the bulbocavernosus/ischiocavernosus.

muscle fibers of the urethra, most prominently in the lower third, are simple tubular and are lined by columnar epithelium. Their ducts enter directly into the lumen of the urethra except in the lower third, where they may open externally.

As stated previously, the musculature of the urethra is both smooth and striated in nature. The striated "voluntary sphincter" is composed of the encircling fibers of the bulbocavernosus and ischocavernosus. This sphincter may only voluntarily close, not open. The smooth muscle of the urethra consists of an inner longitudinal layer continuous with the corresponding layer of the bladder. The distribution is asymmetrical, with more bundles anteriorly than laterally and with increasing density close to the bladder. It is postulated that shortening of these fibers is significant in urethral opening during micturition. The circular smooth muscle begins in the lower third and gradually increases in the middle and upper thirds, finally intermingling with the longitudinal fibers as they spiral into the bladder. There are no longitudinal striated muscle fibers along the course of the urethra. Continuous with the fibers of the bulbocavernosus and ischocavernosus in the lower third, striated fibers gradually encircle the middle third of the urethra to form the so-called voluntary sphincter (Fig 4). Striated fibers then diminish and are absent except for a few coursing into the vesical neck. Krantz's description of the striated sphincter of the urethra is conceptually consistent with subsequent descriptions by DeLancey[39, 40] and Oelrich.[41] The corresponding elements are: (1) bulbocavernosus decussation = urethrovaginal sphincter, (2) ischocavernosus decussation = compressor urethrae, and (3) striated urethral sphincter = urethral sphincter. The postulated presence of the lissosphincter as described by von Ludinghausen[31] and subsequently by Jeffcoate and Roberts[43] at the vesical neck is interesting, but it is impossible to reconcile with known demonstrable anatomic findings.

The levator ani lies in close proximity inferiorly to the posterior urethral wall in its course from the pubic rami to the coccyx. There were no

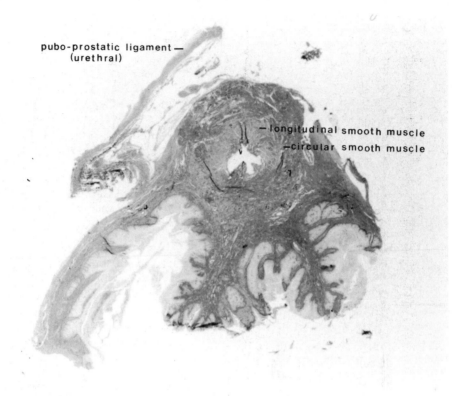

pubo-prostatic ligament —
(urethral)

— longitudinal smooth muscle
— circular smooth muscle

FIGURE 4.

Diagram of a section through C, Figure 2, from a photomicrograph at junction of the middle and inner thirds of the urethra. Note the pubourethral ligaments. The striated muscle is about to end as the inner third of the urethra is reached. An outer circular and inner longitudinal smooth muscle is noted surrounding the urethral lumen.

connections to the urethra noted in Krantz's study, possibly secondary to its well-developed fascia.

The bladder wall and urethral musculature are inseparable, and although there may be suggestions of layers in postmortum specimens, there are no distinguishable layers. The bladder is covered by a thin connective tissue layer continuous with the fascia endopelvina. The dome of the bladder is supplied by branches of the superior vesical artery, and the base is supplied by the inferior vesical. Venous drainage is via a nonspecific plexus that may cause troublesome bleeding at the time of pelvic dissection.

The nerve supply arises from the hypogastric and pelvic plexi. There are numerous parasympathetic ganglia in the loose connective tissue surrounding the bladder. Both myelinated and unmyelinated elements are found. The neurophysiology of incontinence will be discussed in a later section.

The anterior vaginal wall is separate both grossly and histologically from the bladder and urethra except in the lower two thirds of the urethra. Loose connective tissue surrounds the vagina. There is no "pubovesical fascia" so often alluded to by numerous authors. The blood supply to the vaginal wall is similar to that of the urethra. The upper and middle thirds are supplied by branches of the inferior vesical artery. The nerves are similar to those of the bladder. The vagina is lined by stratified squamous epithelium surrounded by an inner circular and outer longitudinal muscle layer. In the middle third of the urethra, circular muscle fibers surround the urethra and may interlace with occasional longitudinal fibers. In the upper third, the urethral and vaginal muscles are distinctly separate.[36]

Four separate components of the nervous system are essential for normal physiologic function of the lower urinary tract. They are (1) the parasympathetic system, (2) the sympathetic system, (3) somatic nerves, and (4) the central nervous system (CNS). Central cognitive and somatic control involves the cerebral cortex, the midbrain, and the lumbosacral spinal centers. The bladder is supplied by sympathetic fibers from T11 to L2 and by parasympathetics originating in S2–4. The hypogastric plexus contains the fibers from the sympathetic system that join the parasympathetics. The vesical neck and the posterior urethra are innervated by the sympathetic system, whereas the detrusor muscle is supplied by parasympathetics. The major function of the sympathetics is regulation of tonus of the vesical neck and posterior urethra. α-Adrenergic stimulation causes contraction of the bladder neck smooth muscle and inhibits parasympathetic-induced detrusor contractions. β-Adrenergic receptors cause bladder relaxation. The sympathetic system is also responsible for the perception of stretch in the bladder. Thus, the sympathetic system functions primarily in the storage and filling phases, and the parasympathetic system functions primarily in voiding.

Somatic innervation is becoming more prominent in discussions of incontinence evaluation and therapy. The bulbocavernosus/ischiocavernosus muscles, whose decussating fibers form the voluntary sphincter, are innervated by the terminal branches of the pudendal nerve. Current theory states that injury to the pudendal nerve during pregnancy, childbirth, or extensive pelvic surgery may predispose individuals to stress incontinence by compromising the sphincter mechanism of these important muscles.

PATHOPHYSIOLOGY

The International Continence Society defines stress urinary incontinence as a (1) symptom, (2) sign, and (3) condition. The *symptom* is the patient's initial complaint of involuntary loss of urine during stress (increasing intra-abdominal pressure). The *sign* denotes observation of loss of urine from the urethra *immediately* upon an increase in abdominal pressure. The *condition* is the loss of urine when the intravesical pressure exceeds the maximal urethral pressure in the absence of detrusor activity.

One of the few points of agreement in old and recent literature is that the primary etiologic factor that produces stress incontinence is the incomplete transmission of abdominal pressure to the urethra secondary to displacement from its normal intra-abdominal position.[44–48] This is generally manifested by anatomic displacement of the normal urethral axis in relation to the anterior vaginal wall and pubic symphysis, as described by Krantz.[34] Other functional and anatomic abnormalities of the urethra may be involved.[49, 50] In simplest terms, a female is continent when bladder pressure is lower than urethral closing pressure. The physiologic mechanism of continence involves a dynamic interplay of (1) mechanical, (2) structural, and (3) neurologic factors. If any of these is sufficiently deficient to allow the intravesical pressure to exceed the static intraurethral pressure, the patient becomes incontinent. The components of the continence mechanism have recently been accurately and succinctly summarized by Summitt and Bent[44] and by Staskin et al.[51] These components involve (1) the internal urethral "sphincter," (2) the extrinsic urethral "sphincter," (3) proper anatomic support of the urethrovesical junction, and (4) intact innervation to these components[51] (Table 3).

The internal urethral "sphincter" mechanism involves four structures for maintaining a urethral closing pressure and a mucosal seal. First, the urethral mucosa helps to provide a watertight seal by coaptation secondary to folds of the urethral surface. Second, the vascular supply of the submucosa acts as a further framework of spongy tissue that supplements urethral pliability.[51] Third, the smooth muscle fibers of the urethra maintain constant tonus, dependent on neurologic modulation of their response. The urethra has an autonomic supply and is especially rich in sympathetic fibers.[52] This is the site of possible damage secondary to multiple incontinence operations (i.e., shortening the urethra, damage to the periurethral vascular plexus, other extensive pelvic surgical procedures, and childbirth). Finally, the elastic and connective tissue of the urethral

---

TABLE 3.

Factors Involved in Intrinsic Continence Mechanism

Internal urethral "sphincter" mechanism
  Urethral mucosa seal
  Elastic and connective tissue of the urethral wall
  Smooth muscle of the urethral wall
  Submucosal vascular plexus
Extrinsic urethral sphincter
  Bulbocavernosus
  Ischiocavernosus
  Midurethral striated muscle
Neurologic control
  α-Adrenergic receptors
  Somatic nerve control
Anatomic support
  Childbirth
  Aging
Bladder mechanism
  Detrusor instability
  Capacity

wall contributes to the overall pliability and coaptation of the mucosal lining. These four structures, like the vaginal epithelium, are estrogen sensitive. Distinct estrogen receptors have been demonstrated in both lower animals and human females. Estrogen administration both orally and vaginally increases proliferation and maturation of atrophic epithelium, which widens the vascular lumen and increases vascular pulsation in the urethral bed.[51] The internal urethral sphincter mechanism is probably the mechanism involved in those studies that demonstrate improvement in stress incontinence following estrogen therapy alone.[53] Lack of estrogen (i.e., menopause) obviously leads to the opposite result.

It is important to note that urethral length may be functional or anatomic. Although some studies have demonstrated improvement in incontinence with urethral lengthening, many patients with short anatomic urethras are functionally continent for a given bladder volume. Functional urethral length is defined as the length along which the closure pressure exceeds resting bladder pressure. Indeed, most patients show little change in functional length or closure pressure after retropubic urethropexy.

The role of urethral smooth muscle in the continence mechanism remains controversial. Several authors have described "functional" smooth muscle sphincters.[35, 43, 52] However, these are difficult if not impossible to demonstrate in anatomic specimens.

The external urethral "sphincter" consists of fibers of the bulbocavernosus and ischiocavernosus that decussate over the distal portion of the urethra in three relatively discrete positions. Distally to proximally they are (1) those portions of the bulbocavernosus muscle that course over the distal portion of the urethra, often described as the urethrovaginal sphincter; (2) ischiocavernosus fibers more proximal to those of the bulbocavernosus, referred to as the compressor urethrae; and (3) the periurethral circular striated muscle, or sphincter urethrae. The urethrovaginal sphincter and compressor urethrae originate in the distal third of the urethra, arch over the superior surface, and may blend with fibers of the sphincter urethae. These blended fibers, which have been demonstrated to consist primarily of "fast-twitch" fibers innervated by the pudendal nerve,[54, 55] may contract with increasing intra-abdominal pressure (i.e., sneezing, straining) to increase distal urethral resistance. In fact, they may contract in anticipation of an upcoming increase in intra-abdominal pressure. The sphincter urethrae is thought by some[56] to be primarily composed of "slow-twitch" fibers innervated by the splanchnic nerves and arranged in a circular fashion external to the urethral smooth muscle. These may contribute to overall tonus and may add to overall resistance to flow. The three components of the external urethral sphincter together have been termed the "striated urogenital sphincter" by some authors.[50]

The neurologic control of continence has been studied intensively in recent years.[57, 58] Sympathetic innervation is generally associated with the storage mechanism, and parasympathetic innervation is associated with bladder emptying. Studies have shown varied sympathetic density in the female urethra.[59, 60] Therefore, two opposing theories have been proposed. One involves dense sympathetic innervation, which would imply an active role in urethral closure with sympathetic inhibition of parasympathetic activity at the ganglionic level. The presence of α-adrenergic receptors in the bladder neck is the pharmacologic basis for treatment with "alpha stimulants."

The second theory relies on the fact that the periurethral striated muscle is innervated by terminal branches of the pudendal nerve.[54-56] Damage to the branches that also innervate the pelvic diaphragm during extensive pelvic surgery or childbirth may decrease pelvic support and the potential response to anticipated stress phenomena.[61-64] This may explain so-called urethral instability as described by McGuire[65] and Sand et al.[66] Patients who fail initial surgical therapy may obtain some improvement via methods to increase coaptation as described by Staskin et al.[51]

The anatomic support of the bladder and entire urethral length are considered by most authors, including the present, to be the single most important correctable factor in female stress incontinence. The pubourethral (puboprostatic) ligaments originate along the lateral wall of the urethra at the junction of the middle and upper thirds to form a ligamentous structure that inserts into the pubic ramus bilaterally.[33] These structures are notably deficient in those women noted to have stress urinary incontinence. Histologically, these have been shown to consist of collagen, smooth muscle fibers, and cholinergic nerve fibers. They are not morphologically different in females with and without incontinence.[38, 39]

The levator ani muscles with their fasciae attach laterally to the urethra. Defects in attachment of the muscle to the arcus tendineus form the basis for the "paravaginal defect" described by Richardson et al.[67]

As the bladder fills, the supporting ligaments maintain elevation of the urethra against the symphysis. Thus, the urethra remains in its normal anatomic position. Continued filling elongates the longitudinal fibers of the urethra, and this, coupled with tonus of the periurethral smooth muscles, increases intraurethral pressure. When the bladder is sufficiently full, sensations proceed through spinal afferents, and a cord reflex initiates the desire to void. If bladder emptying is not socially appropriate or if intra-abdominal pressure increases for any reason, a voluntary closure of the striated musculature occurs. When voiding is socially appropriate, cord reflexes with cerebral modulation through the parasympathetic system initiate the voiding response. The intravesical pressure is increased by hydrostatic pressure and increased intra-abdominal pressure. The longitudinal muscles of the urethra contract and displace the external circular smooth muscle and striated muscle. Coupled with relaxation of the pelvic diaphragm, the bladder base descends, funneling of the bladder neck occurs, and the urethral closing pressure decreases below that of the bladder. At the same time, the pelvic diaphragm contracts, and the bladder base and urethra rise. The cessation of voiding may occur in the opposite fashion by voluntary closure of the urethra via the striated sphincter.

In a normally continent female, the bladder and urethra are maintained in an intra-abdominal position, with the urethra forming an angle of approximately 16 degrees with the vagina. When the patient strains, the bladder base may descend, but not below the level of the symphysis, and the urethra maintains its relative position. Therefore, increases in intra-abdominal pressure are equally transmitted to the bladder and urethra. Adequate fixation of the bladder neck via the pubourethral ligaments, coupled with the ability of the "voluntary sphincter" to contract, allows the intraurethral pressure to be consistently maintained above that of the bladder, and the patient remains continent.

To aid in comprehension of this mechanism, this system has been compared with a lever system of the third class by Krantz[34] (Fig 5). As applied to the urethra and bladder, the fulcrum (A) is at the external urethral meatus, and the force (F) is the pubourethral ligaments exerting an upward force on the urethrovesical neck. The load (L) is the capacity (force and vector) of the bladder. Normally the functional lengths AL/AF are the same, and the angle of function (urethra to anterior vaginal wall) is approximately 16 degrees. By whatever mechanism (aging, childbirth, etc.), the urethra becomes detached (pubourethral ligaments decrease function; F decreases), and the ratio of load (L) to force (F) becomes greater than 1. With either increased intra-abdominal pressure or contraction with detrusor instability adding to the load, urine is expressed and incontinence occurs.

Phrased in a different fashion, loss of anatomic support allows downward and posterior rotation of the bladder neck and proximal segment of the urethra from their normal intra-abdominal position and prevents equal transmission of abdominal pressure to the urethra and bladder. This results in funneling of the urethra, loss of the normal valvular mechanism, and subsequent incontinence[68] (Fig 6).

Most women who demonstrate this urethral mobility will be cured by operations that correct this positioning defect. The surgeon is advised to exercise caution lest the patient have concomitant detrusor instability.

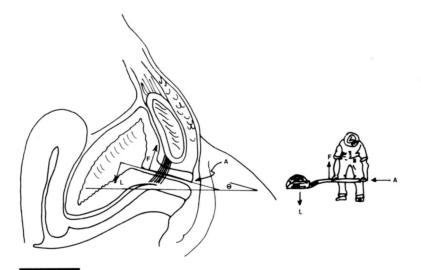

FIGURE 5.

Analogy of the urethra and its attachments to a lever system of the third order as described by Krantz. A = fulcrum at the external urethral meatus; F = upward stabilizing force by the pubourethral ligaments; L = expulsive forces of the bladder plus abdominal pressure. (Adapted from Krantz K: Anatomy, physiology, and embryological development of the urethro-vesical junction, in Slate W (ed): *Disorders of the Urethra.* Baltimore, Williams & Wilkins, 1978.)

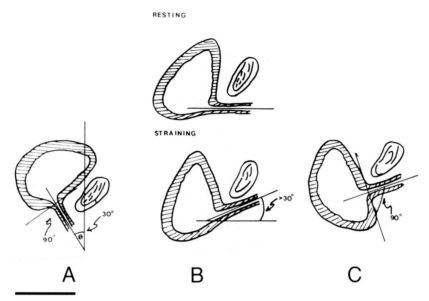

RESTING

STRAINING

A   B   C

FIGURE 6.
A, normal bladder and urethral relationships. **B,** relationship of the bladder and urethra with detachment and stress incontinence. **C,** relationship of the bladder and urethra with detachment and cystocele. Note maintenance of the urethrovesical angle and increased excursion of the urethra greater than 30 degrees. (Adapted from Bhatia NN: Pelvic relaxation and urinary problems, in Hacker NF, Moore JG (eds): *Essentials of Obstetrics and Gynecology,* ed 2. Philadelphia, WB Saunders Co, 1992.)

This point will be discussed in more detail later and in the section in this chapter on surgical repair.

The presence of a superimposed cystocele presents a special case for consideration. With rotational descent of the urethrovesical junction and subsequent descent of the bladder base to a further degree, the relationship of the urethra to the bladder is relatively reestablished and results in continence with an increase in intra-abdominal pressure. Indeed, the patient may be unable to void completely and may demonstrate significant residual urine and/or recurrent infection. Correction of the cystocele without concomitant repair and restoration of the urethrovesical angle may therefore result in subsequent incontinence. This condition has been more than amply demonstrated by the inadequacy of anterior repair (Kelly plication for long-term correction of stress incontinence).[69-74] In the case of a superimposed cystocele it is important to correct both the anterior vaginal wall defect as well as the urethrovesical defect to optimize success.

Finally, intrinsic bladder dysfunction may mimic genuine stress incontinence and/or complicate its diagnosis and therapy. This dysfunction may take the form of (1) detrusor instability (DI), (2) detrusor hyperreflexia, or (3) disturbances in bladder-filling mechanics. Detrusor instability is defined as a bladder shown to objectively contract spontaneously or on provocation during the filling phase while the patient is attempting to inhibit micturition. Contractions may be asymptomatic or interpreted by the patient as a normal desire to void. These are usually phasic in type and do not necessarily imply a neurologic disorder. Detrusor hyperreflexia is overactivity resulting from disturbance of the nervous control mechanisms. This term should only be used when there is objective evidence of a neurologic disorder.[75] Disturbances in bladder filling, e.g., overdistension, may also mimic stress incontinence. It is important for the clinician to avoid mistaking these disturbances for genuine stress incontinence. Although full discussion of these parameters is beyond the intended scope of this chapter, numerous references are available.[76, 77]

EVALUATION

Urinary continence depends on a complex interplay of multiple factors, including (1) adequate anatomic support of the urethra and bladder, (2) intact urethral "sphincteric" (smooth muscle) capability, (3) normal function of the bladder relative to the urethra, (4) absence of other pathology mistaken for urinary incontinence, and (5) intact higher control centers. Therefore, like patients with other complex medical disorders, evaluation of a complaint (symptom) of urinary incontinence must systematically include each of these components to narrow the differential diagnosis and select appropriate surgical or nonsurgical therapy. The emphasis of this section is the proper identification and differentiation of the patient with genuine stress incontinence who will respond to surgical therapy from the patient with detrusor instability or other disorders that should be treated nonsurgically.

The differential diagnosis of urinary incontinence must include both genitourinary and nongenitourinary causes, recently reviewed by Walters and others[44, 78–80] (Table 4). Genitourinary problems include the intrinsic problems of bladder filling and storage and anatomic defects. Other considerations may include fistulas or congenital anomalies. Nongenitourinary disorders are common in older patients and may include immobility, neurologic, and pharmacologic factors.

Genuine stress incontinence by definition is the loss of urine when the increase in intra-abdominal pressure exceeds the intraurethral pressure in the absence of a spontaneous detrusor contraction. *Idiopathic detrusor instability*, on the other hand, is defined as detrusor overactivity in the absence of a neurologic disorder. Detrusor activity caused by aberrant neurologic control is termed *detrusor hyperreflexia*. Genuine stress incontinence accounts for approximately 50% to 70% of urinary incontinence and must be differentiated primarily from detrusor instability, which accounts for 20% to 40% of cases seen by the urogynecologist. The most troublesome to diagnose are mixed disorders of stress incontinence and detrusor instability or other disorders, which account for 24% to 61%.[78] Overflow incontinence is defined as involuntary loss of urine associated with bladder overdistension[75] and may be associated with postsurgical obstruction, diabetes, and various neurologic disorders.

The proper evaluation of a patient with the complaint of urinary incontinence requires a systematic approach, with several components (Table 5) depending on the patient's symptoms. Patient history remains the main source of information to limit the differential diagnosis and lead to appropriate confirmatory studies. However, accuracy of the history

TABLE 4.
Differential Diagnosis*

Genitourinary
  Filling/storage disorders
  Detrusor hyperreflexia
  Detrusor instability
  Genuine stress incontinence
  Mixed incontinence
  Overflow incontinence
  Fistula
  Congenital anomalies
Nongenitourinary
  Cognitive
  Environmental
  Functional
  Metabolic
  Mood
  Neurologic
  Pharmacologic

*From Walters MD: *Contemp Rev Obstet Gynecol* 1992; 9–21. Used by permission.

alone as a predictor of diagnostic accuracy has recently been called into question. Farrar[81] et al. found the history to be quite accurate; it predicted 96.4% of women with only stress incontinence and 89% of women with urge incontinence, with or without stress incontinence, as having detrusor instability. Others, including Sand et al.[82] and Webster et al.,[83] found the history to be a suggestive but not an accurate predictor of diagnosis when other objective testing was performed. In addition, Cardozo and Stanton[77] found that 49% of women who had a complaint of stress incontinence had unstable detrusors.

The history should include an accurate description of the patient's loss of urine. *Stress incontinence* is associated with "stress" phenomena, e.g., lifting, laughing, coughing, and exercises. *Urge incontinence* is asso-

TABLE 5.
Evaluation of Incontinence

History and physical examination
Laboratory
Q-tip testing (urethral mobility)
Cystometrography
Urethrocystometry
Urethra pressure profile

ciated with feelings of urgency and statements like "unable to reach the bathroom," even with a partially filled bladder. *Overflow incontinence*, on the other hand, may be characterized by dribbling or loss of urine associated with an overfilled bladder. Other pathologic phenomena may mimic true incontinence. For example, urethral diverticuli may be seen as intermittent urine loss associated with stress phenonema. Continuous urinary leakage may result from an ectopic ureter, a fistula, or even vaginal discharge alone.

The duration, age at onset, and volume of urine lost should be noted. A consideration of frequency, dysuria, nocturia, and hematuria may lead to the diagnosis of urinary tract infection (UTI).

Patient questionnaires and diaries may be useful to help pinpoint the diagnosis[78, 79] (Table 6). Questions 1 through 9 help differentiate stress from urge incontinence and indicate detrusor instability. Questions 11 through 13 screen for UTI and neoplasia, and 14 through 17 screen for bladder dysfunction. Diaries may reveal problems of excessive fluid intake, infrequent voiding schedules, and small bladder capacity, which may be corrected by nonsurgical means.

A history of possible use of prescription and nonprescription drugs, especially those with sympathomimetic and anticholinergic properties, must be elicited. Anticholinergics may promote urinary retention and subsequent overflow incontinence. Over-the-counter decongestants and

---

TABLE 6.
Incontinence Questions*

1. Do you leak urine when you cough, sneeze, or laugh?
2. Do you ever have such an uncomfortably strong need to urinate that if you don't reach the toilet, you will leak?
3. If "yes" to No. 2, do you ever leak before you reach the toilet?
4. How many times during the day do you urinate?
5. How many times do you void during the night after going to bed?
6. Have you wet the bed in the past year?
7. Do you develop an urgent need to urinate when you are nervous, under stress, or in a hurry?
8. Do you ever leak during or after sexual intercourse?
9. Do you find it necessary to wear a pad because of your leaking?
10. How often do you leak?
11. Have you had bladder, urine, or kidney infections?
12. Are you troubled by pain or discomfort when you urinate?
13. Have you had blood in your urine?
14. Do you find it hard to begin urinating?
15. Do you have a slow urinary stream?
16. Do you have to strain to pass your urine?
17. After you urinate, do you have dribbling or a feeling that your bladder is still full?

*From Walters MD, Realini JP: *J Am Board Fam Pract* 1992; 5:289–301. Used by permission.

antihistamines, especially those containing adrenergic agents, may also lead to urinary retention[79] (Table 7).

Finally, a history of diseases affecting the central nervous system should be sought. Parkinson's disease, strokes, and senile dementia may all affect bladder stability. Diseases affecting the spinal cord and peripheral nervous system, such as spina bifida, multiple sclerosis, and diabetes, may lead to lower tract dysfunction with symptoms of incontinence.

Physical examination should include a pelvic examination, especially of the introitus and vagina, and a neurologic examination emphasizing S2–4.[84] Vaginal discharge alone has led to initial complaints of urinary incontinence.[85] In addition, atrophic vaginitis and genital prolapse may have a significant influence on the manifestation of urinary incontinence. The lower third of the vagina and urethra are of the same embryologic origin, and some cases of incontinence may respond to estrogen therapy alone. One must rule out pelvic masses (ovarian, uterine, and gastrointestinal), which may lead to an erroneous diagnosis of incontinence, by performing a thorough bimanual and rectovaginal examination.

The neurologic examination should center on S2–4 and include both motor and sensory components. Flexion of the hip, knee, and ankle will test motor function. The strength of the bulbocavernosus/ischiocavernosus should be tested by voluntary vaginal outlet contraction because these indirectly contribute to the external urethral sphincter. The lower deep tendon reflexes, including patellar, ankle, and plantar, should be evaluated. The anal reflex may be tested by stroking the skin near the anus to cause reflex contraction. Bulbocavernosus contraction may be tested by tapping the clitoris.

Finally, urinary loss should be objectively confirmed. A small loss immediately after stress points to genuine stress, whereas loss occurring several seconds later may indicate either detrusor pathology alone or combined incontinence. The standing position gives more consistent results (84%) than does the supine position (40%). There is no significant corre-

TABLE 7.
Medications Affecting Lower Urinary Tract Function*

Type of Medication	Lower Urinary Tract Effects
Diuretic	Polyuria, frequency, urgency
Anticholinergic	Urinary retention, overflow incontinence
Psychotropic	
Antidepressant	Anticholinergic actions, sedation
Antipsychotic	Anticholinergic actions, sedation
Sedative-hypnotic	Sedation, muscle relaxation
α-Adrenergic blocker	Stress incontinence
α-Adrenergic agonist	Urinary retention
β-Adrenergic agonist	Urinary retention

*From Walters MD, Realini J: *J Am Board Fam Pract* 1992; 5:289–301. Used by permission.

lation between the severity of incontinence and the degree of anatomic abnormality.[86] For example, patients with severe cystorectoceles may be entirely continent.[87]

Q-tip testing, originated by Crystle et al.[88] and reported in 1971, has been widely used to evaluate urethral mobility as a factor in stress incontinence. The test was discovered by accident while anesthetizing the urethra of a patient for a bead chain cytourethrogram. The patient strained, and the degree of axis rotation of the chain and urethra by radiography correlated with rotation of the free end of the applicator stick. The currently used form of the test requires a sterile cotton swab to be inserted through an anesthetized urethra and the change in angle upon straining to be measured. Angles of change greater than 35 to 40 degrees are considered abnormal. Multiple studies using this test during the past 20 years have yielded mixed results. In 1986, Montz and Stanton[89] found that 32% of patients with a positive test had pure detrusor instability or sensory urgency and 29% of patients with a negative test had pure stress incontinence. The test was more likely to be positive in younger persons without previous surgery. Bergman et al.,[90] in a study of 105 patients, found that more than 90% of patients with stress urinary incontinence and no previous surgery had a positive test; however, 33% of patients with bladder instability and 50% with pelvic relaxation and no incontinence also had a positive test. If the patient giving a history of incontinence demonstrates a negative Q-tip test, a stable bladder, and no history of incontinence surgery, the diagnosis is in doubt, and the patient should be considered for a sling procedure because of the high failure rate for retropubic surgery.[91] Fantl et al.[92] found no significant difference in the urethral axis and excursion in a group of continent vs. incontinent females, and Walters and Shields[93] concluded that the Q-tip test added no additional information to the history and physical examination. The current consensus appears to be that the Q-tip test is a simple, inexpensive, office-based test that may accurately quantify the mobility of the bladder neck and proximal portion of the urethra in women with and without pelvic relaxation.[94] A positive test may be somewhat predictive in that most women with stress urinary incontinence do have a mobile urethrovesical angle. If the test is negative, indicating a lack of urethral mobility, the diagnosis of stress urinary incontinence should be questioned.[95] The success of a standard retropubic operation for stress incontinence will be limited, and other procedures, e.g., sling, should be considered.

Laboratory tests include the obvious urinalysis and culture to evaluate the patient for cystitis. If the patient has hematuria and no evidence of cystitis, further evaluation for upper tract disease, stones, and/or neoplasia should be performed. Voided volume and the amount of residual urine provide an estimate of bladder capacity and the ability to empty, which may prove useful in postoperative management. A patient with a large capacity or residual may have problems voiding. In addition, patients with a large amount of residual urine may have deficient detrusor tonus and/or an anatomic defect that should be corrected at the time of surgery.

Cystometry plays an integral role in the evaluation of incontinence and should be used in all patients to help diagnose detrusor instability, especially in older patients and patients with previous surgery. The method varies from simple, inexpensive water cystometry, which may be performed at the bedside or office, to complex multitransducer procedures combined with videocystometry, which require expensive physiologic monitors and radiography.

Single-channel cystometry may be done orthograde with a diuretic or (more commonly) retrograde with CO_2 or H_2O. The simplest system is constructed with a water manometer, standard intravenous tubing, and a catheter[96] (Fig 7). The Foley catheter is placed after noting the volume voided with a full bladder to indicate capacity and residual. Water is introduced retrograde at 50 mL/min, stopping every minute to assess measured pressure. During normal bladder filling, bladder pressure should not increase by more than 14 to 15 cm H_2O before maximum capacity is reached. Provocative measures such as heel bouncing may be used to evaluate for detrusor instability.[97] Accuracy should approach 75% to 90% and is considered useful in those settings where more complex urodynamic evaluation is not readily available.[98–100] One should observe for proper perception of temperature sensation and fullness. Lack thereof may be the first sign of multiple sclerosis or amyotropic lateral sclerosis.

Subtracted cystometry techniques have been the standard in major

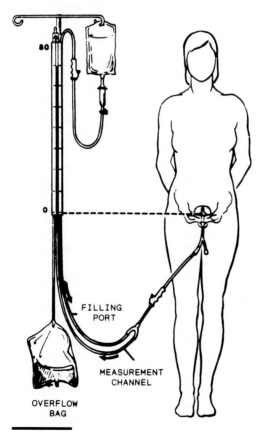

FIGURE 7.

Simple standing cystometry. (From Brubaker L, Sand PK: *Clin Obstet Gynecol* 1990; 33:315–324. Used by permission.)

hospitals. In this technique, abdominal pressure is measured by use of a transducer catheter placed in the vagina or rectum and another transducer placed within the bladder. The bladder is filled retrograde and the patient asked to note filling, fullness, and maximal capacity. Abdominal pressure is electronically subtracted and a curve constructed. Detrusor instability is diagnosed by detrusor pressures greater than 15 cm H_2O over baseline obtained either spontaneously or with provocative maneuvers. Electromyography in addition to cystometry may help to differentiate urethral instability from voluntary contractions of the pelvic floor.

Urethrocystometry or video urethrocystometry further improves the accuracy of simple and subtracted cystometry by measuring intravesical, abdominal, and urethral pressures simultaneously. Urethrocystometry offers the best urodynamic evaluation today and should be used for complex conditions or patients with previous failed incontinence surgery. In this technique, a dual-transducer catheter is placed so that one transducer is in the bladder and another is in the urethra along with an intravaginal transducer measuring abdominal pressure. In this fashion, the urethral closure pressure (difference between the urethral and bladder pressure) may be measured. Low bladder compliance is signaled by detrusor pressure increases greater than 15 cm H_2O in the presence of low bladder volume. In addition, urethral pressure changes greater than 15 cm H_2O indicate a so-called unstable urethra that may result in urinary leakage without involuntary bladder contraction.

Urethral pressure profilometry uses the same equipment as cystometry: a dual-transducer catheter in the urethra and bladder and another to measure intra-abdominal pressure. The urethral/bladder catheter is withdrawn at a predetermined rate while intraurethral and intravesical pressure are maintained, and the urethral closure pressure profile is computed and drawn. The functional urethral length (the length over which the urethral pressure exceeds bladder pressure) and the maximum urethral closure pressure are determined. By using these techniques, Bhatia and Ostergard[101] demonstrated a significant decrease in functional urethral length and urethral pressure profile in women with stress urinary incontinence. Van Geelen et al.[102] demonstrated that functional urethral length and urethral closure pressure in response to stress do not change during pregnancy. Likewise, hormonal changes and engagement of the presenting part did not alter these parameters. However, urethral length and pressure profiles were decreased postpartum in patients undergoing vaginal delivery as compared with cesarean section and nulliparous patients.

Although cystometrographic studies are widely accepted, controversy continues regarding the usefulness of the urethral pressure profile, especially in the diagnosis of stress incontinence. Problems include reproducibility, both between patients and between occasions. In addition, the urethral pressure profile may be affected by position and bladder filling.[86, 102] In this context, genuine stress incontinence is defined as urinary loss when the urethral pressure is less than or equal to bladder pressure in the absence of detrusor activity. Low maximum urethral closure pressures have been shown to correlate with surgical outcome. Patients with low pressure often fail standard stress urinary incontinence operations, presumably because of a noncompliant urethra, and may benefit from a sling procedure.[49]

Uroflowmetry is used mainly to evaluate patients for possible outflow obstruction.[103] A patient with a full bladder voids through a device standardized to measure flow. Maximum flow rates in normal individuals should measure greater than 20 mL/sec, and average flow rates should measure greater than 10 mL/sec.[104]

Parameters shown to affect the results of evaluation studies include the route of filling, the medium used, and position. In general, retrograde flow appears to be the most practical method of evaluation. Carbon dioxide urethrocystoscopy, originally developed by Robertson,[105] is commonly used and is not messy; however, CO_2 is irritating to the bladder and is obviously not physiologic.[106] The supine position is the least sensitive for detecting detrusor instability[98] and may cause misdiagnosis of a significant number of cases. The best position is standing, but this may not be possible for elderly patients.

In summary, evaluation of incontinence requires the classic history and physical examination. These are relatively good predictors in the majority of patients who have stress urinary incontinence, but additional studies including laboratory testing, cystoscopy, and cystometry should be used to maximize diagnostic accuracy. The most sophisticated electronic measurements should be used for patients who are elderly, have failed previous operations, and/or have the diagnosis called into question for other reasons.

NONSURGICAL MANAGEMENT

Although the majority of patients seen with the complaint of stress urinary incontinence will be helped by surgical therapy, there remain those patients with other types of incontinence not amenable to anatomic alteration. In addition, the advent of "managed care" and government control will mandate wider use of nonsurgical therapy as the first line of treatment for patients. Nonsurgical therapy addresses patients with urge incontinence, detrusor instability, overflow incontinence, and decreased cognition. Nonsurgical therapies fall into several broad categories, including (1) nonspecific therapy, (2) behavioral therapy, (3) physiotherapy, and (4) pharmacologic therapy (Table 8). A full discussion of all parameters is beyond the intended scope of this section, and the reader is referred to appropriate references for detailed discussion.

Nonspecific management, including the use of pads or other absorbent garments, is the most common method of management of urinary incontinence[107] and accounts for $1.5 billion dollars annually.[23]

Behavioral techniques include (1) bladder training, (2) timed voiding, and (3) prompted voiding. These obviously have no side effects and do not limit future options, but they require motivated patients and/or care givers. Bladder training introduces a voiding schedule with progressively increased intervals between mandatory voidings together with relaxation techniques.[23] The program requires the patient to avoid voiding off schedule and may use bladder distension techniques.[108] The initial voiding interval is 2 to 3 hours, and treatment may last several months. Fantl et

TABLE 8.
Nonsurgical Therapy for
Stress Incontinence

Nonspecific
Behavioral training
  Bladder training
  Habit training
  Prompted voiding
Physiotherapy
  Pelvic muscle exercises
  Vaginal cases
  Biofeedback
  Electrical stimulation
Pharmacologic therapy
  Anticholinergics
  Calcium-based blockers
  Antidepressants
  α-Adrenergic agonists
  Estrogen therapy

al.[109] reported that 12% of patients so treated were cured and that 75% were improved by at least 50%. Introduced initially to control urge incontinence, the technique may also help stress incontinence.[110]

Habit training is scheduled toileting on a planned basis. There is no effort to delay voiding and resist urge. Jarvis demonstrated an 86% improvement in his study of 51 nursing home patients using this technique.[111]

Prompted voiding may be effective in some nursing home patients as a supplement to habit training and requires monitoring on a regular basis, prompting the patient to use the toilet, and positive reinforcement.

Pelvic muscle exercises (Kegel exercises), first described by Arnold Kegel[112] in 1949, involve active exercise of the bulbocavernosus, ischiocavernosus, and levator. Unfortunately, the exercises are often taught postpartum at a time when they may not be most useful.[113] In addition, the exercises are frequently performed incorrectly with resultant gluteal contraction. If used correctly and for a sufficient length of time, 30% to 70% of patients may improve.[114] Exercises may employ weighted vaginal cones as a gauge for contraction strength.

Biofeedback uses electrical or mechanical devices to provide feedback and allow patients to gauge change in physiologic responses that mediate bladder control.[23] Biofeedback is used in conjunction with other behavioral techniques and depends on the knowledge and skill level of the physician. Studies report a range of improvement from 54% to 95% of selected patient groups.

Electrical stimulation of the pelvic viscera, muscles, and nerve supply may aid certain patients. Stimulation of afferent fibers may increase storage capabilities, and stimulation of efferent fibers may induce bladder contraction. Patient discomfort presently limits these techniques, and they are not widely used.

Pharmacologic therapy is widely used for the treatment of bladder storage disorders and has been recently summarized by several authors.[115, 116] Propantheline is an anticholinergic-like agonist but has fewer central effects. Five adequately controlled trials were reviewed.[23] Some trials used doses of 15 to 30 mg four times daily, which caused significant side effects, and incontinence frequency decreased by only 13% to 17%. Other trials concluded that less impaired patients may tolerate higher doses and have higher success rates.

Oxybutynin (Ditropan) is an antispasmodic with anticholinergic and direct smooth muscle relaxant properties. The drug proved superior to placebo in five studies[23] and reduced incontinence by 15% to 56%.

Calcium channel blockers may favorably influence detrusor instability by blocking the calcium influx necessary for contraction. At this time, these agents are not recommended for general use.

Tricyclic antidepressants have been used in three randomized controlled studies.[23] Documented decreases in incontinence frequency occurred. Side effects included fatigue, xerostomia, dizziness, and blurred vision. Doses of 10 to 25 mg one to three times a day are usually adequate. In general, although the aforementioned drugs are beneficial for patients with detrusor instability, the degree of improvement is not large, and cures are uncommon. They should be used in cooperation with a voiding regimen or other behavioral therapy to achieve the most improvement.

α-Adrenergic agents such as phenylpropanolamine (PPA) are thought to improve urinary incontinence secondary to improvement in urethral sphincter tonus mediated by action in the α-adrenergic receptors present in the bladder neck, base, and proximal segment of the urethra. Eight prospective studies were reviewed,[23] and 31% to 45% of patients had decreased incontinence. Side effects include nausea, dry mouth, rash, and itching. Overall, few cures (0% to 14%) are reported, but 30% to 60% of patients may improve. Caution must be used in those patients with hypertension and other cardiac problems.

Finally, since the urethra and lower third of the vagina are of the same embryologic origin, they both experimentally improve in tonus and vascularity with the use of exogenous estrogens administered both orally and vaginally. In the experimental animal, Batra and Iosif[117] were able to demonstrate estradiol receptors in the cytoplasm and nuclear fraction of the urethra and bladder. Both estriol and estradiol (Estrace) derivatives have been used with some success. Kinn and Lindskog[118] used PPA and estriol, alone and in combination, and noted that measured leakage was reduced by both estriol and PPA as a single treatment (28%) and as a combined technique (40%). In addition, initial low urethral pressures were increased. Hilton[119] also demonstrated increased maximum urethral closure pressures but no objective change in urethral pressure profiles. A reduction in the severity of symptoms of stress urinary incontinence, urgency, and voiding difficulties was noted. Karram et al.[120] concluded that estrogen alone, in the absence of age and other precipitating factors for stress incontinence, is of minimal importance. On the other hand, Bhatia et al.[121] studied 11 postmenopausal women with stress urinary incontinence and found that 54.5% were cured or improved and 45% were unchanged.

SURGICAL THERAPY

The operative approach to stress urinary incontinence was introduced approximately 130 years ago by Baker Brown[122] and others in the 1860s. Review of the historical literature in the 1860s reveals elaborate surgical patterns covering the anterior and posterior vaginal wall to repair injuries sustained at childbirth. The modern era of therapy for the cure of incontinence began with Kelly and Dumm's report in 1914.[123] Since that time, three main schools of thought have developed, each with their own proponents and detractors, all claiming to be very successful (Table 9). The result, aptly described by Richardson,[124] is "to wade through a voluminous urogynecological literature, inundated with contradictions, unsubstantiated opinions, speculative assertions, and modification upon modification." For example, the definition of "cure" varies considerably from one paper to another depending on subjective vs. objective urodynamic assessment. At the University of Kansas, our bias for proper procedure is based on extensive experience with the Marshall-Marchetti-Krantz (MMK) procedure in greater than 5,000 cases performed by one of the original authors. This chapter will present a detailed description of the MMK procedure as it is presently used at the University of Kansas. Only a brief description of other well-described procedures will follow. For further details, the reader is referred to the extensive literature that is available.

TABLE 9.
Surgical Therapy for Stress Incontinence

Vaginal vesicourethropexy
  Kelly plication and
  Kelly/Kennedy modification
  Vaginal retropubic procedures
Retropubic urethropexy
  Burch
  Paravaginal defect
  Marshall-Marchetti-Krantz
Needle urethropexy
  Pereyra
  Stamey
  Gittes
  Raz
Combination and repairs for special conditions
  Abdominal anterior repair and retropubic urethropexy
  Sling procedures
  Artificial sphincters

In 1914, Kelly and Dumm[123] described their procedure for the therapy of women with urinary incontinence "without manifest injury to the bladder" characterized by "gushes of urine following coughing, sneezing, laughing, stooping, and walking." Previous procedures included creating an artificial channel into which a catheter was placed,[122] closure of the urethra and creation of a vesicoabdominal fistula,[125] and creation of a rectovaginal fistula with vaginal closure.[126] Even fairly sophisticated periurethral injections had been attempted, similar to those presented in some recent reports.

Kelly and Dumm[123] reported 20 patients, 90% of whom were cured or improved in the short term. The purpose of the operation they described was to repair the injured sphincter muscle at the level of the urethrovesical junction. The Kennedy[127] modification freed the urethra from the vaginal wall with subsequent plication of the "sphincter." For many years, these operations were the standard of comparison and the first choice of treatment, especially for those patients with an accompanying cystorectocele. Recently these procedures have been criticized for lack of concomitant short-term and long-term success by several authors. Even in Kelly and Dumm's original series, only 65% of patients experienced long-term cures. It should also be pointed out that there is no evidence of a urethral sphincter as described by Kelly and others of the time. Beck and McCormick[69] have recently reported success with a vaginal retropubic procedure; however, there are few long-term data regarding this procedure.

Forerunners of retropubic operations to correct incontinence date to Hepburn,[128] who described retropubic cystopexy for the treatment of urethral prolapse in 1927 and who was subsequently reviewed by Miller.[129] The success of all operations, whether MMK, Burch, or paravaginal defect, depends on the degree of restoration of the urethrovesical junction to its original retropubic location. The Burch[130] procedure was originally developed in 1961 when he sought a satisfactory location to anchor sutures during an MMK procedure. The procedure is widely used and has proved to be reasonably successful in short- and long-term studies.[131] The procedure may fail in patients with low urethra closure pressures and shorter urethral functional lengths[132] and is superior to the modified Pereyra operation.[133]

Paravaginal defect is a relatively new development in retropubic repairs.[134] The repair is based on correction of defects in the pelvic fascia resulting in pelvic relaxation and cystourethrocele. When compared with the Burch procedure, the paraurethral tissues are attached to the lateral pelvic wall at the level of the iliopectineal line rather than Cooper's ligament. A recent review of the procedure in 149 patients by Shull and Baden[135] reports 97% success rates. The authors found that the incidence of postoperative urinary retention is decreased with this procedure when compared with MMK and Burch procedures.

Needle retropubic urethropexy was developed as a response to blood loss and hospital stay reported for transabdominal retropubic procedures. Pereyra[136] first described the vaginal procedure in 1959. It has since been modified by him and others.[137] One of the many variations is that of Stamey,[138] who introduced urethrocystoscopic control and Dacron bolsters to help prevent suture pull-through. Others, including Gittes and Loughlin[139] and Raz,[140] have all introduced modifications reported to give at least good initial success rates. These repairs apparently increase the proximal urethra pressure transmission ratios, but to a lesser degree than do retropubic procedures. A recent review demonstrated an overall success rate of 85%.[141] Figure 8 compares and contrasts these procedures.

Combination repairs of stress incontinence and cystocele have taken several forms and are used in this institution on a frequent basis. As described by Macer,[142] the procedure was successful in 92% of cases. Advantages of combination repairs currently employed are that they allow one to avoid vaginal procedures when a cystocele is present and they combine cystocele repair with retropubic repair of incontinence for possibly greater success.

Sling procedures have used multiple materials and are reserved primarily for patients who fail initial repair, who have a functionless urethra, or who demonstrate low urethral closure pressure. Many materials, including fascia lata,[143, 144] polytetrafluoroethylene,[145, 146] lyodura,[147] polyglactin 910,[148] and Silastic[149] have been used by credible authors with varied success.

Artificial sphincters are reserved for failures and work by increasing urethral resistance with an inflatable pump. Success rates are relatively high; however, complications of the procedure and foreign body reactions have occurred.

The MMK procedure, perhaps the most widely used operation for primary treatment of stress incontinence, was reported by Marshall, Marchetti, and Krantz[150] in 1950. Ironically, the initial operation was performed for male incontinence following an abdominoperineal resection. The most recent 1,000 cases of these 5,000 performed by one of the original authors are the subject of a report in progress.[2] The technique has been modified somewhat since the original paper and is presented in its current form following[151] (Fig 9).

The patient is placed in the dorsal lithotomy position with the knees flexed. The abdomen and the vagina are prepared in standard fashion. In

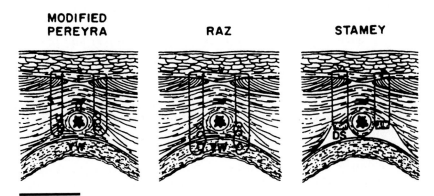

FIGURE 8.

Comparison of various needle procedures used in surgical therapy for stress incontinence. (From Karram MM, Bhatia NN: *Obstet Gynecol* 1989; 73:906–914. Used by permission.)

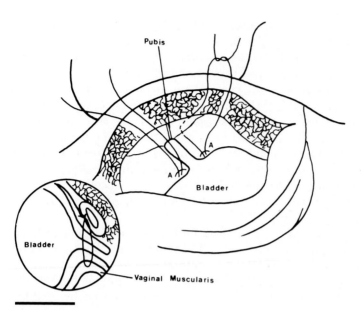

FIGURE 9.

The Marshall-Marchetti-Krantz procedure as currently performed at the University of Kansas. Note the single suture in each side and attachment to the symphysis in the midline. (Adapted from Krantz KE: Vesicovaginal fistula and Marshall-Marchetti-Krantz procedure, in Masterson BJ (ed): *Manual of Gynecologic Surgery.* Berlin, Springer-Verlag, 1979.)

the past, a no. 18 Foley catheter with a 5-mL bulb was inserted and the bladder filled with 150 mL of dilute indigo carmine. In the present-day version, a Kish catheter[152] is inserted and the bladder filled with 50 mL of normal saline. Utilization of the Kish catheter greatly aids delineation of the urethrovesical junction and the leading edge of the bladder. This is especially true for those patients in whom previous surgery has distorted the tissue planes. A Pfannenstiel incision is made 2 cm anterior to the symphysis pubis and carried to the conjoined fascia, which is divided. The rectus abdominis muscles are separated in the midline. If hysterectomy is to be performed, this procedure is carried out before the MMK procedure. In addition, an abdominal cystocele repair may be performed, thus obviating the need for a vaginal anterior repair and possible disruption of urethral integrity. The space of Retzius is entered and the transversalis fascia stripped in a lateral movement from the midline under the rectus muscles. The space of Retzius is now visible with the bladder in the midline. The surgeon introduces the first two fingers of the left hand into the vagina and palpates the urethrovesical junction as defined by the Foley bulb. The left-hand index finger elevates the vagina at the urethrovesical junction of the patient's right side. An open sponge is then used to gently strip the bladder from the anterior vaginal wall. This procedure is critical for proper suture placement. Indeed, most of the repeat procedures referred to this institution have failed secondary to incorrect suture placement resulting in bladder trauma, inadequate elevation of the urethrovesical junction, etc. A Deaver retractor is used to hold the bladder in position so that sutures may then be placed. At this time, one nonabsorbable suture (2-0 Mersilene double armed on an intestinal needle) is placed at the urethrovesical junction on each side. Sutures should be placed at right angles to the axis of the urethra. The suture is lifted and the second bite taken as shown (Fig 9,A). This ensures that the sutures will not pull through and gives a theoretical 4:1 advantage over a single suture. A similar procedure is then performed on the left side. The point of fixation to the symphysis is determined by gently elevating the point of suture placement with the fingers in the vagina. The point of contact is where the sutures should be placed. With a gentle clockwise action of the wrist, the needle is placed in the cartilaginous septum at the mid-point of the symphysis. It should be noted that a noncutting needle is used. Use of this particular needle and careful placement in the cartilage minimize the risk of osteitis pubis. Elevation of the suture will produce a notable tenting of the vaginal epithelium at the fold of Shaw, which may be palpated by fingers in the vagina. Inadvertent entry into the bladder will be indicated by spill of H_2O (or by spill of indigo carmine if the un-modified technique is used). When the Kish catheter is used, bladder entry can usually be avoided in all but the most difficult of dissections. Despite routine use of drains by others, we have not found it advantageous to routinely drain the space of Retzius, and hematoma formation has not been a problem. The fascia is closed with a 2-0 polyglycolic suture and skin with 4-0 or 5-0 suture. The Kish catheter is replaced with a standard no. 18 Foley catheter placed to drain by gravity. An iodophor gauze pack is placed in the vagina to help protect the repair for the first 24 hours.

Postoperatively, the catheter is removed on day 1 or 2. Superpubic catheters have not been necessary in our experience because of the short duration of catheterization. The longest catheter maintenance in a recent review of 150 cases was 3 weeks. Most patients are able to pass a voiding trial (less than 150 mL residual) on the second or third day. The patient may then be discharged to home care or to return to the clinic for a catheter trial if necessary. In the event of incidental bladder entry, the catheter should remain until urine is clear of red blood cells and may then be removed. The patient may resume normal activities within 3 to 4 weeks, but should be cautioned against heavy lifting and straining.[153]

A recent review of 56 articles[154] reporting on the MMK procedure by others revealed only three large series.[155–157] Favorable results occurred in 92% of primary procedures and 84% of repeat operations. Evaluation of our current series reveals success rates of approximately the same magnitude or better.

A few caveats are in order. Although the history and physical examination may give good hints toward diagnosis, a 20% to 40% chance of inaccuracy is incurred if the diagnosis relies on history alone. The Marshall and/or Bonney tests are frequently used successfully; however, Bergman and Bhatia[158] have recently shown the Marshall test to be occlusive in function and to have limited utility. A similar result was noted by Bhatia and Ostergard in evaluation of the Bonney test.[159] Urodynamic evaluation of patients thought to have stress incontinence has long been the standard in this institution, and our findings are in agreement with others in the literature. Studies[160] have shown a significant decrease in functional urethral length and closure pressure when compared with patients without stress incontinence. The same authors[161] demonstrated increases in functional length and closure pressure in patients following a Burch procedure, and Peters and Roemer[162] reported similar findings in a group of 88 patients who underwent MMK surgery.

It is especially important to evaluate those patients who may have detrusor instability. Approximately 30% of patients with detrusor instability and stress incontinence will fail urethropexy, and idiopathic detrusor instability may develop in an additional 7% with a stable detrusor.[163] On the other hand, Langer et al.[164] demonstrated a reduction in detrusor instability from 24% to 9% in a group of 92 patients and development of detrusor instability in 27% of patients with only stress incontinence. Indeed, many of these patients may be improved by medical therapy.[165] In summary, patients should be carefully evaluated for the presence of detrusor instability, and patients with detrusor instability should be offered medical therapy as an alternative to surgery. Although detrusor instability may develop after urethropexy, the incidence is low.

SUMMARY

Urinary incontinence in general and stress incontinence in particular are significant problems for many women. The condition affects a great number of people, especially the elderly, and costs an enormous amount of money yearly. Many persons accept incontinence as a normal part of aging and do not discuss it with their physician.

Stress incontinence is the result of a combination of factors that may affect the aging female, including incomplete abdominal pressure transmission, urethral hypermobility, and intrinsic urethral and/or bladder pathology.

Although the history and physical examination are mainstays of evaluation, modern urodynamic techniques supplement and increase accuracy and should be used. Multiple procedures have been described for correction of stress incontinence, and all report a high degree of success in elevation of the urethrovesical junction to a relatively normal position.

As more research and clinical data are collected, perhaps the confusion and controversy regarding proper evaluation and treatment of this fascinating condition will be eliminated and the Gordian knot of urinary incontinence untied.

REFERENCES

1. Snyder T: Do gynecologists really understand urinary incontinence? In preparation.
2. Snyder T: The University of Kansas approach to stress incontinence. The MMK: Review of 1000 cases. In preparation.
3. Bates P, Bradley WE, Glen E, et al: The standardization of terminology of lower urinary tract function. *J Urol* 1979; 121:551–554.
4. Ouslander JG, Kane RL, Abrass IB: Urinary incontinence in elderly nursing home patients. *JAMA* 1982; 248:1194–1198.
5. Campbell AJ, Reinken J, McCosh L: Incontinence in the elderly: Prevalence and prognosis. *Age Aging* 1985; 14:65–70.
6. Tobin GW, Brocklehurst JC: The management of urinary incontinence in local authority residential homes for the elderly. *Age Aging* 1986; 15:292–298.

7. Diokno AC, Brock BM, Brown MB, et al: Prevalence of urinary incontinence and other urological symptoms in the noninstitutionalized elderly. *J Urol* 1986; 136:1022–1025.

8. Brink CA, Wells TJ, Diokno AC: Urinary incontinence in women. *Public Health Nurs* 1987; 4:114–119.

9. Holst K, Wilson PD: The prevalence of female urinary incontinence and reasons for not seeking treatment. *N Z Med J* 1988; 101:756–758.

10. Francis WJA: Disturbances of bladder function in relation to pregnancy. *J Obstet Gynaecol Br Emp* 1960; 67:353–366.

11. Stanton SL, Kerr-Wilson R, Harris VV: The incidence of urological symptoms in normal pregnancy. *Br J Obstet Gynaecol* 1980; 87:897–900.

12. Snooks SJ, Setchell M, Swash M, et al: Injury to innervation of the pelvic floor sphincter musculature in childbirth. *Lancet* 1984; 2:546–550.

13. Yarnell JWG, Voyle GJ, Richards CJ, et al: The prevalence and severity of urinary incontinence in women. *J Epidemiol Community Health* 1981; 35:71–74.

14. Resnick NM: Urinary incontinence in the elderly. *Hosp Pract* 1986; 21:80C–80Z.

15. Wyman JF, Harkins SW, Choi SC, et al: Psychosocial impact of urinary incontinence in women. *Obstet Gynecol* 1987; 70:378–381.

16. Walters MD, Taylor S, Schoenfeld LS: Psychosexual study of women with detrusor instability. *Obstet Gynecol* 1990; 75:22–26.

17. Hafner RJ, Stanton S, Guy S: A psychiatric study of women with urgency incontinence. *Br J Urol* 1977; 49:211–214.

18. Morrison LM, Eadie AS, McAlister ES, et al: Personality testing in 226 patients with urinary incontinence. *Br J Urol* 1986; 58:387–389.

19. Thiede HA: The prevalence of urogynecologic disorders. *Obstet Gynecol Clin North Am* 1989; 16:709–716.

20. Hu TW: Impact of urinary incontinence on health care costs. *J Am Geriat Soc* 1990; 38:292–295.

21. Brazda JF: Washington report. *Nation Health* 1983; 13:3.

22. Hu TW, Gabelko K, Weis KA, et al: Urinary incontinence: Treatment patterns, costs, and clinical guidelines, in *Urinary Incontinence in Adults. Clinical Practice Guideline.* Rockville, Md, US Department of Health and Human Services, 1992, p 98.

23. *Urinary Incontinence in Adults: Clinical Practice Guideline.* Rockville, Md, US Department of Health and Human Services, 1992.

24. Ullery J: *Stress Incontinence in the Female.* New York, Grune & Stratton, 1953, pp 1–45. (Cited from Laut's L'Histoire de l'anatomie.)

25. Spiegel A: *De Humani Corporis Fabrica . . .* Pub Basil, Joannis Oporini. 1543, p 512.

26. Cowper W: *Anatomia Corporum Humanorum . . .* Ultrachet, Germany, Nicolaum Muntendam, 1750.

27. Griffith J: Anatomie of the bodie of man. *J Anat & Physiol* 1891; 25:534–49.

28. Vesalius A: *D corp hum fab lib LV.* 1542, p 399.

29. Bell C: *Trans Med Chir Soc Lond,* vol 1. 1809.

30. Kennedy WT: The muscle of micturition. *Am J Obstet Gynecol* 1946; 52:206–47.

31. Von Ludinghausen M: Gynecological operations and topographical anatomy. *Z Gesamt Anat* 1931; 97:257.

32. Bonney V: On diurnal incontinence of urine in women. *J Obstet Gynaecol Br Emp* 1923; 30:358–365.

33. Krantz K: The anatomy of the urethra and anterior vaginal wall. *Am J Obstet Gynecol* 1951; 62:374–386.

34. Krantz K: Anatomy, physiology, and embryological development of the urethro-vesical junction, in slate W (ed): *Disorders of the Urethra*. Baltimore, Williams & Wilkins, 1978.

35. Ullery JC: *Stress Incontinence in the Female*. New York, Grune & Stratton, 1953, pp 1–45.

36. Zacharin RF: *Stress Incontinence of Urine*. New York, Harper & Row, 1972.

37. Wilson PD, Dixon JS, Brown ADG, et al: Posterior pubourethral ligaments in normal and genuine stress incontinent women. *J Urol* 1983; 130:802–805.

38. Milley PS, Nichols DH: The relationship between the pubo-urethral ligaments and the urogenital diaphragm in the human female. *Anat Rec* 1970; 170:281–284.

39. DeLancey JOL: Anatomy and embryology of the lower urinary tract. *Obstet Gynecol Clin North Am* 1989; 16:717–731.

40. DeLancey JOL: Correlative study of paraurethral anatomy. *Obstet Gynecol* 1986; 68:91–97.

41. Oelrich TM: The striated urogenital sphincter muscle in the female. *Anat Rec* 1983; 205:223–232.

42. Deleted in proof.

43. Jeffcoate TNA, Roberts H: Observations on stress incontinence of urine. *Am J Obstet Gynecol* 1952; 64:721–738.

44. Summitt RL Jr, Bent AE: Genuine stress incontinence: An overview, in Ostergard DR, Bent AE (eds): *Urogynecology and Urodynamics. Theory and Practice*, ed 3. Baltimore, Williams & Wilkins, 1991, pp 393–403.

45. Hilton P, Stanton SL: Urethral pressure measurement by microtransducer. The results in symptom free women and those with genuine stress incontinence. *Br J Obstet Gynaecol* 1983; 90:919–933.

46. Enhorning GE: Simultaneous recording of intravesical and intraurethral pressure. A study of urethral closure pressure in normal and stress incontinent women. *Acta Chir Scand* 1961; 276:1–68.

47. McGuire EJ, Lytton B, Pepe V, et al: Stress urinary incontinence. *Obstet Gynecol* 1976; 47:255–264.

48. Anderson RS: A neurogenic element to urinary genuine stress incontinence. *Br J Obstet Gynaecol* 1984; 91:41–45.

49. Sand PK, Bowen LW, Panganiban R, et al: The low pressure urethra as a factor in failed retropubic urethropexy. *Obstet Gynecol* 1987; 69:399–402.

50. DeLancey JOL: Structural aspects of the intrinsic continence mechanism. *Obstet Gynecol* 1988; 72:296–301.

51. Staskin DR, Zimmern PE, Hadley HR, et al: The pathophysiology of stress incontinence. *Urol Clin North Am* 1985; 12:271–278.

52. Lapides J: Structure and function of the internal vesical sphincter. *J Urol* 1958; 80:341–353.

53. Schiff I, Tulchinsky D, Ryan KJ: Vaginal absorption of estrone and 17β-estradiol. *Fert Steril* 1977; 28:1063–1066.

54. Snooks SJ, Badenoch DR, Tiptaft RC, et al: Perineal nerve damage in genuine stress incontinence: An electrophysiological study. *Br J Urol* 1985; 57:422–426.

55. Gosling J: The structure of the bladder and urethra in relation to function. *Urol Clin North Am* 1979; 6:31–38.

56. Gosling JA, Dixon JS: Light and electron microscopic observations of the human external urethral sphincter. *J Anat* 1979; 129:216–220.

57. Ostergard DR: The neurological control of micturition and integral voiding reflexes. *Obstet Gynecol Surv* 1979; 34:417–423.

58. Ostergard DR: Neurological control of micturition and integral voiding reflexes, in Ostergard DR, Bent AE (eds): *Gynecologic Urology and Urodynam-*

ics. Theory and Practice, ed 2. Baltimore, Williams & Wilkins, 1985, pp 29–41.

59. Gosling JA, Dixon JS: The structure and innervation of smooth muscle in the wall of the bladder neck and proximal urethra. *Br J Urol* 1975; 47:549–558.

60. Sundin T, Dahlstrom A, Norlen L, et al: The sympathetic innervation and adrenoreceptor function of the human lower urinary tract in the normal state and after parasympathetic denervation. *Invest Urol* 1977; 14:322–328.

61. Beck RP, Hsu N: Pregnancy, childbirth, and the menopause related to the development of stress incontinence. *Am J Obstet Gynecol* 1965; 91:820–823.

62. Tapp A, Cardozo L, Versi E, et al: The effect of vaginal delivery on the urethral sphincter. *Br J Obstet Gynaecol* 1988; 95:142–146.

63. Iosif CS, Ingemarsson I: Prevalence of stress incontinence among women delivered by elective cesarian section. *Int J Gynaecol Obstet* 1982; 20:87–89.

64. Allen RE, Hosker GL, Smith ARB, et al: Pelvic floor damage and childbirth: A neurophysiological study. *Br J Obstet Gynaecol* 1990; 97:770–779.

65. McGuire EJ: Reflex urethral instability. *Br J Urol* 1978; 50:200–204.

66. Sand PK, Bowen LW, Ostergard DR: Uninhibited urethral relaxation: An unusual cause of incontinence. *Obstet Gynecol* 1986; 68:645–648.

67. Richardson AC, Lyon JB, Williams NL: A new look at pelvic relaxation. *Am J Obstet Gynecol* 1976; 126:568–573.

68. Bhatia NN: Pelvic relaxation and urinary problems, in Hacker NF, Moore JG (eds): *Essentials of Obstetrics and Gynecology*, ed 2. Philadelphia, WB Saunders, 1992.

69. Beck RP, McCormick S: Treatment of urinary stress incontinence with anterior colporrhaphy. *Obstet Gynecol* 1982; 59:269–274.

70. Park GS, Miller EJ Jr: Surgical treatment of stress urinary incontinence: A comparison of the Kelly plication, Marshall-Marchetti-Krantz, and Pereyra procedures. *Obstet Gynecol* 1988; 71:575–579.

71. Iosif CS: Results of various operations for urinary stress incontinence. *Arch Gynecol* 1983; 233:93–100.

72. Beck RP, McCormick S, Nordstrom L: A 25-year experience with 519 anterior colporrhaphy procedures. *Obstet Gynecol* 1991; 78:1011–1018.

73. Bergman A, Ballard CA, Koonings PP: Comparison of three different surgical procedures for genuine stress incontinence: Prospective randomized study. *Am J Obstet Gynecol* 1989; 160:1102–1106.

74. Bergman A, Koonings PP, Ballard CA: Primary stress urinary incontinence and pelvic relaxation: Prospective randomized comparison of three different operations. *Am J Obstet Gynecol* 1989; 161:97–101.

75. Abrams P, Blaivas JG, Stanton SL, et al: The standardisation of terminology of lower urinary tract function. *Scand J Urol Nephrol* 1988; 114(suppl):5–19.

76. Hirsch LB, Montella JM, Bent AE: Detrusor instability, in Ostergard DR, Bent AE (eds): *Urogynecology and Urodynamics. Theory and Practice*, ed 3. Baltimore, Williams & Wilkins, 1991, pp 363–367.

77. Cardozo LD, Stanton SL: Genuine stress incontinence and detrusor instability—a review of 200 patients. *Br J Obstet Gynaecol* 1980; 87:184–190.

78. Walters MD: Steps in evaluating the incontinent woman. *Contemp Obstet Gynecol* 1992; 9–21.

79. Walters MD, Realini JP: The evaluation and treatment of urinary incontinence in women. A primary care approach. *J Am Board Fam Pract* 1992; 5:289–301.

80. McCarthy TA: Differential diagnosis of urinary incontinence, in Ostergard DR, Bent AE (eds): *Urogynecology and Urodynamics. Theory and Practice*, ed 3. Baltimore, Williams & Wilkins, 1991, pp 83–86.

81. Farrar DJ, Whiteside CG, Osborne JL, et al: A urodynamic analysis of micturition symptoms in the female. *Surg Gynecol Obstet* 1975; 141:875–881.

82. Sand PK, Hill RC, Ostergard DR: Incontinence history as a predictor of detrusor stability. *Obstet Gynecol* 1988; 71:257–260.

83. Webster GD, Sihelnik SA, Stone AR: Female urinary incontinence. The incidence, identification and characteristics of detrusor instability. *Neurourol Urodynam* 1984; 3:235–342.

84. Stanton SL: Introduction to preoperative evaluation of the incontinent patient, in Ostergard DR, Bent AE (eds): *Gynecologic Urology and Urodynamics. Theory and Practice*, ed 2. Baltimore, Williams & Wilkins, 1985, pp 69–78.

85. Julian TM: Pseudoincontinence secondary to unopposed estrogen replacement in the surgically castrate premenopausal female. *Obstet Gynecol* 1987; 70:382–383.

86. Khan Z, Mieza M, Bhola A: Relative usefulness of physical examination, urodynamics and roentgenography in the diagnosis of urinary stress incontinence. *Surg Gynecol Obstet* 1988; 167:39–44.

87. McGuire EJ, Lytton B, Pepe V, et al: Stress urinary incontinence. *Obstet Gynecol* 1976; 47:255–264.

88. Crystle CD, Charme LS, Copeland WE: Q-tip test in stress urinary incontinence. *Obstet Gynecol* 1971; 38:313–315.

89. Montz FJ, Stanton SL: Q-tip test in female urinary incontinence. *Obstet Gynecol* 1986; 67:258–260.

90. Bergman A, McCarthy TA, Ballard CA, et al: Role of the Q-tip test in evaluating stress urinary incontinence. *J Reprod Med* 1987; 32:273–275.

91. Bergman A, Koonings PP, Ballard CA: Negative Q-tip test as a risk factor for failed incontinence surgery in women. *J Reprod Med* 1989; 34:193–197.

92. Fantl JA, Hurt WG, Bump RC, et al: Urethral axis and sphincteric function. *Am J Obstet Gynecol* 1986; 155:554–558.

93. Walters MD, Shields LE: The diagnostic value of history, physical examination, and the Q-tip cotton swab test in women with urinary incontinence. *Am J Obstet Gynecol* 1988; 159:145–149.

94. Walters MD, Diaz K: Q-tip test: A study of continent and incontinent women. *Obstet Gynecol* 1987; 70:208–211.

95. Karram MM, Narender NB: The Q-tip test: Standardization of the technique and its interpretation in women with urinary incontinence. *Obstet Gynecol* 1988; 71:807–811.

96. Brubaker L, Sand PK: Cystometry, urethrocystometry, and videocystourethrography. *Clin Obstet Gynec* 1990; 33:315–325.

97. Mainprize TC: Diagnosis of urinary incontinence. *Clin Obstet Gynecol* 1990; 33:308–314.

98. Sand PK, Hill RC, Ostergard DR: Supine urethroscopic and standing cystometry as screening methods for the detection of detrusor instability. *Obstet Gynecol* 1987; 70:57–60.

99. Ouslander J, Leach G, Abelson S, et al: Simple versus multichannel cystometry in the evaluation of bladder function in an incontinent geriatric population. *J Urol* 1988; 140:1482–1486.

100. Sand PK, Brubaker LT, Novak T: Simple standing incremental cystometry as a screening method for detrusor instability. *Obstet Gynecol* 1991; 77:453–457.

101. Bhatia NN, Ostergard DR: Urodynamics in women with stress urinary incontinence. *Obstet Gynecol* 1982; 60:552–559.

102. Van Geelen JM, Lemmens WAJG, Eskes TKAB, et al: The urethral pressure profile in pregnancy and after delivery in health nulliparous women. *Am J Obstet Gynecol* 1982; 144:636–649.

103. Bergman A, Bhatia NN: Uroflowmetry: Spontaneous versus instrumented. *Am J Obstet Gynecol* 1984; 150:788–790.

104. Cholhan HJ: Urodynamic studies: When, what, and why. *Contemp Obstet Gynecol* 1992; 25–39.

105. Robertson JR: Dynamic urethroscopy, in Ostergard DR, Bent AE (eds): *Urogynecology and Urodynamics. Theory and Practice*, ed 3. Baltimore, Williams & Wilkins, 1991, pp 115–121.

106. Wein AJ, Hanno PM, Dixon DO, et al: The reproducibility and interpretation of carbon dioxide cystometry. *J Urol* 1978; 120:205–206.

107. Herzog R, Fultz N, Normolle D, et al: Methods used to manage urinary incontinence by older adults in the community. *J Am Geriatr Soc* 1989; 37:339–347.

108. Keating JC, Schulte EA, Miller E: Conservative care of urinary incontinence in the elderly. *J Manipulative Physiol Ther* 1988; 11:300–308.

109. Fantl JA, Wyman JF, McClish D, et al: Efficacy of bladder training in older women with urinary incontinence. *JAMA* 1991; 265:609–613.

110. Burgis KL, Whitehead WE, Engel BT: urinary incontinence in the elderly: Bladder-sphincter biofeedback and toilet skills training. *Ann Intern Med* 1985; 103:507–515.

111. Jarvis GJ: A controlled trial of bladder drill and drug therapy in management of detrusor instability. *Br J Urol* 1981; 53:565–566.

112. Kegel A: Progressive resistance exercise in the functional restoration of the perineal muscles. *Am J Obstet Gynecol* 1948; 56:238–248.

113. Bo K, Larsen S, Oseid S, et al: Knowledge about and ability to correct pelvic floor muscle exercises in women with urinary stress incontinence. *Neurourol Urodynam* 1988; 7:261.

114. Wells T: Pelvic floor muscle exercise. *J Am Geriatr Soc* 1990; 38:333–337.

115. Norton PA: Nonsurgical management of stress urinary incontinence. *Contemp Obstet Gynecol* 1992; 63–78.

116. Luber KM, Bent AE: Clinical management of urge incontinence in women. *Female Patient* 1992; 17:67–71.

117. Batra SC, Iosif CS: Female urethra: A target for estrogen action. *J Urol* 1983; 129:418–420.

118. Kinn AC, Lindskog M: Estrogens and phenylpropanolamine in combination for stress urinary incontinence in postmenopausal women. *Urology* 1988; 32:273–280.

119. Hilton P: The use of intravaginal oestrogen cream in genuine stress incontinence. *Br J Obstet Gynaecol* 1983; 90:940–944.

120. Karram MM, Yeko TR, Sauer MV, et al: Urodynamic changes following hormonal replacement therapy in women with premature ovarian failure. *Obstet Gynecol* 1989; 74:208–211.

121. Bhatia NN, Bergman A, Karram MM: Effects of estrogen on urethral function in women with urinary incontinence. *Am J Obstet Gynecol* 1989; 160:176–181.

122. Baker Brown: Diseases of women remediable by operation. *Lancet* 1864, March 5, pp 263–266.

123. Kelly HA, Dumm WM: Urinary incontinence in women, without manifest injury to the bladder. *Surg Gynecol Obstet* 1914; 18:444–450.

124. Richardson DA: The evaluation of differential surgical procedures, in Ostergard DR, Bent AE (eds): *Urogynecology and Urodynamics. Theory and Practice*, ed 3. Baltimore, Williams & Wilkins, 1991, pp 413–421.

125. Rutenberg: *Wien Med Wochenschr* 1875, No 37.

126. Pepin EA: Pathogenie et traitement operatoire de l'incontinence urethrale d'urine chez la femme (these). Paris, Steinheil, 1893, p 42.

127. Kennedy WT: Incontinence of urine in the female, the urethral sphincter

mechanism, damage of function, and restoration of control. *Am J Obstet Gynecol* 1937; 34:576−587.

128. Hepburn TN: Prolapse of the urethra in female children. *Surg Gynecol Obstet* 1927; 44:400−401.

129. Miller JR: Prolapse of the urethra treated by the Hepburn operation. *Am J Obstet Gynecol* 1945; 49:591−595.

130. Burch JC: Urethrovaginal fixation to Cooper's ligament for correction of stress incontinence, cystocele, and prolapse. *Am J Obstet Gynecol* 1961; 81:281−290.

131. Milani R, Scalambrino S, Quadri G, et al: Marshall-Marchetti-Krantz procedure and Burch colposuspension in the surgical treatment of female urinary incontinence. *Br J Obstet Gynaecol* 1985; 92:1050−1053.

132. Bowen LW, Sand PK, Ostergard DR, et al: Unsuccessful Burch retropubic urethropexy: A case-controlled urodynamic study. *Am J Obstet Gynecol* 1989; 160:452−458.

133. Bhatia NN, Bergman A: Modified Burch versus Pereyra retropubic urethropexy for stress urinary incontinence. *Obstet Gynecol* 1985; 66:255−261.

134. Richardson AC, Edmonds PB, Williams NL: Treatment of stress urinary incontinence due to paravaginal fascial defect. *Obstet Gynecol* 1981; 57:357−362.

135. Shull BL, Baden WF: A six-year experience with paravaginal defect repair for stress urinary incontinence. *Am J Obstet Gynecol* 1989; 160:1432−1440.

136. Pereyra JA: A simplified surgical procedure for the correction of stress incontinence in women. *West J Surg Obstet Gynecol* 1959; Jul-Aug:223−226.

137. Pereyra AJ, Lebherz TB: The modified Pereyra procedure, in Buchsbaum H, Schmidt JD (eds): *Gynecologic and Obstetric Urology*, ed 1. Philadelphia, WB Saunders, 1978, pp 259−277.

138. Stamey TA: Endoscopic suspension of the vesical neck for urinary incontinence. *Surg Gynecol Obstet* 1973; 136:547−554.

139. Gittes RF, Loughlin KR: No-incision pubovaginal suspension for stress incontinence. *J Urol* 1987; 138:568−570.

140. Raz S: Modified bladder neck suspension for female stress incontinence. *Urology* 1981; 17:82−85.

141. Karram MM, Bhatia NN: Transvaginal needle bladder neck suspension procedures for stress urinary incontinence: A comprehensive review. *Obstet Gynecol* 1989; 73:906−914.

142. Macer GA: Transabdominal repair of cystocele, a 20 year experience, compared with the traditional vaginal approach. *Am J Obstet Gynecol* 1978; 131:203−207.

143. Wheeless CR Jr, Wharton LR, Dorsey JH, et al: The Goebell-Stoeckel operation for universal cases of urinary incontinence. *Am J Obstet Gynecol* 1977; 128:546−549.

144. Parker RT, Addison WA, Wilson CJ: Fascia lata urethrovesical suspension for recurrent stress urinary incontinence. *Am J Obstet Gynecol* 1979; 135:843−852.

145. Summitt RL Jr, Bent AE, Ostergard DR, et al: Stress incontinence and low urethral closure pressure. *J Reprod Med* 1990; 35:877−880.

146. Horbach NS, Blanco JS, Ostergard DR, et al: A suburethral sling procedure with polytetrafluoroethylene for the treatment of genuine stress incontinence in patients with low urethral closure pressure. *Obstet Gynecol* 1988; 71:648−652.

147. Iosif CS: Operative treatment of women with prolapse and genuine primary stress incontinence. *Urol Int* 1983; 38:199−202.

148. Fianu S, Soderberg G: Absorbable polyglactin mesh for retropubic sling operations in female urinary stress incontinence. *Gynecol Obstet Invest* 1983; 16:45−50.

149. Stanton SL: Silastic sling for urethral sphincter incompetence in women. *Br J Obstet Gynaecol* 1985; 92:747–750.

150. Marshall VF, Marchetti AA, Krantz KE: The correction of stress incontinence by simple vesicourethral suspension. *Surg Gynecol Obstet* 1950; 88: 509–518.

151. Krantz KE: Vesicovaginal fistula and Marshall-Marchetti-Krantz procedure, in Masterson BJ (ed): *Manual of Gynecologic Surgery*. Berlin, Springer-Verlag, 1979.

152. Snyder TE: Utilization of the Kish urethral illuminating catheter for improved urethrovesical visualization in the Marshall-Marchetti-Krantz procedure. In preparation.

153. Krantz KE: Marshall-Marchetti-Krantz procedure for stress urinary incontinence, in Fitzpatrick J (ed): *Perspectives in Gynecology*, vol 1. New York, Pfizer Laboratories, 1980, pp 1–11.

154. Mainprize TC, Drutz HP: The Marshall-Marchetti-Krantz procedure: A critical review. *Obstet Gynecol Surv* 1988; 43:724–729.

155. Giesen JE: Stress incontinence. A review of 270 Marchetti operations. *Aust N Z J Obstet Gynaecol* 1974; 14:216.

156. Lee RA, Symmonds RE, Goldstein RA: Surgical complications and results of modified Marshall-Marchetti-Krantz procedure for urinary incontinence. *Obstet Gynecol* 1979; 53:447–450.

157. Riggs JA: Retropubic cystourethopexy: A review of two operative procedures with long-term follow-up. *Obstet Gynecol* 1986; 68:98–105.

158. Bergman A, Bhatia NN: Urodynamic appraisal of the Marshall-Marchetti test in women with stress urinary incontinence. *Urology* 1987; 29:458–462.

159. Bhatia NN, Bergman A: Urodynamic appraisal of the Bonney test in women with stress urinary incontinence. *Obstet Gynecol* 1983; 62:696–699.

160. Bhatia NN, Ostergard DR: Urodynamics in women with stress urinary incontinence. *Obstet Gynecol* 1982; 60:552–559.

161. Bhatia NN, Ostergard DR: Urodynamic effects of retropubic urethropexy in genuine stress incontinence. *Am J Obstet Gynecol* 1981; 140:936–941.

162. Peters FD, Roemer VM: Urodynamic findings following surgery in women with urinary stress incontinence. *Arch Gynecol* 1981; 230:299–306.

163. Sand PK, Bowen LW, Ostergard DR, et al: The effect of retropubic urethropexy on detrusor stability. *Obstet Gynecol* 1988; 71:818–822.

164. Langer R, Ron-El R, Newman M, et al: Detrusor instability following colposuspension for urinary stress incontinence. *Br J Obstet Gynaecol* 1988; 95:607–610.

165. Karram MM, Bhatia NN: Management of coexistent stress and urge urinary incontinence. *Obstet Gynecol* 1989; 73:4–7.

Editor's Comment

Dr. Snyder provides an excellent discussion of urinary incontinence, with concise but germane treatments of anatomy, neurology, evaluation of the patient, and management. The discussion on patient evaluation should be very helpful to the practitioner since it contains numerous clinical "pearls" in evaluating the patient with urinary incontinence. The discussion is especially helpful in assisting the reader in understanding and determining the various conditions that contribute to incontinence.

Equally significant is the treatment of both nonsurgical and surgical management of the incontinent patient. One must emphasize that medical management should be attempted initially since up to 70% of patients may note improvement. The author describes in detail the MMK procedure as performed at the University of Kansas Medical Center. Several helpful hints are given, such as use of the Kish catheter and placing indigo carmine in the bladder. However, I do not understand the use of an iodophor vaginal pack and how this will help protect the repair.

Overall, Dr. Snyder provides the reader with valuable tools in evaluating the patient with incontinence. The diagrams are very helpful in understanding the anatomic defects leading to incontinence.

Sebastian Faro, M.D., Ph.D.

Vaginal Vault Prolapse—Prevention and Surgical Management

STEPHEN H. CRUIKSHANK, M.D.

S upporting the vaginal cuff at the time of an abdominal or vaginal hysterectomy is essential for preventing vaginal vault prolapse. Vault prolapse is an infrequent yet tragic complication to gynecologic surgery, and its prevention should be one of the primary goals of reconstructive pelvic surgery. Using the uterosacral and cardinal ligament complexes to support the vaginal vault is a recommended step in both transvaginal and transabdominal hysterectomy. Any successful repair restores the normal anatomy and restores a functioning vagina.

During hysterectomy various principles of vaginal fixation can be used to prevent vaginal vault prolapse. This chapter will discuss attaching the vagina to the pelvic supportive structures, correcting or preventing an obvious or potential enterocele, and colpopexy, either vaginal or abdominal.

This chapter also pictorially represents procedures performed routinely and adjunctly to help prevent posthysterectomy prolapse. Strict attention must be paid to attaching the uterosacral and cardinal ligaments to the vaginal membrane. Techniques to close the cul-de-sac of Douglas to prevent enterocele formation are also discussed.[1, 2]

ANATOMY

The normal vaginal axis lies almost horizontal superior to the levator plate.[3] The vagina lies parallel to the levator ani and not directly over the genital hiatus. At a time of increased intra-abdominal pressure, the levator plate and the endopelvic fascia (especially the cardinal/uterosacral complex) hold the cervix and upper part of the vagina in their proper positions.

Stretching and laceration of the supportive structures can result in uterine and/or vaginal prolapse. The etiologic factors include trauma, menopausal atrophy and attenuation, and possibly pudendal neuropathy, with loss of levator and endopelvic fascia integrity. The uterus and vagina then overlie the genital hiatus, which leads to prolapse of these organs.

Advances in Obstetrics and Gynecology, vol 1
© 1994, Mosby–Year Book, Inc.

PREVENTING VAGINAL PROLAPSE AT THE TIME OF HYSTERECTOMY

During transvaginal hysterectomy care must be taken to reattach the uterosacral/cardinal ligament complex to the vagina. The following steps can be performed at the beginning or finish of the procedure. Performing these steps in the beginning of a transvaginal hysterectomy will ensure that (1) the sutures are not cut by mistake later in the operation and (2) these steps are not forgotten should the procedure become difficult or complicated.

After the anterior and posterior cul-de-sacs are entered, the uterosacral and cardinal ligaments are cut and ligated. If these supporting structures are not frail or attenuated, the pedicles should be immediately sutured to the vaginal membrane (Fig 1). By securing these to the lateral angles of the vagina, the vault is supported, and the lateral angles of the vaginal cuff, a common source of postoperative bleeding, are readily su-

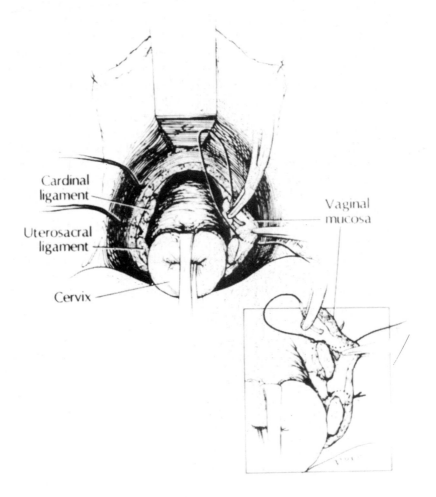

FIGURE 1.

Uterosacral-cardinal ligaments attached to the vaginal membrane. (From Cruikshank SH: *Am J Obstet Gynecol* 1987; 156:1433–1440. Used by permission.)

tured. These steps are completed during any transvaginal hysterectomy. If the indication for hysterectomy includes uterovaginal prolapse, any laxity in these ligaments will require shortening. Shortening can be accomplished at the beginning of the procedure if the anterior cul-de-sac has been entered and the bladder retracted. This step elevates the bladder and ureters out of harm's way. When the uterosacral/cardinal ligaments need shortening but the hysterectomy must be performed without being in the anterior cul-de-sac, the shortening steps should be done after the uterus is extirpated and the bladder and ureters are elevated. A recent study shows that in all patients except those with severe uterovaginal prolapse and/or procidentia, the ureters are actually protected by cutting the car-

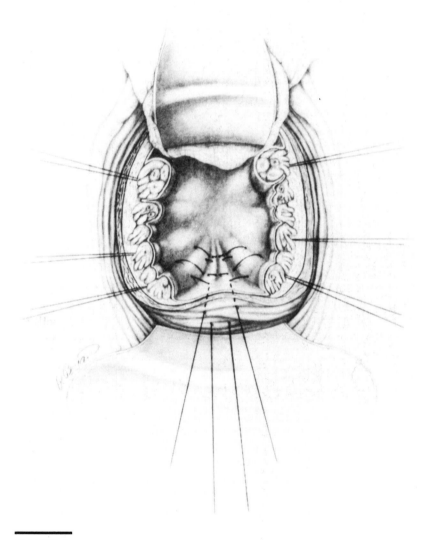

FIGURE 2.

Modified McCall cul-de-plasty. (From Thompson JD, Rock JA (eds): *Telinde's Operative Gynecology*. Philadelphia, JB Lippincott, 1992, p 720. Used by permission.)

dinal ligaments at the start of the procedure.[4] This step allows the ureters to fall laterally and to retract toward the lateral pelvic sidewall.

The McCall "cul-de-plasty" or its modification is another means of supporting the vaginal cuff during transvaginal hysterectomy.[5, 6] This procedure incorporates the uterosacral and cardinal ligaments to the peritoneal surface. The sutures are attached so that when they are tied, the uterosacral/cardinal ligaments are drawn toward the midline to help close off the cul-de-sac. When the sutures are tied, they also draw the posterior vaginal apex up to the supporting structures and elevate it to a normal position. This can be performed with one or several sutures (Fig 2). The only drawback to this type of culdeplasty is a theoretical increased incidence of kinking or ligating the ureter because of its proximity to the uterosacral ligament.

Any modification of these two procedures that attaches the supporting structures to the vagina will work. The important point to remember is that these steps should be accomplished during a transvaginal hysterectomy. During an abdominal hysterectomy, the cardinal and uterosacral ligaments should also be attached to the vaginal cuff. As soon as the uterus and cervix are removed, the cardinal and uterosacral pedicles should be sewn to the lateral angles of the vagina either as part of the lateral angle stitch or separately. There is no need to incorporate the round ligaments to the cuff since they do not aid in cuff suspension and in fact may draw the ovaries to a position overlying the vaginal apex and thus predispose to dyspareunia.

Prolapse of the vagina is due to a loss of normal pelvic supports or to omission of the steps using these pelvic support tissues during hysterectomy. This complication occurs after either transvaginal or transabdominal hysterectomy. Hysterectomy will not by itself cure uterovaginal prolapse. Hysterectomy permits the pelvic surgeon to visualize and use the supportive structures and attach them to the vaginal membrane.

As mentioned, several methods of vaginal fixation at the time of hysterectomy are recognized today. Regardless of the particular method chosen, posthysterectomy prolapse can be prevented in most cases by using the cardinal/uterosacral complex as described.

PREVENTING ENTEROCELE

Another step that helps prevent complications following transvaginal or transabdominal hysterectomy is caring for the cul-de-sac of Douglas. Whether a normal cul-de-sac, a deep cul-de-sac, or an obvious enterocele is found, every attempt should be made to avert future enterocele formation and to identify and correct an obvious one.

Closure of the abdominal peritoneum should be performed during vaginal hysterectomy in an attempt to prevent enterocele formation. Closure of peritoneum itself is unnecessary for proper healing. However, a deep cul-de-sac or obvious enterocele left unrepaired will lend itself to future enterocele formation and possible vaginal vault prolapse.

At the time of transvaginal hysterectomy it is preferable to close the cul-de-sac as follows: Beginning at the 12 o'clock position, a full-length, long-acting absorbable or permanent suture is placed through the ante-

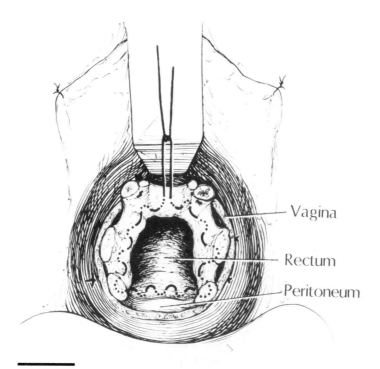

FIGURE 3.

Closing the cul-de-sac and peritoneal cavity during vaginal hysterectomy. (From Cruikshank SH: *Am J Obstet Gynecol* 1987; 156:1433–1440. Used by permission.)

rior peritoneum (Fig 3). In a clockwise direction (counterclockwise for the left-handed), a running purse-string suture is placed in the peritoneum. At the level of the uterosacral and cardinal ligaments, a bite is taken through each proximal to the ligature connecting the pedicle to the vagina. The suture is then passed through the anterior rectal serosa about 3 to 4 cm above the level of the peritoneal reflection. The suture is carried around to meet the free end of the tie and is drawn and tied to ensure adequate and *high* abdominal peritoneal closure (Fig 4). The suture is then held and sewn to the vagina at the level of the cardinal ligaments as the vaginal cuff is closed.

Two of the several other methods that have been described to care for the posterior cul-de-sac of Douglas in both transvaginal and transabdominal hysterectomy will be presented.[5-9] All of the methods vary only slightly in technique, but the goal remains the same: to prevent or repair an enterocele.

The Halban cul-de-sac closure[10] is a vertical-type closure of the peritoneum that was first described for abdominal procedures (Figs 5 and 6). By incorporating the peritoneal sutures vertically, ureteral damage is averted and a potential, deep, or obvious enterocele sac is closed. This procedure is good for transvaginal surgery as well (Fig 7). It repairs the cul-de-sac and places no sutures near the ureters. It also accomplishes high peritoneal ligation, an important step in closing a deep cul-de-sac.

The Moschcowitz procedure was first described as a method to close off a deep cul-de-sac in conjunction with prolapse of the rectum. It has

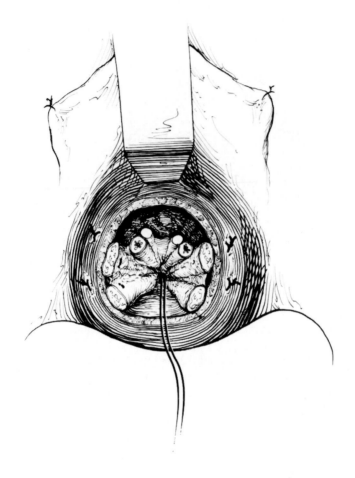

FIGURE 4.

Peritoneal closure complete. (From Cruikshank SH: *Am J Obstet Gynecol* 1987; 156:1433–1440. Used by permission.)

since been modified and heralded as a technique to close the cul-de-sac during various abdominal procedures (i.e., hysterectomy, abdominal sacrocolpopexy, abdominal procedures for genuine stress incontinence). The Moschcowitz procedure uses a circumferential suture (Fig 8) to close the cul-de-sac. The anterior portion of this ligature is attached to the posterior side of the lower uterine segment if the uterus is left in situ or to the posterior vaginal wall peritoneum after hysterectomy. The first method of cul-de-sac closure described above for transvaginal hysterectomy is in essence a modification of the abdominal Moschcowitz suture. Whether performed abdominally or vaginally, care must be taken to avoid

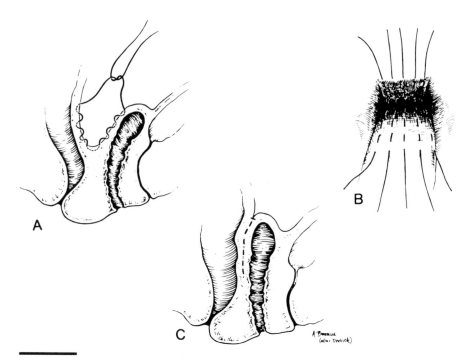

FIGURE 5.
A–C, Halban cul-de-sac closure (abdominal, uterus extirpated). (From Nichols DH: *Vaginal Surgery.* Baltimore, Williams & Wilkins, 1989, p 326. Used by permission.)

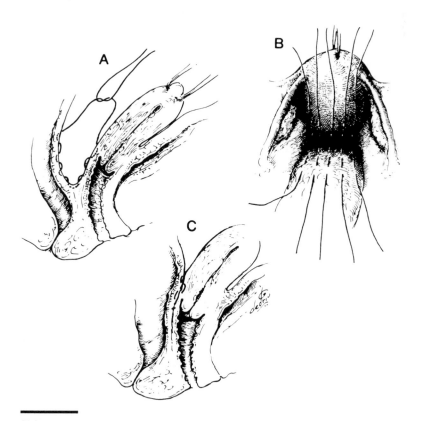

FIGURE 6.
A–C, Halban-type cul-de-sac closure (abdominal, uterus in situ). (From Nichols DH: *Vaginal Surgery.* Baltimore, Williams & Wilkins, 1989, p 325. Used by permission.)

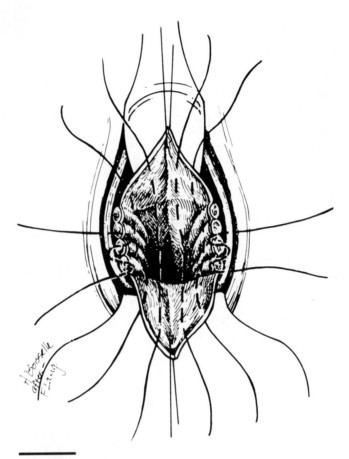

FIGURE 7.

Halban-type closure—vaginal. (From Nichols DH: *Vaginal Surgery*. Baltimore, Williams & Wilkins, 1989, p 324. Used by permission.)

the ureter as it proximates the uterosacral ligaments. This can be done by direct palpation and identification[11] of these structures while placing the cul-de-sac plicating ligatures.

Enterocele formation is more common than is generally recognized. Ranny[7] reported an incidence of 18.1% in patients undergoing major gynecologic operations. Failure to close a deep cul-de-sac at the time of hysterectomy or other procedure can result in hernia formation. Whether repairing or preventing an obvious or potential enterocele, the objectives are the same: (1) to restore function and anatomy, (2) to prevent recurrences, and (3) to use an appropriate procedure.

Transvaginal hysterectomy or transperitoneal abdominal procedures are appropriate times to evaluate the cul-de-sac and prevent an enterocele. High peritoneal ligation using the anterior rectal wall will help prevent enterocele. Either a circumferential or vertical obliterative technique of the cul-de-sac may be used.

ADJUNCT SUPPORT TO THE VAGINAL CUFF

In most transvaginal hysterectomies performed the patients already have some degree of uterovaginal descensus. At times the primary indication

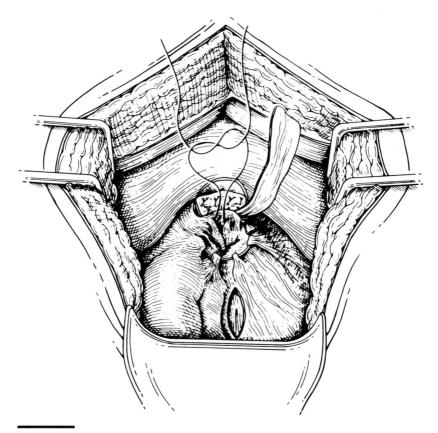

FIGURE 8.

Moschcowitz procedure to close the deep cul-de-sac during an abdominal colpo-sacropexy. (From Thompson JD, Rock JA (eds): *Telinde's Operative Gynecology*. Philadelphia, JB Lippincott, 1992, p 882. Used by permission.)

for the hysterectomy is symptomatic pelvic relaxation. In cases of moderate or severe uterovaginal prolapse, adjunct vaginal apex support may be necessary. Moderate uterovaginal prolapse is defined as the presentation of the cervix past the midportion of the vagina or to the introitus with Valsalva's maneuver. Severe uterovaginal prolapse is defined as the presentation of the cervix past the introitus with or without Valsalva's maneuver[12] (Figs 9 and 10). If these degrees of relaxation are present before surgery, these patients may be candidates for more than just utero-sacral/cardinal ligament complex attachment to the vaginal membrane. Moreover, there will be patients who do not present preoperatively in this manner but who, after vault support and plastic vaginal repairs, will have the vaginal vault pulled to or past the introitus. Both preoperative and intraoperative evaluation of pelvic support must be performed in order to repair all defects present.

Traditionally, sacrospinous fixation of the vagina and abdominal sacrocolpopexy have been regarded as therapeutic tools to be used only for the repair of vaginal vault prolapse and/or certain types of entero-celes.[13, 14] However, these procedures may also be used as an adjunct to prevent posthysterectomy vault prolapse. Not every hysterectomy patient is a candidate. If there is a loss of the pelvic supportive structures (utero-

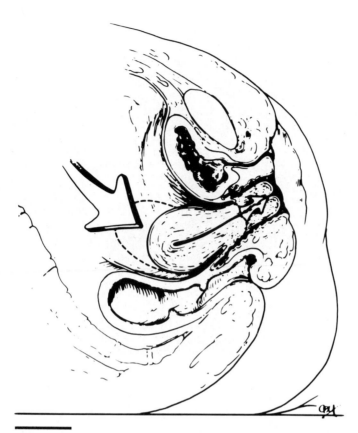

FIGURE 9.

Moderate uterovaginal prolapse. (From Cruikshank SH, Cox DW: *Am J Obstet Gynecol* 1990; 162:1611−1619. Used by permission.)

sacral/cardinal ligament complex) at the time of vaginal hysterectomy, an attempt to use their remnants should be made. Sacrospinous fixation of the vagina as an adjunct to this reconstruction will prevent further vault prolapse. If an abdominal hysterectomy is indicated in someone with uterovaginal prolapse, abdominal sacrocolpopexy can be performed as an adjunct.

If preoperative or intraoperative evaluation during transvaginal hysterectomy reveals the need for adjunct vaginal support, a sacrospinous fixation of the vagina is easy to perform after hysterectomy. The sacrospinous ligament fixation procedure is performed as follows: (1) The posterior vaginal wall is opened to the apex and the rectovaginal space entered. (2) This space is dissected with the operator's finger to the level of the ischial spines. (3) At that time the descending rectal septum (pillar) is perforated, and the pararectal space is opened (Fig 11). (4) With additional blunt dissection, the ischial spine and coccygeus muscle/sacrospinous ligament complex are palpated and identified visually. (5) Long-acting absorbable sutures or monofilament permanent sutures are placed through the ligament. (6) These sutures are held and left untied until any additional reconstructive procedures are finished. (7) Ligament fixation is carried out with both safety and pulley stitches (Fig 12). If for some

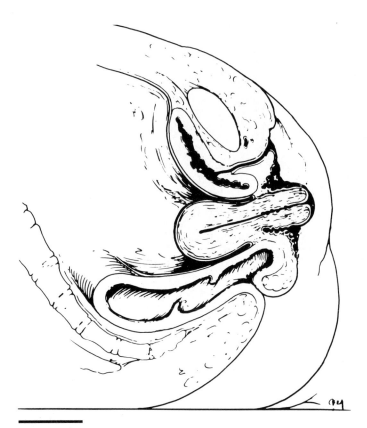

FIGURE 10.

Severe uterovaginal prolapse. (From Cruikshank SH, Cox DW: *Am J Obstet Gynecol* 1990; 162:1611–1619. Used by permission.)

reason an abdominal hysterectomy is indicated in spite of the presence of uterovaginal prolapse, an abdominal sacrocolpopexy can be performed.

This discussion will be limited to a modification of two of the several methods of abdominal sacrocolpopexy.[15, 16] (1) An incision is made in the peritoneum in the hollow of the sacrum from the sacral promontory downward as far posteriorly as possible. (2) The cul-de-sac is obliterated by the Moschcowitz operation. (3) Three to five permanent sutures are placed in the periosteum approximately 1 cm apart. These sutures are used to hold one end of the graft (Teflon, Mersilene, Goretex, or homologous fascia) to the sacrum. (4) The other end of the graft is sutured to the posterior wall of the exposed vaginal vault. (5) The graft is sewn to the vaginal vault and sacral promontory periosteum. At that time the graft is secured to the underlying serosa of the sigmoid with two or three 2-0 nonabsorbable sutures (Fig 13).

In summary, the literature is replete with attempted nonsurgical and surgical management of genital prolapse. Over 1,500 articles exist on the management of prolapse. Before the 20th century most therapies were partial or had serious drawbacks. This short discussion summarizes only a few anatomically correct operations for supporting the vaginal vault. Others exist, and their omission here is not meant to slight. Various principles of vaginal fixation during hysterectomy are recognized today. It is

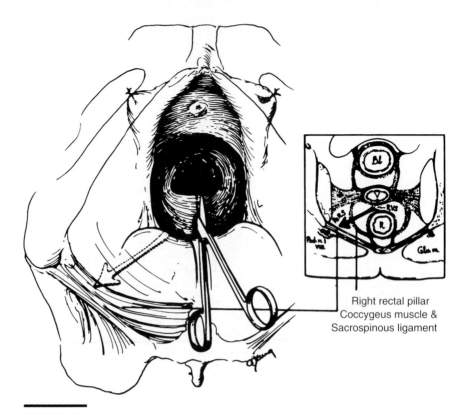

Right rectal pillar
Coccygeus muscle &
Sacrospinous ligament

FIGURE 11.
Dissecting rectovaginal and pararectal spaces. (From Cruikshank SH, Cox DW: *Am J Obstet Gynecol* 1990; 162:1611–1619. Used by permission.)

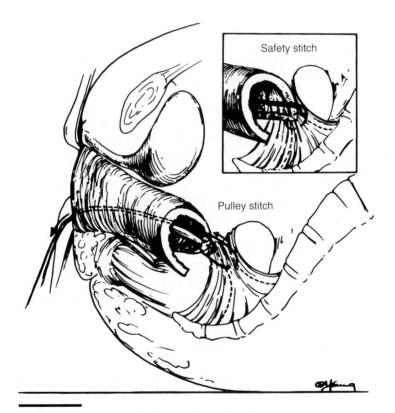

Safety stitch

Pulley stitch

FIGURE 12.
Fixation demonstrating pulley and safety stitches. (From Cruikshank SH, Cox DW: *Am J Obstet Gynecol* 1990; 162:1611–1619. Used by permission.)

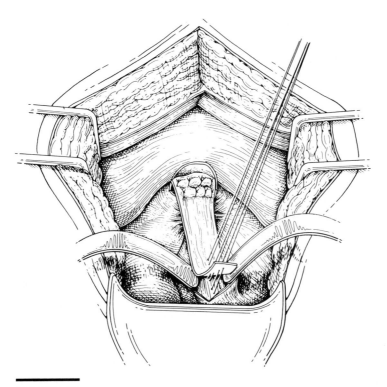

FIGURE 13.

Abdominal sacrocolpopexy. (From Thompson JD, Rock JA: *Telinde's Operative Gynecology*. Philadelphia, JB Lippincott, 1992, p 883. Used by permission.)

of paramount importance that the surgeon evaluate the laxity of the supporting structures and attempt the necessary repairs during the initial operation. Hysterectomy offers a good opportunity to evaluate all anatomic aspects of pelvic support and to prevent future vaginal prolapse. Attaching the pelvic supportive structures to the vagina, repairing an obvious or potential enterocele, and using adjunct procedures when needed are all part of the surgical armamentaria to support the vaginal cuff.

VAGINAL VAULT PROLAPSE

Vaginal vault prolapse poses quite a challenge to the gynecologic surgeon, as is evidenced by the more than 40 procedures proposed for its surgical repair. Few of these have reconstructed the vagina in its normal anatomic position, a result that is of utmost importance. When a successful reconstruction is accomplished, the anatomy is not distorted, the anatomy does not predispose to enterocele formation, and the vagina has normal function. With any reconstructive procedure there will be some incidence of operative failure. Some of these factors are unpredictable, but such factors as age, poor tissue, scar tissue, increased abdominal pressure, and neuropathies may prevent optimal reconstruction and lead to less than a perfect result. Every attempt should be made to restore the anatomy to its normal position at all times. The two previously described methods of attaching the vagina by abdominal sacrocolpopexy or by vaginal sacrospinous fixation represent two methods of good anatomic restoration.

Each patient must be treated individually. If good support and good function of the vagina are to be the result of an operative repair of post-hysterectomy prolapse, a considerable variation in technique from patient to patient may be required. However, the goals in each case will be restoring the vagina to its normal anatomic position and preventing recurrence. Recurrences are frequently due to four factors: (1) An enterocele sac was ignored. (2) The vaginal vault was suspended in a much too anterior position—possibly to the anterior rectus abdominal wall—thereby predisposing to a rapid recurrence of enterocele. (3) Both of the aforementioned factors may be present. (4) The procedure was performed incorrectly.

One of the most important factors in selecting the procedure of choice is whether or not the patient will remain sexually active. In today's world women are maintaining their sexual function longer and longer, and if an obliterative technique is to be performed, it is of paramount importance that the woman be sure that she thereafter will not be sexually active. Recent studies on the Neugebauer-Le Fort operation[17] for vaginal prolapse have reported good results. Nevertheless, every effort should be made to preserve vaginal function, length, and axis.

Three major categories have evolved from the 40 plus procedures described over the last century for vaginal vault prolapse: (1) complete obliteration (colpocleisis); (2) abdominal sacrocolpopexy or vaginal sacrospinous fixation (or a modification thereof); and (3) anterior abdominal wall/ventral fixation, which is rarely used because of the lack of restoration of normal anatomy. The remaining anatomically correct procedures for vaginal vault prolapse are those that have already been described: sacrospinous fixation of the vagina and abdominal sacrocolpopexy with the use of either an artificial type of graft or an analogous fascial-type graft.

It is not intended that this section describe every type of repair that has been described in the past for this tragic complication of hysterectomy. However, a partial review of the different types of abdominal repairs and vaginal repairs can be found in the reference section.[12–22] Suffice it to say that the most important aspect of all of these is that normal anatomy is restored and that the specific site or sites of damage are properly reconstructed.

It has been demonstrated both clinically and anatomically that the suspensory fibers that attach to the vaginal vault are the site of damage that results in vaginal vault prolapse.[23] These include the fibers that make up the endopelvic fascia of the cardinal and uterosacral ligament complex. When these are destroyed, surgically lax, or not used for prevention of posthysterectomy prolapse at the time of hysterectomy, vaginal vault prolapse can result. Therefore, every effort should be made to use these fibers at the time of hysterectomy and reattach them to the vaginal vault to prevent posthysterectomy prolapse.[24] Theoretically, this should work in almost every case to prevent prolapse. However, a diminution in the suspensory fibers, menopausal atrophy, or a loss of the neural supply to this area for some reason may still result in vaginal vault prolapse, and one of the anatomic repairs for vault prolapse will have to be used.

Traditionally, transvaginal sacrospinous fixation has been regarded as a therapeutic tool to be used only for vaginal vault prolapse. The procedure can also be used as an adjunct against posthysterectomy vault prolapse. Not every vaginal hysterectomy patient will be a candidate. However, if there is a loss of the pelvic supportive structures (uterosacral/cardinal ligament complex) noted at the time of hysterectomy, an attempt should be made to use their remnants. Sacrospinous fixation of the vagina as an adjunct will prevent further vault prolapse and restore normal anatomy. If for some reason the abdominal approach is used, then abdominal sacrocolpopexy should be used if the vaginal apex's suspensory fibers are surgically lax.

SUMMARY

It is obvious from the numerous attempts noted in the literature that repair of vault prolapse is a significant problem for the gynecologic surgeon. However, careful reconstruction of anatomy at the time of hysterectomy will ideally prevent a large majority of cases of posthysterectomy prolapse. Should prolapse occur, restoration of the normal anatomic relationships should be attempted either transvaginally or transabdominally. In addition, each and every other defect should be corrected at the same time. It is emphasized that treatment of only the vaginal vault prolapse, without taking care of a cystocele, an enterocele, a rectocele, or a paravaginal defect, can result in recurrence of other anatomic hernias and failure of the initial repair. An anatomic vaginal or abdominal repair can be accomplished in this group of patients without any reduction in vaginal depth, diameter, or function.

REFERENCES

1. Symmonds RE, Williams TJ, Lee RA, et al: Posthysterectomy enterocele and vaginal vault prolapse. *Am J Obstet Gynecol* 1981; 140:852.
2. Kaser O, Ikg FA, Hirsch HA: *Atlas of Gynecologic Surgery*, ed 2. New York, Thieme-Stratton, 1985, 6.1–6.9.
3. Nichols DH, Milley PS, Randall CL: Significance of restoration of normal vaginal depth and axis. *Obstet Gynecol* 1970; 36:251–256.
4. Cruikshank SH, Kovac SR: Role of the uterosacral-cardinal ligament in protecting the ureter during transvaginal hysterectomy. *Int J Gynaecol Obstet* 1993, in press.
5. McCall ML: Posterior culdeplasty. *Obstet Gynecol* 1957; 10:595–602.
6. Thompson JD, Rock JA (eds): *Telinde's Operative Gynecology*. Philadelphia, JB Lippincott, 1992, pp 720–723.
7. Ranny B: Enterocele, vaginal prolapse, pelvic hernia: Recognition and treatment. *Am J Obstet Gynecol* 1981; 140:852–859.
8. Torpin R: Excision of the cul-de-sac of Douglas—for surgical care of hernias through the female caudal wall, including prolapse of uterus. *J Int Coll Surg* 1955; 24:322–330.
9. Moschcowitz AV: The pathogenesis, anatomy, and cure of prolapse of the rectum. *Surg Gynecol Obstet* 1912; 15:7.
10. Halban J: *Gynakologische Operations*. Berlin, Urban & Schwarzenberg, 1932, pp 171–172.
11. Cruikshank SH, Pixley RL: Surgical method of identifying the ureters during total vaginal hysterectomy. *Obstet Gynecol* 1986; 67:277–280.
12. Cruikshank SH, Cox DW: Sacrospinous fixation at the time of transvaginal hysterectomy. *Am J Obstet Gynecol* 1990; 162:1611–1619.

13. Randall CL, Nichols DH: Surgical treatment of vaginal inversion. *Obstet Gynecol* 1971; 38:327–332.

14. Morley GW, DeLancey JOL: Sacrospinous ligament fixation for eversion of the vagina. *Am J Obstet Gynecol* 1988; 158:872–881.

15. Lansman HA: Posthysterectomy vault prolapse: Sacral colpopexy with dura matter graft. *Obstet Gynecol* 1984; 63:577–581.

16. Feldman GB, Birnbaum SJ: Sacral colpopexy for vaginal vault prolapse. *Obstet Gynecol* 1979; 53:399–401.

17. Ahranjani M, Nora E, Rexai P, et al: Neugebauer–Le Fort operation for vaginal prolapse. *J Reprod Med* 1992; 37:959–964.

18. Ridley JH: A composite vaginal vault suspension using fascia lata. *Am J Obstet Gynecol* 1976; 126:590–596.

19. Stanton SL, Cardozo CA: Results of the colposuspension operation for incontinence and prolapse. *Br J Obstet Gynaecol* 1979; 86:693–697.

20. Lee RA, Symmonds RE: Surgical repair at posthysterectomy vault prolapse. *Am J Obstet Gynecol* 1972; 112:953–956.

21. Langmade CF, Oliver JA, White JS: Cooper ligament repair of vaginal vault prolapse twenty-eight years later. *Am J Obstet Gynecol* 1978; 131:134–142.

22. Palma PCR, Pinotti JA: Endoscopic suspension of vaginal prolapse. *Int J Gynaecol Obstet* 1988; 27:451–454.

23. Delancey JOL: Anatomic aspects of vaginal eversion after hysterectomy. *Am J Obstet Gynecol* 1992; 166:1717–1728.

24. Cruikshank SH: Preventing posthysterectomy vaginal vault prolapse and enterocele during vaginal hysterectomy. *Am J Obstet Gynecol* 1987; 156:1433–1440.

Editor's Comment

Dr. Cruikshank has presented an excellent discussion of a very difficult subject. The prevention and treatment of vaginal vault prolapse is important to every gynecologist who performs hysterectomies. The section on anatomy, although brief, is very helpful. The diagrams are clear and detailed and facilitate understanding of the discussion.

The author presents alternate approaches to preventing vaginal vault prolapse while performing a vaginal hysterectomy. Care is taken to point out that while performing a hysterectomy, especially in a patient with a deep cul-de-sac, the posterior cul-de-sac must be addressed if an enterocele is to be prevented. Failure to do so will eventually, in a large number of patients, lead to vaginal vault prolapse. All too often, especially in training programs, the entire operative procedure (hysterectomy and management of vaginal support) is not taught, and as a result posthysterectomy patients return with vaginal vault prolapse. There are various approaches to preventing the development of an enterocele, which can lead to vaginal vault prolapse, e.g., McCall, Moschcowitz, or Halbans culdoplasty or some variation of these classic approaches. The author carefully points out that these procedures can be employed whether one is performing a vaginal or abdominal hysterectomy. Care is also taken to emphasize which of these techniques is likely to compromise the ureters. This is a valuable discussion on an important subject that the author has presented in a very concise and clear manner.

Sebastian Faro, M.D., Ph.D.

Reproductive Endocrinology

Menopause—A Deficiency Disease

JOSEPH W. GOLDZIEHER, M.D.

I n 1966, after several decades of experience in treating menopausal women with estrogen, Robert A. Wilson, a board-certified gynecologist from New York, wrote a popular book entitled *Feminine Forever*. In it, he stated that the entire menopausal syndrome is a preventable disease that can be treated by lifetime estrogen replacement therapy (ERT). Except for a few technical details, his writings are as up-to-date as the current publications that are proclaiming the value of this approach. In fact, Germaine Greer, in her 1992 book on menopause, states that "one is obliged to question the morality of withholding estrogen, rather than the wisdom of prescribing it." Recognizing that his ideas ran counter to contemporary medical opinion, Wilson anticipated the sort of establishment outcry that had met the pioneering work of Jenner, Semmelweiss, and Pasteur. Nevertheless, he was overwhelmed by the virulence of the attacks leveled against him by the medical profession. Were he alive today and able to read the current Food and Drug Administration (FDA) mandated package insert for estrogens, which still says, "The majority of women do not need estrogen replacement therapy for longer than 6 months," he undoubtedly would say that the medical profession is *still* being dragged, kicking and screaming, to the viewpoint that menopause is, purely and simply, a *deficiency disease* that may extend over a third of a woman's lifetime.

The basis for this establishment intransigence is a complex of conscious and subconscious cultural, religious, and sexist attitudes in a male-dominated specialty, many of whose practicing members never received a thorough grounding in reproductive endocrinology and consequently regard sex hormones with insecurity and misgivings. The outward manifestation of this attitude is usually expressed as a concern about estrogen-induced carcinogenesis or a statement to the effect that the perceived symptoms are likely to be transitory (i.e., the FDA statement) and therefore trivial.

Of course, the most serious hazards of this deficiency disease are not immediately perceived but nevertheless have an enormous impact. Cardiovascular disease accounts for nearly 50% of female deaths (compared with 4% from breast cancer). There are reasons to believe, as will be discussed later, that cardiovascular mortality can be cut in half by ERT. In 1988 it was estimated that the costs associated with osteoporotic fractures exceeded 8 billion dollars a year, not a trivial sum. Thus, for health care

Advances in Obstetrics and Gynecology, vol 1
© 1994, Mosby–Year Book, Inc.

savings by preventive intervention, if not for our mission to optimize individual health and quality of life, it is time to reassess our professional attitudes.

REPLACEMENT THERAPY

One problem in achieving consensus on appropriate replacement therapy is the fragmentation of interests of various investigators. "Bone people" appear to think that estrogen replacement is not necessary if there is no osteoporosis or that whatever dose is recommended for bone protection is sufficient in general. "Heart people" look at the problem from their limited perspective. Practitioners who seek to relieve symptoms of estrogen deficiency, such as hot flashes, think the job is done when relief is gained. These short-term perspectives permeate bureaucratic and medical/residency policies such as the FDA-mandated package insert; somewhere, the holistic approach seems to have been lost. It may sound offensively elementary, but it is necessary to state that we treat *people*, not symptoms or organs.

ANDROGENS

The functioning ovary secretes substantial amounts of a proandrogen, androstenedione, which is readily converted to testosterone by the addition of a single proton. Precisely what role androstenedione plays in the endocrine milieu of women has been poorly defined, and when we discuss "replacement therapy" in menopause management, its role is never mentioned. Androstenedione is a simple molecule, chemically somewhat similar to progesterone, dirt cheap, unpatentable, and therefore of no interest to the pharmaceutical industry even though it is unlikely that the FDA would require 10-year dog and monkey studies for the filing of a new drug application (NDA). Formulation for clinical use presents much the same problems as progesterone, which is also commercially uninteresting. The availability of prescription androgens is extremely limited. Methyltestosterone is not a very good androgen; fluoxymesterone (Halotestin) has virtually disappeared from mention in the *Physicians' Desk Reference* (PDR). There are some oral estrogen/androgen combinations on prescription, but the available ratios are very limited. Injectable androgens are far too concentrated and have a poor pharmacokinetic profile. Several decades ago, the World Health Organization undertook a sophisticated and intensive chemical synthesis program to develop long-acting androgens (for other purposes), and a number of interesting agents with good pharmacokinetic profiles were produced. None of them are currently available. Androgens are the wasteland of pharmaceutical interest in the United States.

The relationship of endogenous androgen levels to libido is complex but well recognized: loss of libido after oophorectomy in reproductive-age women is typical. Menopausal women, *if asked*, will commonly admit—and complain about—a loss of libido. To assume that this is due entirely to a decrease in endogenous androgen levels is, of course, simplistic in the extreme. A certain amount of routineness or other factors in her life may contribute. A menopausal woman is not likely to be "turned on" by the addition of a little testosterone to her estrogen-replacement regimen. There are physicians who are enthusiastic about the results achieved with testosterone supplementation, but there are also many women who initially reject the suggestion of any hormone therapy at all because they have heard that they will grow a mustache. Obviously, there is a great deal of individual variation in response, psychological, social, and physical, in terms of unwanted androgenicity. One suggested alternative has been to apply testosterone ointment to the clitoral area to improve vasculature and sensitivity. There are no controlled clinical studies on this modality. In short, improvement in sexual function in the older couple is not limited to the relief of dyspareunia; counseling and a judicious trial of androgens should not be forgotten.

ESTROGENS AND PROGESTINS

Since menopause, whether spontaneous, radiational, or surgical, is an estrogen deficiency state leading to estrogen deficiency diseases, the rationale of its management is obvious. The details, however, are complex. Every tissue that has estrogen receptors (and that includes a lot of territory) is entitled to its fair share of estrogen. But tissues differ very widely in their estrogen sensitivity, and it has not been demonstrated that the log dose/response curves of tissues A to Z are parallel, a requirement for precise comparisons of dosage and potency. Moreover, the time required for tissue responses to reach a plateau (if they do) is also variable. How nature strikes a balance among all these competing requirements is an interesting question; some women are less impressed with nature's success than are others. At a point where the response of liver cells in synthesizing certain serum proteins may be nearly maximal, the autonomic nervous system may still be complaining bitterly, in sweats and flashes, of inadequate ERT. Epidemiologic data concerning the minimum level of ERT that is cardioprotective are accumulating, but much remains to be done. The same is true with respect to prevention of osteoporosis. Data concerning management of immediate deficiency symptoms are almost entirely lacking. Experienced physicians will be well aware that proper ERT requires more individualization than virtually any other common medication. This is due in part to the issue of tissue responsiveness and in part to the fact that estrogens undergo enterohepatic recirculation, a phenomenon known to be associated with great interindividual and intraindividual variability. With the ethinyl estrogens, probably the most intensively studied of all the estrogens, the coefficient of variation of plasma levels among individuals may be as much as ±40%, a huge number. Autonomic symptoms may be well controlled by small doses of estrogen in one individual whereas another is not relieved by larger doses that are producing symptoms of excess dosage elsewhere—breast tenderness, for example. This dilemma is a common one, and it is precisely when the addition of progestational compounds such as medroxyprogesterone acetate, 20 to 30 mg/day orally, or 100 mg of Depo-Provera intramuscularly, should be used. These compounds will have a profound effect on the autonomic nervous system without the need to go to uncomfortable estrogen levels. Another example is the initiation of ERT in an elderly woman who has been estrogen deficient for many years. Starting therapy with a daily dose of 0.625 mg of conjugated equine estrogens is likely to produce an angry telephone call about mastalgia within a week. A more appropriate initiation would be 1 tablet once during the first week, 2 tablets equally spaced during the second week, and so on, to give the tissues a chance to regenerate estrogen receptors. Young, oophorecto-mized women may require 3.7 mg of conjugated equine estrogens or 6 to 8 mg of micronized estradiol daily for full replacement. As is well known, the level of plasma follicle-stimulating hormone (FSH) is *not* a suitable criterion of dosage adequacy. To repeat Sir William Osler's dictum: *listen* to the patient.

The psychic and somatic relief that is obtained by elimination of the estrogen deficiency state is enormously gratifying both to the patient and physician. Management over the long term to ensure that side effects (such as menstrual bleeding), cancerophobia, gossip, or media misinfor-mation do not cause discontinuation is the challenge that must be met. Every television spectacular exploiting "new information" about hor-mones and breast cancer in the latest issue of the *New England Journal of Medicine* or *JAMA* will generate phone calls; these must be met con-scientiously, and many women who do not bring up the matter sponta-neously will nevertheless harbor new fears that must be assuaged. In that regard it is important, before discussing or initiating ERT with a patient, to determine what her store of information, misinformation, or concerns may be. This communication with the patient probably will be a deter-mining factor in her future compliance.

Both the dose and the route of administration can and should be in-dividualized. In general, as long as a satisfactory plasma level of estrogen is achieved, it should make little difference how the estrogen got there. However, many women who have tried estrogens and had untoward ex-periences with one type or route of estrogen administration may be per-suaded to try alternatives (micronized estradiol instead of conjugated es-trogens, transvaginally or transdermally instead of by the oral route, etc.). Transdermal estradiol application has the theoretical advantage of pro-viding fairly stable levels of plasma estradiol that can be measured and adjusted appropriately; vaginal creams not only have local restorative ef-fects[1] but also can provide significant blood levels.[2] Whether the hepatic effects of orally administered estrogens (vs. other routes) have any clini-cal significance is debatable.

The benefits of ERT to various tissues and organ systems have been extensively covered in the literature. This discussion will be confined to two areas of life-and-death importance: cardiovascular disease and osteo-porosis; the benefit/risk assessment will be in this context.

Cardiovascular Effects

Presumably by analogy to the issue of thromboembolic disease attributed to oral contraceptive use, concerns have been expressed about the possi-bility of such hazards from ERT. An intensive search of the world litera-ture has failed to produce any evidence of such a hazard,[3] and a recent case-control study[4] has come to the same conclusion. Studies of hormone-induced changes in coagulation factors, as in the case of hormonal contraceptives, shed no light on this matter.[5]

There is no longer any question that ERT protects against atherogenic cardiovascular disease; estimates of the reduction in relative risk range from 0.34 to 0.80.[6–8] Sullivan et al.[9, 10] reported that never-users who had more than 70% coronary stenosis had a 60% 10-year survival rate vs. a 97% survival rate among ever-users. Hong et al.[11] have stated that absence of estrogen use was the most powerful independent predictor of the presence of coronary artery disease in postmenopausal women undergoing coronary angiography. And yet in a review that acknowledged the virtually unanimous conclusions of over 20 studies on cardiovascular effects, Goldman and Tosteson[12] still state: "It is disappointing that we in medicine collectively have not made more progress *toward resolving the clinical conundrum* of postmenopausal estrogen replacement" [italics added]. Evidently no amount of data will persuade the estrophobes.

In regard to the issue of atherogenesis, the beneficial effect of estrogens on the lipoprotein profile is acknowledged. There is much concern, however, whether this benefit is attenuated by the "adverse " effects on the profile of added progestins.[9, 10] Just as with oral contraceptives, where it was shown that adverse lipid profiles do not diminish the protective effect of estrogen against coronary atheromatosis, studies of menopausal regimens in cynomolgus monkeys have shown that the beneficial effect of estrogen is primarily exerted at the level of the coronary artery wall[13–15] and that the impact of alterations in plasma lipoproteins is much less significant. Thus the concerns about progestins appear to be red herrings; the protective estrogen effect *ipso facto* persists.

Risks of Estrogen Use

BREAST CANCER.—In 1939 Lacassagne, a French investigator, injected mice with estrogen and produced breast tumors. Subsequent investigation showed that this result required (1) special strains of mice, (2) their infection with a mouse mammary tumor virus, and (3) the presence of prolactin, which was adduced by the fact that the tumors did not appear in hypophysectomized infected animals. Estrogen given to pregnant rodents of several species produced in the offspring a multiplicity of tumors, few of which have any correlates in humans. With this start, the "hormones cause cancer" scare was off and running, and these three words have been embedded in the public consciousness for the past 50 years despite our improved understanding of estrogens as promoters, not proximate carcinogens. For more than 30 years we have had epidemiologic studies, from Bergqvist to Ziel, without a clear resolution of the problem. Recent studies have shown no increased relative risk,[16, 17] and meta-analyses have shown no increased risk or a risk in the region of 1.3 with confidence limits of 1.2 to 1.6,[18] almost exactly the same as the increase in breast cancer risk from obesity.[19] This is clearly not the place to discuss so controversial an issue; the important point is that the public has been thoroughly frightened about ERT without having the breast cancer risk put in perspective. About 4% of women die of breast cancer, and a 30% to 50% increase raises this to 6%. *Fifty* percent of women die of cardiovascular diseases; if ERT reduces the relative risk by half, the proportionate benefit is obvious, and we have not even mentioned the deaths avoided by the prevention of osteoporotic fractures.

The issue that frequently arises is whether to use ERT in a woman who has had or develops breast cancer. Oncologists adamantly aver that ERT should not be used. However, as Creasman[20] has repeatedly pointed out, there are simply *no data* to support the position that estrogens cannot be used. Survival analysis of never users, past users, and current users failed to show statistically significant differences.[21] Nevertheless, medicolegal concerns enter into the decision process. We should engage in a detailed discussion of risks vs. benefits with the patient (along with the spouse or partner, if possible) to ensure that she (or they) are comfortable with their state of knowledge. The patient must then provide a handwritten note of her decision, which will then be followed with regard to the use or nonuse of ERT.

ENDOMETRIAL CARCINOMA.—Endometrial carcinoma is a favorite concern of the estrophobes. There is no question that prolonged, uninterrupted administration of estrogen can lead to endometrial changes that are interpreted as carcinoma. However, the degree of malignancy and prognosis of estrogen-associated endometrial carcinoma is quite different from the spontaneous variety.[22, 23] The late R.B. Greenblatt carried out an interesting study (personal communication) on six women diagnosed as having estrogen-induced endometrial carcinoma on biopsy. Before hysterectomy they were treated intensively with intramuscular progesterone. In none of the surgical specimens could the pathologist find any evidence of malignancy.

It is well established that therapy with progestational agents in sufficient amount and duration prevents hyperplasia and subsequent metamorphosis and is an essential part of ERT regimens in women with uteri. This puts an end to the endometrial carcinoma concern. Statistics such as those of Cauley et al.[24] indicate that 10.9% of women over the age of 64 years take estrogen only, but the proportion who had had a hysterectomy was not stated.

The most important issue is how to administer the progestin to confer protection against adverse endometrial changes. The classic regimens of oral progestin for 10 to 14 days per month serve the purpose but induce monthly bleeding, which at some point becomes an unacceptable inconvenience to many women and is a major cause of discontinuation. In an attempt to solve this problem, some have advocated the initiation of progestin exposure every 3 months instead of at monthly or other intervals. This issue needs further exploration. In perimenopausal women who may ovulate occasionally and are therefore at potential risk of conception, the use of low-dose monophasic oral contraceptives is an important option. For many years, some European and American clinicians have been prescribing two or three 21-day packages back-to-back to produce 49- or 70-day cycles, which are very well accepted.

The classic 25-day estrogen regimen, with its monthly bleeding, is being rapidly replaced by continuous estrogen administration. Instead of the short course of relatively high-dose progestin (10 mg/day of medroxyprogesterone acetate for 10 to 14 days, for example), concomitant continuous progestin at low dosage (2.5 mg medroxyprogesterone acetate or 0.5 to 1.0 mg norethindrone, for example) offers several advantages. For the rare woman who has adverse reactions to progestational compounds, the reduction in dosage may be a solution to the problem. More important, about two thirds of women (after an interval of several months of irregular spotting/bleeding) become amenorrheic, and this is a highly desirable outcome.[25] In the event of a bleeding episode in previously amenorrheic women receiving this regimen, the likelihood is that this is occurring from an atrophic endometrium (which is the characteristic histologic appearance with a continuous/combined regimen), often due to omission of the daily estrogen dose. There are several options. One may continue the regimen and see whether this event recurs, or one may discontinue both agents, allow a menstrual period to occur, and wait a few weeks to see whether there is any further bleeding. If further bleeding does occur, biopsy may be performed with a small-caliber instrument, and/or a transvaginal sonogram may be obtained. (The accuracy and sensitivity of sonographic examination of the endometrium needs further development). Dilatation and curettage (D&C) are not indicated. Physicians who perform endometrial biopsies too freely in these older women are likely to see them go elsewhere for their gynecologic care. Finally, there are a few patients who, for unknown reasons, cannot tolerate progestin therapy in any form. In these instances, estrogen must be withheld at some point to make certain by plasma estrogen determination that there are no significant endogenous sources of estrogen. A transvaginal sonogram will help to determine the thickness of the endometrium, and in due course, ERT may be resumed.

The issue of ERT for the woman who has had endometrial carcinoma is similar to that for breast cancer (see earlier). Again, there are simply no data to justify withholding of ERT.[26]

OSTEOPOROSIS

Osteoporosis is one of the major hazards of estrogen deficiency, whether it be from oophorectomy, "exercise amenorrhea," anorexia nervosa, hypothalamic or hypopituitary hypogonadism, or menopause. Menopause-induced osteoporosis currently affects 35 million American women and in 1988 cost the United States *$27 million a day*. Surely, at a time when spiraling health care costs are a top-priority item on the federal agenda and when an outpouring of publications attests to the potential of various preventive and therapeutic interventions, the use of these interventions should demand our utmost attention. To bring this into a human perspective, there is, in an article on the late General Douglas MacArthur in *National Geographic Magazine*, a full-page color photograph of his widow, fragile of limb and literally bent double by vertebral crush fractures, bravely bemedalling one by one a line of full-dress, ramrod-straight military men. Whoever turns that page without moisture in the eyes is *very* tough.

As is so well summarized by Ettinger et al.,[27] estrogen-dependent bone loss follows a predictable pattern. At first, trabecular bone may be lost at a rate of 5% to 8% and cortical bone at a rate of 1% to 3% annually. After a decade or so of estrogen deficiency this rate slows, but by that time a third to a half of maximum bone mass may have been lost. At this point even minimal trauma will cause radial or vertebral fractures. It is estimated that over half of 50-year-old women will sustain osteoporosis-related fractures during the remainder of their lives. In another decade, the hip fracture rate begins to climb. Twelve percent to 20% of hip fracture patients will die within a year (a prognosis far worse than that of patients with breast cancer), and most of the survivors will require permanent nursing or custodial care.

Since the time of Fuller Albright, type I (postmenopausal) osteoporosis has been distinguished from type II or "senile" osteoporosis (whatever "senile" is supposed to mean). Type II bone loss proceeds at the same rate in elderly men and women. The nature and rank order of the mechanisms responsible for this process are in debate, but it is becoming increasingly clear that many of the elderly population are in a marginal or frankly deficient state of calcium balance and active vitamin D availability, for reasons discussed below.

The various risk factors that predispose to osteoporosis are well known. Another risk factor, overmedication with thyroid hormone, has recently been emphasized.[28] However valuable this knowledge may be epidemiologically or in research stratagems, it should not lead us to make (let alone act upon) risk estimates *in any particular individual*.

LABORATORY WORKUP

For proper evaluation, we have a wealth of diagnostic modalities available. Without doubt, modern radiographic technology has revolutionized the diagnosis and therapeutic supervision of osteoporosis. Dual-energy x-ray densitometry and quantitative computer tomography (CT) have the precision necessary to evaluate the degree of osteoporosis and changes in status over time. Quantitative CT still requires a fairly heavy radiation dosage, which no doubt will decrease with new technology. Single-beam densitometry for certain bones may be adequate. Since bone remodeling is a very slow event, it is rarely necessary (except for investigative purposes) to make measurements more often than every 2 years. Even less frequent monitoring is reasonable in women who enter menopause with good bone mineral density and receive appropriate therapy. Bone densitometry is advisable in every perimenopausal or postmenopausal woman if at all possible. This gives a much more objective basis for planning preventive care than does a list of risk factors. Moreover, the procedure itself has power to improve compliance with the planned regimen, and compliance is certainly one of the major problems in the effective management of menopause. If initial bone density is excellent, the patient should be met with enthusiasm and encouragement to keep it that way; if there are already signs of bone mineral loss, this should be presented to the patient as an incentive for developing lifelong commitment to changes in lifestyle and therapeutic compliance.

The degree of bone mineral activity can be evaluated by standard measurements of serum calcium, phosphate, and alkaline phosphatase. Evaluation with the high-sensitivity thyroid-stimulating hormone (TSH) assay of the level of thyroid activity (especially in women receiving thyroid replacement) is important. Calcium turnover can be roughly assessed by the urinary calcium/creatinine ratio. Bone alkaline phosphatase isoenzyme, ionized serum calcium level, and occasionally, serum protein electrophoresis may be informative in idiopathic osteoporosis. More sophisticated and very useful measures of bone turnover are urinary bone γ-linolenic acid (GLA) protein (osteocalcin) and hydroxyproline excretion. A recently developed assay for pyridinoline and deoxypyridinoline (markers of collagen resorption) correlates with bone resorption as measured by iliac crest bone biopsy.

THERAPEUTIC INTERVENTION

Exercise

Although the harmful effect of physical inactivity on bone mass is well documented, studies of the effect of exercise are less clear cut, leaving aside trials in world-class athletes and the like. Recently, a 1-year walking program (1 hour, four times a week, to 75% to 80% of the measured maximum heart rate), together with an 800-mg/day calcium supplement, prevented a 7% decrease in lumbar spine density seen in sedentary controls, increased femoral-neck density by 2% vs. a loss of 1% in controls receiving moderate calcium intake, but had no effect on distal-radius or total-body calcium[29, 30] in a study of women with a mean age of 82 years; it was found that even very mild activity slowed bone loss and resulted in accretion over a 3-year period. Aloia et al.[31] found that exercise was helpful in retarding bone loss even in the acute stage of postmenopausal loss.

In addition to the stimulant effect on bone itself, exercise is highly important in maintaining muscle strength and consequently equilibrium, thereby lessening the tendency to falling. Finally, exercise of adequate intensity will produce release of endorphins and a feeling of well being that may be of considerable psychological importance.

Calcium and Vitamin D

It is well established that bone mineral loss starts in the early or mid 40s in women, accelerates during menopause, and continues at a slower rate into old age. The efficiency of intestinal calcium absorption declines by about 40% from age 20 to age 80 in spite of increasing levels of parathyroid hormone. There is evidence that most Americans in the postmenopausal years have a marginal or inadequate calcium intake. Additionally, low vitamin D intake and lessened exposure to sun cause levels of vitamin D to decrease,[32] a phenomenon most apparent in women with osteoporosis. The low levels of vitamin D tend to increase parathyroid hormone levels and produce a secondary hyperparathyroidism and consequent decrease in vertebral bone density.[33] The American diet is also relatively high in phosphate and sodium, both of which tend to increase renal calcium loss. Lactose intolerance and low-cholesterol, low-calorie diets tend to limit calcium intake. Further, with increasing age the efficiency of calcium absorption at low intake levels is decreased. There is additionally an age- and estrogen deficiency–related decrease in formation of the active vitamin D metabolite calcitriol, either because of a decreased response of renal vitamin D 1α-hydroxylase to the stimulus of parathyroid hormone[34] due in part to the estrogen deficiency or because there may be an increased intestinal resistance to the action of 1,25-dihydroxyvitamin D.[35] However, Riggs and Nelson[36] feel that insufficient endogenous production of calcitriol is the major cause of decreased calcium absorption in postmenopausal women.

The addition of calcium to the diet, at least 1,000 to 1,500 mg of elemental calcium per day, is recommended.[37] However, in the early menopausal years calcium replacement alone does not retard bone loss[38, 39] as it does in later years.[37] Although calcium carbonate has the highest calcium content per unit weight, it may be poorly absorbed by the 10% or so of older people who have achlorhydria.[40] Calcium citrate shows 20% to 60% better absorption[39]; the citrate may also exert some anti–nephrolith-forming activity.

Vitamin D enhances calcium absorption, stimulates matrix formation, and increases osteoclast activity. A dose of 50,000 units every 15 to 30 days is recommended; this presumes that despite any enzymatic derangements, enough calcitriol will be generated. In recent years, the use of calcitriol itself has been recommended at a total daily dose of about 0.6 to 0.8 μg in two or three divided doses.[41, 42] Aside from the inconvenience of such multiple dosage, which is likely to produce problems with compliance, close monitoring to prevent hypercalcemia is required. Daily urinary calcium excretion should be maintained at less than 400 mg/day. Some investigators have found that such therapy, over the long term, decreases the vertebral fracture rate, whereas others have not.[43]

Franz[44] has raised the issue of the role of magnesium deficiency in causing osteoporosis; Silverberg et al.[45] do not concur with this hypothesis, but point out that virtually nothing is known about how dietary magnesium may protect against bone loss, if indeed it does. The possibility that boron may also be important in osteoporosis has also been raised.[46, 47]

Estrogen

Estrogen, by inhibiting bone resorption, reduces bone loss at all skeletal sites.[48] The effect persists as long as the estrogen deficiency is corrected, and bone loss accelerates promptly once estrogen replacement is stopped. Estrogen replacement is therefore a lifetime intervention. The classic randomized crossover studies of Christiansen et al.[49, 50] showed that estrogen/progestin therapy in early menopause not only maintained bone mineral density but actually increased it, in contrast to immediate and progressive loss in the placebo group. Positive effects of estrogen have been demonstrated in women at least to the age of 70.

The response of bone to estrogen is related to dose (and duration).[27] Several studies have shown that less than 0.625 mg of conjugated equine estrogen is ineffective (although the patient numbers per age group are small); unfortunately this has been taken to mean that this dose is adequate in general.[51] On the one hand, very elderly women may not tolerate this dose because of mastalgia and other side effects, and we do not know whether their increased sensitivity in these parameters is or is not reflected in the responsiveness of their bones. On the other hand, an understanding of the pharmacology of estrogens as substances that undergo enterohepatic recycling clearly indicates that there will be a very large interindividual variability in response, and there is no reason to believe that bone response will be an exception. Quigley et al.[52] showed that 0.625 mg of conjugated equine estrogen is approximately equivalent to 1 mg of micronized estradiol; both retarded the rate of bone loss by about two thirds regardless of age. Lindsay et al.[51] found no difference between 0.625- and 1.25-mg conjugated equine estrogen doses, but the number of subjects per group was not stated, and in any event the statistical sensitivity of the study was very poor. Mandel et al.[53] found the action of 10 µg of ethinyl estradiol to be equivalent to 1.25 mg of conjugated equine estrogens, whereas Horsman et al.[54] did not find a net gain of bone at doses below 25 µg ethinyl estradiol, at which level there was significant improvement, including endosteal bone improvement. Estrogen given vaginally or transdermally achieves significant blood levels, and when estradiol is the administered agent, blood assays are a convenient way to assess the adequacy of the delivery system. Vaginal estradiol cream (2 g), for example, produces plasma estradiol levels of about 60 ± 20 pg/mL at 12 hours and remains in this same range after 15 days' use.[55] Although progestin therapy is recommended primarily for endometrial protection, it has significant effects on bone mineral density. Lobo et al.[56] in a study of urinary calcium parameters found 150 mg of medroxyprogesterone acetate (Depo-Provera) every 3 months to have an effect equivalent to 0.625 mg of conjugated equine estrogens daily. Mandel et al.[57] found 20 mg of oral medroxyprogesterone acetate (which was much more potent than megestrol acetate) to have a positive effect on urinary calcium parameters, whereas Gallagher et al.[58] and McNeeley et al.[59] found it merely to be synergistic with administered estrogen. Christiansen et al.[60] had earlier found that progestins alone may prevent bone loss without reducing bone resorption (i.e., by increasing formation) and that this action was synergistic with estrogen. Others have used 1 mg norethindrone as the progestin with apparently similar results. Many studies using transdermal estradiol delivery with cyclic progestin addition have documented the effectiveness of this route of administration on bone turnover.[61]

Fluoride

Sodium fluoride has been repeatedly shown to increase bone mineral density in the lumbar spine in at least 70% of patients taking this compound.[62] This is accomplished by direct induction of bone formation (osteoblastic stimulation) along the quiescent bone surface, bypassing the normal resorption/formation remodeling sequence. The lack of resorption is attributed to the greater resistance of fluoride-treated bone to mineral dissolution. It has been shown that concomitant calcium and vitamin D supplementation is necessary to avoid secondary hyperparathyroidism and osteomalacia. No diminution of effectiveness occurs for at least 4 and possibly for 10 or more years of treatment. For unknown reasons, about 20% to 35% of patients do not respond.[63] The effect of fluoride on the appendicular skeleton is unclear. Current evidence is contradictory, with some studies showing improvement[64] or no effect and others claiming an accelerated rate of cortical bone loss and hip fracture.[65] The Mayo

Clinic study,[66] using 60 to 90 mg on alternate days with 1,500 mg of calcium daily, found cumulative increases of 35% for the lumbar spine and 12% for the femoral neck, and a 4% reduction in the radial shaft. The 15% reduction in new crush fractures in the fluoride-treated group did not attain statistical significance. The Henry Ford study[67] used the same fluoride regimen but did not find a difference in the new vertebral fracture rate after 4 years of therapy.

A considerable number of European countries have approved the use of fluoride. A 1988 consensus report by Heaney et al.[68] based on the world literature concluded that fluoride was an effective treatment for osteoporosis because it improved bone mass and reduced the incidence of spinal fractures.

Oral fluoride therapy is associated with significant side effects, chiefly gastrointestinal, in up to 30% of patients. These can be minimized with enteric-coated preparations or slow-release formulations.[69] Transient lower extremity pain syndrome may occur in up to 50% of patients; fluoride therapy but not calcium supplementation should be temporarily interrupted. The therapeutic window of plasma fluoride concentration should be maintained at 95 to 180 ng/mL (25 mg of slow-release formulation twice daily), and treatment should be continued for 1 to 2 years before a significant decrease in vertebral crush fractures can be expected.

One study[70] examined the concomitant effect of fluoride and estrogen. Vertebral density increased 3.2% with fluoride and 7.3% with added estrogen. However, a decrease in femoral neck density was seen with both regimens.

Calcitonin

There is substantial literature on calcitonin and its use in osteoporosis.[71] In the United States it is available as an injectable (salmon calcitonin [Calcimar], human calcitonin [Cibacalcin]). Elsewhere, a nasal spray of salmon calcitonin is also available.[72] Calcitonin inhibits osteoclasts,[73] which serves to lower serum calcium levels (thus at least 1,000 mg of elemental calcium should be used during treatment), which in turn increases parathyroid hormone production, which in turn stimulates the synthesis of calcitriol with resultant improvement in intestinal calcium absorption. Since calcitonin itself inhibits gastric acid secretion, which is necessary for the absorption of calcium carbonate, it is best injected at bedtime. Calcium is given with meals. Recent studies with a reduced dosage of calcitonin (120 units/wk instead of 50 to 100 units/day) together with large doses of vitamin D (150,000 units/wk) over a period of 2 to 6 years seemed to overcome the usual plateauing of the beneficial calcitonin effect at 18 to 24 months.[74] There was increased trabecular bone mass and no decrease in cortical bone mass, and possible calcitonin nonresponders (i.e., low-turnover osteoporosis) became responders.

Subcutaneous calcitonin at 100 units/day (optimum dosage regimens have not been worked out) produces an increase in bone calcium of about 1.5% per year (vs. continuing loss in controls), although values ranging from 2.3% to 13% have been reported.[71] It is important to note that increases in femoral and radial bone density as well as improvements in vertebral trabecular bone were observed. However, only high-turnover osteoporosis (as determined by urinary GLA-protein or hydroxyproline excretion) seems to be improved; this represents perhaps one third of cases of osteoporosis.[75] Macintyre et al.[76] studied the effect of percutaneous estrogen/progestin therapy with and without added calcitonin and observed no change from addition of the latter over a 2-year period.

Calcitonin treatment is especially useful in women who cannot or will not take estrogen and is noteworthy for its effect on bone pain, which begins to improve by the second week of calcitonin therapy. Indeed, one of the causes of compliance failure is the disappearance of pain, whereupon the patient often discontinues injection therapy. In patients receiving glucocorticoid therapy (for rheumatoid arthritis, for example) drug-induced bone loss may be curtailed, and the added alleviation of pain (by stimulation of β-endorphin production by calcitonin) may permit a reduction in glucocorticoid dosage.

The side effects of calcitonin are not insignificant. Pain at the site of injection may be minimized by subcutaneous rather than intramuscular injection. Gastrointestinal (nausea, vomiting) and vascular (flushing) symptoms may occur in 10% to 20% of patients, although these symptoms will be mitigated with time. Diuresis may occur in 10% of patients. Finally, the cost of the medication is not insignificant.

Biphosphonates

The effectiveness of this class of compounds in Paget's disease naturally directed attention to the possibility of affecting the bone remodeling cycle[77, 78] to prevent or reverse the changes of osteoporosis. Biphosphonates are poorly absorbed—1% at 5 mg/kg to 6% at 20 mg/kg (this is a promising area for improvement for an expensive drug)—and excreted unchanged. Biphosphonates (the only one currently available in the United States is etidronate) adsorb to the mineralizing surface of bone, especially to active turnover areas, and exert physicochemical effects that disrupt crystal growth of new hydroxyapatite. They also affect nearby cells by inactivating osteoclasts involved in bone remodeling.[79] The first attempt to influence and synchronize areas of bone remodeling involved a cyclic regimen comprised of three steps: (1) Withhold calcium and supply a high phosphate load for several days to stimulate parathyroid hormone secretion and to activate osteoblasts; (2) administer biphosphonate, calcium, and vitamin D for 14 days to inhibit resorption; and (3) follow with calcium/vitamin D for a period of 3 months to uncouple osteoblastic and osteoclastic activity, with the latter under prolonged inhibition. This three-step cycle would then be repeated. Subsequent studies[80] showed no apparent benefit of the initial high-phosphate phase.

The results of this therapy are at present controversial. Storm et al.[81] observed a significant increase in vertebral bone mineral and a decrease in the vertebral fracture rate after 150 weeks of etidronate therapy. Papapoulos et al.[79] found an increase in trabecular bone over a period of 3 years, stabilization for 2 years, and a decreased vertebral fracture rate. Smith et al.[82] studied bone turnover in women undergoing surgical menopause and found that daily etidronate suppressed the changes initiated by acute estrogen withdrawal. On the other hand, Pacifici et al.[83] found that etidronate was less effective than estrogen/progestin therapy on vertebral bone and did not prevent axial bone loss. Biphosphonates may be particularly useful in glucocorticoid-associated bone loss. Availability of other biphosphonates and further studies make this a promising area for improvement in the treatment of osteoporosis. When estrogen therapy cannot be used, this modality with its absence of toxicity certainly commends itself.

Thiazides

In 1986 Wasnich et al.[84] reported that thiazides (typically, 25 mg of hydrochlorothiazide) diminished bone resorption. The effect at four bone sites was similar to that of estrogen, and users of both together had the highest bone mineral content levels.

Androgens, Anabolic Steroids, and Progestins

In determining peak trabecular bone density in young adulthood, androgens exert a significant effect.[85] Androgen levels decline after menopause, and their anabolic effect is diminished or lost. Efforts to dissociate the androgenic from the anabolic effect have produced a number of compounds such as stanozolol or ORG OD-14, which have been examined briefly for their potential in osteoporosis,[86, 87] but careful prospective trials and evaluations of toxicity remain to be carried out. Several studies of nandrolone decanoate are in progress.[88] Many progestational compounds (17-hydroxyprogestrone caproate, norethindrone, medroxyprogesterone acetate) decrease urinary calcium excretion and thus may have some positive bone effects, but no systematic evaluation is available. Greco et al.[89] examined acute changes in calcium metabolism induced by 200 mg of Depo-Provera in patients with glucocorticoid-induced osteoporosis and found that changes in osteocalcin, skeletal alkaline phosphatase, and calcitonin indicated a stimulation of osteoblastic activity. Concern (probably unjustified) about the effect of progestins on the lipid profile has dampened investigative enthusiasm.

Antiestrogens

Current management of breast cancer includes the use of antiestrogens such as tamoxifen (clomiphene is another antiestrogen). Large numbers of women are therefore going to be exposed to these agents, whether or not they have endogenous estrogen production. In 1984 Beall et al.[90] reported a protective effect of clomiphene against osteoporosis in experimental animals, which was subsequently confirmed by Stewart and Stern.[91] A preliminary clinical trial[92] observed a reduction in bone turnover by measurement of serum osteocalcin and a decrease in bone loss as measured by densitometry. Future research with these mixed estrogen agonists/antagonists may turn out to be very important.

SUMMARY

It is necessary to have an operational perspective on the condition of menopause, viewing it as a persistent deficiency which produces subjective and objective symptomatology and in the long run accelerates atherogenic cardiovascular disease and osteopenia, both of which can shorten life expectancy. The basic philosophy and practical details of replacement therapy are discussed, together with important nonhormonal interventions. As in many other situations, *prevention* of the complications of long-term estrogen deficiency is the optimum approach. The benefit/risk evaluation of estrogen replacement therapy must be made and shared clearly with the intended recipient.

REFERENCES

1. Semmens JP, Tsai JCC, Semmens EC, et al: Effects of estrogen therapy in vaginal physiology during menopause. *Obstet Gynecol* 1985; 66:15–18.
2. Martin PL, Yen SSC, Burnier AM, et al: Systemic absorption and sustained effects of vaginal estrogen creams. *JAMA* 1979; 242:2699–2700.
3. Young RL, Goepfert AR, Goldzieher JW: Estrogen replacement therapy is not conductive of venous thromboembolism. *Maturitas* 1991; 13:189–192.
4. Devor M, Barrett-Connor E, Renvall M, et al: Estrogen replacement therapy and the risk of venous thrombosis. *Am J Med* 1992; 92:275–282.
5. Mammen EF: Oral contraceptives and blood coagulation: A critical review. *Am J Obstet Gynecol* 1982; 142:781–790.
6. Petitti DB, Perlamn JA, Sidney S: Noncontraceptive estrogens and mortality: Long-term follow-up of women in the Walnut Creek Study. *Obstet Gynecol* 1987; 70:289–293.
7. Bush TL, Barrett-Connor E, Cowan LD, et al: Cardiovascular mortality and noncontraceptive use of estrogen in women: Results from the Lipid Research Clinics Program Follow-up Study. *Circulation* 1987; 75:1102–1109.
8. Henderson BE, Paganini-Hill A, Ross RK: Decreased mortality in users of estrogen replacement therapy. *Arch Int Med* 1991; 151:75–78.
9. Sullivan JM, Vander Zwaag R, Lemp GF, et al: Postmenopausal estrogen use and coronary atherosclerosis. *Ann Intern Med* 1988; 108:358–363.
10. Sullivan JM, Vander Zwaag R, Hughes JP, et al: Estrogen replacement and coronary artery disease. *Arch Intern Med* 1990; 150:2557–2562.
11. Hong MK, Romm PA, Reagan K, et al: Effects of estrogen replacement therapy on serum lipid values and angiographically defined coronary artery disease in postmenopausal women. *Am J Cardiol* 1992; 69:176–178.
12. Goldman L, Tosteson ANA: Uncertainty about postmenopausal estrogen. *N Engl J Med* 1991; 325:800–802.
13. Wagner JD, Clarkson TB, St. Clair RW, et al: Estrogen and progesterone replacement therapy reduces low density lipoprotein accumulation in the coronary arteries of surgically postmenopausal cynomolgus monkeys. *J Clin Invest* 1991; 88:1995–2002.
14. Wagner JD, St. Clair RW, Schwenke DC, et al: Regional differences in arterial low density lipoprotein metabolism in surgically postmenopausal cynomolgus monkeys. *Arterioscler Thromb* 1992; 12:717–726.
15. Williams JK, Adams MR, Klopfenstein HS: Estrogen replacement modulates constrictor responses of atherosclerotic (AS) coronary arteries in vivo. *Circulation* 1988; 78(Suppl 2):45.
16. Wingo PA, Layde PM, Lee NC, et al: The risk of breast cancer in postmenopausal women who have used estrogen replacement therapy. *JAMA* 1987; 257:209–215.
17. Palmer JR, Rosenberg L, Clarke EA, et al: Breast cancer risk after estrogen replacement therapy: Results from the Toronto Breast Cancer Study. *Am J Epidemiol* 1991; 134:1386–1395.
18. Steinberg KK, Thacker SB, Smith SJ, et al: A meta-analysis of the effect of estrogen replacement therapy on the risk of breast cancer. *JAMA* 1991; 265:1985–1990.

19. Harris RE, Namboodire KK, Wynder EL: Breast cancer risk: Effects of estrogen replacement therapy and body mass. *J Natl Cancer Inst* 1992; 84:1575–1582.

20. Creasman WT: Estrogen replacement therapy: Is previously treated cancer a contraindication? *Obstet Gynecol* 1991; 77:308–312.

21. Strickland DM, Gambrell D Jr, Butzin CA, et al: The relationship between breast cancer survival and prior postmenopausal estrogen use. *Obstet Gynecol* 1992; 80:400–404.

22. Chu J, Schweid AI, Weiss NS: Survival among women with endometrial cancer: A comparison of estrogen users and nonusers. *Am J Obstet Gynecol* 1982; 143:569–573.

23. Collins J, Allen LH, Donner A, et al: Oestrogen use and survival in endometrial cancer. *Lancet* 1980; 2:961–963.

24. Cauley JA, Cummings SR, Black DM, et al: Prevalence and determinants of estrogen replacement therapy in elderly women. *Am J Obstet Gynecol* 1990; 163:1438–1444.

25. Leather AT, Studd JWW: Can the withdrawal bleed following oestrogen replacement therapy be avoided? *Br J Obstet Gynaecol* 1990; 97:1071–1079.

26. Creasman WT, Henderson D, Hinshaw W, et al: Estrogen replacement therapy in the patient treated for endometrial cancer. *Obstet Gynecol* 1986; 67:326–330.

27. Ettinger B, Genant HK, Cann CE: Long term estrogen replacement therapy prevents bone loss and fractures. *Ann Intern Med* 1985; 102:319–324.

28. Wartofsky L: Osteoporosis: A growing concern for the thyroidologist. *Thyroid Today* 1988; 11:1–11.

29. Nelson ME, Fisher EC, Dilmanina FA, et al: A 1-yr walking program and increased dietary calcium in postmenopausal women: Effects on bone. *Am J Clin Nutr* 1991; 53:1304–1311.

30. Smith EL, Reddan W: Physical activity—a modality for bone accretion in the aged. *Am J Radiol* 1976; 126:1297.

31. Aloia JF, Cohn SH, Ostuni JA, et al: Prevention of involutional bone loss by exercise. *Ann Intern Med* 1978; 89:356–358.

32. Francis RM, Peacock M, Storer JH, et al: Calcium malabsorption in the elderly: The effect of treatment with oral 25-hydroxyvitamin D_3. *Eur J Clin Invest* 1983; 13:391–396.

33. Villareal DT, Civitelli R, Chines A, et al: Subclinical vitamin D deficiency in postmenopausal women with low vertebral bone mass. *J Clin Endocrinol Metab* 1991; 72:628–634.

34. Slovik DM, Adams JS, Neer RM, et al: Deficiency production of 1,25-dihydroxyvitamin D in elderly osteoporotic patients. *N Engl J Med* 1981; 305:372–374.

35. Gennari C, Agnusdei D, Nardi P, et al: Estrogen preserves a normal intestinal responsiveness to 1,25 dihydroxyvitamin D_3 in oophorectomized women. *J Clin Endocrinol Metab* 1990; 71:1288–1293.

36. Riggs BL, Nelson KI: Effect of long term treatment with calcitriol on calcium absorption and mineral metabolism in postmenopausal osteoporosis. *J Clin Endocrinol Metab* 1985; 61:457–461.

37. Dawson-Hughes B, Dallal GE, Krall EA, et al: A controlled trial of the effect of calcium supplementation on bone density in postmenopausal women. *N Engl J Med* 1990; 323:878–883.

38. Ettinger B, Genant HK, Cann CE: Postmenopausal bone loss is prevented by treatment with low-dosage estrogen with calcium. *Ann Intern Med* 1987; 106:40–45.

39. Nicar MJ, Pak CYC: Calcium bioavailability from calcium carbonate and calcium citrate. *J Clin Endocrinol Metab* 1985; 61:391–393.

40. Recker RR: Calcium absorption and achlorhydria. *N Engl J Med* 1985; 313:70–73.

41. Gallagher JC, Goldgar D: Treatment of postmenopausal osteoporosis with high doses of synthetic calcitriol. *Ann Intern Med* 1990; 113:649–655.

42. Aloia JF: Role of calcitriol in the treatment of postmenopausal osteoporosis. *Metabolism* 1990; 39:35–38.

43. Gallagher JC, Jerpbak CM, Jee WSS, et al: 1,25 dihydroxyvitamin D: Short- and long-term effects on bone and calcium metabolism in patients with postmenopausal osteoporosis. *Proc Natl Acad Sci U S A* 1982; 79:3325.

44. Franz KB: Abnormalities in parathyroid hormone secretion and 1,25-dihydroxyvitamin D_3 formation in women with osteoporosis. *N Engl J Med* 1989; 320:1697–1698.

45. Silverberg SJ, Shane E, de la Cruz L, et al: Reply to the editor. *N Engl J Med* 1989; 320:1698.

46. Nielsen FH: Boron—an overlooked element of potential nutritional importance. *Nutr Today* 1988; 1:4–7.

47. Nielsen FH, Hunt CD, Mullen LM, et al: Effect of dietary boron on mineral, estrogen and testosterone metabolism in postmenopausal women. *FASEB J* 1987; 1:;394–397.

48. Ettinger B: Prevention of osteoporosis: Treatment of estradiol deficiency. *Obstet Gynecol* 1988; 72(suppl):12–17.

49. Christiansen C, Christensen MS, McNair P, et al: Prevention of early postmenopausal bone loss: Controlled 2-year study in 315 normal females. *Eur J Clin Invest* 1980; 10:273.

50. Christiansen C, Christensen MS, Transbol I: Bone mass in postmenopausal women after withdrawal of oestrogen/progestogen replacement therapy. *Lancet* 1981; 1:459.

51. Lindsay R, Hart DM, Clark DM: The minimum effective dose of estrogen for prevention of postmenopausal bone loss. *Obstet Gynecol* 1984; 63:759–763.

52. Quigley MET, Martin PL, Burnier AM, et al: Estrogen therapy arrests bone loss in elderly women. *Am J Obstet Gynecol* 1987; 156:1516–1523.

53. Mandel FP, Geola FL, Lu JKH, et al: Biologic effects of various doses of ethinyl estradiol in postmenopausal women. *Obstet Gynecol* 1982; 59:673–679.

54. Horsman A, Jones M, Francis R, et al: The effect of estrogen dose on postmenopausal bone loss. *N Engl J Med* 1983; 309:1405–1407.

55. Martin PL, Yen SSC, Burnier A, et al: Systemic absorption and sustained effects of vaginal estrogen creams. *JAMA* 1979: 242:2699–2700.

56. Lobo RA, McCormick W, Singer F, et al: Depo-medroxyprogesterone acetate compared with conjugated estrogens for the treatment of postmenopausal women. *Obstet Gynecol* 1984; 63:1–5.

57. Mandel FP, Davidson BJ, Erlik Y, et al: Effects of progestins on bone metabolism in postmenopausal women. *J Reprod Med* 1982; 27:511–514.

58. Gallagher JC, Kable WT, Goldgar G: Effect of progestin therapy on cortical and trabecular bone: Comparison with estrogen. *Am J Med* 1991; 90:171–178.

59. McNeeley SG Jr, Schinfeld JS, Stovall TG, et al: Prevention of osteoporosis by medroxyprogesterone acetate in postmenopausal women. *Int J Gynaecol Obstet* 1991; 34:253–256.

60. Christiansen C, Nilas L, Riis BJ, et al: Uncoupling of bone formation and resorption by combined oestrogen and progestagen therapy in postmenopausal osteoporosis. *Lancet* 1985; 2:800–801.

61. Lufkin EG, Wahner HW, O'Fallon WM, et al: Treatment of postmenopausal osteoporosis with transdermal estrogen. *Ann Intern Med* 1992; 117:1–9.

62. Kleerekoper M, Balena R: Fluorides and osteoporosis. *Annu Rev Nutr* 1991; 11:309–324.

63. Pitt P, Berry H: Fluoride treatment in osteoporosis. *Postgrad Med J* 1991; 67:323–326.

64. Dure-Smith BA, Kraenzlin ME, Farley SM, et al: Fluoride therapy for osteoporosis: A review of dose-response, duration of treatment, and skeletal sites of action. *Calcif Tissue Int* 1991; 49(suppl):64–67.

65. Hedlund RL, Gallagher JC: Increased incidence of hip fracture in osteoporotic women treated with sodium fluoride. *J Bone Miner Res* 1989; 4:223–225.

66. Riggs BL, Hodgson SF, O'Fallon WM, et al: Effect of fluoride treatment on the fracture rate in postmenopausal osteoporosis. *N Engl J Med* 1990; 320:802–809.

67. Kleerekoper M, Peterson E, Phillips E, et al: Continuous sodium fluoride therapy does not reduce vertebral fracture rate in postmenopausal women. *J Bone Miner Res* 1989; 4(suppl):376.

68. Heaney RP, Baylink DJ, Johnston CC Jr, et al: Fluoride therapy for the vertebral crush fracture syndrome: A status report. *Ann Intern Med* 1989; 111:678–680.

69. Pak CYC, Sakhaee K, et al: Attainment of therapeutic fluoride levels in serum without major side effects using a slow-release preparation of sodium fluoride in postmenopausal osteoporosis. *J Bone Miner Res* 1986; 1:563–571.

70. Raymakers JA, Van Pijke CF, Hoekstra A, et al: Monitoring fluoride therapy in osteoporosis by dual photon absorptiometry. *Bone* 1987; 8:143–148.

71. McDermott MT, Kidd GS: The role of calcitonin in the development and treatment of osteoporosis. *Endocrinol Rev* 1987; 8:377–390.

72. Overgaard K, Riis BJ, Christiansen C, et al: Nasal calcitonin for treatment of established osteoporosis. *Clin Endocrinol* 1989; 30:435–442.

73. Gruber HE, Ivey JL, Baylink DJ, et al: Long-term calcitonin therapy in postmenopausal osteoporosis. *Metabolism* 1984; 33:295–303.

74. Palmieri GMA, Pitcock JA, Brown P, et al: Effect of calcitonin and vitamin D in osteoporosis. *Calcif Tissue Int* 1989; 45:137–141.

75. Civitelli R, Gonnelli S, Zacchei F, et al: Bone turnover in postmenopausal osteoporosis. Effect of calcitonin treatment. *J Clin Invest* 1988; 82:1268–1274.

76. Macintyre M, Whitehead L, Banks LM, et al: Calcitonin for prevention of postmenopausal bone loss. *Lancet* 1988; 1:900.

77. Canalis E: The hormonal and local regulation of bone formation. *Endocrinol Rev* 1983; 4:62–77.

78. Raisz LG: Local and systemic factors in the pathogenesis of osteoporosis. *N Engl J Med* 1988; 318:818–828.

79. Papapoulos SE, Landman JO, Bijvoet OLM, et al: The use of biphosphonates in the treatment of osteoporosis. *Bone* 1992; 13(suppl):41–49.

80. Steiniche T, Hasling C, Charles P, et al: The effect of etidronate on trabecular bone remodeling in postmenopausal spinal osteoporosis: A randomized study comparing intermittent treatment and an ADFR regimen. *Bone* 1991; 12:155–163.

81. Storm T, Thamsborg G, Steiniche T, et al: Effect of intermittent cyclical etidronate therapy on bone mass and fracture rate in women with postmenopausal osteoporosis. *N Engl J Med* 1990; 322:1265.

82. Smith ML, Fogelman I, Hart DM, et al: Effect of etidronate disodium on bone turnover following surgical menopause. *Calcif Tissue Int* 1989; 44:74–79.

83. Pacifici R, McMurtry C, Vered I, et al: Coherence therapy does not prevent axial bone loss in osteoporotic women: A preliminary comparative study. *J Clin Endocrinol Metab* 1988; 66:747.

84. Wasnich RD, Ross PD, Heilbrun LK, et al: Differential effects of thiazide and estrogen upon bone mineral content and fracture prevalence. *Obstet Gynecol* 1986; 67:457–462.

85. Buchanan JR, Myers C, Lloyd T, et al: Determinants of peak trabecular bone

density in women: The role of androgens, estrogen and exercise. *J Bone Miner Res* 1988; 3:673–680.

86. Chesnut CH, Ivey JL, Gruber HE, et al: Stanozolol in postmenopausal osteoporosis: Therapeutic efficacy and possible mechanism of action. *Metabolism* 1983; 32:571–580.

87. Vaishnav R, Beresford JN, Gallagher JA, et al: Effects of the anabolic steroid stanozolol on cells derived from human bone. *Clin Sci* 1988; 74:455–460.

88. Gennari C, Agnusdei D, Gonnelli S, et al: Effects of nandrolone decanoate therapy on bone mass and calcium metabolism in women with established postmenopausal osteoporosis: A double-blind placebo-controlled study. *Maturitas* 1989; 11:187–197.

89. Greco EO, Simmons R, Baylink DJ, et al: Effects of medroxyprogesterone acetate on some parameters of calcium metabolism in patients with glucocorticoid-induced osteoporosis. *Bone Miner* 1991; 13:153–161.

90. Beall PT, Misra LK, Young RL, et al: Clomiphene protects against osteoporosis in the mature ovariectomized rat. *Calcif Tissue Int* 1984; 36:123.

91. Stewart PJ, Stern PH: Effects of the antiestrogens tamoxifen and clomiphene on bone resorption in vitro. *Endocrinology* 1986; 118:125–131.

92. Mazess RB, Barden HS, Love RR, et al: Tamoxifen reduces bone loss in women with breast cancer. Presented at the Third International Symposium on Osteoporosis, Copenhagen, October 1990.

Editor's Comment

Dr. Goldzieher has given us a unique discussion on the management of the menopausal patient. He delivers with great insight the philosophy of caring for the whole patient and urges us not to focus on individual areas such as vasomotor instability or osteoporosis.

The discussion on androgens and their significance for well-being is to the point. The warning issued in this section is important, especially when providing care for the patient who has had an oophorectomy. He points out that when managing the patient with decreased libido, the entire answer does not reside in the prescription of testosterone alone. Testosterone may be of benefit but should be used in conjunction with proper counseling.

This philosophy is carried through on the discussion of estrogen replacement therapy. The reader is encouraged to understand that the many different tissues of the body requiring estrogen do not all have similar dosage requirements. The physician must evaluate the dosage employed for each patient with regard to this widespread effect of estrogen. It is important to remember that along with the beneficial effects there may be unwanted effects such as breast tenderness, water retention, weight gain, etc. The point is that patients of differing ages may have differing dosage requirements.

Dr. Goldzieher briefly and matter-of-factly puts to rest the concern of estrogen causing thromboembolic disease. He is not suggesting that an individual who has experienced repeated thromboembolic episodes receive estrogen replacement therapy. The discussion does summarize the literature on the benefits of estrogen as it protects against atherogenic cardiovascular disease. The significance of the relationship of estrogen and its protective effect against coronary atheromatosis should not be lost in the debate over the effect of progestins on lipoproteins.

The relationship of estrogen to breast cancer is discussed and the pertinent literature capsulized. This is an important discussion because it underscores the fact that estrogen replacement therapy need not be withheld from the patient who has had breast cancer. No solution is offered to this dilemma, but a technique in management is given.

Osteoporosis has a variety of etiologies and is not due solely to estrogen deficiency secondary to oophorectomy or menopause. In fact, "exercise amenorrhea" may play a significant role as more and more women undertake rigid exercise routines. Osteoporosis is a major problem worldwide with respect to morbidity, quality of life, and costs. There is a good discussion on the laboratory tests available and their usage in prevention and management of osteoporosis. The author explains simple treatment regimens to prevent osteoporosis. There is a more-than-adequate discussion on various estrogens and inhibition of bone reabsorption.

Sebastian Faro, M.D., Ph.D.

The Role of Gonadotropin-Releasing Hormone Agonists in Gynecology

R. IAN HARDY, M.D., Ph.D.

ANDREW J. FRIEDMAN, M.D.

G onadotropin-releasing hormone (GnRH) agonists have become one of the most versatile classes of drugs for gynecologic disorders since oral contraceptives were introduced in 1960. In order to understand how GnRH agonists may be used to treat various disorders, one must have a knowledge of their pharmacology and mechanism of action. This chapter will review the physiology and the pharmacology of GnRH agonists and discuss the multitude of clinical uses for this new class of drugs. Because GnRH antagonists are not yet commercially available for gynecologic disorders, the clinical applications for GnRH agonists will not be addressed.

BIOCHEMISTRY, PHARMACOLOGY, AND DRUG INFORMATION

Gonadotropin-releasing hormone is a hypothalamic decapeptide that stimulates the release of gonadotropic hormones from the anterior lobe of the pituitary gland. The amino acid sequence and synthesis of porcine GnRH were first reported by Matsuo et al.[1] in 1971. Independently, Burgus et al.[2] characterized ovine GnRH and found the sequence to be identical with that of porcine GnRH. The structure of the decapeptide Glu-His-Trp-Ser-Tyr-Gly-Leu-Arg-Pro-Gly-NH$_2$, is common to all mammalian species that have been investigated. Since 1971, more than 2,000 analogues of GnRH have been synthesized.[3] A list of some of the commonly used GnRH agonists and their relative potencies is presented in Table 1.

STRUCTURE AND ACTIVITY

A simple understanding of the chemical structure of GnRH is useful to appreciate its physiologic activity. Modifications of this structure have produced numerous analogues with different half-lives, binding affinities, and intrinsic activity. The GnRH molecule assumes a hairpin configuration that leaves amino acids 5 to 6 and 6 to 7 vulnerable to cleavage by pituitary peptidases (Fig 1). Mechanisms for rapid inactivation are important for regulation of any circulating hormone. Peptidases account for the short 2- to 8-minute half-life of GnRH. By inserting a D-amino acid in position 6, protection from degradation is provided, and potency is mark-

TABLE 1.
Dose, Route of Administration, Potency, and Structure of Gonadotropin-Releasing Hormone Agonists Available Worldwide*

Agonist	Structure	Route	Dose (mg)	Potency (GnRH = 1)
Leuprorelin	D-Leu^6, Pro^9-NHEt	Subcutaneous	0.5–1.0	15–100
		Intramuscular, depot	3.75–7.5†	
Buserelin	D-Ser(Bu)^6, Pro^9-NHEt	Subcutaneous	0.2	100
		Intranasal	0.9–1.2	
Histrelin	D-His(Bz)^6, Pro^9-NHEt	Subcutaneous	0.1	100
Nafarelin	D-[Na(2)^6]	Intranasal	0.4–0.8	200
Triptorelin	D-Trp^6	Intramuscular, polymer	2–4†	100
Goserelin	D-Ser(tBu)^6, aza-Gly^{10}	Subcutaneous, implant	3.6†	230

*From Dawood MY: *Am J Obstet Gynecol* 1993; 168:679. Used by permission.
†Monthly.

edly enhanced.[4] A second cleavage site is present between amino acids 9 and 10. By removing the tenth amino acid (glycine) and terminating the ninth amino acid (proline) with an ethylamide moiety, potency is further enhanced. As noted in Table 1, most commercial GnRH agonists have both a D-aromatic amino acid in position 6 and a proline residue with an ethylamide moiety at position 9.

The ability of GnRH to induce synthesis and release of pituitary gonadotropins resides in the second and third amino acids. By inserting a D-aromatic amino acid in position 3, a GnRH antagonist with high binding affinity but reduced or absent intrinsic activity is created. Its potency is enhanced by replacing position 2 amino acid (histidine) with a chlorophenylalanine group.

MECHANISM OF ACTION

Continuous high-dose GnRH infusion induces a biphasic response in pituitary gonadotropin release. Leutinizing hormone (LH) and follicle-stimulating hormone (FSH) levels increase initially followed by a progressive and sustained decline.[5] The long half-lives and enhanced potencies of GnRH agonist mimic the action of continuous high-dose GnRH infusion and produce a state of hypogonadotrophic hypogonadism. This paradoxical gonadal suppression may be sustained indefinitely in response to chronic GnRH agonist administration.

The qualitative responses of FSH and LH to treatment with the same GnRH analogue are different. In one study, after GnRH agonist treatment, the immunoreactive (I) and bioactive (B) FSH levels decreased by 92%

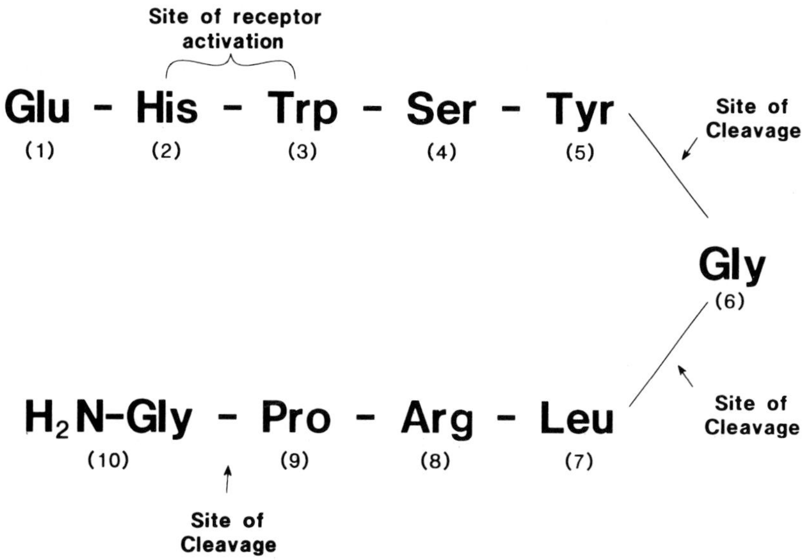

FIGURE 1.

Chemical structure of the hypothalamic decapeptide GnRH. Amino acids 2 and 3 are important for receptor activation. Degradation of GnRH occurs by cleavage of the decapeptide between amino acids 5 and 6, 6 and 7, and 9 and 10. (From Friedman AJ: The biochemistry, physiology, and pharmacology of gonadotropin releasing hormone (GnRH) and GnRH analogs, in Barbieri RL, Friedman AJ (eds): *Gonadotropin Releasing Hormone Analogs—Applications in Gynecology*, New York, Elsevier, 1991, p 2. Used by permission.)

and 83%, respectively, but the B/I ratio significantly increased. Immunoreactive LH decreased by 92% and B-LH by 93%. No changes in the B/I ratios of LH were found.[6] In a separate study[7] in which B-LH was reduced after GnRH agonist therapy, LH-α was elevated at least 10-fold over baseline, whereas LH-β decreased to less than 35% of pretreatment level. The effective loss of LH bioactivity, therefore, is likely related to decreased LH-β subunits. These studies suggest that gonadotropins secreted after chronic GnRH agonist therapy are biologically altered.

The cDNA of human pituitary GnRH receptor has been isolated.[8] Binding studies of the cloned receptor demonstrate high affinity and pharmacologic properties similar to those of the native human pituitary GnRH receptor. Northern blot and reverse transcriptase/polymerase chain reaction (PCR) analysis reveal that its mRNA is expressed in the pituitary, ovary, testis, breast, and prostate. Gonadotropin-releasing hormone receptors have been isolated in human granulosa cells at a late stage of follicular maturation.[9] The ovarian GnRH receptor may play a role as an intraovarian regulator. During sexual maturation in the rat, the GnRH binding capacity of the ovary began to rise at 7 days of age to a peak at 28 days and declined during the prepubertal period.[10] Treatment of hypophysectomized rats with GnRH agonist results in a decrease in FSH-inducible type 1 insulin-like growth factor (IGF-1) binding to isolated granulosa cells.[11]

BIOAVAILABILITY AND DELIVERY SYSTEMS

The physiologic availability of an orally administered drug is dependent on its ability to be absorbed and its resistance to digestion or breakdown. The high peptidase activity of the gastrointestinal tract results in rapid degradation of GnRH, even with the D-aromatic amino acid substitutions of GnRH agonists. The large size of the nondegraded peptide is also poorly absorbed across the intestinal mucosa. This accounts for the low bioavailability (0.01% to 0.1%) of orally administered GnRH agonist. The need for parenteral administration has resulted in the development of intravenous, intranasal, subcutaneous, depot, and transdermal formulations.

Bioavailability with intranasal administration is greater than with oral administration but is still only in the range of 2% to 5% because of enzymatic degradation and poor absorption.[12] Nafarelin acetate is an intranasal GnRH agonist with a D-alanine-D-naphthyline substitution at position 6. Nafarelin's low bioavailability is adequate to achieve a therapeutic effect because of its inherent high biological potency, estimated to be 200 times greater than native GnRH potency. The time to maximum concentration is approximately 18 minutes with intranasal administration vs. 2 minutes with intravenous administration.[13] Neither rhinitis nor decongestant therapy substantially affects the nasal absorption of nafarelin.[14] The half-life of nafarelin is 4.3 hours. A metered dose nebulizer delivers 200 μg with each 100 μL of spray. The recommended dose is 200 μg twice daily, alternating nostrils with each administration. If this dose fails to achieve adequate hypoestrogenism, it may be increased to 400 μg twice daily. Intranasal administration of GnRH agonist offers the distinct advantage of allowing rapid termination of therapy. This may be important if intolerable side effects (see later) develop. Many clinicians recommend initiating long-term GnRH agonist therapy with either intranasal or subcutaneous administration and then switching to the depot formulation after the first month of therapy.

Subcutaneous administration of GnRH agonist has a bioavailability profile similar to that provided by intravenous delivery. Most premenopausal women treated daily with 0.5 mg/day of leuprolide acetate will have serum estradiol (E_2) levels of less than 30 pg/mL. Leuprolide acetate is packaged in vials containing 2.8 mL (5 mg/mL). For a patient receiving 0.5 mg (0.1 mL) subcutaneously daily, one vial should last 28 days. Leuprolide can be self-administered with a low-dose insulin syringe (10 units = 0.1 mL = 0.5 mg). Tuberculin syringes should not be used because some of the drug is lost in the hub of the syringe. Dose adjustments in 0.1-mg increments can be based on serum E_2 levels. Increased dosing may be required in obese patients; effective decreased dosing will reduce cost to the patient.

Depot formulations release GnRH agonist at a constant rate over time and provide the advantage of infrequent administration and increased compliance. A 3.75-mg intramuscular injection of depot leuprolide acetate maintains a therapeutic level (0.5 to 1 ng/mL) for 4 weeks. Plasma levels of leuprolide are undetectable 8 weeks after intramuscular injection (Fig 2). Long-acting GnRH agonist implants designed to be effective for 3 months are being tested in patients with endometriosis.[15] One-centimeter rods containing slowly biodegradable polylactide/glycolide

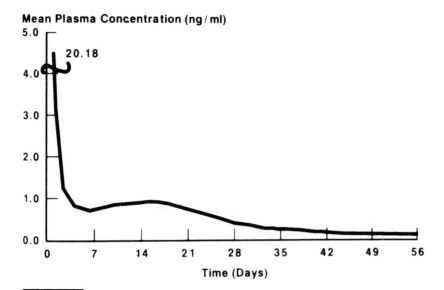

Mean Plasma Concentration (ng / ml)

FIGURE 2.

Within hours of an intramuscular injection of leuprolide acetate depot, 7.5 mg, a plasma concentration of approximately 20 ng/mL is achieved. The concentration drops rapidly to therapeutic levels (0.5 to 1.0 ng/mL) and remains stable for approximately 2½ weeks. A gradual decline in plasma levels is noted after 2½ weeks, and leuprolide is usually undetectable 8 weeks after injection. (From Friedman AJ: GnRH agonists: Patient selection, drug information, monitoring, and side effects, in Barbieri RL, Friedman AJ (eds): *Gonadotropin Releasing Hormone Analogs—Applications in Gynecology*, New York, Elsevier, 1991, p 25. Used by permission.)

with either 3.3 or 6.6 mg buserelin were implanted subcutaneously. Current use is limited by the excessive variation in the return of ovarian function, which ranged from 100 to 194 days (median, 118) in the 3.3-mg group and 79 to 290 days (median, 178) in the 6.6-mg group.

Transdermal administration of peptides has been limited by the barrier properties of the skin. Transdermal vs. subcutaneous administration of leuprolide has been compared experimentally by using electrically powered transdermal patches delivering a current of 0.22 μA.[16] The area under the curve for LH response, maximum LH response, and time to maximum LH response was similar for both transdermal and subcutaneous administration. Transdermal GnRH agonists are not currently being commercially marketed.

INITIATION AND MONITORING OF THERAPY

Gonadotropin-releasing hormone agonist therapy should be initiated any time from the mid to late luteal phase (cycle days 21 to 28) until the early follicular phase (cycle days 1 to 3). Although initiation at the midluteal phase may lead to a more prompt suppression of ovarian estrogen production,[17] a major disadvantage of luteal phase administration is the uncertainty about a possible pregnancy. Several studies have demonstrated a blunted agonist phase when GnRH agonists were administered in either the very early follicular phase or midluteal phase as compared with

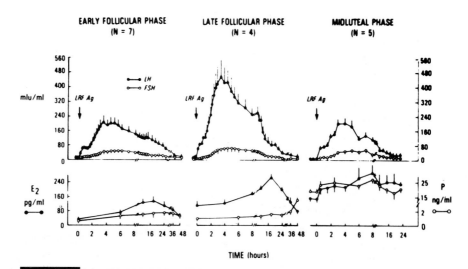

FIGURE 3.

Changes in leutinizing hormone (LH), follicle-stimulating hormone (FSH), estradiol (E_2), and progesterone (P) concentrations (mean $\pm$ SE) in the early follicular phase, late follicular phase, and midluteal phase in response to a subcutaneous 50-g dose of the GnRH agonist (D-Trp, Pro-NEt)-GnRH over a 48-hour period. *LRF = leutinizing hormone–releasing factor.* (From Sheehan KL, Casper RF, Yen SSC: *Am J Obstet Gynecol* 1979;135:760. Used by permission.)

the late follicular phase[18] (Fig 3). High initial doses of GnRH agonist are more successful than lower doses at achieving rapid, more complete inhibition of pituitary-ovarian function.[19] Treatment with very low doses may prolong the agonist response.

All patients should have a documented sex steroid–dependent disorder (e.g., ultrasound for uterine fibroids, laparoscopy for endometriosis, subjective daily logs for premenstrual syndrome [PMS]). There are few if any circumstances in which it is appropriate to initiate GnRH agonist therapy for presumed endometriosis diagnosed by symptoms alone. During treatment, a patient's symptoms and bleeding history should be recorded. Most women will be amenorrheic by 6 to 8 weeks of therapy. If amenorrhea does not occur by 8 weeks of therapy, consideration may be given to increasing the dose of GnRH agonist in the absence of a positive serum βhCG. A serum E_2 assay should be repeated after 4 to 6 weeks to confirm a hypoestrogenic response ($E_2 < 30$ pg/mL).

Menses usually return approximately 6 weeks after the last subcutaneous injection of GnRH agonist therapy (range 2 to 24 weeks) or 10 weeks after the final depot injection (range, 5 to 30 weeks). If the return of menses is delayed greater than 3 months, serum FSH should be measured to assess ovarian function and βhCG to rule out pregnancy.

SIDE EFFECTS

Menopausal Symptoms

The most common side effects of GnRH agonist therapy reflect the induced hypoestrogenic state and include hot flushes, sleep disturbance, vaginal dryness, and dyspareunia. Infrequent idiopathic reactions include palpitations, headache, depression, peripheral edema, chloasma, rash, hair loss, lactation, breast engorgement, and arthralgia. Asymptomatic adverse effects of GnRH agonist include lipid profile changes and osteoporosis. The frequency of side effects is summarized in Table 2.

Lipoprotein Profiles

Estrogen replacement in the postmenopausal patient is known to induce favorable changes in the lipoprotein profile. Studies have been conducted to determine whether the hypoestrogenic state induced by GnRH agonist therapy is associated with significant lipid changes. In one study,[20] after 1 month of therapy, GnRH agonist paradoxically induced a significant elevation in high-density lipoprotein (HDL) cholesterol (by 31.4%), in HDL_2 cholesterol (24.6%), and in HDL_3 cholesterol (45.7%), but no significant change in low-density lipoprotein (LDL) cholesterol or in apolipoprotein (Apo) A-I and Apo B. The lipoprotein changes had a favorable effect on the atherogenic index (total cholesterol/HDL cholesterol) and Apo A-I/Apo B ratio. In a separate study,[21] after 12 months of GnRH agonist therapy and a 6-month follow-up, a sustained increase in HDL_3 choles-

TABLE 2.

Temporal Onset of Adverse Effects in 102 Women Treated with Leuprolide Acetate Depot*

Effect	1	2	3	4	5	6	7	8	9	10	11	12	Total†
Hot flushes	8	12	28	26	11	4	2	1	1	0	0	0	93(91)
Insomnia	2	6	12	6	4	4	16	2	2	1	1	0	56(55)
Mood lability	6	6	10	6	2	0	4	2	0	4	6	0	46(45)
Menorrhagia/ hypermenorrhea	7	14	11	4	2	1	1	2	1	1	0	0	44(42)
Headaches	2	8	14	6	0	0	6	4	0	0	0	0	40(39)
Vaginal dryness	0	4	6	6	3	1	12	2	1	1	2	0	38(37)
Arthralgias/myalgias	0	0	12	0	0	0	5	1	0	0	6	2	26(25)
Hair loss	0	2	4	0	2	0	2	2	1	3	2	0	18(18)
Mastalgia	3	1	5	0	1	1	0	0	2	0	0	1	14(14)
Peripheral edema	2	0	6	0	0	0	0	2	0	1	1	0	12(12)
Depression	2	1	3	0	2	0	0	0	0	1	0	0	9 (9)
Fatigue	0	2	2	0	0	0	0	0	0	0	3	1	8 (8)
Skin rash	2	0	2	0	1	1	0	1	0	0	0	0	7 (7)
Short-term memory loss	0	0	0	0	0	0	2	0	0	0	3	1	6 (6)
Decreased libido	0	0	0	2	0	1	0	0	2	1	0	0	6 (6)
Acne	2	0	1	1	0	0	0	0	0	0	0	0	4 (4)
Increased libido	3	0	0	0	0	0	0	0	0	0	0	0	3 (3)
Decreased appetite	2	0	1	0	0	0	0	0	0	0	0	0	3 (3)
Blurred vision	0	0	0	0	0	0	1	0	0	0	1	0	2 (2)

*From Friedman AJ, Juneaw-Norcross M, Rein MS: *Fertil Steril* 1993; 59:449. Used by permission.
†Values in parentheses are percentages.

terol levels and a small increase in LDL cholesterol were seen. Apo B levels rose significantly and there were marginal increases in Apo A-I and A-II. All changes and trends were reversed after cessation of treatment.

Bone Density

Postmenopausal estrogen deprivation is associated with accelerated resorption of trabecular bone and osteoporosis. Numerous studies with conflicting results have addressed the effect of GnRH agonist on bone mass. These studies are well summarized in a recent review.[22] One could argue that the discrepancy in results may stem from the techniques used for bone density measurements. Trabecular bone (as opposed to cortical bone) is most affected by the hypoestrogenic state. In the adult female, only 24% of the vertebral body is made up of trabecular bone,[23] and the wrist has an even lower proportion of trabecular bone. However, when confining the review of previous studies to those using similar measurements of vertebral bone with dual-photon absorptimetry (as opposed to quantitated computed tomography), some studies[24, 25] reported no change in bone mass after GnRH agonist therapy, whereas others demonstrated significant bone loss that was both reversed[26–28] and not reversed[29] 6 months after completion of treatment. In those studies demonstrating bone loss, depot preparations produced more marked loss than did intranasal administration. Greater bone loss was also related to higher dosing of GnRH agonist. Nearly all studies show an increase in bone turnover, as indicated by the elevation of alkaline phosphatase and osteocalcin and a secondary decrease in serum intact parathyroid hormone (PTH) and 1,25-dihydroxyvitamin D_3. A positive correlation between the decrease from pretreatment serum 1,25-dihydroxyvitamin D_3 values and the reduction in bone mass during GnRH agonist treatment has been demonstrated.[30]

It has been argued that the magnitude of any persistent residual bone loss is unlikely to be of clinical relevance and the benefits of GnRH agonist therapy should not be withheld on the basis of a possible effect on bone.[31] It is important to individualize therapy. There is a significant degree of individual variation with regard to bone loss from GnRH agonist therapy. Cann et al.[32] found that 35% of their treated patients had less than 5% vertebral bone loss, 35% had 5% to 10% loss, 20% had 10% to 15% loss, and 10% had greater than 15% loss. By identifying those patients at risk for osteoporosis, preventing repetitive GnRH agonist therapies, and considering add-back regimens (see later), the clinical effect of possible bone loss can be minimized.

Central Nervous System Side Effects

Rare neurologic side effects of GnRH agonist therapy have been identified. In 3 of 536 women treated with GnRH agonist, mild transient neurologic symptoms occurred during therapy.[33] Symptoms included severe migraine headaches; numbness and tingling of the face; paresthesia and weakness of the hands, arms, and legs; and sensory ataxia. Neurologic symptoms appeared 8 to 12 days after starting the GnRH agonist and subsided within 3 to 7 days after their onset. Central nervous system (CNS) symptoms only occurred when the long midluteal protocol was used. The mechanism of action is not understood. However, the similarity to transient ischemic attacks (TIAs) has prompted the investigation of constrictive vascular effect as a possible etiology.

Inadvertent Use During Pregnancy

Spontaneous pregnancies associated with inadvertent periconceptional administration of long-acting GnRH agonist have been described. Theoretically, the GnRH agonist should induce luteolysis. Anecdotal reports demonstrate that miscarriage rates are only slightly increased. In a report of 11 pregnancies with inadvertent periconceptional GnRH agonist therapy, all cases exhibited impaired function of the corpus luteum in terms of declining progesterone levels despite rising levels of hCG.[34] Of the 11 pregnancies, 7 ended with a normal live birth, 3 with a preclinical gestation, and 1 with a blighted ovum. In a separate report of inadvertent GnRH agonist therapy during 13 early pregnancies, corpus luteum function was normal in 11 of the 13 pregnancies.[35] None of the term infants showed gross anatomic abnormalities.

Effects on Pituitary Function

No adverse effects on pituitary function have been demonstrated with long-term GnRH agonist therapy. Basal and stimulated values of gonadotropins, prolactin, cortisol, thyroid stimulating hormone, and growth hormone (GH) were normal and unchanged by 6 months of GnRH agonist after resumption of menses.[36] Higher serum prolactin levels have been associated with both higher E_2 levels and use of GnRH agonist but have had no effect on the fertilization rate, embryo quality, or occurrence of pregnancy.[37]

GnRH AGONIST THERAPY FOR UTERINE LEIOMYOMAS

Leiomyomas, commonly known as fibroids, are the most common solid pelvic tumors in women. It is estimated that 20% to 25% of all reproductive-age women have fibroids. In 1983, Filicori et al.[38] reported the use of GnRH agonist for reducing the volume of leiomyomas. Since then, numerous clinical trials have shown a reversible reduction in uterine and leiomyoma volume after GnRH agonist therapy.

In a randomized, double-blind, placebo-controlled multicenter study, the effect of leuprolide depot (3.75 mg intramuscularly every 4 weeks for 24 weeks) was examined in women with leiomyoma uteri.[39] The mean uterine volume decreased by 36% at 12 weeks and 45% at 24 weeks of leuprolide therapy. The mean uterine volume returned to pretreatment size 24 weeks after cessation of leuprolide treatment. The majority of patients had resolution or improvement of their fibroid-related symptoms. Although 95% of women treated with leuprolide acetate experienced some side effects related to hypoestrogenism, only five patients (8%) terminated treatment prematurely.[39]

A German multicenter study showed that maximal diminution of uterine and fibroid size had been nearly completely reached within the first 12 weeks of therapy.[40] By analyzing the time course of the fibroid reduction, the response can be predicted in most cases as early as 4 weeks after the first injection. In one study, retrospective analysis showed that a 50% reduction in fibroid size due to GnRH agonist treatment is preceded by a 35% reduction after 4 weeks in 81% of cases.[41]

MECHANISM OF ACTION

Cell receptors from leiomyomas have been studied in an attempt to decipher the mechanism for the observed effect of GnRH agonist therapy. Leiomyomas are unicellular in origin and are believed to derive from a single myometrial cell. Gonadotropin-releasing hormone agonist treatment is associated with a significant reduction in cell size. No significant change in cell number, fibrosis, edema, or mitotic activity is seen.[42] The effect of GnRH agonist on uterine leiomyomas is probably not mediated by uterine GnRH receptors.[43] Fibroids have estrogen receptors and progesterone receptors. The mean fibroid estrogen and progesterone receptor content is significantly greater than mean myometrial estrogen and progesterone receptor content. Following GnRH agonist therapy, the estrogen receptor content of fibroids increases. Clinically, the significant increase in fibroid estrogen receptor may be an explanation for the rapid regrowth of fibroids observed after the cessation of GnRH agonist therapy.[44] The reduction rate of leiomyomas has been best correlated with the decreased binding capacity of progesterone receptors after GnRH agonist treatment.[45]

Other growth factors may play a role in fibroid physiology.[46, 47] The secretion of IGF-1 and IGF-2 by fibroid explants obtained from women treated with the GnRH agonist was significantly less than the secretion by tissue obtained from placebo-treated controls. In vitro prolactin secretion by fibroids is reduced after in vivo treatment with GnRH agonist, although GnRH agonist in vitro has no effect on fibroid prolactin secretion. Leuprolide acetate–treated patients also demonstrate significant decreases in serum GH and IGF-1 concentrations. It is presently unclear whether these effects are a direct result of GnRH agonist or an indirect effect of GnRH agonist–induced hypoestrogenism.

PREOPERATIVE GnRH AGONIST THERAPY

Hysterectomies are one of the most commonly performed major surgical procedures. Fibroids account for 27% of all hysterectomies, or approximately 175,000 annually in the United States.[48] GnRH agonist has been used as a preoperative adjunct to surgical therapy for fibroids. Reported advantages of preoperative medical therapy include a decrease in intraoperative blood loss, an increase in preoperative hemoglobin concentration, and choice of an abdominal rather than a vaginal approach. Reported disadvantages include a delay in definitive therapy and tissue diagnosis, inappropriate treatment of unsuspected leiomyosarcoma,[49] side effects of GnRH agonist therapy including heavy vaginal bleeding in association with hyaline degeneration of submucous fibroids,[50] and added cost.

In one study, 3 months of GnRH agonist therapy before hysterectomy reduced intraoperative blood loss by 115 mL when compared with untreated controls.[51] Pretreatment with GnRH agonist before myomectomy decreased intraoperative blood loss (390 vs. 189 mL) in women with large leiomyomata uteri ($\geq$600 cm^3).[52] Although these reductions are statistically significant and have been reproduced in other studies, clinically they are not sufficient to support the routine use of preoperative GnRH agonist therapy. Such therapy may be better suited to a symptomatic patient who wishes to delay surgery, e.g., a school teacher with hypermenorrhea in October who prefers to take a leave of absence during the summer months. Patients with enlarged uteri who prefer a vaginal hysterectomy may also benefit from preoperative medical therapy. In a randomized trial, patients receiving GnRH agonist therapy were more likely to undergo vaginal hysterectomy than abdominal hysterectomy and, as expected, had shorter hospitalizations.[53]

Pretreatment with GnRH agonist may increase the "recurrence" rate of leiomyomas after myomectomy since, as previously stated, estrogen receptors of fibroids increase after GnRH agonist treatment. In one small study, induction of a period of hypoestrogenism before myomectomy favored short-term recurrence of uterine myomas, thus limiting the efficacy of surgery.[54] In a separate study, myoma recurrence was not associated with pretreatment or preoperative uterine volume, resected myoma mass, or preoperative medical therapy.[55] After 27 to 38 months of follow-up, the recurrence of myomas was found to be greater when at least four myomas were resected.

GnRH AGONIST THERAPY FOR ENDOMETRIOSIS

Endometriosis was originally described by Von Rokitansky[56] in 1860. Despite hundreds of subsequent studies, there still remain many unanswered questions regarding pathophysiology and patient susceptibility. Endometriosis affects 1 in 15 women of reproductive age and is present in approximately 25% of infertile women.[57] The majority of endometriotic implants contain receptors for estrogen, progesterone, and androgens. A hypoestrogenic state, whether induced by oophorectomy, menopause, or GnRH agonist therapy, leads to atrophy of endometriotic implants.

Several controlled clinical trials of GnRH agonist therapy for symptomatic endometriosis have demonstrated prompt clinical relief and laparoscopically confirmed resolution of endometriotic implants. Although recurrence of endometriosis often occurs after cessation of therapy, symptomatic relief may be sustained over a year after therapy. A multicenter, double-blind, comparative trial of over 200 patients reported an 80% reduction in laparoscopic endometriosis scores.[58] In a separate study of 50 patients, pelvic pain was relieved during GnRH agonist treatment in 87.5% of patients. After a follow-up period of up to 37 months, 24 patients were in clinical remission, and 9 experienced recurrence of endometriosis 7 to 14 months after completing treatment.[59] A multicenter, randomized European study[60] of 307 patients with confirmed endometriosis reported that in those patients with recurrence of symptoms after GnRH agonist therapy, the severity of these symptoms was less than at admission in all cases. A German study[61] of 146 patients with pelvic endometriosis reported that after a 6-month course of GnRH agonist, pelvic symptom scores were reduced by 93% and did not exceed one fifth of the pretreatment value throughout the follow-up period of 48 weeks.

Successful treatment of adenomyosis with long-term GnRH agonists has been anecdotally reported.[62] Uterine volume was reduced by 65% after 4 months of therapy, and size reduction was accompanied by amenorrhea and relief of severe dysmenorrhea.

MECHANISM OF ACTION

Progestins and danazol exert direct suppressive effects on endometriosis, whereas GnRH agonist is thought to suppress growth secondary to the induced hypoestrogenic state. Surrey and Halme[63] analyzed in vitro cell proliferation of endometrial stromal cells isolated from biopsy specimens. Medroxyprogesterone acetate, danazol, or leuprolide was added to nutrient media alone and media supplemented with E_2. Medroxyprogesterone acetate and danazol exerted significant antiproliferative effects on stromal cell proliferation, and these effects were enhanced by an absence of exogenous E_2. Leuprolide exerted no consistent effects.

Gonadotropin-releasing hormone agonist may indirectly affect the natural immune response to endometriosis. The immunology of endometriosis is unclear.[64] Preliminary studies have shown that antiendometrial antibodies are significantly reduced after a 6-month course of nafarelin treatment.[65] Cytotoxic activity of peritoneal macrophages from women with endometriosis was increased in GnRH agonist–treated patients.[66]

GnRH VS. DANAZOL

Danazol was the first hormonal agent approved by the Food and Drug Administration for the treatment of endometriosis. Danazol, an isozazol derivative of 17α-ethinyl testosterone, is effective in the treatment of endometriosis because it creates a hypoestrogenic-hyperandrogenic state that is detrimental to the growth and function of endometriotic tissue.[67] Numerous clinical trials[68–71] have reported equal efficacy of GnRH agonist as compared with danazol in the treatment of endometriosis. The side effect profiles of GnRH agonists differ from those of danazol. GnRH agonist is associated with more hot flushes and headaches and danazol with more weight gain and muscle cramps. Estradiol and LH pulse amplitude is more suppressed by GnRH agonist than by danazol.[72] Compliance was greater with GnRH agonist therapy as compared with danazol.[73]

EFFECTS OF INFERTILITY IN PATIENTS WITH ENDOMETRIOSIS

Although endometriosis is more common in patients with infertility, no convincing evidence is present to suggest that stage I or II endometriosis causes infertility. Mechanical factors associated with stage III or IV endometriosis have been directly linked as causative factors in infertility. Cumulative pregnancy rates after GnRH agonist therapy for endometriosis have been examined, and no controlled clinical trials have demonstrated that treatment of early-stage endometriosis improves fertility. A randomized clinical trial evaluating the efficacy of GnRH agonist therapy for 6 months vs. expectant management in the treatment of infertile women with stage I or II endometriosis showed the 1- and 2-year actuarial overall pregnancy rates to be similar in the two groups.[74] In endometriosis patients receiving in vitro fertilization and embryo transfer (IVF-ET), however, "ultralong" (at least 60 days) suppression with GnRH agonist before ovarian stimulation has been compared favorably with standard midluteal-phase suppression. In one study of 33 patients with varying stages of endometriosis, the E_2 response and the number of retrieved oocytes, fertilized oocytes, cleaved oocytes, and transferred embryos was similar in both groups, but the clinical pregnancy rate per transfer was superior in the ultralong protocol (67% vs. 27%).[75] Similar results were reported with the ultralong protocol in stage I or II endometriosis patients receiving gamete intrafallopian transfer (GIFT).[76]

CA-125 LEVELS AND ENDOMETRIOSIS

Serum CA-125, a cell surface antigen, has been shown to be elevated in concentration in women with advanced endometriosis.[77] Changes in CA-125 levels have been correlated with the clinical course of endometriosis.[78] Serial measurements of CA-125 levels have been advocated to monitor the effectiveness of GnRH agonist therapy for endometriosis. Marana et al.[79] showed that CA-125 levels at initial laparoscopy correlated with endometriosis implant scores but not with adhesion scores. CA-125 levels decreased after GnRH agonist therapy but were not correlated with endometriosis scores at second-look laparoscopy. They concluded that mechanisms other than the change in the extent of the disease may be involved in the CA-125 decrease during therapy and that CA-125 levels may not therefore be a reliable indicator for monitoring the efficacy of GnRH agonist treatment of endometriosis. Contrary to the findings of Marana et al., Franssen et al.[80] showed that pretreatment scores for adhesions and not for implants correlated significantly with CA-125 concentrations.

ENDOMETRIOMAS

In general, GnRH agonist treatment of endometriomas is minimally effective. Gonadotropin-releasing hormone agonist appears to be most efficacious only when endometriomas are less than 1 cm in size.[81] Medical treatment of an adnexal mass delays a definitive pathologic diagnosis. Recurrence of endometriosis is common following surgical cystectomy for endometrioma,[82] and data are lacking as to whether long-term hormonal therapy prevents the repetitive recurrence of endometriomas.

GnRH AGONIST THERAPY FOR OVULATION INDUCTION

OVULATION INDUCTION IN THE PATIENT WITH POLYCYSTIC OVARIES

Polycystic ovarian (PCO) disease is characterized by a spectrum of biochemical abnormalities that include ovarian and adrenal hyperandrogenism, elevated LH concentrations, normal or low FSH concentrations, peripherally sustained estrogenism, and hyperinsulinemia. Clinically, PCO disease is often associated with anovulation, amenorrhea, and hirsutism. The use of GnRH agonist has been proposed to block the cycle of hormonal events that perpetuates PCO disease. Bachus et al.[83] examined the effects of adjunctive luteal-phase GnRH agonist therapy in women with PCO disease undergoing ovulation induction with human menopausal gonadotropin (hMG). They concluded that GnRH agonist therapy does not alter cycle fecundity. Others reported that after at least 12 weeks of GnRH agonist suppression without hMG stimulation for PCO disease, maximal suppression of LH occurred after 6 weeks of treatment. Plasma testosterone and androstenedione fell to normal levels but reached pretreatment levels during the follow-up period. There was no effect on plasma dehydroepiandrosterone sulfate (GnRH agonist does not affect adrenal androgen capacity[84]) or sex hormone–binding globulin. Ovarian size decreased significantly, and after cessation of therapy, there was spontaneous ovulation that occurred within 3 weeks in all subjects.[85]

Ovulation induction with pulsatile GnRH is less effective in patients with PCO disease than in patients with hypogonadotropic hypogonadism.[86] One study, however, reports pulsatile GnRH agonist to be highly effective for ovulation induction in patients with PCO disease when preceded by 4 to 8 weeks of GnRH agonist pituitary-ovarian suppression.[87] Administration of GnRH agonist in patients with PCO disease who are undergoing IVF-ET decreased progesterone and androstenedione production by cultured granulosa cells did not affect IVF results.[88] Obese women with PCO disease show a hyperinsulinemic response to glucose that indicates insulin resistance. Treatment of these women with GnRH agonist produces a hypogonadotropic hypogonadal state but does not change the hyperinsulinemic response to glucose.[89]

USE OF GnRH AGONISTS IN IN VITRO FERTILIZATION–EMBRYO TRANSFER

Gonadotropin-releasing hormone agonists have been used widely as adjuncts to gonadotropins for controlled ovarian hyperstimulation in IVF-ET cycles. Advantages of GnRH agonist use include prevention of a premature LH surge, suppression of endogenous basal LH levels, and recruitment of a larger cohort of follicles. Follicular-phase parameters used for cycle cancellation in hMG-only–stimulated IVF cycles cannot be extrapolated to GnRH agonist/hMG cycles (i.e., pregnancy rates are not necessarily related to the E_2 pattern even when E_2 values fall during hMG administration).[90] Gonadotropin-releasing hormone agonists have been used in different protocols including (1) the long protocol with suppression started in the midluteal phase, (2) the short or flare-up protocol initiated in the early follicular phase with gonadotropins, (3) the ultrashort protocol initiated only during cycle days 1 through 3, and (4) follicular phase downregulation. Figure 4 summarizes these protocols.

Numerous studies have compared IVF-ET cycles with and without GnRH agonist and have compared IVF-ET cycles with different GnRH agonist protocols. A meta-analysis was published of ten trials comparing treatment cycle outcomes after GnRH agonist (n = 914) with other ovulation induction protocols (n = 722) and seven trials comparing outcomes after short flare-up (n = 368) with longer-suppression (n = 476) GnRH agonist protocols.[91] The clinical pregnancy rate per cycle commenced was significantly improved after GnRH agonist use for IVF (common odds ratio [OR], 1.80) and GIFT (common OR, 2.37). Cycle cancellation was decreased, whereas the spontaneous abortion rate was similar with and

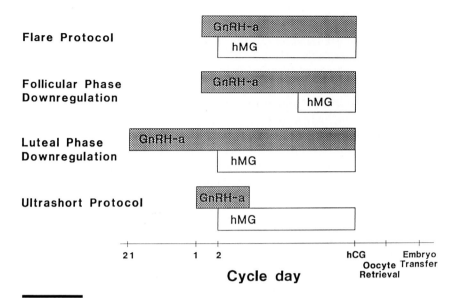

FIGURE 4.

Four different protocols for intravenous fertilization–embryo transfer cycles with gonadotropin-releasing hormone agonist *(GnRH-a)* and human menopausal gonadotropin *(hMG)*.

without GnRH agonist use. Cycle cancellation and pregnancy rates after short flare-up and longer suppression protocols were similar between groups. The selection of one of the GnRH agonist protocols should be individualized for each patient and based on the previous response with gonadotropin stimulation.

Muasher[92] reports little beneficial effect from the use of the long protocol in "low-responder" patients, defined as patients with a basal FSH greater than or equal to 15 mIU/mL. In low-responder patients, the use of the short protocol (GnRH agonist starting on day 2 of the cycle, followed by gonadotropins on day 4 of the cycle) takes advantage of the initial agonistic stimulatory effect of GnRH agonist. Others have recommended starting both GnRH agonist and hMG on cycle day 3 when using the short protocol.[93] In patients with an appropriate response to hMG, San Ramon et al.[94] reported similar fertilization, biochemical, and clinical pregnancy rates in patients receiving either the short or long protocol. However, the short protocol was associated with premature luteinization, hyperandrogenemia, higher spontaneous abortion rates, and poorer pregnancy outcome when compared with the luteal-phase administration of GnRH agonist. The Hallam Medical Centre group reported that the long protocol is superior to the short protocol in terms of significantly greater follicular recruitment, oocyte recovery, fertilization rates, and number of embryos available for transfer.[95] Fewer ampules of hMG are generally needed when the short protocol is used. Use of an ultrashort protocol has been proposed, with cited advantages including decreased cost and inconvenience to the patient. A comparison of the short and ultrashort protocols showed fertilization and pregnancy rates to be similar, but the ultrashort protocol did not always prevent an LH surge.[96]

Comparisons have been made between different GnRH agonists for use in IVF-ET cycles. In one study, patients receiving nafarelin acetate required significantly less hMG and had significantly more embryos frozen for later transfer than those receiving leuprolide acetate.[97] In a separate study comparing buserelin acetate and leuprolide acetate, the number of follicles punctured, the number of oocytes retrieved, the percentage of mature oocytes, and the number of embryos suitable for replacement and cryopreservation were significantly higher in patients receiving leuprolide acetate.[98] Parinaud et al.[99] reported that E_2 levels and the E_2 level per hMG ampule were both significantly lower in IVF-ET cycles with buserelin as compared with leuprolide acetate and triptorelin. The pregnancy per stimulated cycle rate was not significantly different among the groups.

EFFECT ON OOCYTE QUALITY AND GRANULOSA CELL FUNCTION

Human granulosa cells have specific receptors for GnRH and are therefore affected by use of GnRH agonist during IVF-ET cycles. Follicular fluid from IVF patients treated with GnRH agonist has lower E_2 and progesterone concentrations than does follicular fluid of IVF patients receiving gonadotropins alone.[100] Despite the decreased steroidogenesis, normal oocyte maturation occurs. Subsequent embryo development may even occur more rapidly in oocytes obtained during GnRH agonist downregulated cycles.[101] The use of GnRH agonist does not seem to alter the development of embryos after cryopreservation at the pronuclear stage when compared with a similar gonadotropin stimulation treatment without GnRH agonist.[102]

PROGNOSTIC VALUE OF GnRH AGONIST RESPONSE IN IN VITRO FERTILIZATION–EMBRYO TRANSFER CYCLES

The serum E_2 response to GnRH agonist can be used as an indicator of outcome in short-protocol IVF-ET cycles. Padilla et al.[103] described four patterns of serum E_2 response to leuprolide acetate measured during cycle days 2 through 5 before exogenous gonadotropin stimulation (Fig 5). The pattern associated with the highest clinical pregnancy rate had a doubling of the baseline E_2 by cycle day 3 followed by at least a 10% drop by cycle day 4 and elevation thereafter. In a similar study, Winslow et al.[104] used E_2 patterns to predict both the duration and number of hMG ampules required for stimulation.

EFFECTS OF GnRH AGONIST ON ENDOMETRIAL RECEPTIVITY

The use of GnRH agonist in IVF-ET cycles is associated with a 1½-day delay in implantation when compared with IVF-ET cycles using only hMG. Gonadotropin-releasing hormone agonist/hMG–treated pregnancies implant between 7 and 11 days after embryo transfer, whereas hMG-treated pregnancies implant 7 to 9 days after embryo transfer.[105] This larger implantation window may be one factor accounting for the higher pregnancy rates associated with GnRH agonist use in IVF-ET.

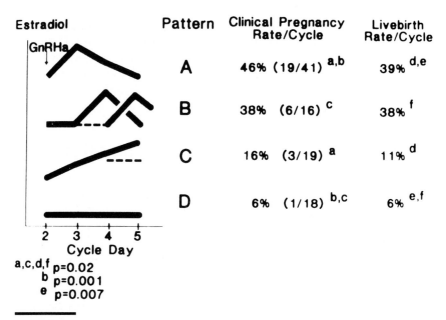

FIGURE 5.

Clinical pregnancy rate and live-birth rate per stimulated cycle for each of the early estradiol patterns after the initiation of leuprolide acetate *(GnRH-a)*. (From Padilla SL, Bayati J, Garcia JE: *Fertil Steril* 1990; 53:291. Used by permission.)

USE OF GnRH AGONIST IN INTRAUTERINE INSEMINATION CYCLES

Because the addition of GnRH agonist to hMG ovarian stimulation seems to improve pregnancy rates in IVF-ET cycles, several studies have addressed adding GnRH agonist to hMG in intrauterine insemination (IUI) cycles. Dodson et al.[106] studied 97 subfertile women who received either hMG alone or hMG following midluteal pretreatment with leuprolide. Cycles that included leuprolide required a larger amount of hMG and more days of stimulation per cycle, but the mean E_2 concentrations and numbers of follicles were not different. Importantly, the cycle fecundity was not different between groups. In a similar study of 321 cycles, Gagliardi et al.[107] concluded that the addition of a GnRH agonist to hMG/IUI improved the pregnancy rate (21.6% vs. 12.8%) without increasing the rate of multiple births or fetal wastage.

USE OF GnRH AGONIST FOR TRIGGERING OVULATION

GnRH agonist administration leading to a surge of endogenous gonadotropins has been reported to be more physiologic than hCG in the triggering of ovulation. In spontaneous cycles both LH and FSH are secreted in a surge at midcycle. Mean serum LH and FSH levels are elevated for 34 hours after GnRH agonist therapy, whereas hCG administration results in elevation of LH-like activity only. Two studies[108, 109] compared the effectiveness of a single midcycle dose of GnRH agonist with hCG on follicular maturation in IVF-ET cycles. In the GnRH agonist–treated group, the mean luteal-phase serum E_2 and progesterone concentrations were lower and luteal-phase length was shortened despite progesterone supplementation in both groups. Pregnancy rates were no different. They concluded that GnRH agonist appears to be an effective alternative to hCG for inducing follicular maturation and that the lower luteal-phase E_2 concentrations may potentially be beneficial in preventing ovarian hyperstimulation and enhancing implantation.

GnRH AGONISTS AND ESTROGEN-PROGESTIN REPLACEMENT THERAPY

Replacement hormonal therapy with estrogens and/or progestins has been proposed for patients receiving GnRH agonists. Studies have addressed the use of "add-back" therapy in patients requiring GnRH agonist therapy for greater than 6 months as well as in patients receiving GnRH agonists for only 3 to 6 months. Although GnRH agonists are effective in the treatment of endometriosis and myomas, the disease recurrence rate after discontinuation of therapy is high. Greater than 6 months of therapy is effective but may not be safe, given the side effects discussed previously. Preliminary evidence suggests that therapy with a GnRH agonist plus low doses of estrogen-progestin is effective in the treatment of endometriosis and fibroids and is associated with few adverse side effects.

PROGESTIN REPLACEMENT THERAPY

Administration of oral medroxyprogesterone acetate has been shown to decrease the incidence of hot flushes in postmenopausal hypoestrogenic women.[110] Early studies evaluated the simultaneous combination treatment of GnRH agonist plus daily oral medroxyprogesterone acetate in women with fibroids.[111] Although menopausal symptoms were markedly reduced, the simultaneous addition of medroxyprogesterone acetate blocked the expected decrease in uterine volume. In a small study of five perimenopausal patients with fibroids, 3 months of therapy with GnRH agonist alone followed by 24 months of GnRH agonist plus cyclic conjugated equine estrogens (0.625 mg on days 1 to 25) and medroxyprogesterone acetate (10 mg on days 16 to 25) resulted in a mean decrease in uterine volume of 49% at 3 months, with no further change in uterine volume over the next 2 years.[112] No changes in bone density were demonstrated.

In patients with endometriosis, simultaneous treatment with GnRH agonist and daily norethindrone (5 to 10 mg) is effective in treating symptomatic endometriosis while ameliorating side effects induced by GnRH agonists alone.[113, 114] The combination therapy is as effective as GnRH agonist alone in reducing circulating gonadotropin and estrogen levels, the extent of visible endometriotic implants, and painful symptoms. Marked vasomotor and vaginal symptoms experienced by patients given GnRH agonist alone are minimized in those receiving GnRH agonist with norethindrone. Lumbar spine bone mineral density loss is significantly reduced and more completely reversed in patients receiving combination therapy.

ESTROGEN REPLACEMENT THERAPY

Estrogen replacement therapy may seem contradictory in a patient with GnRH agonist–induced hypoestrogenism. However, the concentration of E_2 required to reduce hot flushes and protect against bone loss may be less than the concentration of E_2 necessary to cause regrowth of myomas or endometriosis.[115] There is a hierarchy of organ response to E_2 such that calcium metabolism is most sensitive, followed by gonadotropin secretion, vaginal epithelial growth, lipid metabolism, and liver protein production.[116] This "estrogen threshold" hypothesis is shown schematically in Figure 6. Three hypothetical estrogen zones corresponding to different thresholds required for the growth or maintenance of various estrogen-dependent tissues are shown. Zone A encompasses typical concentrations of E_2 seen throughout the menstrual cycle in premenopausal women. Estrogen concentrations in this range will support the growth or maintenance of estrogen-dependent tissues. In zone C, E_2 levels are in the postmenopausal range, similar to estrogen concentrations after GnRH agonist treatment. Estrogen concentrations in this range cannot support growth and lead to regression of most estrogen-dependent tissues. In zone B, E_2 levels are somewhat higher than castrate levels and are similar to those

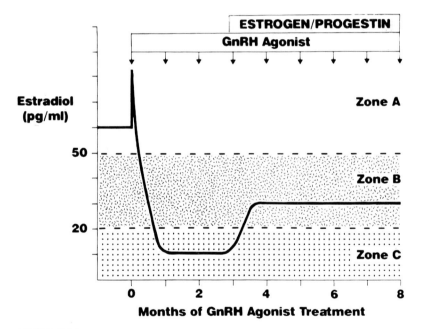

FIGURE 6.

Estrogen threshold hypothesis. Zone A, typical circulating estradiol concentrations in premenopausal women are able to support myometrial-fibroid growth and prevent rapid bone resorption. Zone B, therapeutic window. Myometrial and fibroid volume may decrease at these estradiol levels, but bone resorption is not accelerated. Zone C, hypoestrogenism often attained during gonadotropin-releasing hormone (GnRH) agonist therapy may lead to myometrial-fibroid shrinkage and rapid bone resorption. Note: estradiol values for each zone may differ among patients. (From Friedman AM, Lobel SM, Rein MS, et al: *Am J Obstet Gynecol* 1992; 163:1118. Used by permission.)

found in the early follicular phase. Estrogen concentrations in this range may be high enough to maintain the integrity of some estrogen-dependent tissues (e.g., bone) while causing regression in others (i.e., myomas). The first goal of GnRH agonist hormone add-back therapy would be to control the estrogen-dependent disease process by inducing a hypogonadal state with GnRH agonist treatment. After hypoestrogenism has been achieved and the disease activity has been controlled, small amounts of estrogen, progestin, or both could be added back with the intent of reducing hot flushes and bone loss without causing reinitiation of myoma or endometriotic growth.

EMERGING APPLICATIONS WITH GnRH AGONISTS

The majority of trials evaluating the efficacy of GnRH agonist therapy have focused on its use for leiomyomas, endometriosis, and ovulation induction as discussed above. Other emerging applications of GnRH agonist therapy include its use in premenstrual syndrome (PMS), hirsutism, endometrial ablation, mastalgia, and ovarian, breast, and endometrial cancers.

PREMENSTRUAL SYNDROME

Premenstrual syndrome is an ill-defined collection of psychological, behavioral, and physical changes that are cyclic in nature and occur with increased incidence in the late luteal phase of the menstrual cycle. Numerous etiologies have been proposed, but none have been well proved. Several well-controlled crossover studies have shown subjective benefit from a variety of therapies. Among these is the use of GnRH agonists,[117] which was prompted by the observation that bilateral oophorectomy has been shown to relieve PMS symptoms. Mortola et al.[118] reported on the successful treatment of severe PMS in eight women by combined use of GnRH agonist and estrogen/progestin therapy. Combined sequential administration of conjugated equine estrogen and medroxyprogesterone acetate in addition to GnRH agonist was effective in maintaining the reduced symptom scores seen after GnRH agonist alone and was superior to the addition of conjugated equine estrogen alone, medroxyprogesterone acetate alone, or placebo.

HIRSUTISM

Gonadotropin-releasing hormone agonists are used in the treatment of ovarian androgen excess. Because androgen excess resulting from adrenal hyperplasia is unresponsive to GnRH agonist therapy, it is important to delineate the androgenic source. The ovary is the major source of circulating testosterone and androstenedione in patients with PCO disease. Standard treatment of hirsute patients with or without elevated testosterone levels has included combined estrogen-progestin (oral contraceptive) preparations and spironolactone. This regimen decreases LH secretion, which is required for ovarian androgen production. Gonadotropin-releasing hormone agonists provide an additional mode of therapy that also reduces LH levels. Estrogen replacement can be used in conjunction with a GnRH agonist to extend the duration of therapy for hirsutism and increase steroid hormone binding globulin, thereby decreasing the free androgen concentrations.[119] Rittmaster and Thompson[120] evaluated the effect of leuprolide and dexamethasone on hair growth and hormone levels in hirsute women in order to evaluate the relative importance of the ovary and the adrenal gland in the pathogenesis of hirsutism. After 6 months of GnRH agonist treatment alone, testosterone decreased by 54% in patients with PCO disease and by 36% in patients with idiopathic hirsutism (IH). Androstenedione decreased by 53% in patients with PCO disease and by 31% in patients with IH. Hair growth rates, as assessed by Ferriman-Gallway scores, decreased by 37% in patients with PCO disease and by 14% in patients with IH. The change in hair growth correlated with the change in androstenedione but not with the change in testosterone.

USE OF GnRH AGONISTS BEFORE ENDOMETRIAL ABLATION

Reducing endometrial thickness and vascularity before endometrial ablation has been proved to simplify this hysteroscopic technique and result in increased visualization, decreased bleeding, and decreased endometrial regeneration.[121] Preoperative therapy has classically been the use of either danazol or progestins with their respective side effects. Serden and Brooks[122] compared the preoperative use of progestins, danazol, GnRH agonist, or no treatment in preparation for endometrial ablation. The use of depot leuprolide acetate in a single-dose regimen 4 weeks before surgery resulted in the highest amenorrhea rates with the fewest side effects. The authors also concluded that suppression with depot leuprolide 1 month postoperatively helps to inhibit endometrial regeneration following endometrial ablation.

USE OF GnRH AGONISTS IN FIBROCYSTIC BREAST DISEASE AND MASTALGIA

Symptomatic improvement in women with severe fibrocystic conditions has been reported after danazole use.[123] Using danazol, Gateley and Mansel[124] reported reduced pain in 77% of patients with cyclic mastalgia and 44% with noncyclic mastalgia. Because of a presumed benefit from a hypoestrogenic state, others have used GnRH agonists in patients previously treated with danazol. Monsonego et al.[125] studied hormonal profiles, estrogen receptors, progesterone receptors, and radioultrasonographic and histologic criteria in 66 patients with fibrocystic mastopathy. No characteristic hormonal profile was noted. Estrogen or progesterone receptors were found in only 57% of patients. After depot GnRH agonist therapy of variable duration, a complete symptomatic response was observed in 53% of the patients, and a significant partial response was observed in an additional 45% of the patients. Clinical responses to treatment were independent of hormone receptor status. A separate group reported symptomatic relief after GnRH agonist therapy in 17 of 21 patients with severe recurrent or refractory breast pain.[126] The recurrence of symptoms after stopping GnRH agonist therapy has not been well evaluated.

USE OF GnRH AGONISTS IN OVARIAN, BREAST, AND ENDOMETRIAL CANCERS

Surgical therapy with adjunctive cytostatic chemotherapy or radiotherapy has long been the standard of care in women with gynecologic cancers. With the discovery of both GnRH and estrogen receptors[127] in some of these tumors, several investigators have explored the use of GnRH agonists in these patients.

Treatment with GnRH agonist significantly reduced the growth of human ovarian epithelial carcinoma heterotransplanted in mice as compared with normal control tumors and placebo-treated tumors.[128] Using an ovarian cancer cell line that is estrogen receptor–negative, Thompson et al.[129] showed no increased growth with hMG but decreased growth with GnRH agonists. They concluded that the GnRH agonist effect on ovarian cancer cell proliferation is independent of gonadotropin and steroid levels and may involve a cell cycle regulatory event. In a phase II trial of 30 patients with advanced epithelial ovarian cancer treated with goserelin, disease progression was halted for 6 months or more in 23% of patients.[130]

Antiestrogens such as tamoxifen have been shown to have direct antitumor action and are widely used as adjunctive therapy in breast cancer. Estrogen-sensitive breast tumors have shown a reduction in tumor volume after either GnRH agonist or antagonist therapy.[131, 132] Binding sites for GnRH in human breast carcinomas and breast tumor cell lines have been identified.[133] Neri et al.[134] compared the effects of two different GnRH analogues (decapeptyl, an agonist, and BIM 21009C, an antagonist) and the antiestrogen 4-hydroxytamoxifen on proliferation in antiestrogen-responsive or antiestrogen-resistant human breast cancer cell lines. None of the treatments decreased cell growth, thus suggesting that the direct effect of the GnRH analogues would not be a potent tool for treating antiestrogen-resistant breast tumors. In a study of 75 premenopausal patients with advanced breast cancer treated with long-term GnRH agonist, an objective response was seen in 25 patients (33%), the median duration of which was in excess of 15 months. The response to therapy correlated significantly with the estrogen receptor status of the primary tumor.

Gonadotropin-releasing hormone analogues have a significant antitumor effect in recurrent endometrial cancer. In a recent review, Kullander[135] advocated the use of GnRH agonists in the following circumstances: (1) in pronounced endometrial hyperplasia and adenomatous hyperplasia unresponsive to progestin therapy; (2) in patients with endometrial cancer where surgery is contraindicated or refused; (3) in addition to or as a substitute for radium treatment preoperatively to reduce uterine volume, devitalize the tumor, stop menorrhagia, and improve anemia; (4) in advanced cases as an adjunct to radiotherapy and progestins; and (5) in relapses of endometrial cancer refractory to conventional therapy and in pulmonary metastases. In a phase II trial, Gallagher et al.[136] reported on 17 patients with endometrial cancer that had recurred after surgery, radiotherapy, and progesterone treatment. After depot GnRH agonist therapy, 6 of 17 patients achieved a complete or partial remission that continued for a median of 20 months with no adverse effects.

SUMMARY

In the relatively short history of GnRH agonists, the clinical applications for this powerful class of drugs have expanded tremendously. Today GnRH agonists are commonly used and accepted for the treatment of uterine leiomyomas, endometriosis, and ovulation induction. Current clinical studies hope to clearly define the role of add-back hormonal therapy in patients requiring chronic GnRH agonist therapy. Preliminary studies show promise for the use of GnRH agonists in premenstrual syndrome, hirsutism, endometrial ablation, mastalgia, and gynecologic cancers. Further refinements in GnRH agonists and the introduction of GnRH antagonists will continue to fuel the revolutionary impact of these agents in gynecologic practice and research.

REFERENCES

1. Matsuo H, Baba Y, Nair RM, et al: Structure of the porcine LH- and FSH-releasing hormone. I. The proposed amino acid sequence. *Biochem Biophys Res Commun* 1971; 43:1334–1339.
2. Burgus R, Butcher M, Amoss M, et al: Primary structure of the ovine hypothalamic luteinizing hormone–releasing factor (LRF). *Proc Natl Acad Sci U S A* 1972; 69:278–282.
3. Karten MJ, Rivier JE: Gonadotropin-releasing hormone analog design. Structure-function studies toward the development of agonists and antagonists: Rationale and perspective. *Endocr Rev* 1986; 7:44–66.
4. Stewart JM: Pharmacology of LHRH and analogs, in Zatuchni GI, Shelton JD, Sciarra JJ (eds): *LHRH Peptides as Female and Male Contraceptives.* Philadelphia, Harper & Row, 1981.
5. Belchetz PE, Plant TM, Nakai Y, et al: Hypophyseal responses to continuous and intermittent delivery of hypothalamic gonadotropin-releasing hormone. *Science* 1978; 202:631–633.
6. Matikainen T, Ding YQ, Vergara M, et al: Differing responses of plasma bioactive and immunoreactive follicle-stimulating hormone and luteinizing hormone to gonadotropin-releasing hormone antagonist and agonist treatments in postmenopausal women. *J Clin Endocrinol Metab* 1992; 75:820–825.
7. Lemay A Lourdusamy M: Gonadotropin releasing hormone agonist suppressive treatment of ovarian function decreases serum LH-beta and bioactive LH but maintains elevated levels of LH-alpha. *Clin Endocrinol (Oxf)* 1991; 34:191–196.
8. Kakar SS, Musgrove LC, Devor DC, et al: Cloning, sequencing, and expression of human gonadotropin releasing hormone (GnRH) receptor. *Biophys Res Commun* 1992; 189:289–295.
9. Latouche J, Crumeyrolle-Arias M, Jordan D, et al: GnRH receptors in human granulosa cells: Anatomical localization and characterization by autoradiographic study. *Endocrinology* 1989; 125:1739–1741.
10. Uemura T, Shirasu K, Matsuyama A, et al: Increases in ovarian GnRH receptors by following GnRH treatment. *Endocrinol Jpn* 1984; 31:377–386.
11. Adashi EY, Resnick CE, Vera A, et al: In vivo regulation of granulosa cell type I insulin-like growth factor receptors: evidence for an inhibitory role for the putative endogenous ligand(s) of the ovarian gonadotropin-releasing hormone receptor. *Endocrinology* 1991; 128:3130–3137.
12. Hirai S, Yashiki T, Mima H: Mechanism for the enhancement of nasal absorption of insulin by surfactants. *Int J Pharmacol* 1981; 9:173–175.

13. Chaplin MD: Bioavailability of nafarelin in healthy volunteers. *Am J Obstet Gynecol* 1992; 166:762–765.
14. Henzl MR: Gonadotropin-releasing hormone analogs: Update on new findings. *Am J Obstet Gynecol* 1992; 166:757–761.
15. Fraser HM, Haining R, Cowen GM, et al: Long-acting gonadotropin releasing hormone agonist implant causes variable duration of suppression of ovarian steroid and inhibin secretion. *Clin Endocrinol (Oxf)* 1992; 36:97–104.
16. Meyer BR, Kreis W, Eschbach J, et al: Transdermal versus subcutaneous leuprolide: A comparison of acute pharmacodynamic effect. *Clin Pharmacol Ther* 1990; 48:340–345.
17. Meldrum DR, Wisot A, Hamilton F: Timing of initiation and dose schedule of leuprolide influence the time course of ovarian suppression. *Fertil Steril* 1988; 50:400–402.
18. Sheehan KL, Casper RF, Yen SSC: Effects of a superactive luteinizing hormone–releasing factor agonist on gonadotropin and ovarian function during the menstrual cycle. *Am J Obstet Gynecol* 1979; 135:759–763.
19. Monroe SE, Blumenfeld Z, Andreyko JL: Dose-dependent inhibition of pituitary-ovarian function during administration of a gonadotropin-releasing hormone agonistic analog (nafarelin). *J Clin Endocrinol Metab* 1986; 63:1334–1341.
20. Lemay A, Brideau NA, Forest JC, et al: Cholesterol fractions and apolipoproteins during endometriosis treatment by a gonadotropin releasing hormone (GnRH) agonist implant or by danazol. *Clin Endocrinol (Oxf)* 1991; 35:305–310.
21. Farish E, Fletcher CD, Barnes JF, et al: Reversible menopause induced by the GnRH analogue buserelin: Effects on lipoprotein metabolism. *Acta Endocrinol (Copenh)* 1992; 127:123–126.
22. Dawood MY: Impact of medical treatment of endometriosis on bone mass. *Am J Obstet Gynecol* 1993; 168:674–684.
23. Nottestad SY, Baumel JJ, Kimmel DB, et al: The proportion of trabecular bone in human vertebrae. *J Bone Miner Res* 1987; 2:221–229.
24. Tummon IS, Ali A, Pepping ME, et al: Bone mineral density in women with endometriosis before and during ovarian suppression with gonadotropin releasing hormone agonists or danazol. *Fertil Steril* 1988; 49:792–796.
25. Damewood MD, Schlaff WD, Hesla JS, et al: Interval bone mineral density with long-term gonadotropin-releasing hormone agonist suppression. *Fertil Steril* 1989; 52:596–599.
26. Dodin S, Lemay A, Maheux R, et al: Bone mass in endometriosis patients treated with GnRH agonist implant or danazol. *Obstet Gynecol* 1991; 77:410–415.
27. Johansen JS, Riis BJ, Hassager C, et al: The effects of a gonadotropin-releasing hormone agonist analog (nafarelin) on bone metabolism. *J Clin Endocrinol Metab* 1988; 67:701–706.
28. Devogelaer JP, Nagant de Deuxchaisnes C, Donnez J, et al: LHRH analogues and bone loss. *Lancet* 1987; 1:1498.
29. Nencioni T, Penotti M, Barbieri-Carones M, et al: Gonadotropin releasing hormone agonist therapy and its effect on bone mass. *Gynecol Endocrinol* 1991; 5:49–56.
30. Scharla SH, Minne HW, Waibel-Treber S, et al: Bone mass reduction after estrogen deprivation by long-acting gonadotropin-releasing hormone agonists and its relation to pretreatment serum concentrations of 1,25-dihydroxyvitamin D_3. *J Clin Endocrinol Metab* 1990; 70:1055–1061.
31. Fogelman I: Gonadotropin-releasing hormone agonists and the skeleton. *Fertil Steril* 1992; 57:715–724.

32. Cann CE, Henzl M, Burry K: Reversible bone loss is produced by the GnRH agonist nafarelin, in Cohn DV, Martin TJ, Meunier PJ (eds): *Calcium Regulation and Bone Metabolism, Basic and Clinical Aspects*, vol 9. Amsterdam, Excerpta Medica, 1987, pp 123–127.

33. Ashkenazi J, Goldman JA, Dicker D, et al: Adverse neurological symptoms after gonadotropin-releasing hormone analog therapy for in vitro fertilization cycles. *Fertil Steril* 1990; 53:738–740.

34. Herman A, Ron-El R, Golan A, et al: Impaired corpus luteum function and other undesired results of pregnancies associated with inadvertent administration of a long-acting agonist of gonadotrophin-releasing hormone. *Hum Reprod* 1992; 7:465–468.

35. Smitz J, Camus M, Devroey P, et al: The influence of inadvertent intranasal buserelin administration in early pregnancy. *Hum Reprod* 1991; 6:290–293.

36. Cedars MI, Steingold KA, Lu JH, et al: Pituitary function before, during, and after chronic gonadotropin-releasing hormone agonist therapy. *Fertil Steril* 1992; 58:1104–1107.

37. Meldrum DR, Cedars MI, Hamilton F, et al: Leuprolide acetate elevates prolactin during ovarian stimulation with gonadotropins. *J Assist Reprod Genet* 1992; 9:251–253.

38. Filicori M, Hall DA, Loughlin JS, et al: A conservative approach to the management of uterine leiomyoma: Pituitary desensitization by a luteinizing hormone–releasing hormone analogue. *Am J Obstet Gynecol* 1983; 147:726–727.

39. Friedman AJ, Hoffman DI, Comite F, et al: Treatment of leiomyomata uteri with leuprolide acetate depot: A double-blind, placebo-controlled, multicenter study. The Leuprolide Study Group. *Obstet Gynecol* 1991; 77:720–725.

40. Cirkel U, Ochs H, Schneider HP, et al: Experience with leuprorelin acetate depot in the treatment of fibroids: A German multicentre study. *Clin Ther* 1992; 14(suppl A):37–50.

41. Hackenberg R, Gesenhues T, Deichert U, et al: The response of uterine fibroids to GnRH-agonist treatment can be predicted in most cases after one month. *Eur J Obstet Gynecol Reprod Biol* 1992; 45:125–129.

42. Upadhyaya NB, Doody MC, Googe PB: Histopathological changes in leiomyomata treated with leuprolide acetate. *Fertil Steril* 1990; 54:811–814.

43. Neuman M, Langer R, Golan A, et al: Gonadotropin-releasing hormone (GnRH) action on uterine leiomyomata is not mediated by uterine GnRH receptors. *Fertil Steril* 1991; 56:364–366.

44. Rein MS, Friedman AJ, Stuart JM, et al: Fibroid and myometrial steroid receptors in women treated with gonadotropin-releasing hormone agonist leuprolide acetate. *Fertil Steril* 1990; 53:1018–1023.

45. Uemura T, Mori J, Yoshimura Y, et al: Treatment effects of GnRH agonist on the binding of estrogen and progesterone, and the histological findings of uterine leiomyomas. *Asia Oceania J Obstet Gynaecol* 1991; 17:315–320.

46. Rein MS, Friedman AJ, Pandian MR, et al: The secretion of insulin-like growth factors I and II by explant cultures of fibroids and myometrium from women treated with a gonadotropin-releasing hormone agonist. *Obstet Gynecol* 1990; 76:388–394.

47. Rein MS, Friedman AJ, Heffner LJ: Decreased prolactin secretion by explant cultures of fibroids from women treated with a gonadotropin-releasing hormone agonist. *J Clin Endocrinol Metab* 1990; 70:1554–1558.

48. National Center for Health Statistics: *Hysterectomies in the United States 1965–1984*. Washington, DC, Vital and Health Statistics, Series 13, No 92, Publication No (PHS) 88–1753, Public Health Service, Government Printing Office, 1987.

49. Meyer WR, Mayer AR, Diamond MP, et al: Unsuspected leiomyosarcoma: Treatment with a gonadotropin-releasing hormone analogue. *Obstet Gynecol* 1990; 75:529–532.

50. Friedman AJ: Vaginal hemorrhage associated with degenerating submucous leiomyomata during leuprolide acetate treatment. *Fertil Steril* 1989; 52:152–154.

51. Lumsden MA, West CP, Baird DT: Goserelin therapy before surgery for uterine fibroids. *Lancet* 1987; 1:36–37.

52. Friedman AJ, Rein MS, Harrison-Atlas D, et al: A randomized placebo-controlled, double-blind study evaluating leuprolide acetate depot treatment before myomectomy. *Fertil Steril* 1989; 52:728–733.

53. Stovall TG, Ling FW, Henry LC, et al: A randomized trial evaluating leuprolide acetate before hysterectomy as treatment for leiomyomas. *Am J Obstet Gynecol* 1991; 164:1420–1425.

54. Fedele L, Vercellini P, Bianchi S, et al: Treatment with GnRH agonists before myomectomy and the risk of short-term myoma recurrence. *Br J Obstet Gynaecol* 1990; 97:393–396.

55. Friedman AJ, Daly M, Juneau-Norcross M, et al: Recurrence of myomas after myomectomy in women pretreated with leuprolide acetate depot or placebo. *Fertil Steril* 1992; 58:205–208.

56. Von Rokitansky C: Ueber uterusdrusen-neubildung in uterus and ovarial-sarcomen. *Zkk Gesellschaft Aerzte Wien* 1860; 37:577.

57. Jones HW Jr, Rock JA: Regulation of female infertility, In Diczfalusy E (ed): *Regulation of Human Fertility*. Moscow, WHO Symposium, Scriptor, 1977.

58. Henzl MR, Corson SL, Moghissi K, et al: Administration of nasal nafarelin as compared with oral danazol for endometriosis. *N Engl J Med* 1988; 318:485–489.

59. Zorn JR, Mathieson J, Risquez F, et al: Treatment of endometriosis with a delayed release preparation of the agonist D-Trp6-luteinizing hormone–releasing hormone: Long-term follow-up in a series of 50 patients. *Fertil Steril* 1990; 53:401–406.

60. Nafarelin for endometriosis: A large-scale, danazol-controlled trial of efficacy and safety, with 1-year follow-up. The Nafarelin European Endometriosis Trial Group (NEET). *Fertil Steril* 1992; 57:514–522.

61. Reichel RP, Schweppe KW: Goserelin (Zoladex) depot in the treatment of endometriosis. Zoladex Endometriosis Study Group. *Fertil Steril* 1992; 57:1197–1202.

62. Grow DR, Filer RB: Treatment of adenomyosis with long-term GnRH analogues: A case report. *Obstet Gynecol* 1991; 78:538–539.

63. Surrey ES, Halme J: Direct effects of medroxyprogesterone acetate, danazol, and leuprolide acetate on endometrial stromal cell proliferation in vitro. *Fertil Steril* 1992; 58:273–278.

64. Hill JA: Immunology and endometriosis (editorial). *Fertil Steril* 1992; 58:262–264.

65. Kennedy SH, Starkey PM, Sargent IL, et al: Antiendometrial antibodies in endometriosis measured by an enzyme-linked immunosorbent assay before and after treatment with danazol and nafarelin. *Obstet Gynecol* 1990; 75:914–918.

66. Braun DP, Gebel H, Rotman C, et al: The development of cytotoxicity in peritoneal macrophages from women with endometriosis. *Fertil Steril* 1992; 57:1203–1210.

67. Barbieri RL, Ryan KJ: Danazol: Endocrine, pharmacology and therapeutic applications. *Am J Obstet Gynecol* 1981; 141:453–463.

68. Kennedy SH, Williams IA, Brodribb J, et al: A comparison of nafarelin ac-

etate and danazol in the treatment of endometriosis. *Fertil Steril* 1990; 53:998–1003.

69. Rolland R, van der Heijden PF: Nafarelin versus danazol in the treatment of endometriosis. *Am J Obstet Gynecol* 1990; 162:586–588.

70. Henzl MR, Kwei L: Efficacy and safety of nafarelin in the treatment of endometriosis. *Am J Obstet Gynecol* 1990; 162:570–574.

71. Wheeler JM, Knittle JD, Miller JD: Depot leuprolide versus danazol in treatment of women with symptomatic endometriosis. I. Efficacy results. *Am J Obstet Gynecol* 1992; 167:1367–1371.

72. Hickok LR, Burry KA, Cohen NL, et al: Medical treatment of endometriosis: A comparison of the suppressive effects of danazol and nafarelin on reproductive hormones. *Fertil Steril* 1991; 56:622–627.

73. Shaw RW: An open randomized comparative study of the effect of goserelin depot and danazol in the treatment of endometriosis. Zoladex Endometriosis Study Team. *Fertil Steril* 1992; 58:265–272.

74. Fedele L, Parazzini F, Radici E, et al: Buserelin acetate versus expectant management in the treatment of infertility associated with minimal or mild endometriosis: A randomized clinical trial. *Am J Obstet Gynecol* 1992; 166:1345–1350.

75. Nakamura K, Oosawa M, Kondou I, et al: Menotropin stimulation after prolonged gonadotropin releasing hormone agonist pretreatment for in vitro fertilization in patients with endometriosis. *J Assist Reprod Genet* 1992; 9:113–117.

76. Remorgida V, Anserini P, Croce S, et al: Comparison of different ovarian stimulation protocols for gamete intrafallopian transfer in patients with minimal and mild endometriosis. *Fertil Steril* 1990; 53:1060–1063.

77. Barbieri RL, Niloff JM, Bast RC Jr, et al: Elevated serum concentrations of CA-125 in patients with advanced endometriosis. *Fertil Steril* 1986; 45:630–634.

78. Pittaway DE, Fayez JA: The use of CA-125 in the diagnosis and management of endometriosis. *Fertil Steril* 1986; 46:790–795.

79. Marana R, Muzii L, Muscatello P, et al: Gonadotrophin releasing hormone agonist (buserelin) in the treatment of endometriosis: Changes in the extent of the disease and in CA 125 serum levels after 6-month therapy. *Br J Obstet Gynaecol* 1990; 97:1016–1019.

80. Franssen AM, van der Heijden PF, Thomas CM, et al: On the origin and significance of serum CA-125 concentrations in 97 patients with endometriosis before, during, and after buserelin acetate, nafarelin, or danazol. *Fertil Steril* 1992; 57:974–979.

81. Schenken RS: Gonadotropin-releasing hormone analogs in the treatment of endometriomas. *Am J Obstet Gynecol* 1990; 162:579–581.

82. Barbieri RL, Evans S, Kistner RW: Danazol in the treatment of endometriosis: Analysis of 100 cases with a 4-year follow-up. *Fertil Steril* 1982; 37:737–746.

83. Bachus KE, Hughes CL Jr, Haney AF, et al: The luteal phase in polycystic ovary syndrome during ovulation induction with human menopausal gonadotropin with and without leuprolide acetate. *Fertil Steril* 1990; 54:27–31.

84. Gonzalez F, Hatala DA, Speroff L: Adrenal and ovarian steroid hormone responses to gonadotropin-releasing hormone agonist treatment in polycystic ovary syndrome. *Am J Obstet Gynecol* 1991; 165:535–545.

85. Macleod AF, Wheeler MJ, Gordon P, et al: Effect of long-term inhibition of gonadotrophin secretion by the gonadotrophin-releasing hormone agonist, buserelin, on sex steroid secretion and ovarian morphology in polycystic ovary syndrome. *J Endocrinol* 1990; 125:317–325.

86. Mais V, Melis GB, Strigini F, et al: Adjusting the dose to the individual response of the patient during the induction of ovulation with pulsatile gonadotropin-releasing hormone. *Fertil Steril* 1991; 55:80–85.

87. Filicori M, Flamigni C, Campaniello E, et al: Polycystic ovary syndrome: Abnormalities and management with pulsatile gonadotropin-releasing hormone and gonadotropin-releasing hormone analogs. *Am J Obstet Gynecol* 1990; 163:1737–1742.

88. Dor J, Shulman A, Pariente C, et al: The effect of gonadotropin-releasing hormone agonist on the ovarian response and in vitro fertilization results in polycystic ovarian syndrome: A prospective study. *Fertil Steril* 1992; 57:366–371.

89. Dale PO, Tanbo T, Djoseland O, et al: Persistence of hyperinsulinemia in polycystic ovary syndrome after ovarian suppression by gonadotropin-releasing hormone agonist. *Acta Endocrinol (Copenh)* 1992; 126:132–136.

90. Forman RG, Robinson J, Egan D, et al: Follicular monitoring and outcome of in vitro fertilization in gonadotropin-releasing hormone-agonist–treated cycles. *Fertil Steril* 1991; 55:567–573.

91. Hughes EG, Fedorkow DM, Daya S, et al: The routine use of gonadotropin-releasing hormone agonists prior to in vitro fertilization and gamete intrafallopian transfer: A meta-analysis of randomized controlled trials. *Fertil Steril* 1992; 58:888–896.

92. Muasher SJ: Use of gonadotrophin-releasing hormone agonists in controlled ovarian hyperstimulation for in vitro fertilization. *Clin Ther* 1992; 14(suppl A):74–86.

93. Benadiva CA, Blasco L, Tureck R, et al: Comparison of different regimens of a gonadotropin-releasing hormone analog during ovarian stimulation for in vitro fertilization. *Fertil Steril* 1990; 53:479–485.

94. San Ramon GA, Surrey ES, Judd HL, et al: A prospective randomized comparison of luteal phase versus concurrent follicular phase initiation of gonadotropin-releasing hormone agonist for in vitro fertilization. *Fertil Steril* 1992; 58:744–749.

95. Tan SL, Kingsland C, Campbell S, et al: The long protocol of administration of gonadotropin-releasing hormone agonist is superior to the short protocol for ovarian stimulation for in vitro fertilization. *Fertil Steril* 1992; 57:810–814.

96. Acharya U, Irvine S, Hamilton M, et al: Prospective study of short and ultrashort regimens of gonadotropin-releasing hormone agonist in an in vitro fertilization program. *Fertil Steril* 1992; 58:1169–1173.

97. Penzias AS, Shamma FN, Gutmann JN, et al: Nafarelin versus leuprolide in ovulation induction for in vitro fertilization: A randomized clinical trial. *Obstet Gynecol* 1992; 79:739–742.

98. Balasch J, Jove IC, Moreno V, et al: The comparison of two gonadotropin-releasing hormone agonists in an in vitro fertilization program. *Fertil Steril* 1992; 58:991–994.

99. Parinaud J, Oustry P, Perineau M, et al: Randomized trial of three luteinizing hormone–releasing hormone analogues used for ovarian stimulation in an in vitro fertilization program. *Fertil Steril* 1992; 57:1265–1268.

100. Brzyski RG, Hofmann GE, Scott RT, et al: Effects of leuprolide acetate on follicular fluid hormone composition at oocyte retrieval for in vitro fertilization. *Fertil Steril* 1990; 54:842–847.

101. Keenan D, Cohen J, Suzman M, et al: Stimulation cycles suppressed with gonadotropin-releasing hormone analog yield accelerated embryos. *Fertil Steril* 1991; 55:792–796.

102. Oehninger S, Toner JP, Veeck LL, et al: Performance of cryopreserved pre-

embryos obtained in in vitro fertilization cycles with or without a gonadotropin-releasing hormone agonist. *Fertil Steril* 1992; 57:620–625.

103. Padilla SL, Bayati J, Garcia JE: Prognostic value of the early serum estradiol response to leuprolide acetate in in vitro fertilization. *Fertil Steril* 1990; 53:288–294.

104. Winslow KL, Toner JP, Brzyski RG, et al: The gonadotropin-releasing hormone agonist stimulation test—a sensitive predictor of performance in the flare-up in vitro fertilization cycle. *Fertil Steril* 1991; 56:711–717.

105. Tur-Kaspa I, Confino E, Dudkiewicz AB, et al: Ovarian stimulation protocol for in vitro fertilization with gonadotropin-releasing hormone agonist widens the implantation window. *Fertil Steril* 1990; 53:859–864.

106. Dodson WC, Walmer DK, Hughes CL Jr, et al: Adjunctive leuprolide therapy does not improve cycle fecundity in controlled ovarian hyperstimulation and intrauterine insemination of subfertile women. *Obstet Gynecol* 1991; 78:187–190.

107. Gagliardi CL, Emmi AM, Weiss G, et al: Gonadotropin-releasing hormone agonist improves the efficiency of controlled ovarian hyperstimulation/intrauterine insemination. *Fertil Steril* 1991; 55:939–944.

108. Gonen Y, Balakier H, Powell W, et al: Use of gonadotropin-releasing hormone agonist to trigger follicular maturation for in vitro fertilization. *J Clin Endocrinol Metab* 1990; 71:918–922.

109. Segal S, Casper RF: Gonadotropin-releasing hormone agonist versus human chorionic gonadotropin for triggering follicular maturation in in vitro fertilization. *Fertil Steril* 1992; 57:1254–1258.

110. Schiff I, Tulchinsky D, Cramer D, et al: Oral medroxyprogesterone in the treatment of postmenopausal symptoms. *JAMA* 1980; 244:1443–1445.

111. Friedman AJ, Barbieri RL, Doubilet PM, et al: A randomized, double-blind trial of gonadotropin-releasing hormone agonist (leuprolide) with or without medroxyprogesterone acetate in the treatment of leiomyomata uteri. *Fertil Steril* 1988; 49:404–409.

112. Friedman AJ: Treatment of leiomyomata uteri with short-term leuprolide followed by leuprolide plus estrogen-progestin hormone replacement therapy for 2 years: A pilot study. *Fertil Steril* 1989; 51:526–528.

113. Surrey ES, Judd HL: Reduction of vasomotor symptoms and bone mineral density loss with combined norethindrone and long-acting gonadotropin-releasing hormone agonist therapy of symptomatic endometriosis: A prospective randomized trial. *J Clin Endocrinol Metab* 1992; 75:558–563.

114. Judd HL: Gonadotropin-releasing hormone agonists: Strategies for managing the hypoestrogenic effects of therapy. *Am J Obstet Gynecol* 1992; 166:752–756.

115. Friedman AJ, Lobel SM, Rein MS, et al: Efficacy and safety considerations in women with uterine leiomyomas treated with gonadotropin-releasing hormone agonists: The estrogen threshold hypothesis. *Am J Obstet Gynecol* 1990; 163:1114–1119.

116. Barbieri RL: Hormone treatment of endometriosis: The estrogen threshold hypothesis. *Am J Obstet Gynecol* 1992; 166:740–745.

117. Muse K: Hormonal manipulation in the treatment of premenstrual syndrome. *Clin Obstet Gynecol* 1992; 35:658–666.

118. Mortola JF, Girton L, Fischer U: Successful treatment of severe premenstrual syndrome by combined use of gonadotropin-releasing hormone agonist and estrogen/progestin. *J Clin Endocrinol Metab* 1991; 72:252.

119. Adashi EY: Potential utility of gonadotropin-releasing hormone agonists in the management of ovarian hyperandrogenism. *Fertil Steril* 1990; 53:765–779.

120. Rittmaster RS, Thompson DL: Effect of leuprolide and dexamethasone on hair growth and hormone levels in hirsute women: The relative importance of the ovary and the adrenal in the pathogenesis of hirsutism. *J Clin Endocrinol Metab* 1990; 70:1096–1102.

121. Goldrath MH, Fuller TA, Segal S: Laser photo vaporization of endometrium for the treatment of menorrhagia. *Am J Obstet Gynecol* 1981; 140:14–19.

122. Serden SP, Brooks PG: Preoperative therapy in preparation for endometrial ablation. *J Reprod Med* 1992; 37:679–681.

123. Dogliotti L, Fioretti P, Mebs GB, et al: Current status of therapy of fibrocystic breast disease. *Ann N Y Acad Sci* 1986; 464:350–363.

124. Gateley CA, Mansel RE: Management of the painful and nodular breast. *Br Med Bull* 1991; 47:284–294.

125. Monsonego J, Destable MD, De Saint Florent G, et al: Fibrocystic disease of the breast in premenopausal women: Histohormonal correlation and response to luteinizing hormone releasing hormone analog treatment. *Am J Obstet Gynecol* 1991; 164:1181–1189.

126. Hamed H, Caleffi M, Chaudary MA, et al: LHRH analogue for treatment of recurrent and refractory mastalgia. *Ann R Coll Surg Engl* 1990; 72:221–224.

127. Emons G, Ortmann O, Pahwa GS, et al: Intracellular actions of gonadotropic and peptide hormones and the therapeutic value of GnRH-agonists in ovarian cancer. *Acta Obstet Gynecol Scand Suppl* 1992; 155:31–38.

128. Peterson CM, Zimniski SJ: A long-acting gonadotropin-releasing hormone agonist inhibits the growth of a human ovarian epithelial carcinoma (BG-1) heterotransplanted in the nude mouse. *Obstet Gynecol* 1990; 76:264–267.

129. Thompson MA, Adelson MD, Kaufman LM: Lupron retards proliferation of ovarian epithelial tumor cells cultured in serum-free medium. *J Clin Endocrinol Metab* 1991 72:1036–1041.

130. Lind MJ, Cantwell BM, Millward MJ, et al: A phase II trial of goserelin (Zoladex) in relapsed epithelial ovarian cancer. *Br J Cancer* 1992; 65:621–623.

131. Yano T, Korkut E, Pinski J, et al: Inhibition of growth of MCF-7 MIII human breast carcinoma in nude mice by treatment with agonists or antagonists of LH-RH. *Breast Cancer Res Treat* 1992; 21:35–45.

132. Nicholson RI, Walker KJ, Bouzubar N, et al: Estrogen deprivation in breast cancer. Clinical, experimental, and biological aspects. *Ann N Y Acad Sci* 1990; 595:316–327.

133. Harris N, Dutlow C, Eidne K, et al: Gonadotropin-releasing hormone gene expression in MDA-MB-231 and ZR-75-1 breast carcinoma cell lines. *Cancer Res* 1991; 51:2577–2581.

134. Neri C, Berthois Y, Schatz B, et al: Compared effects of GnRH analogs and 4-hydroxytamoxifen on growth and steroid receptors in antiestrogen sensitive and resistant MCF-7 breast cancer cell sublines. *Breast Cancer Res Treat* 1990; 15:85–93.

135. Kullander S: Treatment of endometrial cancer with GnRH analogs. *Recent Results Cancer Res* 1992; 124:69–73.

136. Gallagher CJ, Oliver RT, Oram DH, et al: A new treatment for endometrial cancer with gonadotrophin releasing-hormone analogue. *Br J Obstet Gynaecol* 1991; 98:1037–1041.

Editor's Comment

Andrew Schally and Roger Guillemin received the Nobel Prize in Medicine for the discovery of GnRH. Not only was this of basic importance to our understanding of the hypothalamic-pituitary-ovarian/endometrial axis, but it has also provided us with a powerful tool to control ovarian steroid-dependent diseases. This complete review by Drs. Hardy and Friedman covers basic concepts and accepted as well as "emerging" clinical applications. One of the more exciting "emerging" applications is "add-back" therapy. Low-dose estrogen and progestin are used to reduce hot flashes and protect against bone loss. Although this appears contradictory, the "estrogen threshold" hypothesis proposed by Friedman et al. suggests a hierarchy of organ response, with bone metabolism being most sensitive. Since this progestin alone vs. estrogen/progestin has shown little increase in the size of myomas with estrogen/progestin. However, after 3 months of add-back therapy with progestin, the uterus attained more than 90% of its original size (Friedman et al., *J Clin Endocrinol Metab*, June 1993). This is an important and interesting study not only because there is now evidence for an acceptable form of long-term therapy but also because it teaches us something interesting about the biology of these tumors. Mounting data suggest that progesterone as opposed to estrogen may be an important mediator for growth of these very common tumors. We await further studies on these "emerging" indications for this class of drug.

Ana A. Murphy, M.D.

Basic and Clinical Concepts in Ovulation Induction

L. MICHAEL KETTEL, M.D.

GREGORY F. ERICKSON, PH.D.

U nderstanding the processes used in ovulation induction requires a basic understanding of the process of ovulation. The fundamentals of normal ovarian physiology and folliculogenesis form a framework around which the clinician can develop an understanding of the possible manipulations that may influence this process. Surgical, hormonal, and pharmacologic methods have been developed to perturb the female reproductive system and result in ovulation.

The science of ovulation induction began as a technique to provide treatment for women whose hypothalamic-pituitary-ovarian-endometrial axis failed to function properly. Infertility, irregular vaginal bleeding, and endometrial hyperplasia often develop in anovulatory women. Treatment strategies to reverse the state of anovulation can lead to resolution or prevention of these disorders.

Although most ovulation induction regimens were developed for the treatment of anovulation, these are now commonly used to stimulate ovulation in ovulatory women. Under most circumstances, the process of normal folliculogenesis results in the ovulation of a single oocyte from a selected dominant follicle. By administering hormonal medications this process can be altered to induce the development of multiple follicles with multiple ovulations. This process, known as superovulation, has found widespread utility in the treatment of infertile couples. Thus, ovulation induction has a role in both ovulatory and anovulatory women.

This review will focus on advances in the induction of ovulation from two perspectives. Advances in the basic understanding of folliculogenesis will be followed by an update and review of clinical ovulation induction regimens under a variety of physiologic and pathophysiologic conditions.

BASIC ADVANCES IN OVULATION INDUCTION

The purpose of this section is to discuss new advances in our understanding of how ligands interact with receptors in the granulosa and theca cells to cause selection and atresia. Knowledge and understanding of this subject are important because it holds promise for future progress in the field of ovulation induction. The functional role of the hormones follicle-stimulating hormone (FSH) and luteinizing hormone (LH) is well charac-

Advances in Obstetrics and Gynecology, vol 1
© 1994, Mosby–Year Book, Inc.

terized. Their ligand-bound receptors generate intracellular signals via G protein-cyclic adenosine monophosphate protein kinase A (cAMP)-PKA signaling pathways leading to the induction of specific biological responses, most notably estradiol synthesis. This principle, which is the underlying basis of successful ovulation induction, is called the two-gonadotropin/two-cell concept. In the past few years, a large number of intrinsic regulatory proteins have been found in healthy and atretic follicles, including the five families of growth factors. These proteins are ligands that interact with the follicle compartment to modulate signal transduction by FSH and LH. An interesting and important theory to emerge is that growth factors, either "selectogenic" or "atretogenic," act as the mediators of FSH and LH action in promoting selection or atresia, respectively. Here we will examine the relationship between hormones, growth factors, and folliculogenesis.

A central question in ovarian physiology is how one follicle is selected to become a dominant preovulatory follicle that secretes its egg into the oviducts to be fertilized.[1, 2] In women, this process, termed folliculogenesis, is very long (Fig 1). It begins when a cohort of primordial follicles is recruited to initiate growth. Successive recruitments give rise to cohorts of developing follicles (primary, secondary, tertiary, and graafian) present in the ovaries. The dominant follicle in each cycle originates from a primordial follicle that was recruited to grow about 1 year earlier (Fig 1). Selection is the last step in this long sequence of events. The actual decision to select the dominant follicle is made near the end of the luteal phase of the cycle.[3, 4] At this time, each ovary contains a cohort of small graafian follicles (2 to 5 mm), all of which are rapidly growing; it is from this cohort that the dominant follicle is selected.[2] After selection, the mi-

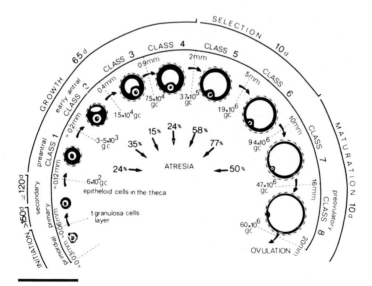

FIGURE 1.

The temporal pattern of human folliculogenesis. The time (d = days) and stages of follicle growth (classes 1 to 8) and percent atresia are shown. The number of granulosa cells (gc) and follicle diameter are indicated. (From Gougeon A: *Hum Reprod* 1986; 1:81. Used by permission.)

totic activities of the granulosa and theca cells increase markedly.[3, 5] The sustained capacity for rapid growth and cell division is the sine qua non of a dominant follicle. Those follicles that lose this property die by apoptosis or programmed cell death,[6] a process called *atresia*. To understand what determines selection and atresia, we must understand the signal processing mechanisms that are coupled to these cellular responses.

THE STRUCTURE OF THE FOLLICLE COMPARTMENT

The graafian follicle is composed of several different tissues (see Fig 1). These include the oocyte, granulosa, theca interna, and theca externa. The granulosa cells develop as a pseudostratified epithelium that is bound peripherally by a basal lamina. The basal lamina is an extracellular matrix of collagen, laminin, and fibronectin fibrils to which the membrana granulosa cells are attracted. By virtue of the basal lamina, the granulosa cells (and egg) develop within an avascular microenvironment termed the *antrum*. The antral or follicular fluid is an exudate of plasma plus various hormones, growth factors and other molecules, some of which are produced by the follicle itself.[1, 2] The latter molecules are ligands that regulate follicle growth and development by endocrine, autocrine, and paracrine mechanisms. The granulosa cells (Fig 2) exist as three subgroups of cells: (1) the corona radiata, which makes contact with the egg and zona pellucida; (2) the cumulus, which makes contact with both the corona and membrana granulosa cells; and (3) the membrana, which makes direct contact with the basal lamina and Call-Exner bodies. It is well known that in animals these subgroups of granulosa cells respond differently to FSH stimulation. That is, despite the fact that all granulosa cells have FSH receptors, only those in the membrana granulosa layer respond to FSH action by expressing $P450_{arom}$, $P450_{scc}$, and LH receptors.[1, 7] These specific FSH responses appear causal to the relative position of the granulosa in the follicle compartment; how this occurs is unknown. The theca interna (Fig 2) is a loose connective tissue containing five to eight layers of highly differentiated theca interstitial cells. LH receptors are present in all theca interstitial cells and control their metabolic, endocrine, and developmental functions.[8] The theca externa contains smooth

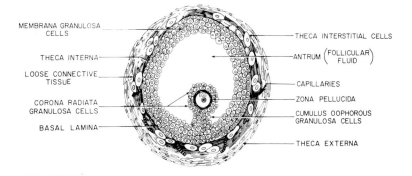

FIGURE 2.

Anatomy of the graafian follicle. (From Erickson GF: The ovary: Basic principles and concepts. In Felig P, Baxter JD, Broadus AE, et al (eds): *Endocrinology and Metabolism*, ed 2. New York, McGraw-Hill, 1987. Used by permission.)

muscle cells that are innervated by autonomic nerves.[2] We know almost nothing about the ligand signal processing mechanisms that modulate cellular responses in the theca externa.

THE TWO-GONADOTROPIN/TWO-CELL CONCEPT

The ability of graafian follicles to grow and develop is dependent on appropriate concentrations of FSH and LH. Classic experiments have demonstrated that interaction of the follicle compartment with FSH and LH leads to the synthesis of steroid hormones, most notably 17β-estradiol. This is the two-gonadotropin/two-cell concept (Fig 3). In this process, FSH and LH interact with transmembrane receptors in the granulosa and theca interstitial cells, respectively, and the binding events are transduced into intracellular signals by heterodimeric G proteins (Fig 3). The LH-bound receptor is coupled to the $\alpha G_{stimulatory}$ (αG_s)-cAMP-PKA pathway and leads to the stimulation of $P450_{scc}$ and $P450_{17\alpha}$ in theca interstitial cells.[9] This results in de novo C_{19} androgen synthesis, especially androstenedione. The FSH-bound receptor activates the αG_s-cAMP-PKA pathway in membrana granulosa cells, and this leads to the stimulation of $P450_{arom}$. $P450_{arom}$ causes the aromatization of androstenedione to estrogen (Fig 3). The obligatory role of FSH in follicle selection is clear. In-

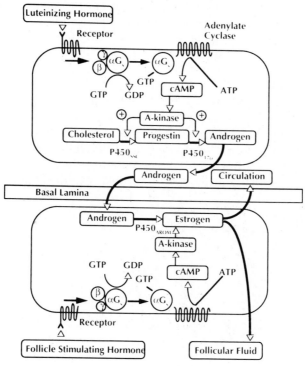

FIGURE 3.

The two-gonadotropin/two-cell mechanism of follicle estrogen biosynthesis. (Adapted from Erickson GF: *Clin Obstet Gynecol* 1978; 21:31.)

deed, only those follicles that concentrate FSH in their microenvironment during the follicular phase escape atresia and mature to the preovulatory stage (Fig 4). There is a large body of evidence in rodents demonstrating that estrogen interacts with nuclear receptors in granulosa cells to promote their growth and differentiation. In women, however, estradiol-bound receptors do not appear to have an obligatory role in the selection process.[10]

THE GROWTH FACTOR CONCEPT

Work carried out in the rat and human has provided important new information about how FSH and LH generate cellular responses in the follicle. All the evidence has led to the novel theory that the actions of FSH and LH may be mediated by intrinsic growth factors produced by the follicle itself. This theory is illustrated in Figure 5.

Growth factors are regulatory proteins that control a wide variety of proliferative and developmental functions. All are ligands that interact with specific receptors on target cells, and the binding events generate signal transduction pathways that modulate cellular responses to endocrine hormones (Fig 5). With respect to the ovary, the search for intrinsic growth factors has been very productive, especially in the rat. All of the growth factors share the property of "modulators." That is, they either increase or decrease the responsiveness of the follicle cells to gonadotropin stimulation. The results of a large number of studies have demonstrated that all five families of growth factors are expressed in the rat follicle, and there is increasing evidence for growth factors in the human ovary (Table 1). The results of these and other experiments have

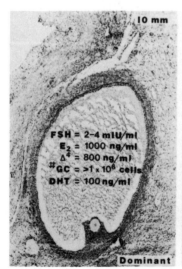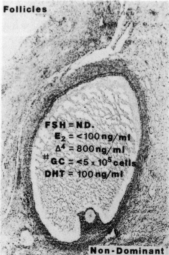

FIGURE 4.

The causal connection between the concentration of FSH and the levels of estradiol CE_{12}) in the follicular fluid. High and low concentrations of FSH lead to the formation of dominant and nondominant (atretic) follicles, respectively. GC-granulosa cells; DHT-dihydrotestosterone (From Erickson GF, et al: *Semin Reprod Endocrinol* 1984; 2:231–243. Used by permission.)

ENDOCRINE SYSTEM

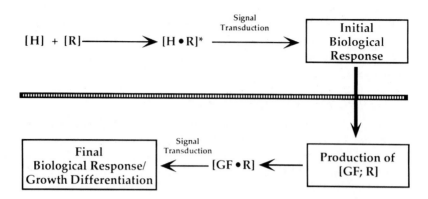

AUTOCRINE/PARACRINE SYSTEM

FIGURE 5.

Current theory of the functional role of growth factors as autocrine/paracrine mediators of the endocrine system. H = hormone; R = receptor; $[H \cdot R]^*$ = active H · R complex after allosteric shape change; GF = growth factor.

led to the concept that growth factors regulate folliculogenesis by autocrine/paracrine mechanisms. For the purpose of limiting the scope of this section, we will focus our attention on recent advances in the basic biology of the ovarian insulin-like growth factor (IGF) system as it relates to the regulation of granulosa cytodifferentiation in the rat and human.

TABLE 1.

The Five Families of Growth Factors Expressed in the Rat Follicle, With Some of the Ligands Listed

	References	
The Autocrine/Paracrine Control Systems*	**Rat**	**Human**
IGF family (GHRH, GH, IGF-1, IGFBPs)	11,12	13
TGFβ family (TGFβ, PDGF, MIS, activin, inhibin; follistatin)	14–16	17–21
EGF/TGFα family (EGF, TGFα)	22	23–26
FGF family (basic FGF, acid FGF)	27	27
Cytokine family (IL, TNF, CSF, interferon)	28	29–31

*IGF = insulin-like growth factor; GHRH = growth hormone–releasing hormone; GH = growth hormone; IGFBP = IGF binding protein; TGF = transforming growth factor; PDGF = platelet-derived growth factor; MIS = meiosis-inducing substance; EGF = epidermal growth factor; FGF = fibroblast growth factor; IL = interleukin; TNF = tumor necrosis factor; CSF = colony-stimulating factor.

THE OVARIAN INSULIN-LIKE GROWTH FACTOR SYSTEM EXAMPLE

There is compelling evidence for a complete IGF system in the graafian follicle[11–31] (Table 2). For example, rat granulosa cells express the growth hormone–releasing hormone (GHRH) ligand[32] and contain specific high-affinity GHRH receptors in their plasma membranes.[32, 33] Exogenous GHRH amplifies FSH-stimulated cAMP and estradiol production,[33] and FSH upregulates the concentration of GHRH receptors in the granulosa cells.[34] Thus, GHRH-bound receptors mediate activation of granulosa cytodifferentiation similar to that found during follicle selection. In human ovaries, immunoreactive GHRH has been detected.[35] Human follicles are apparently able to interact with GHRH because GHRH administered to infertile patients has been found to amplify the ability of exogenous FSH to promote the formation of preovulatory follicles.[36] Thus, intrinsic GHRH in human ovaries might have a direct effect on follicle selection.

Growth hormone receptors appear to be widely distributed in the rat ovary and are present in oocytes, granulosa, theca, and corpora lutea.[37] The growth hormone (GH)-bound receptor in rat granulosa cells amplifies FSH-stimulated estradiol and progesterone production.[38] Similar results have been reported with human granulosa cells.[39, 40] Thus, GH enhances FSH signal transduction in granulosa cells in a manner similar to GHRH. The question of whether the GH responses are dependent on local GHRH production/action is unknown.

Granulosa cells in healthy, but not atretic, rat follicles synthesize IGF-1, and there is evidence that GH stimulates its production.[11–13] IGF-1 receptors are present in the follicle compartment,[41, 42] and the ligand-bound IGF-1 receptor acts in synergy with FSH to stimulate maximal levels of granulosa cell estradiol, LH receptor, and progesterone production.[11] The IGF-1 receptors are present in human follicle cells,[43, 44] and IGF-1 has been found to be a potent stimulator of human granulosa cytodifferentiation.[23, 45–47] Based on all the evidence, the conclusion is emerging that the ovarian IGF system (the ligands GHRH, GH, IGF-1, their receptors, and their biological responses) is functionally coupled to follicle selection, i.e., it acts in synergy with FSH to stimulate granulosa cytodifferentiation.

TABLE 2.

Expression of the IGF System in the Rat Follicle

	References	
The IGF System	**Rat**	**Human**
Growth hormone–releasing hormone: GHRH, GHRH receptor	32–34	35,36
Growth hormone: GH, GH receptor	37,38	39,40
Insulin-like growth factors: IGF-1, IGF-2 (insulin)	11,12	13
IGF receptors: Type 1, Type 2 (insulin)	41,42	43
IGF binding proteins: IGFBP-1, -2, -3, -4, -5, -6	12	41

In this regard, there are six IGF binding proteins, (IGFBP-1, -2, -3, -4, -5, and -6) that can specifically bind the IGF ligands.[48] Both rat[12] and human ovaries[44] express the IGFBPs in a tissue-specific manner. In the rat, IGFBP-2 is found predominantly in the theca and secondary interstitial cells, IGFBP-3 is found in corpora lutea, IGFBP-4 and -5 are found in atretic granulosa cells, and IGFBP-6 is found in the theca externa.

We are beginning to obtain evidence for a most exciting and important function of the IGFBPs. In rodents, the IGFBPs present in follicular fluid have been shown to function as antigonadotropins, i.e., they block FSH-dependent cytodifferentiation.[12][13] Significantly, the mechanism by which IGFBPs inhibit FSH action is by binding IGF-1 produced by the granulosa cells. These results have led to the exciting and important conclusion that intrinsic IGF-1 is an obligatory mediator of FSH action in rat granulosa cells (Fig 6). In this connection, IGFBP-4 and -5 produced by granulosa cells have been shown to block the cell interaction of IGF-1 with its receptor and inhibit the positive effects of FSH on the granulosa cells.[49] Thus, the activation of IGFBP-4 and -5 expression might initiate, facilitate, or complete the process of atresia in rat ovaries. It remains unclear how the different IGFBPs function to regulate folliculogenesis in the human.

It is premature to predict what role, if any, the other families of growth factors (see Table 1) could play in regulating folliculogenesis. Nonetheless, the results so far show a clear indication that granulosa, theca, oocyte, and corpora luteal function can be regulated directly by the other four families of growth factors. Thus, in addition to the IGF family, the transforming growth factor β (TGF-β), TGF-α, fibroblast growth factor (FGF), and cytokine growth factor families can modify ovarian function.

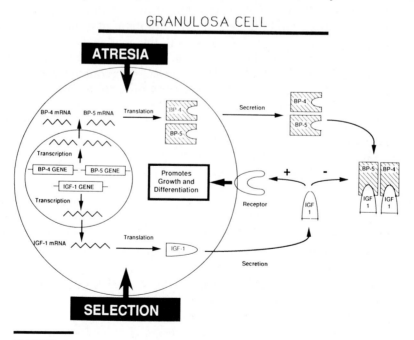

FIGURE 6.

Interactions of IGF-1 and the IGFBPs in causing selection and atresia.

The current challenges are to understand how specific growth factor systems regulate folliculogenesis and how these interactions are integrated into the overall pattern of follicular and luteal regulation during the cycle. Such knowledge might afford new therapeutic benefits for ovulation induction and treatment of human disease.

CLINICAL ADVANCES IN OVULATION INDUCTION

Advances in our understanding of the regulation of ovarian folliculogenesis have been directly applied to clinical techniques in ovulation induction. In fact, the addition of GH to ovulation induction regimens has found recent success. In the next section, a description of recent advances using our expanding basic knowledge of the mechanisms of ovulation will be presented.

HUMAN MENOPAUSAL GONADOTROPINS

Human menopausal gonadotropin (hMG) is a combination of LH and FSH isolated and purified from the urine of postmenopausal women. The first reports of successful induction of ovulation with exogenous gonadotropins were published in the late 1950s. Initial use of hMG was restricted to the anovulatory woman. With the advent of in vitro fertilization and superovulation as treatment modalities for infertility, hMG use has greatly increased.

Exogenous gonadotropin administration bypasses the normal feedback processes that regulate folliculogenesis and stimulates the ovulation of multiple follicles. This can result in multiple pregnancy and ovarian hyperstimulation. Because of these risks, treatment with hMG requires special monitoring and is expensive.

Commercial preparations of hMG include a 1:1 mixture of LH and FSH (Pergonal; Serono, Randolph, Mass) and a purified product of FSH alone (Metrodin; Serono, Randolph, Mass). Purified FSH contains negligible amounts (<1 IU) of LH and was initially developed as a product that might be used in conditions of LH excess such as polycystic ovary syndrome (PCO). There are several reports demonstrating the efficacy of purified FSH in a variety of clinical conditions.[50, 51] However, comparison of purified FSH (Metrodin) to a mixture of LH/FSH (Pergonal) showed no significant advantage to either product.[51, 52]

SUPEROVULATION

Controlled ovarian hyperstimulation, or superovulation, is the result of pharmacologic administration of hormonal agents to induce the development of multiple ovarian follicles. A variety of ovarian stimulation protocols have been developed to control the events that occur in the process of superovulation. Superovulation for the assisted reproductive technologies (ARTs) (in vitro fertilization [IVF], gamete intrafallopian transfer [GIFT], zygote intrafallopian transfer [ZIFT]) is quite different from a regimen of hMG/intrauterine insemination used for other patients in the treatment of infertility.

Ovulation induction protocols for the ART procedures have evolved tremendously since the first successful pregnancy after in vitro fertilization.[53] It became clear that pregnancy success in the ART procedures increases proportionally to the number of embryos replaced. Currently, with techniques for cryopreservation of extra embryos commonly available, stimulation regimens for ART are designed to provide as many oocytes as is safely possible.

Most ART centers use a combination of hMG with gonadotropin-releasing hormone (GnRH) agonist for ovulation induction (Fig 7). GnRH agonist treatment induces a condition of pituitary and gonadal suppression. Bioactive LH is effectively suppressed,[54] which allows full maturation of the follicles while minimizing the possibility of premature luteinization.[55] The combination GnRH agonist/hMG results in the prevention of premature LH surges, improved response, and a decrease in cancellation rate from 30% to only 10%.[56]

The timing of GnRH agonist in combination with hMG has been investigated. Ovarian suppression is usually prompt and consistent when GnRH agonist treatment is begun in the midluteal phase of the cycle.[57] More recently, GnRH agonist has been administered concurrently with hMG in the follicular phase of the cycle.[58] This short regimen uses the gonadotropin flare-up that accompanies the uses of GnRH agonists to promote follicular development. Although the flare-up regimens may save drug costs and shorten stimulation intervals, there are conflicting reports on clinical success. Frydman and colleagues[59] reported similar ovarian responses, ongoing pregnancies, and spontaneous abortion rates when short and long protocols were compared, whereas San Ramon et al.[60] reported that follicular-phase GnRH agonist administration was associated with evidence of premature luteinization, hyperandrogenemia, and poorer pregnancy outcomes as compared with luteal-phase GnRH agonist regimens.

HUMAN MENOPAUSAL GONADOTROPIN COTREATMENT WITH GROWTH HORMONE

Investigations into the process of folliculogenesis have demonstrated that IGF-1 is an important regulator of granulosa cell function.[61] The relationship of GH as the most important regulator of IGF-1 led Homburg and colleagues[62] to study the effect of cotreatment of hMG and GH in ovulation induction regimens.

Growth hormone cotreatment increases serum and follicular fluid IGF-1 levels when compared with standard hMG regimens without GH.[63, 64] Although cotreatment appears to decrease the total amount of

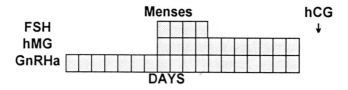

FIGURE 7.

Typical stimulation protocol for assisted reproductive technologies. *hMG* = human menopausal gonadotropins; *hCG* = human chorionic gonadotropin; *GnRHa* = gonadotropin releasing hormone agonist.

hMG required,[63] it does not appear to improve the clinical response in normal women.[64] The ultimate role for cotreatment may be in women who have previously responded poorly to hMG regimens. In one small study,[65] women who had previously responded very poorly to a standard GnRH agonist/hMG protocol received GH cotreatment in a subsequent ART cycle. The investigators reported a significant decrease in the number of days of hMG as well as the total dose of hMG. They also reported an increase in the number of oocytes collected and several pregnancies with this ovulation induction protocol. The small number of subjects (10) precluded statistical significance but demonstrated encouraging findings. In another study of 20 women with previous suboptimal responses to standard ovulation induction regimens, cotreatment with GH and hMG did not change the clinical response unless the woman had ultrasonically diagnosed polycystic ovaries.[66] In this subgroup, cotreatment resulted in an increase in the number of follicles that developed and the number of oocytes collected at retrieval. An interesting variation on this concept was reported by Hughes et al.,[67] who used GHRH in cotreatment with hMG in 12 women with a previous poor response. They reported a significant increase in urinary and plasma GH concentrations with a slight increase in recruited follicles, retrieved oocytes, and follicular fluid IGF-1 levels (statistical significance not reported).

PULSATILE GONADOTROPIN-RELEASING HORMONE

Gonadotropin-releasing hormone is a ten−amino acid protein that is synthesized and released from the arcuate nucleus of the hypothalamus. It is released in discrete secretory bursts into the portal circulation and acts to release both LH and FSH. When delivered in pulses, exogenous GnRH acts in a physiologic manner to stimulate gonadotropin release and activate cyclic reproductive function. Conversely, when delivered in a continuous fashion, GnRH treatment results in a downregulation of pituitary gonadotropin release and suppression of gonadal function. The first report of pulsatile GnRH to restore ovulatory function in humans was published by Leyendecker and colleagues[68] in 1990.

Several studies have established the safety and efficacy of pulsatile GnRH for the treatment of anovulation.[69, 70] Pulsatile GnRH is delivered by means of a small infusion pump that can be programmed to deliver a small bolus (1 to 20 μg) every 60 to 90 minutes. Technology in pulsatile delivery pumps has improved, and devices about the size of a credit card are now available (Fig 8). The medication can be delivered either subcutaneously or intravenously. Although success has been reported with either delivery system, the intravenous route of administration appears to be more effective.[71]

GnRH pump therapy has been used in a variety of clinical conditions but is most effective for women with hypothalamic amenorrhea. Filicori et al.[72] have recently published a review of their experience with pulsatile GnRH in a variety of endocrine disorders. The success of GnRH pump therapy was highest for hypothalamic disorders, (approximately 90% ovulation rate) and lowest in women with PCO (only 43% ovulating). The poor response of women with PCO to GnRH pump therapy has been described previously.[73, 74] Attempts have been made to improve the re-

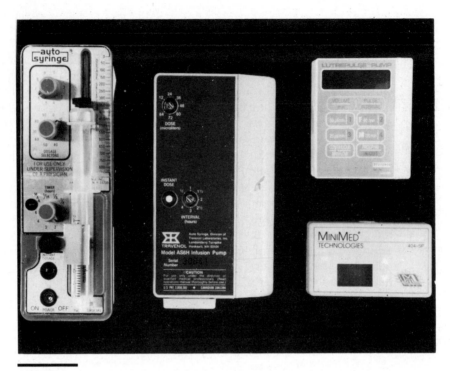

FIGURE 8.
The evolution of pulsatile delivery pumps for GnRH therapy in the induction of ovulation. The first-generation pump is on the *left* and the newest, smallest pumps are on the *right*.

sponse of patients with PCO to pulsatile GnRH by pretreating with long-acting GnRH agonist therapy. By inducing a temporary condition of hypogonadotropic hypogonadism, the dysfunctional gonadotropin secretory patterns and hyperandrogenism associated with PCO are reversed.[75] If pulsatile GnRH therapy is started immediately after completion of an 8-week course of GnRH agonist suppression, the ovulatory success rate greatly improves.[73, 76] In these reports the ovulatory rate approached that expected for patients with hypothalamic amenorrhea. In another report, Surrey and colleagues[77] confirmed that agonist pretreatment induces a condition of hypogonadism, but they were unable to demonstrate a change in response to pulsatile GnRH treatment.

PREMATURE OVARIAN FAILURE

Premature ovarian failure (POF) is a poorly understood condition that results in hypergonadotropic amenorrhea. There are many anecdotal reports of spontaneous ovulation and pregnancy in this group of women, especially while receiving cyclic estrogen/progestin replacement therapy. There are several studies of attempted ovulation induction with hMG in these patients,[78, 79] most of which have reported very poor results. In the last few years, several groups have attempted to improve the results of ovulation induction regimens in this group of patients by suppressing the chronically high circulating levels of gonadotropins before administering hMG. The underlying hypothesis is that the high level of LH and FSH results in ovarian theca and granulosa cell receptor downregulation, thereby rendering any potential remaining follicles unresponsive to stimulation. The most encouraging results have been reported by Check and Chase.[80] They administered exogenous ethinyl estradiol until a rise in serum estradiol levels was detected and then began hMG treatment. With this protocol they described a 60% ovulation rate and a 40% pregnancy rate. Unfortunately, these results could not be duplicated by Surrey and Cedars,[81] who failed to induce ovulation in any subject with exogenous estrogen as a tool to suppress gonadotropin levels. In the only patient who ovulated, they used a GnRH agonist before hMG. Gonadotropin-releasing hormone agonist–induced gonadotropin suppression has also been used as a pretreatment to hMG. A small case report by Rosen and colleagues[82] described success in two patients who received GnRH agonist. One subject received GnRH agonist alone, and the other received GnRH agonist followed by hMG. All of these studies must be interpreted with caution. The clinical syndrome of POF often includes intermittent, unpredictable return of ovarian function. This may explain the discrepancy seen between groups of patients studied.

OVARIAN ABLATION IN POLYCYSTIC OVARY DISEASE

Ovarian wedge resection was originally described as treatment for PCO by Stein and Leventhal[83] in 1935. Since then there have been well-documented successes with a variety of different techniques of ovarian ablation, including operative laparoscopy. Restoration of cyclic menses in up to 95% of patients and pregnancy in 85% of patients have been reported.[84] The major disadvantages of ovarian ablation are the formation of postoperative adhesions and the expense and risk of surgery. Although the procedure is designed to restore fertility in most patients, the resulting adhesions could actually impede the process dramatically.[85, 86] Because of this, most patients are now treated with hormonal medications such as clomiphene citrate, hMG, or pulsatile GnRH.

Recent advances in operative techniques have allowed ovarian ablation to be performed laparoscopically. Ovarian tissue can be destroyed by electrocautery, laser, or wedge resection. These techniques are equally successful in restoring ovarian function with ovulation rates of approximately 90%. However, these techniques may vary in terms of postoperative adhesion formation. Unfortunately, this issue has not been adequately assessed. A recent report by Gürgan et al.[87] reported that adhesions developed in 82% of patients following either electrocautery or Nd:YAG laser ovarian ablation. The subsequent pregnancy rates for the two treatment types were 57% and 40%, respectively. Second-look laparoscopy has been proposed as a useful technique to reduce the amount of adhesions resulting from ovarian ablation. In one report, no advantage to second-look laparoscopy could be identified.[88]

SUMMARY

There have been striking basic science and clinical advances in our understanding of the process of folliculogenesis and, ultimately, ovulation. Our evolving understanding of growth factors in the process of selection and atresia has been applied in the clinic with the development of ovulation induction regimens employing GH to improve outcome. Despite these advances there remain several unanswered questions about the process that determines recruitment and selection. Continued expansion of our understanding of these processes will ultimately lead to improvement in our ability to regulate and control ovulation in clinical medicine.

REFERENCES

1. Hodgen GD: The dominant ovarian follicle. *Fertil Steril* 1982; 38:281–300.
2. Erickson GF: Follicular growth and development, in Sciarra JJ, Droegemueller W (eds): *Gynecology and Obstetrics*, vol 5. Philadelphia, JB Lippincott, 1991, pp 1–24.
3. Gougeon A: Dynamics of follicular growth in the human: A model from preliminary results. *Hum Reprod* 1986; 1:81.
4. Nilsson L, Wikland M, Hamberger L: Recruitment of an ovulatory follicle in the human following follicle-ectomy and luteectomy. *Fertil Steril* 1982; 37:30–34.
5. McNatty KP, Smith DM, Osathanondh R, et al: The human antral follicle: Functional correlates of growth and atresia. *Ann Biol Anim Physiol* 1979; 19:1547–1558.
6. Hurwitz A, Adashi EY: Ovarian follicular atresia is an apoptotic process: A paradigm for programmed cell death in endocrine tissues. *Mol Cell Endocrinol* 1992; 84:19.
7. Whitelaw PF, Smyth CD, Howels CM, et al: Cell-specific expression of aromatase and LH receptor mRNAs in rat ovary. *J Mol Endocrinol* 1992; 9:309.
8. Erickson GF, Magoffin DA, Dyer CA, et al: The ovarian androgen producing cells: A review of structure/function relationships. *Endocr Rev* 1985; 6:371–399.
9. Erickson GF: Normal regulation of ovarian androgen production. *Semin Reprod Endocrinol* 1993, in press.
10. Couzinet B, Lestrat N, Brailly S, et al: Stimulation of ovarian follicular maturation with pure follicle stimulating hormone in women with gonadotropin deficiency. *J Clin Endocrinol Metab* 1988; 66:552–556.
11. Adashi EY, Resnick CE, Hurwitz A, et al: Insulin-like growth factors: The ovarian connection. *Hum Reprod* 1991; 6:1213.
12. Erickson GF, Nakatani A, Liu X-J, et al: The role of IGF-1 and the IGFBPs in folliculogenesis, in Findlay JK (ed): *Cellular and Molecular Mechanisms in Female Reproduction* New York, Academic Press, in press.
13. Giudice LC: Insulin-like growth factors and ovarian follicular development. *Endocr Rev* 1992; 13:641.
14. Knecht M, Feng P, Catt KT: Transforming growth factor-β: Autocrine, paracrine, and endocrine effects in ovarian cells. *Semin Reprod Endocrinol* 1989; 7:12.
15. Ying S-Y: Inhibins, activins and follistatins: Gonadal proteins modulating the secretion of follicle-stimulating hormone. *Endocr Rev* 1988; 9:267–293.
16. Findlay JF: An update on the roles of inhibin, activin, and follistatin as local regulators of folliculogenesis. *Biol Reprod* 1992; 48:15.
17. Hillier SG: Regulatory functions for inhibin and activin in human ovaries. *J Endocrinol* 1991; 131:171–175.
18. Voutilainen R, Miller WL: Human müllerian inhibitory factor messenger ribonucleic acid is hormonally regulated in the fetal testis and adult granulosa cells. *Mol Endocrinol* 1987; 1:604–608.

19. Kim JH, Seibel MM, MacLaughlin DT, et al: The inhibitory effects of müllerian-inhibiting substance in epidermal growth factor induced proliferation and progesterone production in human granulosa-luteal cells. *J Clin Endocrinol Metab* 1992; 75:911–917.

20. Mulheron GW, Bossert NL, Lapp JA, et al: Human granulosa-luteal and cumulus cells express transforming growth factors—Beta type 1 and type 2 mRNA. *J Clin Endocrinol Metab* 1992; 74:458–460.

21. Chegini N, Flanders KC: Presence of transforming growth factor-β and their selective cellular localization in human ovarian tissue of various reproductive stages. *Endocrinology* 1992; 130:1705–1715.

22. May JV, Schomberg DW: The potential relevance of epidermal growth factor (EGF) and transforming growth factor alpha (TGFα) to ovarian physiology. *Semin Reprod Endocrinol* 1989; 7:1.

23. Steinkampf MP, Mendelson CR, Simpson ER: Effects of epidermal growth factor and insulin-like growth factor 1 on the levels of mRNA encoding aromatase P450 of human ovarian granulosa cells. *Mol Cell Endocrinol* 1988; 59:93–99.

24. Richardson MC, Gadd SC, Masson GM: Augmentation by epidermal growth factor of basal and stimulated progesterone production by human luteinized granulosa cells. *J Endocrinol* 1989; 121:397–402.

25. Chegini N, Williams RS: Immunocytochemical localization of transforming growth factors (TGFs) TGF-α and TGF-β in human ovarian tissues. *J Clin Endocrinol Metab* 1992; 74:973–980.

26. Maruo T, Ladiness-Llave CA, Samoto T, et al: Expression of epidermal growth factor and its receptor in the human ovary during follicular growth and regression. *Endocrinology* 1993; 132:924–931.

27. Gospodarowicz D, Ferrara N, Schweigere L, et al: Structural characterization and biological functions of fibroblast growth factor. *Endocr Rev* 1987; 8:95.

28. Adashi EY: The potential relevance of cytokines to ovarian physiology: The emerging role of resident ovarian cells of the white blood cell series. *Endocr Rev* 1990; 11:454.

29. Roby KF, Weed J, Lyles R, et al: Immunological evidence for a human ovarian tumor necrosis factor-α. *J Clin Endocrinol Metab* 1990; 71:1096–1102.

30. Wang L, Robertson S, Seamark RF, et al: Lymphokines, including interleukin-2, alter gonadotropin-stimulated progesterone production and proliferation of human granulosa-luteal cells in vitro. *J Clin Endocrinol Metab* 1991; 72:824–831.

31. Fukuoka M, Yasuda K, Emis M, et al: Cytokine modulation of protgesterone and estradiol secretion in cultures of luteinized human granulosa cells. *J Clin Endocrinol Metab* 1992; 72:254–258.

32. Bagnato A, Moretti C, Ohnishi J, et al: Expression of the growth hormone–releasing hormone gene and its peptide production in the rat ovary. *Endocrinology* 1992; 130:1097.

33. Moretti C, Bagnato A, Solan N, et al: Receptor-mediated actions of growth hormone releasing factor in granulosa cell differentiation. *Endocrinology* 1990; 127:2117.

34. Bagnato A, Moretti C, Frajese G, et al: Gonadotropin-induced expression of receptors for growth hormone releasing factor in cultured granulosa cells. *Endocrinology* 1991; 128:2889–2894.

35. Moretti C, Fabbri A, Gnessi L, et al: Immunohistochemical localization of growth hormone releasing hormone in human gonads. *J Endocrinol Invest* 1990; 13:301–309.

36. Moretti C, Fabbri A, Gnessi L, et al: GHRH stimulates follicular growth and amplified FSH-induced ovarian folliculogenesis in women with anovulatory infertility, in Frajese G, Steinberg E, Rodriguez-Rigan LJ (eds): *Reproductive*

Medicine: Medical Therapy. Proceedings of the Second International Symposium on Reproductive Medicine. New York, Elsevier, 1989, pp 103–112.

37. Lobie PE, Breipohl W, Garcia J, et al: Cellular localization of the growth hormone receptor/binding protein in the male and female reproductive systems. *Endocrinology* 1990; 126:2214.

38. Hutchinson LA, Findlay JK, Herington AC: Growth hormone and insulin-like growth factor-I accelerate PMSG-induced differentiation of granulosa cells. *Mol Cell Endocrinol* 1988; 55:61–69.

39. Carlsson B, Bergh C, Bentham J, et al: Expression of functional growth hormone receptors in human granulosa cells. *Hum Reprod* 1992; 7:1205–1209.

40. Mason HD, Martikainen H, Beard RW, et al: Direct gonadotropic effect of growth hormone on oestradiol production by human granulosa cells in vitro. *J Endocrinol* 1990; 126:1–4.

41. Zhou J, Chin E, Bondy C: Cellular pattern of insulin-like growth factor-I (IGF-I) and IGF-I receptor gene expression in the developing and mature ovarian follicle. *Endocrinology* 1991; 179:3281–3288.

42. Levy MJ, Hernandez ER, Adashi EY, et al: Expression of the insulin-like growth factor (IGF)-I and -II and the IGF-I and -II receptor genes during postnatal development of the rat ovary. *Endocrinology* 1992; 131:1202–1206.

43. Hernandez ER, Hurwitz A, Vera A, et al: Expression of the genes encoding the insulin-like growth factors and their receptors in the human ovary. *J Clin Endocrinol* 1992; 74:419–425.

44. Zhou J, Bondy C: Anatomy of the human ovarian insulin-like growth factor system. *Biol Reprod* 1993; 48:467.

45. Erickson GF, Garzo VG, Magoffin DA: Insulin-like growth factor 1 (IGF-I) regulates aromatase activity in human granulosa and granulosa luteal cells. *J Clin Endocrinol Metab* 1989; 69:716–724.

46. Erickson GF, Magoffin DA, Cragun JR, et al: The effects of insulin and insulin-like growth factors I and II on estradiol production by granulosa cells of polycystic ovaries. *J Clin Endocrinol Metab* 1990; 70:894–902.

47. Erickson GF, Garzo VG, Magoffin DA: Progesterone production by human granulosa cells cultured in serum free medium: Effects of gonadotropins and insulin like growth factor 1 (IGF-I). *Human Reprod* 1991; 6:1074–1081.

48. Shimasaki S, Ling N: Identification and molecular characterization of insulin-like growth factor binding proteins (IGFBP-1,-2,-3,-4,-5,-6). *Prog Growth Factor Res* 1991; 3:243.

49. Liu X-J, Malkowski M, Guo Y-L, et al: Development of specific antibodies to rat insulin-like growth factor binding proteins (IGFBP-2 to -6): Analysis of IGFBP production by rat granulosa cells. *Endocrinology* 1993; 132:1176–1183.

50. Claman P, Seibel MM: Purified human follicle stimulating hormone for ovulation induction: A critical review. *Semin Reprod Endocrinol* 1986; 4:277–283.

51. Venturoli S, Paradisi R, Fabbri R, et al: Induction of ovulation in polycystic ovary: Human menopausal gonadotropin or human urinary follicle stimulating hormone? *Int J Fertil* 1987; 32:66–70.

52. Anderson RE, Cragun JM, Chang RJ, et al: A pharmacodynamic comparison of human urinary follicle stimulating hormone and human menopausal gonadotropin in normal women and polycystic ovary syndrome. *Fertil Steril* 1989; 52:216–220.

53. Steptoe PC, Edwards RG: Birth after reimplantation of a human embryo. *Lancet* 1978; 2:336–337.

54. Cedars MI, Surrey E, Hamilton F, et al: Leuprolide acetate lowers circulating bioactive luteinizing hormone and testosterone concentrations during ovarian stimulation for oocyte retrieval. *Fertil Steril* 1990; 53:627–631.

55. Meldrum DR: Ovulation induction for in vitro fertilization procedures. *Semin Reprod Endocrinol* 1990; 8:213–218.

56. Meldrum DR: GnRH agonists as adjuncts for in vitro fertilization. *Obstet Gynecol Surv* 1989; 44:314–318.

57. Meldrum DR, Wisot A, Hamilton F, et al: Routine pituitary suppression with leuprolide before ovarian stimulation for oocyte retrieval. *Fertil Steril* 1989; 51:455–459.

58. Garcia JE, Padilla SL, Bayati J, et al: Follicular phase gonadotropin-releasing hormone agonist and human gonadotropins: A better alternative for ovulation induction in in vitro fertilization. *Fertil Steril* 1990; 53:302–305.

59. Frydman R, Belaisch-Allart J, Parneix I, et al: Comparison between flare up and down regulation effects of luteinizing hormone–releasing hormone agonists in in vitro fertilization program. *Fertil Steril* 1988; 50:471–475.

60. San Ramon GA, Surrey ES, Judd HL, et al: A prospective randomized comparison of luteal phase versus concurrent follicular phase initiation of gonadotropin-releasing hormone agonist for in vitro fertilization. *Fertil Steril* 1992; 58:744–749.

61. Adashi EY, Resnick CE, Hernandez ER, et al: Insulin-like growth factor 1 as an intraovarian regulator: Basic and clinical implications. *Ann N Y Acad Sci* 1991; 626:161–168.

62. Homburg R, Eshel A, Abdalla HI, et al: Growth hormone facilitates ovulation induction by gonadotropins. *Clin Endocrinol (Oxf)* 1988; 29:113–116.

63. Homburg R, West C, Torresani T, et al: Cotreatment with human growth hormone and gonadotropins for induction of ovulation: A controlled clinical trial. *Fertil Steril* 1990; 53:254–260.

64. Hughes SM, Huang ZH, Matson PL, et al: Clinical and endocrinological changes in women following ovulation induction using buserelin acetate/human menopausal gonadotrophin augmented with biosynthetic human growth hormone. *Hum Reprod* 1992; 7:770–775.

65. Ibrahim ZH, Matson PL, Buck P, et al: The use of biosynthetic human growth hormone to augment ovulation induction with buserelin acetate/human menopausal gonadotropin in women with a poor ovarian response. *Fertil Steril* 1991; 55:202–204.

66. Owen EJ, West C, Mason BA, et al: Co-treatment with growth hormone of sub-optimal responders in IVF-ET. *Hum Reprod* 1991; 6:524–528.

67. Hughes JN, Torresani T, Herve F, et al: Interest of growth hormone–releasing hormone administration for improvement of ovarian responsiveness to gonadotropins in poor responder women. *Fertil Steril* 1991; 55:945–951.

68. Leyendecker G, Wildt L, Hansman M: Pregnancies following chronic intermittent (pulsatile) administration of GnRH by means of a portable pump ("Zyklomat")—a new approach to the treatment of infertility in hypothalamic amenorrhea. *J Clin Endocrinol Metab* 1980; 51:1214–1216.

69. Hurley DM, Brian R, Outch K, et al: Induction of ovulation and fertility in amenorrheic women by pulsatile low-dose gonadotropin-releasing hormone. *N Engl J Med* 1984; 310:1069–1074.

70. Homburg R, Eshel A, Armar NA, et al: One hundred pregnancies after treatment with pulsatile luteinizing hormone releasing hormone to induce ovulation. *BMJ* 1989; 298:809–812.

71. Reid RL, Sauerbrei E: Evaluation of techniques for induction of ovulation in outpatients employing pulsatile gonadotropin-releasing hormone. *Am J Obstet Gynecol* 1984; 148:648–651.

72. Filicori M, Flamigni C, Merriggiola MC, et al: Endocrine response determines the clinical outcome of pulsatile gonadotropin-releasing hormone ovulation induction in different ovulatory disorders. *J Clin Endocrinol Metab* 1991; 72:965–972.

73. Filicori M, Flamigni C, Campaniello E, et al: The abnormal response of polycystic ovarian disease patients to exogenous pulsatile gonadotropin-releasing hormone: Characterization and management. *J Clin Endocrinol Metab* 1989; 69:825–831.

74. Echel A, Abdulwahid NA, Armar NA, et al: Pulsatile luteinizing hormone–releasing hormone therapy in women with polycystic ovary syndrome. *Fertil Steril* 1988; 49:956–960.

75. Chang RJ, Laufer LR, Meldrum DR, et al: Steroid secretion in polycystic ovarian disease after ovarian suppression by a long acting gonadotropin-releasing hormone agonist. *J Clin Endocrinol Metab* 1983; 56:897–903.

76. Filicori M, Campaniello E, Michelacci L, et al: Gonadotropin-releasing hormone (GnRH) analog suppression renders polycystic ovarian disease patients more susceptible to ovulation induction with pulsatile GnRH. *J Clin Endocrinol Metab* 1988; 66:327–333.

77. Surrey ES, Chang RJ, DeZeigler D, et al: Effects of gonadotropin-releasing hormone (GnRH) agonist on pituitary and ovarian responses to pulsatile GnRH therapy in polycystic ovarian disease. *Fertil Steril* 1989; 52:547–552.

78. Johnson TR, Peterson EP: Gonadotropin-induced pregnancy following "premature ovarian failure." *Fertil Steril* 1979; 31:351–353.

79. Tanaka T, Sakuragi N, Fujimoto S, et al: HMG-HCG therapy in patients with hypergonadotropic ovarian anovulation: One pregnancy case report and ovulation and pregnancy rate. *Int J Fertil* 1982; 27:100–103.

80. Check JH, Chase JS: Ovulation induction in hypergonadotropic amenorrhea with estrogen and human menopausal gonadotropin therapy. *Fertil Steril* 1984; 42:919–921.

81. Surrey ES, Cedars MI: The effect of gonadotropin suppression on the induction of ovulation in premature ovarian failure patients. *Fertil Steril* 1989; 52:36–41.

82. Rosen GF, Stone SC, Yee B: Ovulation induction in women with premature ovarian failure: A prospective, crossover study. *Fertil Steril* 1992; 57:448–449.

83. Stein IF, Leventhal ML: Amenorrhea associated with bilateral polycystic ovaries. *Am J Obstet Gynecol* 1935; 29:181–191.

84. Stein IF: Duration of fertility following ovarian wedge resection—Stein-Leventhal syndrome. *Obstet Gynecol Surv* 1965; 20:124–127.

85. Toaff R, Toaff ME, Peyser MR: Infertility following wedge resection of the ovaries. *Am J Obstet Gynecol* 1976; 124:92–96.

86. Adashi EY, Rock JA, Guzick D, et al: Fertility following bilateral ovarian wedge resection: A critical analysis of 90 consecutive cases of the polycystic ovary syndrome. *Fertil Steril* 1981; 36:320–325.

87. Gürgan T, Kişnişçi H, Yarali H, et al: Evaluation of adhesion formation after laparoscopic treatment of polycystic ovarian disease. *Fertil Steril* 1991; 56:1176–1178.

88. Gürgan T, Urman B, Aksu T, et al: The effect of short-interval laparoscopic lysis of adhesion on pregnancy rates following Nd-YAG laser photocoagulation of polycystic ovaries. *Obstet Gynecol* 1992; 80:45–47.

Editor's Comment

This chapter is an excellent example of the advances made in clinical medicine that may be attained when our understanding of physiologic processes is more complete. The role of growth factors as modulators of gonadotropin-mediated events is just beginning to be better understood. As is usually the case, these physiologic processes are complicated and many times redundant. At present, this is best exemplified by the IGF family including IGF-I and its receptor, IGF-II and its receptor, the six IGF binding proteins, and insulin and its receptor. As the name implies there is crossover between these ligands and their respective receptors. This family also includes GnRH, which stimulates IGF-I. GnRH has been used clinically with some success. This ubiquitous family is sure to continue to challenge us as we study their roles in the ovary as well as other reproductive tissues such as the endometrium and myometrium.

Ana A. Murphy, M.D.

Current Concepts in Assisted Reproductive Technology

JOHN S. HESLA, M.D.

T he first human birth following embryo transfer of an oocyte fertilized in a laboratory setting occurred on July 25, 1978.[1] The widespread application of this therapy for infertility has allowed a greater understanding of human reproduction and provided the impetus for major advances in technology that continue to expand the horizons of assisted reproduction. The average delivery rate achieved through in vitro fertilization–embryo transfer (IVF-ET) in the United States and Canada during 1991, the last year of reporting by the national registry, was 15.2% (Table 1). Several facets of this treatment modality will be reviewed.

CONTROLLED OVARIAN HYPERSTIMULATION FOR IN VITRO FERTILIZATION

The first successful IVF-ET pregnancy arose from the fertilization of a single oocyte recovered from a dominant follicle in the natural menstrual cycle.[1] Disadvantages associated with the use of the spontaneous menstrual cycle have included the need for frequent testing for luteinizing hormone (LH) surges as well as a lack of flexibility in scheduling oocyte retrieval for the patient, surgeon, and laboratory personnel. Further experience with this new technology revealed that pregnancy rates were improved by increasing the number of embryos available for transfer through controlled ovarian hyperstimulation.[2] As a result, the vast majority of IVF programs have replaced follicular aspiration in an unstimulated cycle with treatment protocols incorporating controlled ovarian hyperstimulation, although the former approach has recently received renewed interest in selected patient populations.[3]

Rapid follicular enlargement to the graafian follicle stage has been reported to occur over a 4- to 5-day period in natural cycles as well as during ovarian stimulation cycles.[4] The corresponding changes in steroidogenesis are reflected by an exponential increase in peripheral estrogen from basal to preovulatory peak levels. Hence, useful clinical criteria to establish patient response to therapy include frequent assays of plasma estradiol or total urinary estrogen and ultrasonographic measurement of developing follicles.

TREATMENT SCHEDULES

Healthy, normally cycling women of similar weights may have highly variable ovarian responses to a uniform regimen of human menopausal

TABLE 1.

Comparison of Reported Outcomes for All Assisted Reproductive Technology Procedures*

Outcome	IVF†	GIFT†	ZIFT†	Donor‡	Cryopreserved ETs†§
Cycles/procedures¶	24,671	5,452	2,104	1,107	4,225
Cancellation (%)	15.2	19.2	16.0	5.6	NA†
Retrievals	21,083	4,474	1,808	1,045	NA
Transfers per retrieval (%)	87.1	97.7	83.5	94.1	NA
Pregnancies	4,017	1,515	442	328	559
Pregnancy loss (%)	19.9	21.6	19.2	18.3	22.9
Deliveries	3,215	1,188	357	268	431
Deliveries per retrieval (%)	15.2	26.6	19.7	25.6	10.2
Singleton (%)	70	66	67	67	79
EPs†	223	44	20	7	20
EP per transfer (%)	1.2	1.0	1.3	0.7	NA
Birth defects per neonates delivered (%)‖	1.5	1.1	0.8	2.1	0.8

*From Society for Assisted Reproductive Technology: *Fertil Steril* 1993; 59:956. Used by permission.
†IVF = in vitro fertilization; GIFT = gamete intrafallopian transfer; ZIFT = zygote intrafallopian transfer; ET = embryo transfer; NA = not available; EP = ectopic pregnancy.
‡Donor includes known or anonymous, but not surrogate.
§Cryopreserved embryo transfer cycles not done in combination with fresh ETs and not with donor embryos.
¶Includes all cycles, regardless of age or diagnosis; three programs did not report cycles initiated.
‖Birth defect reporting did not account for all neonatal outcomes.

gonadotropins (hMG, Pergonal); however, the response pattern of the individual is typically repetitive when equivalent doses of menotropins are given in subsequent cycles.[5] Very low or high estradiol growth rates are associated with a significantly greater likelihood of missed oocyte recovery or fertilization failure. Nevertheless, the number of developing follicles can be significantly reduced in high-responder patients by decreasing the amount of hMG administered.[6] This dose-response correlation is markedly diminished in poor-responding patients, although increasing the dose of menotropins during the early follicular phase may prove clinically useful, for this is the time period in the menstrual cycle during which follicles are recruited for ongoing development. When an initial starting dose of 300 vs. 450 IU of gonadotropins was administered to the same group of low responders, there was no difference in cancellation rate, maximal estradiol levels achieved, or the number of embryos transferred, although there was a trend toward an increased pregnancy rate.[7] Increasing the medication dosage after the initial 3 to 4 days of hMG administration may merely promote the development of a secondary cohort of small follicles containing oocytes that are unlikely to lead to conception.

The concentration of circulating follicle-stimulating hormone (FSH) on the third day of the menstrual cycle has been recognized as a marker of ovarian reserve and is an important predictor of ovarian response to hormonal stimulation and IVF outcome. During this time period, FSH is usually less than 20 IU/mL when measured by standard commercial radioimmunoassay kits; higher levels suggest a lack of negative feedback of ovarian steroid products at the level of the pituitary gland and hypothalamus.[8] Women with elevated FSH levels have a high cancellation rate before oocyte retrieval and an increased chance of spontaneous abortion if pregnancy ensues. The ongoing pregnancy rate is correlated with both day 3 FSH levels and patient age (Table 2), but more strongly with the former.[8] In general, increasing the dosage of gonadotropins in this low-response group does not alter the stimulation response appreciably, nor does it improve pregnancy prognosis.

Early follicular estradiol levels may reflect cycle dynamics and the likelihood of conception. The estradiol concentration on cycle day 3 prognosticates the response to stimulation and pregnancy outcome in a manner that is independent of the day 3 FSH level. The number of oocytes collected, cleaving embryos, and embryos transferred declines significantly with increasing concentration of day 3 estradiol.[7] Ongoing pregnancies are extremely unlikely when the day 3 estradiol level is greater than 75 pg/mL. No pregnancies were reported by Rosenwaks in patients with both day 3 estradiol levels greater than 45 pg/mL and FSH concentration greater than 17 mIU/mL.[7]

Premature luteinization may occur during the latter stages of hMG therapy as a consequence of heightened LH release by the pituitary gland. This phenomenon results in poor oocyte quality and the associated sequelae of reduced fertilization and cleavage,[9] embryo fragmentation or degeneration,[10] and a lower chance of pregnancy.[11] In order to diminish the possibility of premature luteinization, analogues of gonadotropin-releasing hormone (GnRHa) have been prescribed to suppress circulating levels of bioactive LH and androgens. The use of these agents in protocols of controlled ovarian hyperstimulation enhances follicular response, reduces cycle cancellation from approximately 30% to 7%,[12, 13] and may improve endometrial receptivity as compared with conventional clomiphene citrate/hMG regimens.[14] During 1990, 97% of all programs participating in the IVF-ET Registry included leuprolide or nafarelin acetate in the treatment regimen that was most commonly prescribed.[15] Nevertheless, the use of GnRHa necessitates the administration of larger quantities of gonadotropins to achieve adequate follicular development as a consequence of suppression of endogenous production of FSH. In addition, these analogues may directly influence ovarian function.

Data from prospective, randomized studies suggest that the reduction of premature luteinization achieved through GnRHa administration will increase pregnancy rates.[16] In hMG-only cycles, human chorionic gonadotropin (hCG) must be given before the onset of premature luteinization when the lead follicles are only 15 to 17 mm in size, whereas in the presence of pituitary suppression, the timing of hCG can be delayed until the

TABLE 2.
Effect of Age and Diagnosis of Male Factor on Outcome for Stimulated 1991 in vitro Fertilization Cycles*

Patient Category	No. of Retrievals	Cancellations,† %	Transfers per Retrieval, %	No. of Pregnancies	No. of Deliveries	Deliveries per Retrieval (%)
Women <40 years, no male factor	13,564	14.1	91.9	3,016	2,448	18.0
Women ≥40 years, no male factor	2,257	25.1	86.8	270	181	8.0
Women <40 years, male factor	4,013	9.1	76.9	633	522	13.0
Women ≥40 years, male factor	739	18.8	71.6	66	41	5.5
1991 totals	20,573	14.7	87.7	3,985	3,192	15.5
1990 totals	16,405	14.0	86.2	3,057	2,345	14

*From Society for Assisted Reproductive Technology: Fertil Steril 1993; 59:956. Used by permission.
†Percentage of cycles that did not proceed to retrieval.

follicle size reaches 18 to 20 mm.[17] Patients with polycystic ovarian disease are particularly benefited by such treatment; oocyte fertilization and pregnancy rates are increased and the spontaneous abortion rate is decreased as compared with cycles in which hMG alone is used.[18]

There are two contrasting methods for employing GnRH agonists in ovarian stimulation protocols. In the "short" schedule, the agonist is introduced in the early follicular phase, usually cycle day 2, which results in a prompt release of endogenous LH and FSH. The circulatory levels of gonadotropins will peak 4 to 6 hours after GnRHa administration at concentrations several times that present during the spontaneous midcycle surge of these hormones.[19] Luteinizing hormone and FSH levels will remain elevated in peripheral blood for approximately 10 hours.[19] This temporary flare in circulating FSH stimulates follicular development. Repeat exposure of the pituitary gland to GNRHa results in a reduction of available GnRH receptors, an impairment of postreceptor mechanisms, and ultimately an unresponsiveness to the pituitary gonadotropin to GnRH. Exogenous gonadotropins are begun on day 3 to 5 of the cycle as endogenous production of FSH declines.

In the second, or "long" protocol, suppression of ovarian activity is achieved by the administration of GnRHa for 7 to 14 days before the introduction of exogenous gonadotropins. The heightened release of FSH and LH by the pituitary gland is blunted when GnRHa is started in the midluteal phase rather than the follicular phase of the menstrual cycle; the high progesterone concentration that is present during this time period inhibits pituitary responsiveness.[20] However, with luteal-phase initiation, corpus luteum steroidogenesis is stimulated, and menses may be delayed up to 6 days beyond the expected time of onset. Because prolonged GnRHa administration leads to downregulation of pituitary GnRH receptors and lack of spontaneous follicular development beyond the small antral stage, hMG administration can begin at any time after the onset of menses. This freedom in timing of therapy facilitates the scheduling of midweek oocyte collection. If leuprolide acetate is begun in the early follicular phase as part of the "long" protocol, more prompt pituitary suppression is achieved if the agonist is administered every 12 hours rather than the usual every 24 hours.[20]

The GnRHa flare technique offers certain advantages over the long schedule, including fewer medication requirements and a briefer duration of administration of drugs. Nevertheless, high amounts of LH are released during the agonist phase of action of the analogue which stimulate ovarian androgen production and progesterone secretion by the involving corpus luteum. These hormones may oppose recruitment of secondary follicles and have an adverse effect on oocyte and endometrial development.[21] In general, fewer oocytes are retrieved when the short protocol is used.[22] Administration of GnRHa in the late luteal phase of the natural cycle inhibits the early developmental asynchrony of follicles that occurs in response to increased secretion of FSH. As a result, menotropin stimulation following GnRH pretreatment generally yields a higher number of preovulatory follicles for IVF.[23]

One large series that compared accumulated data from short and long protocols is a recent report by the French IVF-ET Registry that described a per transfer pregnancy rate of 19.7% in short cycles, 24.9% in long cycles, and 21.4% when no analogue was used ($P < .001$).[24] Nevertheless, persistently high success rates have been reported by one group that employs a short protocol whereby leuprolide is initiated on cycle day 2 and menotropins are begun on cycle day 5.[25] Moreover, Hazout et al.[26] noted a similar number of embryos available for transfer and equivalent ongoing pregnancy rates when comparing the long and short (7-day) GnRHa protocol, although a smaller number of oocytes were retrieved in the latter group of patients.

A third, "ultrashort" protocol involves the administration of GnRHa only on days 2, 3, and 4 of the stimulation cycle, with introduction of daily hMG on cycle day 3. This protocol makes use of the initial release of endogenous gonadotropins to augment follicular recruitment. Endogenous gonadotropin secretion remains suppressed during the late follicular phase because the hypothalamic-pituitary axis does not immediately recover the positive-feedback properties of estradiol on gonadotropins after discontinuation of most GnRHa preparations. Macnamee et al.[27] observed no premature elevation of plasma LH levels with the ultrashort protocol employing the agonist buserelin, whereas Hazout and colleagues[26] did note occasional premature luteinization with the ultrashort protocol using triptorelin.

In a recent study from Bourn Hall Clinic,[28] 312 patients with tubal infertility were prospectively randomized to either the ultrashort or long treatment protocol. The mean number of ampules of hMG was significantly higher in the long protocol, but no significant differences were found between the two groups in the incidence of canceled cycles, failed oocyte recovery, mean number of oocytes recovered per patient, complete failure of fertilization, and the fertilization and embryo cleavage rates. However, the long treatment regimen was associated with a larger number of supernumerary embryos for cryopreservation and a higher delivery rate than was the ultrashort protocol.

One of the most commonly employed ovarian stimulation schedules includes the daily use of leuprolide acetate, 1.0 mg subcutaneously, beginning 8 days after ovulation in order to achieve consistent pituitary suppression. The dose is decreased to 0.5 mg daily after the onset of menstruation and is maintained until the day of hCG administration. The average total daily requirement of hMG is 225 IU/day. Using such a protocol, Meldrum and colleagues[29] noted that the length of the stimulation is increased by approximately 3 days over the short protocol or treatment cycles in which GnRHa is not administered. The dose of hMG is varied depending on the patient's day 3 FSH value, age, ovulatory status, history of ovarian surgery, body weight, and prior response to gonadotropin therapy in order to avoid excessive hyperstimulation and achieve steady follicular growth.

Few comparisons exist of the relative efficacy of the various analogues of GnRH in protocols of controlled ovarian hyperstimulation. The patterns of follicular growth appear to vary among the analogues, although these differences do not significantly correlate with the clinical outcome of IVF.[30] Recent preliminary reports examining leuprolide and nafarelin have demonstrated equivalent pregnancy rates with their use. In one prospective, randomized study, nafarelin, 400 μg, was administered twice daily beginning on day 1 of the cycle until ovarian suppression was achieved, at which time the dose was decreased to 200 μg twice daily.[31] Patient response was compared with a leuprolide regimen of 0.5 mg/day initially followed by 0.25 mg/day, half the dose that is usually prescribed. Three ampules (225 IU) of menotropins were administered to stimulate follicular development. The nafarelin schedule yielded a significantly higher number of collected oocytes (12.7 vs. 9.3) and more cryopreserved embryos, although pregnancy outcomes were equivalent. In another recent randomized study, the use of leuprolide in combination with gonadotropins in ovarian stimulation for IVF resulted in significantly higher numbers of total and mature oocytes as compared with that achieved with the GnRHa buserelin.[32] This may be due to a direct effect of the latter, more potent, analogue on granulosa cell function.

Women who respond poorly to the long GnRHa schedule are frequently found to have an elevated circulating FSH concentration when measured early in the follicular phase (i.e., cycle day 3). These patients have decreased ovarian reserve and should not be treated with the long or luteal-phase GnRHa ovarian stimulation protocol described above because they invariably manifest a poor response.[23] High doses of urinary FSH (Metrodin) can be administered in such circumstances to achieve optimal follicular development.

Exogenous FSH is capable of stimulating multiple follicular development in all categories of patients. No significant differences have been noted in patient response with the use of FSH or hMG, although one study reported the collection of a fewer number of oocytes in women treated with GnRHa/FSH. Since exposure of the follicle to high levels of LH may be associated with detrimental effects on development, and since premature luteinization is possible despite the presence of GnRHa, many programs have limited the total daily dose of exogenous LH present in menotropins to 150 to 225 IU. Any additional gonadotropin is administered in the form of purified FSH.

PROGESTERONE MONITORING

The significance of a mild elevation in serum progesterone on the day of hCG administration is controversial. Radioimmunoassay kits for measurement of very low concentrations of progesterone vary in their accuracy, which confounds the issue. In one retrospective analysis of 133 leuprolide/hMG cycles, pregnancy rates were significantly higher when serum progesterone measured less than 0.5 ng/mL on the day that hCG was given.[33]

The adverse effect of this subtle rise in progesterone production may be on endometrial development rather than oocyte quality. Fanchin et al.[34] noted a decrease in pregnancy rate and a trend for a decrease in embryo implantation rate in patients with plasma progesterone levels greater than 0.9 ng/mL on the day of hCG administration despite a similarity in oocyte number and cleavage as compared with those with lower progesterone levels. Moreover, cryopreserved embryos derived from cycles in which there was a rise in progesterone before hCG administration yielded implantation and pregnancy rates equivalent to frozen-thawed embryos from cycles in which there was no rise in progesterone secretion.[35]

THE LUTEAL PHASE

Menotropins and clomiphene citrate alter the normal physiology of ovarian and endometrial cycles. The development of multiple follicles and the subsequent formation of corpora lutea induce supraphysiologic levels of estrogen and progesterone, which in turn may affect the synthesis or function of growth factors of the luteal endometrium.[36] A decreased receptivity of the endometrium in stimulated cycles may explain the relatively low implantation rates achieved through assisted reproductive technologies.

The traditional method of evaluating endometrial development involves performing a biopsy in the late luteal phase of an ovulatory cycle and dating the endometrium based on a theoretical 28-day cycle. Those specimens classified as out of phase by 2 or more days are considered abnormal and may be associated with an altered receptivity to embryo implantation. Abnormal dating of endometrial samples from stimulated cycles has ranged from 28% to 76% in published series; these figures are much higher than those reported for infertile women undergoing biopsy in natural cycles (3.5% to 20%).[37] Forman et al.[38] proposed that high preovulatory levels of estradiol (>500 pg/mL) and progesterone (>10 ng/mL) are associated with diminished concentrations of both estrogen and progesterone receptors, regardless of the type of ovarian stimulation used. Inadequate or deranged endometrial histology may be caused by exposure to an abnormal ratio of estrogen to progesterone.

Imaging techniques are being used to identify new markers to correlate with endometrial development. The availability of high-resolution ultrasonographic images has prompted many studies relating endometrial echogenicity to endometrial quality. In general, the early follicular-phase endometrium appears as a thin white line. As proliferation transpires, the endometrial echoes widen and become multilayered. During the periovulatory period, the endometrial echoes can be visualized as three distinct layers running along the longitudinal axis of the uterus. The luteal endometrium demonstrates some loss of the hyperechogenicity and three-layered appearance. Vaginal ultrasound has been successfully used to assess the adequacy of endometrial maturation before embryo transfer in those patients undergoing donor oocyte IVF therapy.[39]

MICROMANIPULATION OF EMBRYOS AND GAMETES

Advanced techniques of micromanipulation of preimplantation embryos and gametes have been pioneered through work in lower animals. Animal husbandry scientists have bisected embryos to produce twins, performed nuclear transfer of cells from donor embryos into enucleated oocytes to produce clonal lines, biopsied embryos for sexing and genetic screening, and performed pronuclear microinjection of DNA to introduce new genes into the genome of the embryo. The potential impact of the application of these techniques to human therapy is vast. The techniques of micromanipulation are being increasingly used in three separate areas of clinical laboratory procedure, including blastomere and polar body biopsy, sperm injection, and broaching the zona pellucida to enhance the likelihood of blastocyst hatching and implantation.

PREIMPLANTATION DIAGNOSIS

The detection of genetic defects in embryos that arise through IVF therapy would allow the transfer of unaffected embryos and presumably the establishment of a normal pregnancy. The rationale for disease diagnosis at the preimplantation stage of development is the obviation of elective termination of an affected pregnancy if the diagnosis is established at a later stage of gestation through chorionic villus biopsy or amniocentesis.

To diagnose genetic defects at the DNA level, nuclear DNA must be carefully extracted and amplified by polymerase chain reaction (PCR) technology for accurate analysis. Recently published data indicate that biopsy of one or two blastomeres at the eight-cell stage on the third day postinsemination does not adversely affect preimplantation development (Fig 1).[40] This allows a time interval of approximately 12 hours in which to biopsy the embryos and carry out the genetic analysis before transfer later the same day. Unfortunately, some methods of genetic analysis cannot be accomplished in such a brief period. Biopsy of a quarter of the embryo on day 2 following insemination retards cleavage and alters the inner cell mass:trophectoderm ratio, although it has no adverse effect on embryo viability or the proportion developing to the blastocyst stage by day 5 or 6.[41]

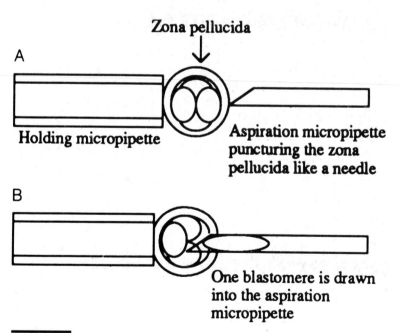

FIGURE 1.

Diagram of the aspiration method for embryo biopsy at cleavage stages. **A,** the glass micropipette punctures the zona pellucida like a needle. **B,** a blastomere is removed by suction. (From Tarín JJ, Handyside AH: *Fertil Steril* 1993; 59:943. Used by permission.)

Preimplantation genetic diagnosis by blastomere biopsy of human embryos was first demonstrated by Handyside and colleagues.[42] Eight couples known to be at risk for transmitting various X-linked diseases were studied, including those who were carriers of X-linked mental retardation, Lesch-Nyan syndrome, adrenoleukodystrophy, retinitis pigmentosa, hereditary sensory motor neuron disease type II, and Duchenne muscular dystrophy. The Y-chromosome–specific sequence was amplified from cells of the biopsy specimen to determine the gender; those diagnosed as females were transferred to achieve a pregnancy. Seventy percent of the manipulated embryos reached blastocyst stage with no significant reduction in cell number or energy substance uptake, suggesting a lack of harm associated with the procedure. Ten of 22 embryos that underwent uterine transfer subsequently implanted, and 7 of these developed to the stage where fetal heart motion could be sonographically detected. Chorionic villus biopsy revealed that 1 of the 7 gestations had been misdiagnosed and was indeed male; this pregnancy was terminated. No abnormalities were detected in the children born through this procedure.

Embryo biopsy for genetic diagnosis of cystic fibrosis, hemophilia A, and other diseases has been described.[43] Cystic fibrosis is caused by mutations in the cystic fibrosis transmembrane regulator gene on chromosome 7. The most common mutation of this gene is a specific three–base pair deletion that causes a loss of a phenylalanine residue at amino acid position 508 (ΔF508). Handyside and colleagues[44] reported the delivery of a homozygous normal child following DNA analysis via nested PCR technology of an embryo derived through IVF. The exact cystic fibrosis mutation in both heterozygous parents must be known for accurate interpretation of the molecular markers.

A high proportion of genetic diseases are caused by abnormalities of chromosome number. Karyotypic analysis of cells removed from early embryos might allow the detection of not only aneuploidy but also structural abnormalities such as deletions, insertions, and translocations. Such analysis, however, requires that the cells be arrested in metaphase and the chromosomes be banded by one of a number of well-established staining methods. Despite numerous attempts, such conventional cytogenetic analysis of human embryos has been only partially successful.[45] Although the majority of nuclei from cleavage-stage embryos cultured overnight in spindle inhibitors will arrest in metaphase, it is difficult to control the spreading of chromosomes. In addition, the chromosomes are typically too short to band effectively. Aneuploidy can sometimes be detected by counting chromosomes, but the chromosomes visualized cannot be identified. An alternative to karyotyping is in situ hybridization of either metaphase or interphase nuclei with probes specific to a given chromosome. One recent report described the use of fluorescent detection of in situ hybridization with a chromosome 18–specific probe for the preimplantation diagnosis of aneuploidy.[46]

Genetic analysis of the multicellular blastocyst may overcome theoretical concerns about the long-term sequelae of micromanipulation of early cleaving embryos. Preimplantation diagnosis via biopsy of the multicellular blastocyst was first reported in animals in 1968 by Gardner and Edwards.[47] In humans as in lower animals, biopsy specimens are taken from trophectoderm cells without affecting the inner cell mass from which the embryo is derived. A slit is made in the zona pellucida opposite the inner cell mass; 12 to 18 hours after this dissection, herniated cells may be collected from the zona surface with a microneedle. In vitro study of the viability of these manipulated blastocysts has not revealed any impairment based upon morphologic criteria and the rate of hCG secretion. As many as 10 to 30 cells have been removed from blastomere masses of more than 100 cells, although none of these human embryos were transferred into the uterus.[48]

The large number of cells obtained from trophectoderm biopsy would clearly improve the reliability of any genetic diagnosis. However, no more than half of normally fertilized embryos reach the blastocyst stage in vitro,[49] and the pregnancy rate after blastocyst transfer is at best no higher than that noted at the cleavage stage. In one recent study of 29 IVF cycles in 18 patients,[50] blastocyst embryo transfer was performed on day 5 after oocyte recovery to determine whether the pregnancy rate significantly differed from that achieved with traditional transfer on day 2. The viable pregnancy rate observed for day 5 transfer was only 10%, less than that achieved through day 2 transfer, which does not support preimplantation genetic diagnosis at the blastocyst stage. Further advances in laboratory technology may facilitate this alternative approach to therapy.

Genetic screening of oocytes or sperm would enable preconception identification of the unaffected allele in carriers of genetic disease. Direct screening of gametes is not possible; however, in the absence of crossing over, the first polar body of the oocyte will be homozygous for the allele not contained in the oocyte and second polar body. If the individual is heterozygotic for an abnormal gene that is found to be present in the first polar body, the diploid embryo that arises following fertilization of that oocyte should be acceptable for uterine transfer to achieve a pregnancy. This procedure assumes that the first polar body does not play a role in embryonic development.

Verlinsky and colleagues[51] reported no decrease in the fertilization and cleavage rate for oocytes that had been subjected to microsurgical polar body removal as compared with that of control oocytes. Puncture of the zona pellucida did not increase the rate of polyspermic fertilization. More than half of the embryos predicted to be affected by the undesired gene developed to the blastocyst stage when cultured in vitro, which suggests that micromanipulation and biopsy had no detrimental effect on preimplantation development.

Polar body analysis is not applicable for gender determination or to assess for autosomal recessive conditions when the carrier state of the mother is not available. Only maternal genetic defects can be detected by analysis of the first polar body. In addition, there is a considerable reduction in the number of embryos available for transfer as a result of the possible crossing over between homologous chromosomes. The genetic analysis that can be performed after removal of the first polar body has relatively low reliability because only a single nucleus is analyzed. Blastomere biopsy is performed in all cases following polar body removal except when the polar body is homozygous for the defective allele; such embryos are suitable for transfer. With this approach, embryos must be biopsied and transferred on day 3, which is the latest day that embryos have been routinely transferred without affecting pregnancy rates.

GAMETE MICROMANIPULATION AS THERAPY FOR MALE INFERTILITY

Artificial opening of the zona pellucida to promote oocyte fertilization was initially accomplished in the mouse model through use of acid Tyrode's solution.[52] Clinical application of this procedure resulted in a high rate of oocyte damage and polyspermic fertilization. Mechanical opening has supplanted zona drilling with acid because of the lower rate of complications. Placement of the oocytes in a medium containing sucrose will shrink the ooplasm and widen the perivitelline space, thereby permitting insertion of the microneedle through the zona without damage to the oolemma. This latter procedure, termed partial zona dissection (PZD), appeared to increase fertilization rates in a selected group of patients with male factor infertility based on moderately abnormal semen profiles.[53] The technique does not appear to be as useful for patients with severe semen alterations. Jean et al.[54] carried out a randomized trial to evaluate the utility of mechanical zona drilling in this patient population who had failed previous attempts at IVF. Although the fertilization rate of the drilled oocytes was significantly higher than control oocytes, the polyspermy rate was so high that the normal fertilization rate after zona drilling remained low and was not statistically different from that of the control oocytes.

Subzonal insertion (SZI), the direct placement of sperm cells into the perivitelline space, has been promoted as more appropriate treatment of severe male factor infertility. Reports of human pregnancy and birth suggest that this technique can result in fertilization even in the most severe cases of abnormal sperm density and motility. More than half of motile sperm placed within the perivitelline space were able to fuse with oolemma in one recent series.[55] Although both PZD and SZI have been shown to be clinically successful either simultaneously or separately, PZD was more beneficial for moderately abnormal semen profiles, whereas SZI appear to be useful particularly in cases of more extreme forms of male infertility.

Fishel et al.[56] described their extensive experience with SZI, which included 225 patients with severe semen defects. Following SZI of 1,003 oocytes, 158 oocytes from 87 patients were fertilized, a significant increase in the number of oocytes fertilized and the number of patients with fertilization as compared with standard in vitro insemination. Twelve clinical pregnancies were established. This study demonstrated a high viability of embryos produced by SZI despite previous concern that SZI may increase the incidence of abnormal embryos owing to avoidance of the natural process of sperm selection at the level of the zona pellucida. Others have reported similar success of subzonal multiple sperm injection in the treatment of patients who previously failed standard IVF.[57]

Nevertheless, these positive results have not been uniformly achieved. The benefit of subzonal sperm microinjection in cases of severe male factor infertility and repeated IVF failure was questioned in a recent report by Sakkas and colleagues.[58] No real improvement was observed in the rate of monospermic fertilization after the injection of up to ten sperm under the zona. In this study, the injection of four sperm was optimal to achieve fertilization without a high rate of polyspermy. Of the 102 embryos transferred, only 3 fetuses (2.9%) developed to the stage at which heart motion could be detected sonographically. A failure of the injected sperm to undergo acrosome reaction may account for a low rate of normospermic fertilization.

Recent developments have been reported in the use of SZI with single sperm and manipulation-assisted sperm adhesion and in the use of direct intracytoplasmic injection (ICSI) in cases of severe oligospermia.[59] In a report of the outcome of 300 cycles of assisted fertilization by ICSI and SZI, Palermo et al.[60] reported normal fertilization of 44% of oocytes following ICSI and 18% following SZI. As a result of using both procedures, 30 patients became pregnant, including 14 after SZI, 8 after ICSI, and 8 after the replacement of embryos following a combination of both techniques.

ASSISTED HATCHING

Despite the fact that microsurgical manipulations may diminish the viability of oocyte and sperm, zona drilling may increase the rate of embryo implantation, even in selected groups of poor-prognosis embryos. A possible impairment of the ability of in vitro cultured embryos to hatch from the zona pellucida after embryo transfer has led to the establishment of a new micromanipulation procedure called assisted hatching.[61] Gaps can be created in the zona pellucida through mechanical dissection, by chemical zona drilling with acid Tyrode's solution, or with laser technique in order to enhance pregnancy rates.[62-64] The precise efficacy of this therapy is still being established. The application of acidic Tyrode's solution creates larger gaps in the zona pellucida than does mechanical dissection; this appears to enhance completion of the hatching process and may be particularly beneficial for embryos with thick zonae.[62]

CRYOPRESERVATION

Embryo cryopreservation plays an important role in augmenting pregnancy rates from each cycle of controlled ovarian hyperstimulation for IVF; nevertheless, some treated couples do not have supernumerary embryos available for storage. Certain patient profiles have been identified that are associated with diminished success through cryopreservation. Toner and colleagues[65] observed that both age and FSH level affect not only the chance to achieve enough embryos for storage but also the outcome of a cryo-thaw cycle. At or above the age of 40 years, the possibility of cryopreservation was decreased by half. Serum FSH levels determined by radioimmunoassay on cycle day 3 also predicted the chance for cryopreservation. No women in the series with levels above 25 mIU/mL were able to have embryos cryopreserved, and fewer than expected were successful with an FSH concentration between 15 and 25 mIU/mL. The chance of a frozen embryo to survive the thawing process bore no relationship to either the age of the woman or to her basal FSH level. Increasing age reduced pregnancy rates mainly through a reduction of embryo quality, whereas increased basal FSH levels reduced pregnancy rates primarily through a reduction in the number of embryos available for cryopreservation and/or transfer.

Embryos are cooled in the presence of cryoprotectants that minimize damage caused by cooling to very low temperatures. The standard technique of equilibrium freezing of pronucleate or early cleavage-stage embryos involves the use of a computer-controlled freezing apparatus and 1,2-propanediol as cryoprotectant. Other cryoprotectants used for embryos include dimethyl sulfoxide (DMSO) and glycerol. High concentrations of these chemicals can be damaging to cells.

Ultrarapid freezing has been recently described as an alternative to the slow cooling technique. This procedure involves a brief, single-step exposure to a relatively high concentration of cryoprotectant that has been precooled to 0°C followed by a simple plunge into liquid nitrogen. Embryos are thawed rapidly, and the cryoprotectant is removed in a single step. One disadvantage to application of the ultrarapid freezing method is the potential toxicity of the high concentrations of cryoprotectant required for this method. Nevertheless, Shaw et al.[66] reported that rapid freezing of mouse two-cell embryos in 4.5M DMSO resulted in greater postthaw embryo viability and reduced chromosome damage when compared with rapid freezing with 1.5M or 3.0M DMSO. In a trial of ultrarapid freezing of 181 4- and 16-cell human embryos, Feichtinger et al.[67] observed that 100 (61%) survived the process and 11 implanted; the overall delivery rate was 7.7%. Although the number of reported pregnancies is small, retrospective comparison with cleavage-stage embryos frozen in 1,2-propanediol and sucrose revealed no significant differences in survival or delivery. Nevertheless, interpretation of the data is compromised because of a lack of information reported regarding the embryo quality before freezing.

Human embryos can be frozen from the pronuclear stage to the expanded blastocyst stage for later uterine placement. The Bourn Hall Clinic[68] reported the outcome of blastocysts frozen in 8% glycerol as cryoprotectant. From 207 cycles of therapy of 198 couples, 379 blastocysts were frozen, and 197 (52.0%) survived following thawing. The resultant clinical pregnancy rate was 9.2% per cycle and 14.2% per transfer. Notably, 38 embryos that were deemed unsuitable for freezing at the early cleavage stage did develop to the blastocyst stage; 22 (57.9%) survived after thawing, and 2 embryos successfully implanted.

In theory, allowing the embryo to develop in vitro to the blastocyst stage before cryopreservation may impair survival because of the greater cell mass. However, Fugger et al.[69] did not detect any difference in survival of embryos frozen as pronuclear zygotes (74.8%) and those frozen at the cleavage stage (70.9%). Although zygote thaw carried a higher pregnancy rate than thaw of cleaved embryos (15.5% vs. 9.7%), this did not attain statistical significance. Menezo and colleagues[70] reported a 21% pregnancy rate per transfer when cocultured human blastocysts were frozen with glycerol after the addition of sucrose. No apparent detrimental effect on embryo survival following micromanipulation and cryopreservation has been observed in the mouse when zona manipulation was performed at the oocyte stage,[71] following blastomere biopsy at the two-cell stage,[71, 72] or when a single blastomere was removed at the eight-cell stage.[73]

Frozen-thawed embryos may be conveniently transferred in the immediate postovulatory period of the natural menstrual cycle or, alternatively, in a simulated natural cycle in which estrogen and estrogen plus progesterone are administered sequentially. The artificial cycle may employ GnRHa suppression to eliminate the possibility of a premature LH surge and untimely rise in progesterone production that might adversely affect endometrial development. Advantages and disadvantages exist for both the natural and simulated cycles. Use of the natural menstrual cycle is generally less expensive because monitoring of the midcycle LH surge can be performed by the patient at home with a urinary test kit. Alternatively, hCG can be administered when the serum estradiol concentration exceeds 180 pg/mL and transvaginal sonography documents appropriate development of the dominant follicle. Transfer is generally performed on cycle day 17 to 19, or 4 days after exposure to hCG/LH. Utilization of treatment cycles in which the endometrium is prepared with exogenous steroids allows an advanced scheduling of transfer. Davies et al.[74] and Muasher et al.[75] have achieved excellent results by performing frozen-thawed embryo transfers in simulated cycles. In the latter series, a 36% pregnancy rate was attained (8 of 22) in anovulatory women undergoing controlled endometrial preparation with leuprolide, transdermal estradiol, and intramuscular progesterone, as compared with a 21% rate per transfer in 144 natural ovulatory cycles. Fugger et al.[69] used clomiphene citrate for their anovulatory patients as a preparation for frozen-thawed embryo transfer. Of 41 clomiphene citrate cycles, 17.3% resulted in conception, which compared well with a 16% pregnancy rate in 121 natural cycles.

Although the cryopreservation of embryos is now an established procedure in human IVF programs worldwide, this therapy has inherent medical, ethical, religious, and legal disadvantages. Cryopreservation of unfertilized oocytes has been attempted as an attractive alternative, for it would circumvent legal and ethical concerns, would provide an option for patients undergoing radiation therapy or chemotherapy for malignancy or extirpative therapy for endometriosis, and might prove useful to the aging woman who wishes to prolong her time span of fertility.

Although there have been reports of survival of cryopreserved preovulatory human oocytes, very few live births have been achieved following uterine transfer of the embryos that have developed from this procedure.[76, 77] Several factors may be involved in the sensitivity of oocytes to cryoinjury. Cooling has been reported to disturb the organization of the meiotic and mitotic spindles of both mouse and human oocytes. Bouquet et al.[78] conducted cytogenetic analysis of 271 frozen-thawed mouse oocytes after IVF and found a significant increase in the rate of triploidy but no increase in aneuploidy by a mechanism that corresponded with retention of the second polar body. The authors also reported a decrease in the fertilization rate after freeze-thaw. Oocyte cryopreservation may cause premature release of cortical granules and result in premature hardening of the zona pellucida.[79] In vitro development of fertilized, thawed oocytes is significantly impaired when compared with controls.[80] No acceptable, reproducible technique of human oocyte cryopreservation has been described to date.

DONOR OOCYTE IN VITRO FERTILIZATION

The earliest employed technique of female gamete donation for the treatment of infertility was adapted from a protocol that has been successfully employed in the reproduction of desirable strains of domestic animals since the 1950s. Intracervical artificial insemination was performed midcycle on normal female volunteers with the sperm of the husband of the infertile woman.[81] Uterine lavage was then conducted during the perinidatory period, and the retrieved blastocyst was subsequently transferred to the uterus of a synchronized recipient. Concerns regarding the spread of infectious diseases, technical difficulties, and the possibility of pregnancy in the donor resulted in the replacement of this procedure with fertilization of donated oocytes in a laboratory setting.

In 1983 Trounson and associates[82] reported the first pregnancy achieved through IVF of donated oocytes in a woman with functional but inaccessible ovaries. The initial report of pregnancy in a woman with ovarian failure occurred in 1984,[83] and the first successful term delivery after egg donation in a natural cycle was described in 1986.[84]

Any woman with ovarian failure who is deemed fit to carry a pregnancy may be considered for donor oocyte IVF-ET. The most common etiology for premature ovarian failure is idiopathic, although individuals with failure because of gonadal dysgenesis, surgical castration, autoimmune factors, or previous chemotherapy or radiation therapy may be candidates. Menopausal women over 45 years of age have successfully delivered infants conceived through this technology.

Others who may benefit include women with decreased ovarian reserve, as characterized by poor response to gonadotropin stimulation and an elevation of serum FSH levels on day 3 of the menstrual cycle, as well as couples with repeatedly poor oocyte and/or embryo quality as judged through prior attempts at IVF. The chance for delivery of a viable infant by an infertile patient over 40 years of age is increased substantially when the oocytes of a younger woman are used; not only is the implantation rate increased, but the usual abortion rate of 60% is reduced to approximately 20% with the use of younger female gametes.[85] Donor oocyte IVF is also applicable for women who wish to avoid transmission of inheritable disorders to their offspring or who have karyotypic abnormalities that preclude normal euploid fertilization.

Potential oocyte donors include relatives or friends of the recipient, anonymous donors, paid donors, and infertile women who wish to donate a portion of their collected oocytes for altruistic reasons or to share the financial burden of assisted reproductive technology therapy. Donors must be in good health and without a medical or family history that would suggest that they may not produce an appropriate number of mature gametes that could lead to the delivery of a healthy infant. The use of donors less than 34 years of age is preferred because of the higher pregnancy rates achieved with the oocytes of a younger woman and in order to reduce the need for genetic counseling of the recipient couple. Oocyte donors generally undergo superovulation with hMG to allow the aspiration of multiple mature follicles. The oocytes are inseminated in the laboratory, and the cultured embryos are subsequently transferred transcervically into the uterus of a hormonally synchronized recipient.

A number of exogenous hormone schedules have been successfully employed to achieve appropriate endometrial development of the donor oocyte recipient. Potential recipients who have intact ovarian function can be rendered temporarily agonadal with the administration of GnRHa before the introduction of exogenous hormone replacement. Estradiol may be administered transdermally, orally, and via polysiloxane-impregnated vaginal rings. Approximately 30% of orally administered estradiol is metabolized before reaching the systemic circulation, thereby effectively reducing the estrogenic effect. Progesterone has been given most frequently by vaginal suppository or intramuscular injection. A lag in early glandular development is frequently seen when endometrial biopsy is performed on cycle day 21 or 22, the anticipated day of implantation. This dyssynchrony in development does not appear to impair the chance for pregnancy as long as stromal maturation proceeds as expected.

The temporal window of endometrial receptivity in humans is restricted to days 16 to 20 of a 28-day cycle, with day 15 being the first day of progesterone administration.[86] Embryo transfer on days 17 to 19 appears to be most favorable for implantation. The length of the recipient's follicular phase is not critical and may be adjusted to accommodate the

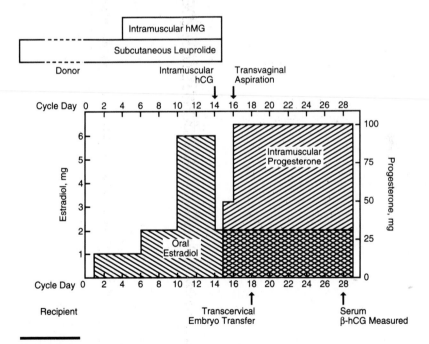

FIGURE 2.

One regimen of ovarian stimulation in the donor and hormone replacement used by recipient in donor oocyte IVF therapy. *hMG* and *hCG* signify human menopausal gonadotropin and human chorionic gonadotropin, respectively. β-hCG is the β-subunit of hCG. (From Sauer MV, Paulson RJ, Lobo RA: *JAMA* 1992; 268:1275. Used by permission.)

duration of the donor's stimulated follicular phase. Progesterone therapy may be initiated on the day before the donor's day of oocyte retrieval, thus permitting appropriate synchronization. One successful protocol of controlled ovarian hyperstimulation and endometrial development is illustrated in Figure 2.

To maintain pregnancy in a woman without functional ovaries and hence a functional corpus luteum, progesterone and estradiol must be administered until placental production of sex steroids is sufficient, usually at 6 to 8 weeks of gestation. Serial hormonal measurements reveal that exogenous supplementation is generally unnecessary beyond 10 to 12 weeks of gestation.[87]

Analysis of the 1,045 donor oocyte IVF cycles reported in the 1991 IVF Registry of the United States and Canada revealed a 31.4% clinical pregnancy rate and a 25.6% delivery rate per retrieval.[88] These statistics compare favorably with the overall IVF clinical and viable pregnancy rates per retrieval of 19.1% and 15.3%, respectively, reported in the same survey. The apparent superiority of ongoing pregnancy rates in the donor oocyte IVF cycles may be attributable to a more favorable uterine environment in the recipient or the transfer of embryos derived from a younger, fertile population as compared with standard IVF therapy.

COCULTURE OF EMBRYOS

Suboptimal laboratory conditions will lead to embryos of reduced viability. Analysis of media obtained from in vitro embryo culture revealed reduced metabolism, accelerated protein turnover, and a functional impairment of metabolite transport systems.[89] Recent studies have reported that as few as 17% of spare embryos that were maintained in vitro progressed to the blastocyst stage.[90] The generally higher pregnancy rates achieved through tubal transfer rather than uterine transfer may be a reflection of the superiority of the tubal environment for embryonic development, the presence of discrete but unidentified tubal factors that improve embryo quality, and improved synchronization of development between the embryo and endometrium at the time that the embryo reaches the uterine cavity.[91]

One approach to mimic the fallopian tube environment is to allow embryos to cleave on a feeder layer of cells obtained from the ampullary fallopian tube, fetal bovine uterus, Vero cells, or other sources.[92, 93] Noncontrolled and nonrandomized studies have suggested that this coculture improves embryo quality and longevity. In one small series of patients, development to the cavitating blastocyst stage was two to three times greater (67%) with coculture than the 17% to 25% observed when spare embryos were grown in culture medium alone.[90, 92] In addition, the rate of blastomere cell division may be increased in embryos cultured on a feeder layer as compared with those cultured in standard media.

Weimer et al.[93] used a fetal bovine uterine coculture system and reported a 35% implantation rate in 40 patients when only two to eight cell embryos were replaced. Others have achieved a pregnancy rate of 31% when at least one blastocyst was transferred.[94] The precise action of the coculture system has not been clearly identified. The zona thinning that occurs in cocultured embryos is thought to lead to a significantly higher likelihood of blastocyst hatching and implantation.[93] The cell line may release embryotrophic factors into the culture medium that have beneficial effects; alternatively, the cells may detoxify the culture medium. Direct apposition of the embryo and cell line may not be necessary; growth of embryos in medium preconditioned by the feeder layer produced a positive coculture effect by yielding 47% cavitating blastocysts as compared with 29% in controls. This beneficial effect of the coculture medium was not as strong as when cells together with medium were used (69% cavitating blastocysts).[95]

TUBAL TRANSFER PROCEDURES

Gamete intrafallopian transfer (GIFT) was originally proposed as a simplified alternative to IVF-ET for couples with nontubal causes of infertility.[96] The theoretical advantages of GIFT include the benefits of in vivo culture within the tubal environment, more appropriate timing of entry of the embryo into the uterine cavity, and the avoidance of endometrial trauma.

The results of GIFT are poor when the procedure is performed as treatment for severe oligoasthenospermia and immunologic infertility[97]; transfer of fertilized oocytes or zygotes into the fallopian tube has been advocated for such cases in which laboratory confirmation of fertilization is considered essential. Tubal transfer performed at the pronuclear stage has been termed pronuclear stage tubal transfer (PROST) or zygote intrafallopian transfer (ZIFT), whereas placement at the two- to eight-cell stage has been termed tubal embryo transfer (TET).

Among the 215 programs submitting data to the United States IVF-ET Registry in 1991, 24,671 cycles initiated for IVF yielded 15.2% deliveries per retrieval.[88] This compared with delivery rates of 26.6% and 19.7% for the 5,452 cycles of GIFT and 2,104 cycles of ZIFT, respectively (see Table 1). The pregnancy loss rate was similar for all three therapies, 19.2% to 21.6%, and the incidence of ectopic pregnancies for both IVF and tubal transfer procedures fell within the range of 1.0% to 1.4% of transfers.

In a report of 399 GIFT cycles, Penzias and colleagues[98] noted that women who received four or more oocytes were three times more likely to achieve pregnancy than those who received three or less. No statistical difference in pregnancy rates was observed in patients who received five, six, seven, or eight oocytes. Weckstein et al.[99] recently reported that transfer of four or five oocytes is optimal with GIFT and recommended that oocytes in excess of five be fertilized in vitro and cryopreserved for future transfer in order to avoid an excessively high multiple pregnancy rate. One center has reported a cumulative pregnancy rate of 52% from one follicular aspiration GIFT/IVF cycle by following this approach. Prior failure of superovulation–intrauterine insemination does not negatively affect the chance of successful pregnancy through GIFT or PROST.[100] The age of the patient may be the most important variable to consider when choosing the number of oocytes to transfer in GIFT. The risk of a multiple gestation in patients over 40 is very low even if ten or more oocytes are transferred. Craft et al.[101] reported only one case of multiple pregnancy of more than twins in 193 GIFT cycles in women age 40 and over even when all oocytes retrieved were transferred.

Transfer of gametes is traditionally performed by cannulation of the fallopian tubes at the time of laparoscopy or minilaparotomy. Transvaginal GIFT is possible through sonographic or hysteroscopic guidance; however, pregnancy rates with transvaginal catheterization were no more than two thirds those of laparoscopic GIFT in one recent series.[102] The major problem of transcervical transfer procedures lies in the lack of reproducibility; this in turn is reflected by the wide range of results that remain no better than those obtained with standard tubal transfer.

Gamete tubal transfer performed at the time of initial screening laparoscopy provides important diagnostic information, enables the surgeon to attempt therapeutic measures, and achieves acceptable pregnancy rates. The first performance of GIFT concurrent with diagnostic laparoscopy was reported in 1989.[103] Eighty-one percent of the patients in this series had appropriate ovarian response to clomiphene citrate, and a pregnancy rate of 24% was achieved. A similar ongoing pregnancy rate of 24.6% was reported by Johns,[104] who used clomiphene citrate to induce ovulation. Gindoff et al.[105] described a pregnancy rate of 24% per cycle at the time of diagnostic laparoscopy through stimulation with hMG. Twenty-one of the 33 patients undergoing concomitant GIFT in their series had adhesions or endometriosis; 19 women received concurrent therapeutic operative endoscopy such as adhesiolysis or fulguration of endometriosis in addition to the oocyte transfer. This combination of a diagnostic and therapeutic procedure should be applied only after having documented patency of the fallopian tubes by hysterosalpingography. Clomiphene citrate–treated ovaries are not as enlarged and highly vascularized as ovaries stimulated by hMG and may provide a more conducive local environment for the surgical treatment of pelvic adhesive disease and endometriosis.

When performing ZIFT, tubal transfer of three or four pronuclear or cleaving embryos provides an optimal chance of pregnancy yet minimizes the possibility of multiple gestation. Some groups recommended transfer of three or fewer embryos,[106] whereas others obtained low numbers of multiple pregnancies even by transferring four zygotes.[107] Negative effects of laboratory conditions on embryos are confirmed by differences in pregnancy rates between GIFT and ZIFT that are accentuated with age. In women over 38 years of age, alterations of the zona pellucida may occur. A thicker zona pellucida is more likely to be detected in this age group; in vitro culture accentuates zona hardening and may interfere with hatching.[108] Hence, the benefits of the tubal environment may be related to the protecting and facilitating effects on the gametes during the process of fertilization and early development.

The debate continues as to whether the difference in pregnancy rates observed between GIFT and IVF cycles is, in fact, significant or is influenced by selection bias. Embryo quality and endometrial receptivity may be more important than the time of entrance of the embryo to the uterine cavity in determining the chances of implantation.[109] Prospective randomized trials comparing GIFT with IVF in unexplained and male infertility did not reveal any difference in pregnancy rates.[97, 110] In a small retrospective analysis by Abdalla et al.,[111] comparable pregnancy rates were obtained after tubal or uterine transfer of frozen-thawed embryos during hormonal replacement. Direct retrospective comparisons conducted by single authors are suspect because the etiology of infertility in patients treated with GIFT may be different from those treated with IVF-ET. Nevertheless, there are few published data from large clinical series to suggest that the implantation rate of embryos is strongly correlated with the specific etiology of the couple's infertility.[91]

Similarly, recent reports suggest that tubal transfer of zygotes is not superior to uterine transfer. Tanbo and colleagues[112] found no statistically significant difference in pregnancy rates following the placement of embryos at similar stages of development in the tubes or uterus of women with non–tubal factor infertility. Comparable results were achieved by Toth et al.,[113] who compared the transfer of pronuclear-stage embryos to the tube vs. cleaving embryos to the uterus. In agonadal women aged 40 and over undergoing oocyte donation in hormonal replacement cycles, fallopian tube transfer did not improve pregnancy rates over those achieved after uterine placement.[109] Moreover, Tournaye and associates[110] reported no therapeutic advantage of ZIFT over IVF–uterine transfer in male factor infertility in terms of reproductive outcome or economic benefit. Large randomized trials are needed to establish with certainty the relative efficacy of tubal vs. uterine transfer.

SUMMARY

Increased understanding of the physiologic processes of gametogenesis and early embryonic development has led to a significant improvement in the clinical pregnancy rates achieved through in vitro fertilization-embryo transfer (IVF-ET) therapy. Controlled ovarian hyperstimulation with exogenous gonadotropins typically yields multiple mature oocytes for insemination. Medical regimens which include concurrent administration of analogues of gonadotropin-releasing hormone are associated with superior outcome, presumably resulting from the inhibition of an endogenous rise in LH secretion, which may occur during the latter stages of folliculogenesis. A subtle increase in ovarian progesterone production during the periovulatory period may adversely affect endometrial development and subsequent embryo implantation. Knowledge of early-pregnancy steroid requirements has led to successful pregnancy in agonadal women through donor-oocyte IVF-ET and estrogen and progesterone replacement therapy.

Major advances in laboratory practices have broadened the possible applications of in vitro fertilization technology. Microsurgical fertilization of oocytes via subzonal sperm insertion and intracytoplasmic sperm injection has resulted in viable embryos and offspring from couples with severe-male-factor infertility. Micromanipulation techniques are also used in embryo and oocyte biopsy for preimplantation diagnosis of genetic diseases, as well as for broaching the zona pellucida to increase the likelihood of embryo hatching. Creating a coculture of embryos with a feeder layer of cells evidently improves the laboratory enviroment for early development. Recent randomized trials have suggested that pregnancy rates achieved through in vitro fertilization approximate those that are achieved through gamete intrafallopian transfer (GIFT) for many categories of infertility. Continuous refinements in laboratory culture methods have made this possible.

REFERENCES

1. Steptoe PC, Edwards RG: Birth after the reimplantation of a human embryo. *Lancet* 1978; 2:366.
2. Wramsby H, Kullander S, Liedholm P, et al: The success rate of in vitro fertilization of human oocytes in relation to the concentrations of different hormones in follicular fluid and peripheral plasma. *Fertil Steril* 1981; 36:448.
3. Paulson RJ, Sauer MV, Francis MM, et al: In vitro fertilization in unstimulated cycles: The University of Southern California experience. *Fertil Steril* 1992; 57:290.
4. Hull ME, Moghissi KS, Magyar DM, et al: Correlation of serum estradiol levels and ultrasound monitoring to assess follicular maturation. *Fertil Steril* 1986; 46:42.
5. Jones HW Jr, Acosta A, Andrews MC, et al: The importance of the follicular phase to success and failure in in vitro fertilization. *Fertil Steril* 1983; 40:317.
6. Benadiva CA, Ben-Rafael Z, Balsco L, et al: Ovarian response of individuals to different doses of human menopausal gonadotropin. *Fertil Steril* 1988; 49:997.
7. Rosenwaks Z: Role of gonadotropin and estradiol levels in predicting IVF results. Assisted Reproductive Technologies Syllabus, The American Fertility Society 25th Annual Meeting, 1992.
8. Scott RT, Toner JP, Muasher SJ, et al: Follicle-stimulating hormone levels on cycle day 3 are predictive of in vitro fertilization outcome. *Fertil Steril* 1989; 51:65.
9. Leung PCS, Lopata A, Kellow GN, et al: A histochemical study of cumulus cells for assessing the quality of preovulatory oocytes. *Fertil Steril* 1983; 39:853.
10. Hartshorne GN: Steroid production by the cumulus: Relationship to fertilization in vitro. *Hum Reprod* 1989; 4:472.
11. Howles CM, Macnamee MC, Edwards RG: Follicular development and early luteal function of conception and nonconception cycles after human in-vitro fertilization: Endocrine correlates. Hum Reprod 1987; 2:17.
12. Meldrum DR, Wisot A, Hamilton F, et al: Routine pituitary suppression with leuprolide acetate before ovarian stimulation for oocyte retrieval. *Fertil Steril* 1989; 51:455.
13. Droesch K, Muasher SJ, Brzyski RG, et al: Value of suppression with a gonadotropin-releasing hormone agonist prior to gonadotropin stimulation for in vitro fertilization. *Fertil Steril* 1989; 51:292.
14. Tummon IS, Daniel SAJ, Kaplan BR, et al: Randomized, prospective comparison of luteal leuprolide acetate and gonadotropins versus clomiphene citrate and gonadotropins in 408 first cycles of in vitro fertilization. *Fertil Steril* 1992; 58:563.
15. Medical Research International, Society for Assisted Reproductive Technology, The American Fertility Society: In vitro fertilization-embryo transfer (IVF-ET) in the United States: 1900 results from the IVF-ET Registry. *Fertil Steril* 1992; 57:15.
16. Ron-El R, Herman A, Golan A, et al: Gonadotropins and combined gonadotropin-releasing hormone agonist–gonadotropins protocols in a randomized prospective study. *Fertil Steril* 1991; 55:574.

17. Cedars MI, Surrey E, Hamilton F, et al: Leuprolide acetate lowers circulating bioactive luteinizing hormone and testosterone concentrations during ovarian stimulation for oocyte retrieval. *Fertil Steril* 1990; 53:627.

18. Homburg R, Levy T, Berkovitz D, et al: Gonadotropin-releasing hormone agonist reduces the miscarriage rate for pregnancies achieved in women with polycystic ovarian syndrome. *Fertil Steril* 1993; 59:527.

19. Rojas FJ, Moretti-Rojas I, Balmaceda JP, et al: Assessment of serum luteinizing hormone during ovarian stimulation with gonadotropins. *Hum Reprod* 1988; 3:207.

20. Meldrum DR, Wisot A, Hamilton F, et al: Timing of initiation and dose schedule of leuprolide influence the time course of ovarian suppression. *Fertil Steril* 1988; 50:400.

21. Loumaye E, Vanbrieken L, Deprester S, et al: Hormonal changes induced by short-term administration of a gonadotropin-releasing hormone agonist during ovarian hyperstimulation for in-vitro fertilization and their consequences for embryo development. *Fertil Steril* 1989; 51:105.

22. Tan S-L, Kingsland C, Campbell S, et al: The long protocol of administration of gonadotropin-releasing hormone agonist is superior to the short protocol for ovarian stimulation for in vitro fertilization. *Fertil Steril* 1992; 57:810.

23. Meldrum DR: GnRH agonists as adjuncts for in vitro fertilization. *Obstet Gynecol Surv* 1989; 44:314.

24. FIVNAT. French national IVF registry: Analysis of 1986 to 1990 data. *Fertil Steril* 1993; 59:587.

25. Garcia JE, Padilla SL, Bayati J, et al: Follicular phase gonadotropin-releasing hormone agonist and human gonadotropins: A better alternative for ovulation induction in in vitro fertilization. *Fertil Steril* 1990; 53:302.

26. Hazout A, de Ziegler D, Cornel C, et al: Comparison of short 7-day and prolonged treatment with gonadotropin-releasing hormone agonist desensitization for controlled ovarian hyperstimulation. *Fertil Steril* 1993; 59:596.

27. Macnamee MC, Howles CM, Edwards RG, et al: Short term luteinizing hormone releasing hormone agonist treatment: Prospective trial of a novel ovarian stimulation regimen for in vitro fertilization. *Fertil Steril* 1989; 52:264.

28. Marcus SF, Brinsden PR, Macnamee M, et al: Comparative trial between an ultra-short and long protocol of luteinizing hormone–releasing hormone agonist for ovarian stimulation in in-vitro fertilization. *Hum Reprod* 1993; 8:238.

29. Meldrum DR, Chetkowski R, Steingold KA, et al: Evolution of a highly successful in vitro fertilization–embryo transfer program. *Fertil Steril* 1987; 48:86.

30. Parinaud J, Oustry P, Perineau M, et al: Randomized trial of three luteinizing hormone–releasing hormone analogues used for ovarian stimulation in an in vitro fertilization program. *Fertil Steril* 1992; 57:1265.

31. Penzias AS, Shamma FN, Gutmann JN, et al: Nafarelin versus leuprolide in ovulation induction for in vitro fertilization: A randomized clinical trial. *Obstet Gynecol* 1992; 79:739.

32. Balasch J, Jové IC, Moreno V, et al: The comparison of two gonadotropin-releasing hormone agonists in an in vitro fertilization program. *Fertil Steril* 1992; 58:991.

33. Schoolcraft W, Sinton E, Schlenker T, et al: Lower pregnancy rate with premature luteinization during pituitary suppression with leuprolide acetate. *Fertil Steril* 1991; 55:563.

34. Fanchin R, de Ziegler D, Taieb J, et al: Premature elevation of plasma progesterone alters pregnancy rates of in vitro fertilization and embryo transfer. *Fertil Steril* 1993; 59:1090.

35. Silverberg KM, Burns WN, Olive DL, et al: Serum progesterone levels pre-

dict success of in vitro fertilization/embryo transfer in patients stimulated with leuprolide acetate and human menopausal gonadotropins. *J Clin Endocrinol Metab* 1991; 73:797.

36. Simmen RC, Simmen FA, Hofig A, et al: Hormonal regulation of insulin-like growth factor gene expression in pig uterus. *Endocrinology* 1990; 127:2166.

37. Cittadini E, Palermo R: The endometrium in human assisted reproduction. *Ann N Y Acad Sci* 1991; 622:230.

38. Forman RG, Eyechenne B, Nessmann C, et al: Assessing the early luteal phase in in vitro fertilization cycles: Relationships between plasma steroids, endometrial receptors, and endometrial histology. *Fertil Steril* 1989; 51:310.

39. Shapiro H, Cowell C, Casper RF: The use of vaginal ultrasound for monitoring endometrial preparation in a donor oocyte program. *Fertil Steril* 1993; 59:1055.

40. Hardy K, Martin KL, Leese HJ, et al: Human preimplantation development in vitro is not adversely affected by biopsy at the 8-cell stage. *Hum Reprod* 1990; 5:708.

41. Tarín JJ, Conaghan J, Winston RML, et al: Human embryo biopsy on the second day after insemination for preimplantation diagnosis: Removal of a quarter of embryo retards cleavage. *Fertil Steril* 1992; 58:970.

42. Handyside AH, Kontogianni EH, Hardy K, et al: Pregnancies from biopsied human preimplantation embryos sexed by Y-specific DNA amplification. *Nature* 1990; 344:768.

43. Handyside AH: Clinical experience in preimplantation diagnosis, in *Abstracts of the International Symposium on Preimplantation Genetics and Assisted Fertilization*. Brussels, Centre for Reproductive Medicine, 1992, p 4.

44. Handyside AH, Lesko JG, Tarín JJ, et al: Birth of a normal girl after in vitro fertilization and preimplantation diagnostic testing for cystic fibrosis. *N Engl J Med* 1992; 327:905.

45. Bongso A, Fong CH, Ng SC, et al: Preimplantation genetics: Chromosomes of fragmented human embryos. *Fertil Steril* 1991; 56:66.

46. Schrurs BM, Winston RML, Handyside AH: Preimplantation diagnosis of aneuploidy using fluorescent in-situ hybridization: Evaluation using a chromosome 18–specific probe. *Hum Reprod* 1993; 8:296.

47. Gardner RL, Edwards RG: Control of the sex ratio at full term in the rabbit by transferring sexed blastocyst. *Nature* 1968; 218:346.

48. Dokras A, Sargent IL, Ross C, et al: Trophectoderm biopsy in human blastocysts. *Hum Reprod* 1990; 5:821.

49. Hardy K: Development of human blastocysts in vitro, in Bavister B (ed): *Preimplantation Embryo Development*. New York, Springer-Verlag, 1993.

50. Bolton VN, Wren ME, Parsons MD: Pregnancies after in vitro fertilization and transfer of human blastocysts. *Fertil Steril* 1991; 55:830.

51. Verlinsky Y, Cieslak J, Evsikov S, et al: Effect of subsequent oocyte and blastomere biopsy on preimplantation development. *Hum Reprod* 1991; 6(suppl 1):136.

52. Gordon JW, Grunfeld L, Garrisi GL, et al: Fertilization of human oocytes by sperm from infertile males after zona pellucida drilling. *Fertil Steril* 1988; 239:347.

53. Malter HE, Cohen J: Partial zona dissection of the human oocyte: A non-traumatic method using micromanipulation to assist zona pellucida penetration. *Fertil Steril* 1989; 51:139.

54. Jean M, Barriere P, Sagot P, et al: Utility of zona pellucida drilling in cases of severe semen alterations in man. *Fertil Steril* 1992; 57:591.

55. Cohen J, Alicani M, Malter HE, et al: Partial zona dissection or subzonal

sperm insertion: Microsurgical fertilization alternatives based on evaluation of sperm and embryo morphology. *Fertil Steril* 1991; 56:696.

56. Fishel S, Timson J, Lisi F, et al: Evaluation of 225 patients undergoing subzonal insemination for the procurement of fertilization in vitro. *Fertil Steril* 1992; 57:840.
57. Imoedemhe DAG, Sigue AB: Subzonal multiple sperm injection in the treatment of previous failed human in vitro fertilization. *Fertil Steril* 1993; 59:172.
58. Sakkas D, Lacham O, Gianaroli L, et al: Subzonal sperm microinjection in cases of severe male factor infertility and repeated in vitro fertilization failure. *Fertil Steril* 1992; 57:1279.
59. Kobayashi K, Okuyama M, Fujimoto G, et al: Subzonal insemination with a single spermatozoon using manipulation assisted sperm adhesion onto the ooplasmic membrane in mouse ova. *Mol Reprod Dev* 1992; 31:223.
60. Palermo G, Joris H, Derde M-P, et al: Sperm characteristics and outcome of human assisted fertilization by subzonal insemination and intracytoplasmic sperm injection. *Fertil Steril* 1993; 59:826.
61. Cohen J, Elsner C, Kort H, et al: Impairment of the hatching process following IVF in the human and improvement of implantation by assisting hatching using micromanipulation. *Hum Reprod* 1990; 5:7–13.
62. Cohen J: Assisted hatching of human embryos. *J In Vitro Fert Embryo Transf* 1991 8:179.
63. Strohmer H, Feichtinger W: Successful clinical application of laser for micromanipulation in an in vitro fertilization program. *Fertil Steril* 1992; 58:212.
64. Tucker MJ, Cohen J, Massey JB, et al: Partial dissection of the zona pellucida of frozen-thawed human embryos may enhance blastocyst hatching, implantation and pregnancy rates. *Am J Obstet Gynecol* 1991; 165:341.
65. Toner JP, Veeck LL, Muasher SJ: Basal follicle-stimulating hormone level and age affect the chance for and outcome of pre-embryo cryopreservation. *Fertil Steril* 1993; 59:664.
66. Shaw JM, Kola I, MacFarlane DR, et al: An association between chromosomal abnormalities in rapidly frozen 2-cell mouse embryos and the ice-forming properties of the cryoprotective solution. *J Reprod Fertil* 1991; 91:9–18.
67. Feichtinger W, Hochfellner C, Ferstl U: Clinical experience with ultrarapid freezing of embryos. *Hum Reprod* 1991; 6:735–736.
68. Hartshorne GM, Elder K, Crow J, et al: The influence of in-vitro development upon post-thaw survival and implantation of cryopreserved human blastocysts. *Hum Reprod* 1991; 6:136.
69. Fugger EF, Bustillo M, Dorfmann AD, et al: Human preimplantation embryo cryopreservation: Selected aspects. *Hum Reprod* 1991; 6:131.
70. Menezo Y, Nicollet B, Herbaut N, et al: Freezing cocultured human blastocysts. *Fertil Steril* 1992; 58:977.
71. Garrisi GJ, Talansky BE, Sapira V, et al: An intact zona pellucida is not necessary for successful mouse embryo cryopreservation. *Fertil Steril* 1992; 57:677.
72. Depypere HT, Carroll JC, Vandekerckhove D, et al: Normal survival and in-vitro development after cryopreservation of zona-drilled embryos in mice. *Hum Reprod* 1991; 6:432.
73. Krzyminska U, O'Neill CO: The effects of cryopreservation and thawing on the development in vitro and in vivo of biopsied 8-cell mouse embryos. *Hum Reprod* 1991; 6:832.
74. Davies DW, Jenkins JM, Anthony FW, et al: Biochemical monitoring during

hormone replacement therapy cycles for transfer of cryopreserved embryos in patients with functional ovaries. *Hum Reprod* 1991; 6:934.

75. Muasher SJ, Kruithoff C, Simonetti S, et al: Controlled preparation of the endometrium with exogenous steroid for the transfer of frozen-thawed pre-embryos in patients with anovulatory or irregular cycles. *Hum Reprod* 1991; 6:443.

76. Chen C: Pregnancy after human oocyte cryopreservation. *Lancet* 1986; 1:884.

77. Van Uem JFHM, Siebzehnrueble ER, Schuh B, et al: Birth after cryopreservation of unfertilised oocytes. *Lancet* 1987; 1:752.

78. Bouquet M, Selva J, Aurous M: The incidence of chromosomal abnormalities in frozen-thawed mouse oocytes after in-vitro fertilization. *Hum Reprod* 1992; 7:76.

79. Vincent C, Pickering SJ, Johnson MH: The zona hardening effect of dimethylsulfoxide requires the presence of an oocyte and is associated with a reduction in the number of cortical granules present. *J Reprod Fertil* 1990; 89:253.

80. Hunter JE, Bernard A, Fuller B, et al: Fertilization and development of the human oocyte following exposure to cryoprotectants, low temperatures and cryopreservation: A comparison of two techniques. *Hum Reprod* 1991; 6:1460.

81. Buster JE, Bustillo M, Thorneycroft IH, et al: Non-surgical transfer of in vitro fertilized donated ova to five infertile women: Report of two pregnancies. *Lancet* 1983; 2:223.

82. Trounson A, Leeton J, Besanka M, et al: Pregnancy established in an infertile patient after transfer of donated embryo fertilized in vitro. *BMJ* 1983; 286:835.

83. Lutjen P, Trounson A, Leeton J, et al: The establishment and maintenance of pregnancy using in vitro fertilization and embryo donation in a patient with primary ovarian failure. *Nature* 1984; 307:174.

84. Rosenwaks Z, Veeck LL, Liu HC: Pregnancy following transfer of in vitro fertilized donated oocytes. *Fertil Steril* 1986; 45:417.

85. Sauer MV, Paulson RJ, Lobo RA: Reversing the natural decline in human fertility: An extended clinical trial of oocyte donation to women of advanced reproductive age. *JAMA* 1992; 268:1275.

86. Navot D, Laufer N, Kopolovic J, et al: Artificially induced endometrial cycles and establishment of pregnancies in the absence of ovaries. *N Engl J Med* 1986; 314:806.

87. Schneider MA, Davies MC, Honour JW: The timing of placental competence in pregnancy after oocyte donation. *Fertil Steril* 1993; 59:1059.

88. Society for Assisted Reproductive Technology: Assisted reproductive technology in the United States and Canada: 1991 results from the Society for Assisted Reproductive Technology generated from The American Fertility Society Registry. *Fertil Steril* 1993; 59:956.

89. Jung T: Protein synthesis and degradation in non-cultured and in vitro culture rabbit blastocysts. *J Reprod Fertil* 1989; 86:507.

90. Bolton V, Hawes SM, Taylor CT, et al: Development of spare human preimplantation embryos in vitro: An analysis of the correlations among gross morphology, cleavage rates and development to the blastocyst. *J In Vitro Fert Embryo Transf* 1989; 6:30.

91. Yovich JL, Yovich JM, Edirisinghe WR: The relative chance of pregnancy following tubal or uterine transfer procedures. *Fertil Steril* 1988; 59:858.

92. Bongso A, Ng SC, Sathananthan H, et al: Improved quality of human embryos when cocultured with human ampullary cells. *Hum Reprod* 1989; 4:706.

93. Weimer KE, Cohen J, Amborski GF, et al: In vitro development and implan-

tation of human embryos following culture on fetal bovine uterine fibroblast cells. *Hum Reprod* 1989; 4:595.

94. Menezo Y, Guerin JF, Czyba JC: Improvement of human early embryo development in vitro by coculture on monolayers of Vero cells. *Biol Reprod* 1990; 42:301.

95. Menezo Y, Hazout A, Dumont M, et al: Coculture of embryos on Vero cells and transfer of blastocysts in humans. *Hum Reprod* 1991; 7(suppl 1):101.

96. Asch RH, Balmaceda JP, Ellsworth LR, et al: Gamete intrafallopian transfer (GIFT): A new treatment for infertility. *Int J Fertil* 1985; 30:41.

97. Leeton J, Rogers P, Caro C, et al: A controlled study between the use of gamete intrafallopian transfer (GIFT) and in-vitro fertilization and embryo transfer in the management of idiopathic and male infertility. *Fertil Steril* 1987; 48:605.

98. Penzias AS, Alper MM, Oskowitz SP, et al: Gamete intrafallopian transfer: Assessment of the optimal number of oocytes to transfer. *Fertil Steril* 1991; 55:311.

99. Weckstein LN, Jacobson A, Galen DI: The role of cryopreservation in gamete intrafallopian transfer and zygote intrafallopian transfer. *Assist Reprod Rev* 1992; 2:2.

100. Robinson D, Syrop CH, Hammitt DG: After superovulation–intrauterine insemination fails: The prognosis for treatment by gamete intrafallopian transfer/pronuclear stage transfer. *Fertil Steril* 1992; 57:606.

101. Craft I, Ah-Moye M, Al-Shawaf T, et al: Analysis of 1071 GIFT procedures: The cases for a flexible approach to the treatment. *Lancet* 1988; 2:1094.

102. Jansen RPS, Anderson JC: Transvaginal versus laparoscopic gamete intrafallopian transfer: A case-controlled retrospective comparison. *Fertil Steril* 1993; 59:836.

103. Pampiglione JS, Bolton VN, Parsons JH, et al: Gamete intrafallopian transfer combined with diagnostic laparoscopy: A treatment for infertility in a distinct hospital. *Hum Reprod* 1989; 4:786.

104. Johns A: Clomiphene citrate–induced gamete intrafallopian transfer with diagnostic and operative laparoscopy. *Fertil Steril* 1991; 56:311–313.

105. Gindoff PR, Hall JL, Nelson LM, et al: Efficacy of assisted reproductive technology during diagnostic and operative infertility laparoscopy. *Obstet Gynecol* 1990; 75:299.

106. Devroey P, Staessen C, Camus M, et al: Zygote intrafallopian transfer as a successful treatment for unexplained infertility. *Fertil Steril* 1989; 52:246.

107. Hammitt DG, Syrop CH, Hahn SJ, et al: Comparison of concurrent pregnancy rates for in-vitro fertilization–embryo transfer, pronuclear stage embryo transfer and gamete intra-fallopian transfer. *Hum Reprod* 1990; 5:947.

108. Malter JE, Cohen J: Blastocyst formation and hatching in vitro following zona drilling of mouse and human embryos. *Gamete Res* 1989; 24:67.

109. Balmaceda JP, Alam V, Rotsztejn DA, et al: Embryo implantation rates in oocyte donation: A prospective comparison of tubal versus uterine transfers. *Fertil Steril* 1992; 57:362.

110. Tournaye H, Devroey P, Camus M, et al: Zygote intrafallopian transfer or in vitro fertilization and embryo transfer for the treatment of male factor infertility: A prospective randomized trial. *Fertil Steril* 1992; 58:344.

111. Abdalla HI, Baber RJ, Kirkland A, et al: Pregnancy in women with premature ovarian failure using tubal and intrauterine transfer of cryopreserved zygotes. *Br J Obstet Gynaecol* 1989; 96:1071.

112. Tanbo T, Dale PO, Åbyholm T: Assisted fertilization in infertile women with patent fallopian tubes. A comparison of in vitro fertilization, gamete intrafallopian transfer and tubal embryo stage transfer. *Hum Reprod* 1990; 5:266.

113. Toth TL, Oehninger S, Toner JP, et al: Embryo transfer to the uterus or the fallopian tube after in vitro fertilization yields similar results. *Fertil Steril* 1992; 57:1110.

Editor's Comment

In the last few years many advances have been made in the assisted reproductive technologies (ART). GnRH analogues used in various ways have improved success rates by decreasing cancellation rates. This point is well made in this excellent chapter, as it is by Drs. Hardy and Friedman in a later chapter. Future research will probably focus on two important areas. The endometrium has been very poorly studied. We are just beginning to understand the concept of endometrial receptivity and those important factors produced by both the endometrium as well as the developing embryo that allow the process of implantation. Another exciting area that will have important implications for ART is preimplantation genetics. With the human genome project under way, many genes associated with human clinical disease will be identified and cloned for the first time. Embryo biopsy will be indicated for sex-linked disorders as well as for those genes that have been identified. In the more distant future, we may look to ART as a means of providing gene therapy.

Ana A. Murphy, M.D.

Oncology

Diagnosis and Contemporary Management of Cervical Intraepithelial Neoplasia

BRUCE PATSNER, M.D.

Papanicolaou and Traut published their classic monograph on microscopic examination of exfoliated cells from the cervix in 1943.[1] That same year, invasive cervical cancer developed in almost 50,000 women in the United States alone. In 1993, 50 years later, invasive cervical cancer will develop in only 13,500 women in the United States, and only one third will die of their disease. Often, those in whom invasive cervical cancer now develops are postmenopausal women who have not had any gynecologic care for many years. The dramatic decline in the incidence of cervical cancer in the United States is one of the finest illustrations in medicine today of the power of screening for malignant disease precursors to alter the natural history of a malignancy. Of all the invasive cancers that may develop in women, only breast cancer and cervical cancer can be effectively screened for, and of these two, only cervical cancer is readily detectable when preinvasive disease is present.

The success thus far achieved in eradicating invasive cervical cancer is due to effective diagnosis and treatment of cervical intraepithelial neoplasia (CIN). Detecting CIN (premalignant disease) and not invasive cancer is the goal of Papanicolaou screening. Remarkably, despite the great success enjoyed thus far with time-honored principles of diagnosis and management of patients with cervical dysplasia, the past several years have generated great controversy. Continuing discussion of proposed new classification systems for exfoliative cytology (the Bethesda system), new technology for diagnosis and treatment (large loop excision of the transformation zone [LLETZ] or the loop electroexcision procedure [LEEP]), the exact role of the human papillomavirus (HPV) in the etiology of genital tract dysplasia, and the proper management of low-grade CIN will all be reviewed in this chapter. We hope to present a thorough discussion of the diagnosis and treatment of patients with abnormal Papanicolaou smears and cervical dysplasia.

EPIDEMIOLOGY AND SCREENING OF CERVICAL DYSPLASIA

Cervical intraepithelial neoplasia, or dysplasia, is a sexually transmitted disease only in the sense that it is rare in celibate women. Any woman who has had (heterosexual) vaginal intercourse at any time is at some risk

Advances in Obstetrics and Gynecology, vol 1
© 1994, Mosby–Year Book, Inc.

for the development of CIN, particularly if coitus occurred during puberty, when squamous metaplasia is at peak activity in the transformation zone of the cervix. (Squamous metaplasia is the "transformation" of
benign columnar into benign squamous epithelium.) Our fundamental
concepts of the natural history or risk factors for the development of dysplasia have altered little over the past decade. Early intercourse, diethylstilbestrol (DES) exposure, multiple sexual partners, lack of prior Papanicolaou smear screening, a previous abnormal Papanicolaou smear, history of sexually transmitted disease, history of prior genital tract
dysplasia, and immunocompromise by acquired immunodeficiency syndrome (AIDS), tuberculosis, or drugs are among the risk factors. The past
decade has, however, seen increased awareness of the existence of the
"high-risk" male partner, recognition of the two to three times greater relative risk[2] for the development of all grades of cervical dysplasia with cigarette smoking, and an enormous literature surrounding the possible role
that HPV infections play in the pathogenesis of cervical dysplasia and
cancer.[3] Because prevention of cervical dysplasia is both difficult at most
and impractical at best, attention has focused instead on detection
(screening) of cervical dysplasia in order to prevent or reduce the incidence of invasive cervical cancer. In this, great success has been achieved,
although questions concerning the ideal screening interval and who
should be screened must still be resolved.

The Papanicolaou smear meets all of the requirements for an effective screening system.[4] It is cost-effective, acceptable to patients, simple
to perform, specific enough to distinguish nonspecific change from disease, and sensitive enough to detect disease in its preinvasive stage (CIN).
The Papanicolaou smear, a test for screening asymptomatic women with
a macroscopically normal cervix, provides us the chance to prevent cancer.

When CIN is detected by a Papanicolaou smear and the patient is appropriately evaluated, treated, and followed, the chance that invasive
squamous cell carcinoma of the cervix will develop in the patient is essentially zero. Even so, mortality from cervical cancer has not been eliminated for four reasons[5]:

1. Screening programs are absent in some areas of the world.
2. Some women are delinquent in obtaining screening or are not
    screened at all. The reasons are various, including high-risk women,
    women who believe that they are "too old" to need screening because
    they are postmenopausal, and women who are unaware of the avail-
    ability of such screening.
3. Errors in sampling or laboratory analysis may occur.
4. Very rarely, patients will experience "rapid progression" from prein-
    vasive to invasive disease over a much shorter time span than usual.

The benefits of cervical cancer screening are limited only to those
women who are actually screened. In places such as British Columbia,
Canada, where organized, centralized Papanicolaou smear screening programs have been implemented, the incidence of invasive cervical cancer
fell by 78% and mortality rates fell by 72% between 1955 and 1985.[6] By

contrast, in Australia, 85% of women who died of invasive cervical cancer in the state of Victoria between 1980 and 1985 had never been screened.[7] Cervical cancer screening programs to detect and treat cervical dysplasia thus have a dramatic impact on the incidence of invasive cervical cancer, provided that specimens are evaluated in cytology laboratories with sufficient expertise and quality control.

HOW OFTEN SHOULD PATIENTS BE SCREENED, AND WHO SHOULD BE SCREENED?

The Canadian Task Force recommended that screening be done at 3-year intervals regardless of risk status and that women aged 60 and over not be screened at all if prior Papanicolaou smears were normal. This approach is economically appealing, but medically it is to be condemned. One of the two major patient populations at risk for the development of cervical or other gynecologic cancers, yet the least likely to be screened, is the lower-income postmenopausal woman. (The second major population at risk is that of sexually active women.) Recent expansion of medicare benefits[8] in the United States to include early cervical cancer detection may significantly improve the general well-being of these patients and can potentially dramatically decrease their incidence of invasive cervical cancer.

The 3-year screening interval for Papanicolaou smears originally proposed by the Walton Report (Canada)[9] in 1974 was later amended in the second Walton Report in 1982[10] to recommend annual screening for women between 18 and 35 years of age and then 5-year screening until age 60 if prior Papanicolaou smears were normal. Both Canadian proposals were rejected by the American College of Obstetricians and Gynecologists (ACOG), which itself recommends annual Papanicolaou smear screening for all women, particularly if they become sexually active before finishing puberty. The Society of Gynecologic Oncologists (SGO) has made a similar recommendation. The controversy over Papanicolaou smear screening intervals persists because no prospective randomized study comparing different Papanicolaou smear screening intervals exists (or is likely to in the United States) and because financial resources for medical care are finite. Nevertheless, American data strongly suggest that regular access to Papanicolaou smear screening on an annual basis will decrease the incidence of invasive cancer for both elderly[11] and younger women.[12] In a study from Washington state, the risk of squamous cell carcinoma was 3.9 times higher for women screened every 3 years than for women screened yearly or every other year. Those patients with invasive cancer whose last Papanicolaou smear was 3 or more years earlier often had more advanced disease.

Annual screening of women to detect preinvasive disease from puberty to past menopause is still the standard of care in the United States. This policy will minimize the likelihood of missed dysplastic lesions because of rapid progression, poor technique, or laboratory or sampling error from a single specimen, and will provide the primary care provider the opportunity to detect other pelvic pathology. Modifications in recommendation for annual Papanicolaou smear screening may be considered if the patient has never been sexually active and has no other risk factors for the development of cervical dysplasia. Improvements in detection of CIN are the result of not only regular annual screening but also greater sophistication in Papanicolaou smear collection techniques that help lessen the possibility that a single Papanicolaou smear screening encounter will miss disease. We address this issue now.

IMPROVEMENTS IN PAPANICOLAOU SMEAR COLLECTION

The cornerstone of proper management of the patient is to obtain a proper specimen. "Adequacy" of Papanicolaou smears is not specifically defined by any current Papanicolaou smear classification system. "Adequacy" may refer to having an arbitrary requisite number of cells on the slide to allow meaningful interpretation by the cytopathologist, or "adequacy" may refer to a smear that contains endocervical cells, thus indicating that "both sides" of the cervical squamocolumnar junction have been sampled. The Bethesda system[13] lists reasons for smear inadequacy, but it does not define what an "adequate" smear is. The Centers for Disease Control concluded that the presence of endocervical cells did not have a major impact on the adequacy of a Papanicolaou smear sample, but the gynecologic literature has for decades emphasized the opposite. Much of the cytologic literature also supports the notion that diagnosis of epithelial abnormalities is improved when the Papanicolaou smear sample contains endocervical cells.[14]

The presence of endocervical cells on a Papanicolaou smear slide is critical for four reasons:

1. There is the potential for lesions to arise de novo in the endocervical canal.
2. Cervical intraepithelial neoplasia arises in the transformation zone, the inner boundary of which is glandular epithelium, where the highest grade of dysplasia is most likely to be found.
3. The squamocolumnar junction in postmenopausal women is often out of range of visualization, and obtaining an adequate smear in this important group of patients is a challenge.
4. The number of epithelial cell abnormalities diagnosed in Papanicolaou smears may be directly related to the presence or absence of endocervical cells.[15]

The "standard" method for obtaining a Papanicolaou smear has been to use a moistened cotton swab for endocervical sampling, followed by a wooden Ayer spatula for the cervix portio. Unfortunately, the cotton swab in particular is not an ideal instrument for exfoliative cytology because the surface often retains too many of the cells that should be transferred to the glass slide. The most significant improvement in Papanicolaou smear collection techniques, and one that ideally will overcome some of the problems with "false negative" smears, is the use of cervical "brush" devices (Cervex Sampler, The Netherlands; Cytobrush, Sweden). Both devices are designed to allow cells loosely attached to the surface of nylon bristles to be readily transferred to a glass slide regardless of the skill of the practitioner and with little or no trauma to the patient or architectural distortion of the cells. Developers of both devices have particularly emphasized the improved ability to obtain endocervical cells.[16] Multiple clinical trials have shown that the Cytobrush is superior to the cotton swab in obtaining endocervical cells.[17,18] The Cytobrush may thus be of particular value in postmenopausal women[19] and women with cervical stenosis.[20] Laboratory trials have also demonstrated that the yield of tumor cells[21] with the cervical brush is 6 to 12 times higher than with a plastic or wooden spatula. The traditional Ayre wooden spatula is not effective in collecting cells for detection of cervical adenocarcinoma.[22] Cervical adenocarcinoma is a malignancy that may be increasing in incidence and is notoriously difficult to detect because of its propensity to arise in the endocervical canal. Any Papanicolaou smear screening system must use collection devices that minimize failure to detect occult cervical pathology, particularly in the endocervical canal. Because it possesses this advantage, the nylon brush sampling device should, at the present time, be considered the method of choice for routine screening for cervical pathology.[23]

Assuming that the Papanicolaou smear has been properly performed with the best cell collecting system, the slides may then be accurately interpreted and any abnormality described. The newest and most widely used nomenclature system for description of cervical cytology is the Bethesda system.

THE BETHESDA SYSTEM

Serious questions regarding quality control of laboratories that do Papanicolaou smear analysis have emerged in the past half decade, generated in part by the realization that some women with invasive cervical cancer were erroneously interpreted to have normal Papanicolaou smears. Because of perceived problems with variations in the reporting of Papanicolaou smear results with the old Papanicolaou system, concerns about quality of laboratory analysis, and concerns about sample adequacy, a 1988 workshop sponsored by the National Cancer Institute published a new set of recommendations and guidelines[24] for reporting the results of genital tract cytology. These have come to be known as the "Bethesda system." The Bethesda system was developed to specifically address the issue of Papanicolaou smear adequacy and improve communication between the cytologist/pathologist and primary health care provider so that clinically important information is not lost. A comparison of this system with the old Papanicolaou system and current World Health Organization (WHO) classification is shown in Table 1.

The impetus for the development of a new classification system for Papanicolaou cytology was the need to eliminate the old Papanicolaou "class system" of reporting, which correlated poorly with histopathology. The Bethesda system presumably would accurately reflect the severity of the squamous epithelial cell abnormalities present. The major change made to obtain good correlation between reported and actual severity was conversion of a three-grade dysplasia categorization (mild to moderate to severe carcinoma in situ [CIS]) to a two-tier system of squamous intra-

TABLE 1.
Comparison of Cervical Cytology Nomenclature Systems

Papanicolaou System	World Health Organization System	Bethesda System
Class I	Normal	Within normal limits
Class II	Atypical	Reactive/reparative change
Class III	Dysplasia	Squamous epithelial cell abnormality
		Atypical squamous cells of undetermined significance
		Squamous intraepithelial lesion
	Mild dysplasia	Low grade SIL* (including HPV*)
	Moderate dysplasia	High-grade SIL
	Severe dysplasia	High-grade SIL
Class IV	Carcinoma in situ	High-grade SIL
Class V	Invasive cancer	Squamous cell carcinoma
		Glandular cell abnormality
		Nonepithelial cell cancer

*SIL = squamous intraepithelial lesion; HPV = human papillomavirus.

epithelial lesion (SIL): (1) low grade (HPV and CIN I together) and (2) high grade (moderate and severe dysplasia).

The Bethesda system also provided a new, separate description for glandular cell abnormalities (e.g., adenocarcinoma) and created new categories for both squamous and glandular cell abnormalities, called atypical (squamous/glandular) cells of undetermined significance (ASCUS and AGCUS), not previously described in any other existing Papanicolaou classification.

The ACOG rejected the Bethesda system, for reasons that will be discussed, in a 1990 editorial published in *Obstetrics and Gynecology*.[25] Unfortunately, the Bethesda system has become so widespread that, like death and taxes, it is probably here to stay. A critical review of the merits and problems of the Bethesda system follows, with the hope that its major deficiencies will be addressed and amended.

WHAT ARE THE MERITS OF THE BETHESDA SYSTEM?

First, the Bethesda system is the only classification to specifically raise the issue of Papanicolaou smear sample adequacy. Unfortunately, its categories (satisfactory, less than optimal, and unsatisfactory) are never defined, and criteria for inclusion of any specimen, based on the number of cells, the presence of endocervical cells, or other distinctions, are not provided but are left instead to the individual reader. That the issue of definition of smear adequacy has been raised is clearly an important step, and the definition will no doubt be refined. Discovering the explanations for less-than-optimal cytology is a critical first step, but the problem of interlaboratory variation remains unsolved in the meantime. Second, the Bethesda system rejects the old Papanicolaou smear system class II (atypical) category as too vague and replaces it in part with a category of reactive and reparative changes that specifically exclude dysplasia to avoid confusion as to whether cells were abnormal enough to require further evaluation (e.g., colposcopy with directed biopsy). Finally, the Bethesda system is the first to specifically direct attention to glandular cell abnormalities, such as adenocarcinoma in situ, which have assumed increasing clinical significance in recent years.

WHAT ARE THE PROBLEMS WITH THE BETHESDA SYSTEM AS IT IS PRESENTLY FORMULATED?

They are significant. First and foremost, the old Papanicolaou system and the current WHO system are time-tested, their terminology is understood, and marked declines in the incidence of invasive cervical cancer can be attributed to their emphasis of diagnosis and treatment of dysplasia. Moreover, current problems in management of patients with CIN and cervical cancer are the result not of the classification systems but of the poor screening of high-risk populations. The utility of the Bethesda system, on the other hand, is totally unproved.

Emphasis on quality control in laboratories is laudable but can and should be a part of any screening classification. The lack of definition of smear adequacy is a glaring omission in a system that developed in the first place because of perceived problems in this area. The category of "less-than-optimal" specimen adequacy is particularly irksome in its lack of clarity. In one recent study reviewing the University of Iowa experience with the Bethesda system, half of the complaints from clinicians concerned difficulties with this category alone.[26] The replacement of three-letter dysplasia-CIS terminology with a two-tier system must under normal circumstances produce fewer interobserver interpretation discrepancies (since three categories are fewer than two), but what the Bethesda system has actually done, in effect, is replace one three-tier system with another: low-grade SIL; high-grade SIL; and atypical cells, squamous or glandular, of undetermined significance. This third category of "atypical" cells is not defined, an omission inherently confusing to a clinician trying to manage a patient and one that is certain to amplify reporting variations between laboratories. For atypical *squamous* cells of undetermined significance, the only question is whether to perform colposcopy on the patient. (The onus of responsibility to rule out significant disease is ultimately the clinician's.) For atypical *glandular* cells of undetermined significance, the practitioner is forced to evaluate the endocervical canal and possibly myometrium as well. Does this mean that *all* patients in this category need conization loop excision and endometrial evaluation? The implications of this undefined category are unknown; either the "atypical cells of undetermined significance" should be precisely defined for the cytologist to allow for a precise recommendation to the clinician, or the category should be eliminated entirely. The category also raises the serious possibility that individuals interpreting the slides will overuse this category to "cover" themselves in the event that significant cervical pathology develops at a later date.

Finally, but most important, the current classification of SIL into a low-grade category with HPV and CIN I together and into a high-grade SIL that includes moderate and severe dysplasia is fraught with difficulties. Not only may it not be an improvement over the previous CIN classification, but it may actually create more problems than it solves. Traditionally, cervical dysplasia was categorized as mild, moderate, or severe, and all patients were treated. There has never been any question that the risk of progression to invasive cancer increases as the severity of dysplasia increases, nor any question that the risk of progression from mild dysplasia to CIS is less than that for moderate dysplasia. Inclusion of moderate and severe dysplasia in the same category occurred in the Bethesda system presumably because there is little literature supporting the notion that moderate dysplasia should not be treated,[27] and there is some debate over whether to treat all patients with CIN I. If, on the other hand, the Bethesda system is intended to reflect risk of progression to cancer, then its high-grade category is arbitrary because the likelihood of moderate dysplasia progressing is significantly less than for severe dysplasia.

Categorizing mild dysplasia with HPV/koilocytosis only is even more problematic. Although in some series the risk of progression to CIS in patients whose Papanicolaou smears show either CIN I or koilocytosis/ HPV only is about the same (15%[28] although distinguishing the two colposcopically may be difficult even for skilled colposcopists), the two entities do look different. There is at present consensus that isolated cervical HPV infection requires no treatment regardless of the HPV subtype or patient risk category. There are many experts who do treat some or all patients with mild dysplasia, however. The controversy over whether patients with mild dysplasia should all be treated is not one that was created by the Bethesda system, but low-grade SIL retains the unfortunate grouping (one for which treatment is never performed and one for which treatment is often performed). Finally, informing patients that SIL is the diagnosis immediately requires an explanation that the virus invariably is sexually transmitted, when the diagnosis may in fact be only mild dysplasia without koilocytosis. Eliminating the CIN I-with-HPV category would give the clinician the flexibility to tell the patient that she has either abnormal cell growth (dysplasia), a viral infection, or both. Treatment issues may then be dealt with accordingly. Because there is some controversy over whether to treat mild dysplasia, it would be wrong to classify Papanicolaou smears and biopsies as simply normal, dysplasia, or cancer. On the other hand, differences in natural history between CIN II and CIS need to be recognized too.

HOW ARE WE TO RESOLVE ALL OF THESE ISSUES?

Ideally, improvements in Papanicolaou smear reporting attributable directly to the Bethesda system—efforts toward quality control and comments on smear adequacy and glandular abnormalities—should be retained and refined. The presently meaningless ASCUS category should be defined or eliminated. The two-tier SIL system is not supported by clinical data, and the low-grade SIL category should be changed so that one may tell the patient that she has mild dysplasia, HPV infection, or both. In addition, clinicians and cytologists alike must acknowledge that some of the failure to detect cervical cancer is the false negative rate of the Papanicolaou smear itself; no classification system will affect this last factor.

These problems with the Bethesda system of classification of abnormal Papanicolaou smears represent a formal confrontation with two of the most confusing and contentious issues in the management of a patient with an abnormal Papanicolaou smear: proper evaluation of the patient with an "atypical" smear and management of the patient with mild cervical dysplasia.

MANAGEMENT OF THE "ATYPICAL" PAPANICOLAOU SMEAR AND CERVICAL INTRAEPITHELIAL NEOPLASIA I

All classification systems for abnormal Papanicolaou smears contain categories that fall between "within normal limits" and a firm diagnosis of dysplasia. This category includes Papanicolaou smears that are described as class II (Papanicolaou classification system), atypical squamous cells of undetermined significance (Bethesda system), and inflammatory, or squamous, atypia. All of these appellations are problematic for the clinician since they are poorly defined, if defined at all, and thus an impediment to the clinician who is looking for guidance as to the proper course of patient management. The critical question to be addressed in evaluating these patients is whether cervical dysplasia (or worse) is already present. In effect, this is the same as asking which patients with "atypical" Papanicolaou smears should undergo colposcopic evaluation. The Bethesda system category of "reactive or reparative changes" represents an excellent effort to eliminate some cytologic abnormalities that were formerly included in these categories.

WHICH PATIENTS WITH "ATYPICAL" PAPANICOLAOU SMEARS SHOULD UNDERGO COLPOSCOPIC EVALUATION?

Recommendations in the current literature for management of patients with "atypical" smears vary greatly. Montz et al.[29] reviewed 632 women with "minimally abnormal" Papanicolaou smears and determined that complete colposcopic and cytologic regression will occur in the majority of women over a short period of time. Follow-up was only over a 9-month period of time, and 2% to 20% of patients did progress to significant dysplasia. The majority of studies published in the last 5 years[30, 31] on patients with atypical smears strongly suggest that at least 10% to 15% of patients will have cervical dysplasia (from 5% to 40%) and that one third or more have evidence of HPV infection, which although not necessarily requiring treatment does indicate that closer follow-up may be necessary. Recent studies by Spitzer et al.[32] and Rader et al.[33] both noted that upward of one third of patients with atypical squamous cells will have colposcopic and biopsy evidence of cervical dysplasia; the study by Rader and colleagues also strongly suggested that colposcopy is the most cost-effective method of evaluation when compared with other methods such as cervicography.

Current recommendation for evaluation of a patient with an "atypical" Papanicolaou smear is colposcopy with directed biopsy; merely repeating the Papanicolaou smear after a discrete interval is a traditional method that is not supported by the vast majority of current literature and is to be avoided. In situations where colposcopy services are limited, HPV DNA testing has been suggested[34] as a way to determine which patients with atypical smears require colposcopy; those patients with HPV positivity are more likely to have biopsy-proved cervical dysplasia on colposcopy. Whether this approach is cost-effective as opposed to simply referring all patients for colposcopy is unknown.

Before the categorization of cervical HPV infection and mild cervical dysplasia into the same category of low-grade SIL, the controversy over treatment of mild dysplasia was limited. Clearly, if the two entities are essentially equivalent and there is concensus that HPV infection alone does not need treatment, the issue of whether CIN I needs to be treated is immediately raised. The Bethesda system raises the specter of *overtreatment* of many patients if one assumes that CIN I does need treatment and all patients with HPV infection are classified in the low-grade SIL category. It is unlikely that the issue will be resolved in the near future. All would agree that even though high-grade lesions are historically more likely to progress than are low-grade lesions, determining the behavior of an individual lesion is impossible. Moreover, 29% or more of "low-grade" CIN lesions are associated with high-risk HPV types 16, 18, or 33,[35] and the distribution of HPV types 6, 11, 18, and 33 in both low- and high-grade SIL was identical in the largest and most controlled series in the literature.[36] Given these facts and the fact that the "preinvasive phase" may be shorter in younger than in older women,[37] the proven efficacy in preventing invasive cervical cancer by treating all CIN should make one approach with great caution any recommendation to not treat CIN I. The recommendation should, in any case, be made only for extremely reliable patients with access to expert follow-up evaluation in a clinical research setting. The current standard, then, is treatment of CIN regardless of degree.

TREATMENT OF CERVICAL INTRAEPITHELIAL NEOPLASIA: EXCISIONAL VS. DESTRUCTIVE METHODS

All methods for treatment of cervical dysplasia are predicated on evidence that suggests the presence of abnormal cells (Papanicolaou smear) followed by evaluation of the cervix (by colposcopy) to identify areas from which the abnormal cervical epithelial cells may have arisen. Endocervical curettage (ECC), or sampling the canal, may or may not be performed on all patients, depending on philosophy, the institution of training, or even the country. Advocates of routine ECC regardless of whether colposcopy is adequate (i.e., the entire cervical abnormality can be seen) claim that occult endocervical cancers will not be overlooked; there is no evidence to support this claim. Moreover, the detection of occult invasive cancer in the canal will still require conization or loop excision to determine whether microinvasive or invasive cancer is present. Endocervical curettage that indicates dysplasia in the absence of extension of disease into the canal colposcopically usually reflects "contamination" from the portio and may invariably be ignored unless ECC products show cells that are markedly more dysplastic than either a Papanicolaou smear or biopsy from the portio. The issue is important since a "positive" ECC is a classic indication for cone biopsy (or loop excision).

WHAT ARE THE THERAPEUTIC OPTIONS, AND WHAT NEW TREATMENTS ARE AVAILABLE?

In most cases the correct approach to appropriate treatment of cervical dysplasia will be based on whether colposcopy is adequate (i.e., the entire lesion can be seen) and whether there is a correlation between the Papanicolaou smear and colposcopic impression. If routine ECC is done, the information it provides should decide the modality of treatment if there is a marked discrepancy (two grades or more) between the findings on ECC and Papanicolaou smear or cervical biopsy. In most other instances, the decision as to whether a destructive procedure or an excisional procedure is acceptable is based on whether the entire abnormal cervical epithelium can be seen.

A cylindrical tissue specimen of cervical epithelium that includes portio and part of the endocervical canal is called a cone biopsy. Such a portion of cervix may be excised by a knife (cold knife conization), by carbon dioxide (laser conization), or by any loop excision instrument (loop conization). Before colposcopy was widely employed, cone biopsy was the standard for treatment of patients with an abnormal Papanicolaou smear and a macroscopically normal cervix. A cone specimen is still necessary in the following circumstances:

1. No other modality of treatment is available.
2. The entire abnormal cervical epithelium extends into the endocervical canal out of range of visualization.
3. The ECC findings are significantly worse than those of biopsy and Papanicolaou smear in the presence of otherwise adequate colposcopy.
4. The Papanicolaou smear is significantly worse than colposcopically directed cervical biopsies.
5. Microinvasive carcinoma is diagnosed by Papanicolaou smear, colposcopy, or biopsy.
6. Invasive cancer is suspected but cannot be confirmed by biopsy.
7. The experience of the colposcopist is limited. This last is a "soft" indication; one might argue that only experienced colposcopists should be evaluating patients with abnormal Papanicolaou smears in the first place.

Two additional indications that have been espoused for excisional procedures are (1) the youth of the patient (if follow-up is a problem and if it is reassuring to have a tissue specimen encompassing the entire lesion and ruling out invasive cancer) and (2) very large CIN 3 lesions. The cure rates for such lesions are high with laser and lower with cryoprobe treatment, presumably because the cryoprobe may not be large enough to freeze the entire lesion. In the absence of these criteria for a tissue specimen, once properly performed colposcopy has established the need, any one of a number of "destructive" treatments is acceptable and has high cure rates and a proven track record.

One area that must be addressed concerning excisional procedures (LEEP, laser, or cold knife cone) for treatment of cervical dysplasia is what to do in the case of a specimen with positive margins (i.e., dysplasia extending to the endocervical and/or exocervical portions of the specimen) or in the case of cautery artifact that precludes final analysis of the adequacy of the specimen. It is tempting for the clinician to "reexcise" the rim of remaining cervical portio or canal, but the overwhelming majority of such patients can simply be followed with repeat Papanicolaou smears and colposcopy in 4 months once the area has fully healed. Virtually all patients with persistent significant dysplasia will be detected within the first year of follow-up, and further therapy can be safely performed at that time.[38]

A wide array of destructive techniques for the treatment of dysplastic epithelium has been described and is in use. In many instances, the procedure of choice is governed by the institution that the patient is being treated in and, in many cases, the country that the patient is from. Use of all techniques is based on proper pretreatment colposcopic evaluation.

All established methods for destructive treatment of CIN are highly successful in skilled hands, and all are currently office-based procedures. In Australia, electrocoagulation diathermy using a ball and needle tip to destroy the entire transformation zone and deep cervical glands has been used to treat CIN for 20 years, with a first-treatment success rate of 98% and a complication rate (e.g., bleeding, stenosis) of under 2%.[39] The vast majority of these patients had CIS, and although the initial series was done under general anesthesia, the procedure is now done in the office under local.[40] This technique is not taught in the United States for reasons that have nothing to do with success rates in eradicating CIN or minimizing short- and long-term patient morbidity.[41]

Standard Bovie (hot) electrocautery has been used for the treatment[42] of CIN under local anesthesia with primary success rates of 86% or greater. Similar results have been obtained in Canada (97% overall cure rate).[43] Semm cold coagulation[44] using multiple applications of a thermal probe heated to 100° C and applied directly to the cervix has a cure rate in excess of 90% and has been used in the office without any anesthesia. In some institutions in Europe, cold knife conization has been extensively used with cure rates in excess of 90% and long-term follow-up of 10 years or more.[45]

In the United States, the two destructive techniques employed for treatment of CIN are cryotherapy and carbon dioxide laser therapy. Cryotherapy employs as refrigerants either nitrous oxide ($-89°$ C) or carbon dioxide ($-65°$ C), which are contained under pressure and which transmit cold to the cervix through special probes applied directly to the cervix. Freezing crystallizes intracellular water with subsequent disruption of the cell and tissue destruction of the superficial layer of cells of the transformation zone. Use of a double-freeze technique (3 minutes on, 5 minutes off, 3 minutes on) improves results,[46] provided that the probe tip selected encompasses the entire abnormality on the portio and the ice ball formed extends 4 to 5 mm beyond the outer margin of abnormal epithelium. Failure to form an appropriate ice ball will result in inadequate depth of freezing and persistence of abnormal epithelium in glandular crypts, which may be 4 to 5 mm deep.

Cryotherapy requires little dexterity, has minimal morbidity, and is fast, inexpensive, and effective. Posttreatment discharge may be watery and profuse for 3 to 4 weeks and constitutes its only major side effect; stenosis is rare and bleeding scant. The technique is clearly not designed for lesions that are larger than available probes or that extend into the endocervical canal. Posttreatment, the squamocolumnar junction may move into the endocervical canal, and evaluation of patients in whom abnormal Papanicolaou smears subsequently develop may be more difficult. Expected success rates are 95% or more with CIN I and II and 80% to 94% with CIS, depending on patient selection.[47, 48] The likelihood of recurrent dysplasia following cryotherapy if Papanicolaou smears every 4 months remain normal for the first year posttreatment is less than 0.5%, based on an enormous series of almost 3,000 patients[49]; this seems to hold true even for patients with CIN III. The majority of cryotherapy failures occur within the first 12 months of treatment,[50] and these cases almost certainly represent persistent rather than recurrent disease. Long-term follow-up of all patients treated with cryotherapy is important, however, because in a very small percentage significant cervical pathology will later develop, often in the endocervical canal and often requiring excisional diagnosis[51] because the portio of the cervix is usually unremarkable. Cryotherapy is unquestionably the most inexpensive, the simplest, and the least cumbersome effective treatment for CIN presently available. The rare reports of invasive cervical cancer shortly after treatment[52] with cryotherapy are invariably a reflection of poor pretreatment evaluation.

Until the advent of loop excision procedures, the carbon dioxide laser was the newest innovation in treatment of genital tract neoplasia. Introduced in the 1970s, the carbon dioxide laser uses a monochromatic beam of light that impacts on the cervical epithelium under direct colposcopic visualization and "vaporizes" tissue by instantaneous boiling of intracellular water. The CO_2 laser offers precision and excellent healing without scarring, watery discharge, or displacement of the squamocolumnar junction; it offers low morbidity in skilled hands (2% incidence of bleeding), has an excellent cure rate for all grades of dysplasia (90% to 98%),[53] and may be used in the office with or without local anesthesia. Results of treatment for CIN have improved as the depth of destruction of tissue has been increased from 5 to 7 mm[54]; higher-energy machines offer increased speed. In skilled hands the procedure takes 5 to 7 minutes at power densities of 1,000 W/cm^2 or higher. Adjustable beams offer great versatility in the treatment of diffuse HPV on the portio and upper part of the vagina, and laser conization may be readily performed if a tissue specimen is needed.

The drawback of CO_2 laser treatment for CIN is cost. Use of the CO_2 laser does require some surgical and colposcopic skills. As with all other forms of therapy for CIN, close short-term (every 4 months for the first year) and long-term follow-up of all patients is essential and a requirement for use of the laser.

Medical therapies for cervical dysplasia have produced consistently disappointing results, and all remain investigational at present. Interferon gel, 5-fluorouracil and folic acid supplements[55] have had little effect in altering the biology of cervical dysplasia.

Hysterectomy (vaginal or abdominal) can no longer be advocated as the treatment of choice for CIS, even in women who have completed childbearing and who desire sterilization,[56] because more conservative treatments are almost as effective (95%+ vs. 100%) and morbidity and mortality are much lower. Women with dysplasia who have other gynecologic conditions (prolapse, intractable menometrorrhagia) and who refuse all other forms of therapy may be offered hysterectomy, as may the occasional patient with high-grade SIL who had recurrent disease despite multiple attempts at conservative therapy. Patients who undergo hysterectomy for CIN still require close follow-up with vaginal Papanicolaou smears since vaginal intraepithelial neoplasia (VIN) will eventually develop in 1% of such patients.

LOOP EXCISION PROCEDURES: THE "NEWEST" DEVELOPMENT

Electrosurgery for the treatment of cervical abnormalities dates back to the 1960s but, although highly effective, was abandoned once cryotherapy was developed. The highest success rates (97%) reported for primary treatment of CIN are the results of the Australian experience with electrocoagulation diathermy[57]; this technique never achieved popularity in the United States, in part because in the past the treatment required a general anesthetic.

For the past 20 years, the literature on treatment of CIN in North America has been focused almost exclusively on either cryosurgery or carbon dioxide laser therapy (either ablation or conization).[58] Loop excision procedures (LLETZ, England; fine loop diathermy, loop conization, or LEEP, United States)[59] are a direct extension of the work of the French colposcopist Rene Cartier and others, who advocated use of a small 5 × 5-mm electrosurgical loop for cervical biopsies. In 1989 Prendiville and Cullimore[60] advanced the technique by using a larger diameter loop to excise the entire transformation zone. This modification allowed simultaneous diagnosis and treatment of abnormal-appearing cervical epithelium in patients with abnormal Papanicolaou smears. This advance in technique—excision of the entire abnormal transformation zone and not just a strip of tissue for biopsy—was made possible by the development of new electrosurgical generators that allowed a precise, varied blend of coagulation and cutting currents at low power output levels. Before 1990 essentially no American literature existed on loop excision procedures despite the fact that a perusal of the current literature on treatment of cervical dysplasia might give the impression that these techniques are the only ones presently suitable for the treatment of CIN. Indeed, a recent review of treatment of CIN by Jones[61] in 1990 failed to mention loop excision procedures at all.

Loop excision involves the use of a high-frequency current from a grounded electrosurgical generator that is passed through a loop-shaped wire attached to a plastic handle. The current may be a cutting waveform alone or a combination of cutting and coagulation waveforms. The cutting is not done by the loop itself but rather by the spark that jumps ahead of the loop, and the unit must be on before the loop contacts the cervix. Lugol's staining of the abnormal cervical epithelium is done, local anesthesia and vasopressin (Pitressin) are instilled, the loop is slowly pushed into the cervix 2 to 3 mm lateral to the lesion down to a depth of 7 to 8 mm and then slowly moved parallel to the surface of the cervix (either in a vertical or horizontal direction) until the opposite side of the cervix is reached, and the loop is pulled out.[62] The power settings will depend on the electrosurgical generator used and may vary from machine to machine; generally, a blend 1 setting on 40 cut and 60 coagulation is used. The specimen size will depend on the size of the loop, and the loop conization may thus tailor the specimen to each patient. Once excised, the specimen is placed in fixative. The base is coagulated with a ball tip, and Monsel's solution is applied. The procedure takes about 5 to 10 seconds once the patient is prepared, and a smaller loop may be used to take a separate sample of endocervical tissue. There is variation in the ideal current setting among different electrosurgical generators, and unintentional patient burns and damage to noncervical tissue are risks. The procedure should be used with great caution, if at all, in patients with cervicitis.

The impetus for the development of loop excision techniques came from England, which has a large backlog of patients (particularly postmenopausal) with abnormal Papanicolaou smears and inadequate colposcopy and which has a lack of manpower and facilities to schedule the requisite number of visits for initial evaluation to perform colposcopy with directed biopsy or to manage subsequent treatment by conization or other methods.[63] These logistic problems do not exist in the United States, and evaluation of loop excision procedures should focus on its role vs. established techniques, e.g., laser and cryotherapy.

A review of the literature in the United States on the role of LEEP/ LLETZ procedures covering only a 2-year period between 1990 and 1993 nevertheless runs the gamut from a simpler alternative to cold knife conization to a one-step diagnosis and treatment for all patients with any degree of atypical cervical cytology.[64, 65] In the latter instance, LEEP might well signify "Let's excise every patient." The proper role for loop excision procedures is certainly somewhere between the two.

Loop excision of the cervix is, in effect, conization of the cervix with a hot wire instead of a knife or laser. The cutting artifact by electric current is comparable to that by laser conization but is less than by knife. The cost of equipment is more than the laser although less than that for cryotherapy. Inconvenience to the patient during the procedure is more than by laser conization and is less than by cryotherapy. Success rates for treatment of all grades of CIN (96%) are comparable to those obtained with the laser (92%) and are slightly higher (85 to 90%) for select patients with CIN III than those obtained with cryotherapy.[66] The difference in success rates is not statistically significant. No data are available on loop excision long-term cure rates for CIN. Nor are any data available on the incidence of cervical stenosis or reproductive performance for comparison with any other method. The complication rate of 2% to 4% for immediate and delayed hemorrhage is comparable to laser treatment and higher than for cryotherapy. Loop conization is comparable in technical difficulty to knife conization but requires less dexterity than CO_2 laser conization does.

Loop excision is certainly a superb alternative to cold knife conization except, perhaps, in cases where any cautery artifact is unacceptable, as in patients with known microinvasive cervical cancer who are undergoing conization to rule out frank invasion. Loop electroexcision procedures produce an otherwise equivalent surgical specimen, are faster[67] and possibly less morbid, and in select patients may be done in the office. When compared with laser or cold knife conization there is no question that office loop excision represents a major advance. Some cautery artifact is unavoidable with loop excision techniques,[68] but it is no worse than that obtained with carbon dioxide laser conization.

Established "ablative," or destructive, techniques such as cryotherapy or laser have enjoyed high success rates. Purported advantages for routine use of loop excision over laser treatment or cryotherapy for known or suspected CIN are as follows[69]:

1. Diagnosis and treatment may be accomplished in one sitting.
2. Occult invasive or microinvasive cervical cancer may be detected that would otherwise be "destroyed."
3. The need for skilled colposcopy, upon which the use of cryotherapy and laser treatment is predicated, is eliminated.
4. The cost is less.

HOW VALID ARE THE REASONS FOR CHOOSING ONE TECHNIQUE OVER ANOTHER?

Cryotherapy and laser ablation do not preserve a surgical specimen except from pretreatment biopsy. On the other hand, if colposcopic evaluation of a patient with an abnormal Papanicolaou smear is done properly, those patients who require an excisional technique (i.e., conization) will be identified before treatment, and another surgical specimen should not be required.

Identification of unsuspected microinvasive or early invasive cervical cancer by loop excision is a theoretical advantage over destructive procedures, but in patients with adequate colposcopy, there are no American data to support the actual advantage. Even evaluation of the cryotherapy literature reveals that during follow-up the incidence of adenocarcinoma (in situ or invasive) is the same for patients with dysplasia whether they were treated with cryotherapy or not.[70] Because adenocarcinoma in situ is often associated with CIN and often occurs deep within the cervical stroma, it is tempting to postulate that nondetection of this entity by destructive therapy would result in a higher incidence of subsequent cervical adenocarcinoma; this is not the case. It is estimated that only 1 in 1,000 (0.1%) patients with CIN will have an unsuspected early invasive cancer that might theoretically be detected were the transformation zone excised.[71] Clearly, many if not all of these microinvasive cancers are adequately treated by destructive methods, and a "high" endocervical lesion might be missed by any technique. Finally, some of the "occult cancers" were obvious, frankly invasive cancers; failure to detect them immediately is human error, not a sufficient reason to abandon established effective methods of therapy.

Advocating loop excision for all patients because it minimizes the potential mistakes made by marginal colposcopy seems to be at odds with another alleged advantage of loop excision, which is to "see and treat" at the same time. Clearly, loop excision allows expert colposcopists evaluating patients with known abnormal Papanicolaou smears to confirm the diagnosis and treat at the same time. Given the difficulties even accomplished clinicians may have in distinguishing metaplasia from HPV infection or mild dysplasia colposcopically, however, the proven approach of establishing dysplasia by colposcopically directed biopsy and then selecting proper treatment is the preferable option. Using loop excision without biopsy-proven disease increases the likelihood that loop conization will be increasingly performed by nonexpert colposcopists for either innocuous cervical lesions or normal/metaplastic squamous epithelium (which, based on the current literature, will be the only pathologic finding in 10% to 25% of excision specimens).[72] This "false negative" rate of 15% or more may be acceptable in England but probably will not be acceptable in the United States—particularly if long-term complications from loop excision prove similar to that of cold knife conization. A loop excision specimen is dramatically larger and, mathematically, should lessen the likelihood that a single punch biopsy by a relatively unskilled examiner will miss significant disease; unfortunately, the potential for unnecessary damage is also greater if loop excision is used to obtain a biopsy specimen.

Complications of secondary infertility (cervical stenosis) or recurrent pregnancy loss due to cervical incompetence resulting from a loop cervical conization are not defensible if the pathologic diagnosis is merely metaplastic squamous epithelium. Competent colposcopy thus is still a requirement for intelligent use of loop excision techniques.

The role, therefore, of loop excision procedures is still evolving. Loop excision is at least equivalent to laser or cold knife conization, has unique advantages, and has already replaced other excision techniques as the procedure of choice when a surgical sample is a necessity. Cold knife conization now has few absolute indications when loop excision is available. For the expert colposcopist who can identify dysplasia colposcopically, loop excision allows diagnosis and treatment at the same sitting. For the practicing clinician, competent colposcopy and biopsy are essential before the use of any method to treat cervical dysplasia. The cure rates for most modalities are essentially equivalent. Patients should be counseled about complication data and the need for long-term follow-up for loop excision procedures. The argument that destructive procedures must be abandoned because occult invasive cancers are routinely being undetected is not borne out by the American literature or by any long-term follow-up data on laser treatment or cryotherapy. The strength of the argument may reflect inadequacies on the part of some of the colposcopists or cytologists participating in the studies from England that do support this contention.[73] Cost analyses neglect to mention that cryotherapy is established and much less expensive than any other technique. Cost comparisons of loop excision with laser therapy fail to use lower cost estimates for newer laser equipment and fail to factor into loop excision costs the price of kits required for each excision procedure or the added cost of pathologic analysis of a cone specimen. Cost analysis data such as these have not yet been published, so the real cost advantage (if any) of loop excision has not been established.

SUMMARY

The diagnosis and effective treatment of CIN based on proper evaluation of a properly obtained Papanicolaou smear is one of the great success stories of contemporary gynecology. Dramatic declines in the incidence of invasive cervical cancer have resulted whenever effective screening of women at risk has been carried out. A new classification system (Bethesda) has been introduced, and a wide array of office-based destructive or excisional treatment modalities is available. Loop excision is the most recently developed of these methods. Much work needs to be done to improve access to Papanicolaou smear screening for both young and post-menopausal women and to improve access to therapy in both the United States and abroad.

REFERENCES

1. Papanicolaou GN, Traut HF: The diagnostic value of vaginal smears in carcinoma of the uterus. *Am J Obstet Gynecol* 1943; 142:193.
2. Trevathan E, Layde P, Webster LA, et al: Cigarette smoking and dysplasia and carcinoma in situ of the uterine cervix. *JAMA* 1983; 250:499–502.
3. Hatch KD: Implications of human papillomavirus in cervical and vulvar cancer. *Curr Opin Obstet Gynecol* 1990; 2:80–84.
4. Wilkinson EJ: Pap smears and screening for cervical neoplasia. *Clin Obstet Gynecol* 1990; 33:817–825.
5. Wain GV, Hacker NF: Pitfalls in the screening and early diagnosis of cervical cancer. *Curr Opin Obstet Gynecol* 1990; 2:74–79.
6. Anderson GH, Boyes DA, Benedet JL, et al: Organization and results of the cervical cytology screening program in British Columbia, 1955–1985. *BMJ* 1988; 296:957–958.
7. Mitchell H: *Med J Aust* 1987; 146:87–91.
8. Mandelblatt J, Schechter C, Fahs M, et al: Clinical implications for cervical cancer screening under Medicare. The natural history of cervical cancer in the elderly: What do we know? What do we need to know? *Am J Obstet Gynecol* 1991; 164:644–651.
9. The Walton Report: Cervical cancer screening programs. *Can Med Assoc J* 1976; 114:1003.
10. The Canadian Task Force on Cervical Cancer Screening Programs: Summary of the 1982 Canadian Task Force Report. *Can Med Assoc J* 1982; 127:581.
11. Nasca PC, Ellish N, Caputo TA, et al: An epidemiologic study of Pap smear screening histories in women with invasive carcinomas of the uterine cervix. *N Y State J Med* 1991; 91:152–156.

12. Shy K, Chu J, Mandelson M, et al: Papanicolaou smear screening interval and risk of cervical cancer. *Obstet Gynecol* 1989; 74:838–843.
13. The 1988 Bethesda System for reporting cervical/vaginal cytologic diagnoses: Developed and approved at a National Cancer Institute Workshop, Bethesda, Maryland, U.S.A. December 12–13. *J Reprod Med* 1989; 34:779–785.
14. Elias A, Linthorst G, Bekker B, et al: The significance of endocervical cells in the diagnosis of cervical epithelium changes. *Acta Cytol* 1983; 27:225.
15. Vooijs GP, Elias A, Graaf van der Y, et al: Relationship between the diagnosis of epithelial abnormalities and the composition of cervical smears. *Acta Cytol* 1985; 29:323–328.
16. Vooijs GP: Endocervical brush device. *Lancet* 1989; 1:784.
17. Laverty CR, Farnsworth A, Thurloe JK, et al: The importance of the cell sample in cervical cytology: A controlled trial of a new sampling device. *Med J Aust* 1989; 150:432–436.
18. Koonings PP, Dickinson K, d'Ablaing G, et al: A randomized clinical trial comparing the Cytobrush and cotton swab for Papanicolaou smears. *Obstet Gynecol* 1992; 80:241–245.
19. Hoffman MS, Finan M, Wallach P, et al: Use of the Cytobrush in postmenopausal women. *J Gynecol Surg* 1991; 7:23–25.
20. Hoffman MS, Gordy LW, Cavanagh D: The use of the Cytobrush sampler in patients with cervical stenosis. *Am J Obstet Gynecol* 1991; 164:52–53.
21. Rubio CA, Kock Y, Stormby N, et al: Studies on the distribution of abnormal cells in cytological smears. VII. Cervical brush versus plastic and wooden spatulas. *Gynecol Oncol* 1990; 39:167–170.
22. Boon ME, de Graaf Guilloud JC, Kok LP, et al: Efficacy of screening for cervical squamous and adenocarcinoma. The Dutch Experience. *Cancer* 1987; 59:862–866.
23. van Erp EJM, Dersjany-Roord MC, Arentz NPW, et al: Should the Cytobrush be used in routine screening for cervical pathology? *Int J Gynaecol Obstet* 1989; 30:139–144.
24. National Cancer Institute Workshop: The 1988 Bethesda System for reporting cervical/vaginal cytologic diagnoses. *JAMA* 1989; 262:931–934.
25. Herbst AL: The Bethesda System for cervical/vaginal cytologic diagnoses: A note of caution. *Obstet Gynecol* 1990; 76:449–450.
26. Bottles K, Reiter RC, Steiner AL, et al: Problems encountered with the Bethesda system: The University of Iowa experience. *Obstet Gynecol* 1991; 78:410–414.
27. Nasiell K, Nasiell M, Vaclavinkova V: Behavior of moderate cervical dysplasia during long-term follow-up. *Obstet Gynecol* 1983; 61:609–614.
28. Syrjanen KR: Current concepts of human papillomavirus infections in the genital tract and their relationship to intraepithelial neoplasia and squamous cell carcinoma. *Obstet Gynecol Surv* 1984; 39:252–265.
29. Montz FJ, Monk BJ, Fowler JM, et al: Natural history of the minimally abnormal Papanicolaou smear. *Obstet Gynecol* 1992; 80:385–388.
30. Pearlstone AJ, Grigsby PW, Mutch DG: High rates of atypical cervical cytology: Occurrence and clinical significance. *Obstet Gynecol* 1992; 80:191–195.
31. Kohan S, Noumoff J, Beckmann EM, et al: Colposcopic screening of women with atypical Papanicolaou smears. *J Reprod Med* 1985; 30:383–388.
32. Spitzer M, Krumholz BA, Chernys AE, et al: Comparative utility of repeat Papanicolaou smears, cervicography, and colposcopy in the evaluation of atypical Papanicolaou smears. *Obstet Gynecol* 1987; 69:731–735.
33. Rader JS, Rosenzweig BA, Spirta R, et al: Atypical squamous cells. A case-series study of the association between Papanicolaou smear results and human papillomavirus DNA genotype. *J Reprod Med* 1991; 36:292–297.
34. Cox JT, Schiffman MH, Winzelberg AJ, et al: An evaluation of human papil-

lomavirus testing as part of referral to colposcopy clinics. *Obstet Gynecol* 1992; 80:389–395.

35. Lungu O, Sun XW, Felix J, et al: Relationship of human papillomavirus type to grade of cervical intra-epithelial neoplasia. *JAMA* 1992; 267:2493–2496.

36. Syrjanen K, Kataja V, Yliskoski M, et al: Natural history of cervical human papillomavirus lesions does not substantiate the biologic relevance of the Bethesda system. *Obstet Gynecol* 1992; 76:675–682.

37. Stanbridge CM, Suleman BA, Persad RV, et al: A cervical smear review in women developing cervical carcinoma with particular reference to age, false negative cytology and the histologic type of the carcinoma. *Int J Gynecol Cancer* 1992; 2:91–100.

38. Buxton EJ, Luelsey DM, Wade-Evans T, et al: Residual disease after cone biopsy: Complications of excision and follow-up cytology as predictive factors. *Obstet Gynecol* 1987; 70:529–532.

39. Chanen W, Rome RM: Electrocoagulation diathermy for cervical dysplasia and carcinoma in situ: A 15-year survey. *Obstet Gynecol* 1983; 61:673.

40. Chanen W: The efficacy of electrocoagulation diathermy performed under local anesthesia for the eradication of precancerous lesions of the cervix. *Aust N Z J Obstet Gynaecol* 1989; 29:189.

41. Hollyock VE, Chanen W, Wein R: Cervical function following treatment of intraepithelial neoplasia by electrocoagulation diathermy. *Obstet Gynecol* 1983; 61:79–81.

42. Nan Schuurmans S, Ohlke ID, Carmichael JA: Treatment of cervical intraepithelial neoplasia with electrocautery: Report of 426 cases. *Am J Obstet Gynecol* 1984; 148:544–546.

43. Deigan EA, Carmichael JA, Ohlke ID, et al: Treatment of cervical intraepithelial neoplasia with electrocautery: A report of 776 cases. *Am J Obstet Gynecol* 1986; 154:255–259.

44. Duncan ID: The Semm cold coagulator in the management of cervical intraepithelial neoplasia. *Clin Obstet Gynecol* 1983; 26:996.

45. Kolstad P, Klem V: Long term follow-up of 1121 cases of carcinoma in situ. *Obstet Gynecol* 1979; 48:125.

46. Creasman WT: Symposium on cervical neoplasia II. Cryosurgery. *Colposc Gynecol Laser Surg* 1985; 1:275–279.

47. Hatch KD, Shingleton HM, Austin JM, et al: Cryosurgery of cervical intraepithelial neoplasia. *Obstet Gynecol* 1981; 57:692–698.

48. Benedet JL, Miller DM, Nickerson KG, et al: The results of cryosurgical treatment of cervical intraepithelial neoplasia at one, five, and ten years. *Am J Obstet Gynecol* 1987; 157:268–273.

49. Richart RM, Townsend DE, Crisp W, et al: An analysis of "long-term" follow-up results in patients with cervical intraepithelial neoplasia treated by cryotherapy. *Am J Obstet Gynecol* 1980; 137:823–826.

50. Stuart GCE, Anderson RJ, Corlett BMA, et al: Assessment of failures of cryosurgical treatment in cervical intraepithelial neoplasia. *Am J Obstet Gynecol* 1982; 142:658–663.

51. Kooning PP, D'Ablaing G, Schlaerth JB, et al: A clinical-pathology review of cervical intraepithelial neoplasia following cryotherapy failure. *Gynecol Oncol* 1992; 44:213–216.

52. Nunez C, Shapiro SP: Invasive carcinoma of the cervix after cryosurgery. Report of three cases. *J Reprod Med* 1981; 26:29–34.

53. Baggish MS: A ten-year experience treating cervical intraepithelial neoplasia with the CO_2 laser. *Am J Obstet Gynecol* 1989; 161:60.

54. Burke L: Is laser surgery superior to cryosurgery for the treatment of high grade CIN? *J Gynecol Surg* 1991; 7:53–55.

55. Butterworth CE, Hatch KD, Soong S-J, et al: Oral folic acid supplementation

for cervical dysplasia. A clinical intervention trial. *Am J Obstet Gynecol* 1992; 166:803–809.

56. van Nagell JR, Hanson MB, Donaldson ES, et al: Treatment of cervical intraepithelial neoplasia III by hysterectomy without intervening conization in patients with adequate colposcopy. *Cancer* 1985; 56:2737–2739.

57. Chanen W: Radical electrocoagulation diathermy, in Coppleson M (ed): *Gynecologic Oncology: Fundamental Principles and Clinical Practice*, vol 2. Edinburgh, Churchill Livingstone, 1981, pp 821–825.

58. Benedet JL, Miller DM, Nickerson KG: Results of conservative management of cervical intraepithelial neoplasia. *Obstet Gynecol* 1992; 79:105–110.

59. Cartier R: *Practical Colposcopy*, ed 2. Paris, Laboratorie Cartier, 1984, pp 139–156.

60. Prendiville W, Cullimore S: Large loop excision of the transformation zone (LLETZ). A new method of management for women with cervical intraepithelial neoplasia. *Br J Obstet Gynaecol* 1989; 96:1054–1060.

61. Jones HW III: Treatment of cervical intraepithelial neoplasia. *Clin Obstet Gynecol* 1990; 33:826–836.

62. Wright TC, Gagnon S, Ferenczy A, et al: Excising CIN lesions by loop electrosurgical procedure. *Contrib Obstet Gynecol* 1991; 3:57–73.

63. Mor-Yosef S, Lopes L, Pearson S, et al: Loop diathermy cone biopsy. *Obstet Gynecol* 1990; 75:884–886.

64. Turner MJ, Rasmussen MJ, Flannelly GM, et al: Outpatient loop diathermy conization as an alternative to inpatient knife conization of the cervix. *J Reprod Med* 1992; 37:314–316.

65. Bigrigg MA, Codling BW, Pearson P, et al: Colposcopic diagnosis and treatment of cervical dysplasia at a single clinic visit: Experience of low voltage diathermy loop in 1000 patients. *Lancet* 1990; 336:229–231.

66. Murdoch JB, Grimshaw RN, Monaghan JM: Loop diathermy excision of the abnormal cervical transformation zone. *Int J Gynecol Cancer* 1991; 1:105–111.

67. Oyesanya OA, Amerisangie CN, Manning EAD: Outpatient excisional management of cervical intraepithelial neoplasia. A prospective, randomized comparison between loop diathermy excision and laser excisional conization. *Am J Obstet Gynecol* 1993; 168:485–488.

68. Wright TC, Richart RM, Ferenczy A, et al: Comparison of specimens removed by CO_2 laser conization and the loop electrosurgical excision procedure. *Obstet Gynecol* 1992; 79:147–153.

69. Schinck J: The loop electrosurgical procedure for evaluation and treatment of cervical dysplasia. *Clin Consult Obstet Gynecol* 1992; 4:126–130.

70. Schmidt C, Pretorius RG, Bonin M, et al. Invasive cervical cancer following cryotherapy for cervical intraepithelial neoplasia or human papilloma-virus infection. *Obstet Gynecol* 1992; 80:797–800.

71. Luesley D: Advances in colposcopy and management of cervical intraepithelial neoplasia. *Curr Opin Obstet Gynecol* 1992; 4:102–108.

72. Murdoch JB, Grimshaw RN, Morgan PR, et al: The impact of loop diathermy on management of early invasive cervical cancer. *Int J Gynecol Cancer* 1992; 2:129–133.

73. Chappatte OA, Byrne DL, Raju KS, et al: Histological differences between colposcopic-directed biopsy and loop excision of the transformation zone (LETZ): A cause for concern. *Gynecol Oncol* 1991; 43:46–50.

Editor's Comment

Dr. Patsner provides us with an excellent summary of the epidemiology, diagnosis, and treatment of cervical intraepithelial neoplasia. Past decades have seen a multitude of changes in this area that often have resulted only in confusion for the practitioner. I concur with Dr. Patsner that the Bethesda system, yet another classification to report cervical cytology, has made it more difficult to manage low-grade lesions when using previous recommendations for cervical intraepithelial neoplasia. This system, despite the several pitfalls outlined by Dr. Patsner, is unfortunately being widely adopted, and the clinician must learn how to interpret the results and recommend appropriate evaluation and treatment intervention.

The majority of this chapter reviews the three most widely accepted methods for treating cervical intraepithelial neoplasia: cryotherapy, laser ablation, and electrocoagulation loop excision. Dr. Patsner provides a step-by-step description of each modality and cites the literature pertaining to each. One of Dr. Patsner's concerns is that electrocoagulation loop excision (LLETZ and LEEP) will be used in situations where ablative therapy is not required. The advantage of LLETZ and LEEP excisions is the addition of a pathologic evaluation equivalent to that produced by cervical conization. I believe that as our experience and comfort level with LLETZ and LEEP grow, cold knife conization will become an outmoded procedure. The ability to obtain a comparable pathologic specimen by loop excision in the practitioner's office will result in significantly reduced cost.

Ira R. Horowitz, M.D.

The Role of Laparoscopy in the Gynecologic Oncology Patient

MARK D. ADELSON, M.D.

Discussion of the role of laparoscopy in gynecologic oncology is germane to all gynecologists and surgeons who use or wish to use this modality. Indications and diseases may vary, but technique and an effort to reduce complications are basic considerations to all operative laparoscopists, who must be fluent in the language of safety before any evaluation of indications can be undertaken.

The primary goal of this chapter, then, is to impress upon the reader the basics, safety, and safeguards of laparoscopy. Advantages, disadvantages, and the uniqueness of laparoscopy will lead this discussion; indications, procedures, and techniques will follow. We will highlight complex laparoscopic procedures that are now applicable to modern state-of-the-art practice and will mention procedures requiring further development. Some of these require prior training and skill in performing their laparotomy counterparts and so will not be a part of the armamentarium of the general obstetrician-gynecologist. The basic safety and technical considerations, however, are of importance to all advanced laparoscopists, whether they be general or subspecialty-trained gynecologists or general surgeons.

Operative video laparoscopy is the descriptive term we have chosen to best encompass this new-wave laparoscopy. Laparoscopy is not new and has been termed abdominoscopy, splanchnoscopy, (operative) pelviscopy, (video) laseroscopy, celioscopy, and peritoneoscopy. Diagnostic laparoscopy dates back to a 1910 report by the Swedish physician Jacobaeus.[1] Poor light delivery, suboptimal optical systems, and the difficulty of operating while bent over a direct-view scope delayed advancements.

The first video endoscopy was performed in 1956, but poor resolution and lack of color limited its use.[2] The Hopkins glass fiber rod lens system introduced in the 1950s provided the needed optical clarity of the laparoscope. This was accomplished by replacing the air spaces within the scope with optical glass.[3] The first CO_2 insufflator was introduced by Semm, and its use was documented in 1966.[4] An automatic insufflator was introduced the following year. The high-intensity light source was introduced in 1969. These advances spurred the development and widespread use of direct-view laparoscopy for diagnostic and simple operative procedures. As long ago as 1973 the first laparoscopic salpingo-oophorectomy was performed by Semm in Germany,[5] and the first salpingectomy for ectopic pregnancy was performed by Shapiro and Adler in the United States.[6]

Color video laparoscopy was first performed in 1974 with bulky equipment and insufficient camera resolution. Circon ACMI (Stamford, Conn) manufactured the first high-resolution color tube in 1984. The development of whiter light sources (e.g., xenon, metal halide), more reliable (high-flow) CO_2 insufflators, and the microprocessor chip (charge coupled device [CCD]) high-resolution camera (1988) ushered in the modern era of video laparoscopy. In that same year, the first laparoscopic lymphadenectomy was performed in France by Querleu et al.[7] The first laparoscopic hysterectomy was reported the following year by Reich et al.[8] The first laparoscopic-assisted radical hysterectomy was reported in 1992 by Nezhat et al.[9]

Key to the safe employment of operative video laparoscopy is an understanding that this is a new technique. The pitfall of assuming that this is merely an updating of older direct-view diagnostic and simple operative techniques learned in residency training must be avoided. If this false assumption gives us the temerity to perform complex procedures without the advanced training that is needed, patient safety will be compromised.

The advantages of operative video laparoscopy are many. Because of the recent introduction of this modality, however, some of these advantages have not yet been documented in the literature. Randomized studies comparing the same operation performed by laparotomy and laparoscopy are scant. Many of these studies should not be performed for ethical reasons because the advantages of laparoscopy are clear. Additionally, since video recording of the procedures is simple, objective documentation of the completeness of the procedures can be presented.

A reduction in overall patient morbidity is observed, even with advanced procedures, when a procedure is done by laparoscopy (as opposed to laparotomy, Table 1). This, of course, assumes sufficient training, experience, and development of skill on the part of the surgeon. Decreased postoperative pain and the reduction or elimination of postoperative narcotics are clear advantages. Resumption of bowel function is rapid. Generally patients are able to eat by postoperative day 1. Hospital discharge

TABLE 1.

Laparoscopic Procedures

Diagnostic
Simple operative
  Tubal ligation, cyst aspiration
Intermediate operative
  Salpingotomy, adhesiolysis
Advanced operative
  Ovarian cystectomy, myomectomy, salpingo-oophorectomy,
    hysterectomy, lymphadenectomy

is rapid, generally by postoperative day 1. Most patients can return to normal activities in 1 to 2 weeks with full recovery of energy level. Cosmesis is greatly improved because the operation can be performed via a 10- to 11-mm infraumbilical incision, with up to three secondary incisions (3 to 12 mm apiece).

Some literature documentation does exist. Levine[10] compared hospital cost and postoperative stay for patients undergoing lysis of adhesions, adnexectomy, or myomectomy. He found that these procedures performed laparoscopically resulted in a savings of $1,600 and 4 hospital days when compared with laparotomy. Zouves et al.[11] and Brumsted and associates[12] demonstrated a statistically significant reduction in postoperative narcotic use, length of surgery, hospital stay, and days to return to work for ectopic pregnancies treated by laparoscopy vs. laparotomy.

Vermesh et al.[13] performed a prospective randomized evaluation of linear salpingostomy for ectopic pregnancy and compared laparoscopy and laparotomy. The laparoscopy group had a statistically significant reduction in estimated blood loss, length of hospital stay, and hospital costs. Postoperative tubal patency and intrauterine and ectopic pregnancy rates did not differ. Baumann et al.,[14] in a nonrandomized prospective cohort study of ectopic pregnancy, demonstrated a statistically significant reduction in hospital stay, weeks until return to domestic and work activities, hospital costs, drug costs, and disability payments. Nezhat and colleagues,[15] in a comparison of ten cases of hysterectomy performed by laparoscopy and ten by laparotomy, showed a reduction in estimated blood loss, hospital stay, and weeks to recovery of normal function.

The disadvantages of laparoscopy result from the difference between operative laparoscopy and laparotomy. Whereas laparotomy is largely guided by tactile sensation, the sense of touch is limited in laparoscopy. Laparoscopy is guided by video viewing, which requires a spatial reorientation. Not only are we not touching the tissue with fingers, we are not even looking directly at the operative site. Additionally, current video systems provide monocular two-dimensional viewing. Even though the operative field is magnified on the high-resolution color monitor, we lose some resolution and must learn the new (and often foreign) techniques of video and remote operation with instruments tethered at the skin like a fulcrum. These differences translate into requirements of greater operator skill, specialized equipment, and increased operative time (for most advanced procedures).

Knowledge of prior surgical procedures and past abdominopelvic inflammatory conditions is essential to avoid injury. Accordingly, the preoperative evaluation must include retrieval of all operative notes of past surgeries. One must also know whether abdominopelvic masses or pregnancy exists. Use of sonography or computed tomography (in the absence of pregnancy) should be liberal, more so than for laparotomy. When a history of major abdominal infection (e.g., peritonitis, ruptured appendicitis, septic cholecystitis), major adhesion-generating surgery (tumor reduction, bowel resection), or radiation exists, one must strongly consider abandoning the closed technique for the open technique. Often the most dense site for abdominal wall adhesion formation is the periumbilical region, so a trocar site may be selected in the upper portion of the abdomen.

Thorough and documented informed consent is also an important preoperative task. Certain risks such as brachial plexopathy may occur with laparoscopy much more commonly than with laparotomy. Numbness, paresthesia, or motor weakness of the hands and arms are usually temporary but are frightening to the patient. All patients undergoing laparoscopy should understand the potential need for and give consent to laparotomy. Indications for laparotomy could be a surgical emergency (e.g., bleeding, perforation of a viscus), anesthetic indication (prohibitively high $Paco_2$ of 60 mm Hg or greater or peak airway pressure of 60 cm H_2O or greater, hypoxia, serious arrhythmia), disease indication (metastatic ovarian cancer or significant adhesive disease), or other technical inability to complete the procedure laparoscopically. The need for laparotomy should be rare, especially in the hands of an experienced operative laparoscopist.

PREOPERATIVE PREPARATION

Preoperative patient preparation is important for laparoscopy, perhaps more so than for laparotomy. Patients must be instructed to avoid medications that may interfere with hemostasis. Aspirin and nonsteroidal anti-inflammatory agents should be avoided for 2 weeks before surgery. Poor hemostasis at surgery reduces visibility by staining tissues and obscuring the field. Even an efficient irrigation-aspiration system (we prefer the Bard Gyne-Flo Irrigator/Aspirator and Pump, C. R. Bard, Inc., Tewksbury, Mass) does not overcome these disadvantages. Patients should be given cathartics (e.g., magnesium citrate) along with clear liquids the night before surgery (and often enemas the morning of surgery) to empty the intestines. Laparoscopic surgery in the confined space of the peritoneal cavity becomes more difficult when distended bowel obscures the field. Patients who have a pelvic mass, suspected ovarian cancer, or suspected severe adhesive disease should be given a formal bowel preparation before surgery. This will reduce the infectious morbidity should intentional or unintended enterotomy or colotomy occur. We prefer to use a polyethylene glycol–based solution (e.g., GoLYTELY, Braintree Laboratories, Inc., Braintree, Mass) for the mechanical preparation since it does not result in water or electrolyte imbalance. We use erythromycin and neomycin for the oral antibiotic preparation. Intravenous prophylactic antibiotics are used for both uncomplicated cases (cefazolin sodium, 1 g, as Kefzol, Eli Lilly and Company, Indianapolis) and for cases in which a bowel preparation is prescribed (cefotetan, 2 g, as Cefotan, Stuart Pharmaceuticals, Wilmington, Del).

POSITIONING

Positioning requirements of operative video laparoscopy result in different or exaggerated physiologic changes when compared with laparotomy. Consideration of these changes permits us to identify relative medical contraindications to laparoscopy. Severe cardiovascular disease is probably the strongest contraindication. The combination of steep Trendelenburg position (20 to 30 degrees), and abdominal distension by CO_2 reduces venous return to the heart and impairs pulmonary mechanics. Patients with ischemic heart disease, mitral valve insufficiency, or congenital/acquired conditions with pulmonary hypertension and decreased or fixed cardiac output may be better candidates for laparotomy. A large diaphragmatic hernia may impair pulmonary function. The lengthy operating time and the frequent need for the lithotomy position may make patients with severe hip immobility (e.g., from arthritis or prosthesis) less-than-optimal laparoscopy candidates.

This discussion of safety will first review the steps to begin and perform laparoscopic surgery. Initially the surgeon should personally check that all equipment is present and working. This includes the video monitor (placed at the foot of the table if one is used or at the sides of the table if two are used), videocassette recorder (VCR), light source, insufflator, monopolar and bipolar cautery units, and laser (if used). Some equipment, such as the camera, bipolar forceps, trocars, and insufflating needle, cannot easily be tested until the patient is under anesthesia and the sterile field has been draped. This responsibility can be delegated to the nursing staff only after sufficient training and familiarity with the equipment has been ensured.

Comfortable positioning that cushions pressure points is very important. The patient is initially supine, centered in the width of the table. The arms should be carefully padded and tucked at the sides, palms up. If necessary, the arms may rest on arm boards placed parallel to and against the table at the patient's sides or supported by metal sleds placed into the sides of the table. We try to avoid using additional supports since they force the surgeon to stand away from the table and cause greater fatigue from arm and back strain. Pressure at the patient's elbow, especially from the edge of the table, must be avoided to prevent ulnar nerve damage. Shoulder braces are usually necessary to keep the patient from sliding cephalad from the steep Trendelenburg position. These must be positioned over the acromial process. Avoiding more medial placement or more lateral placement over the head of the humerus will reduce the risk of brachial plexus injury. Keeping the arms tucked at the sides is essential when shoulder braces are used, or the risk of brachial plexopathy from pressure or stretching may be increased.[16] For the same reason, the head should be kept in the midline and not flexed or turned to the side.

Equal emphasis should be placed on positioning of the legs. We prefer to use the Allen Universal Stirrup (Allen Medical Systems, Cleveland, Ohio), which cradles the foot. The patient's legs will be supported by the balls of her feet (which will be further dorsiflexed by placing pads under the balls and toes of the feet), thereby avoiding nerve injury or venous stasis by avoiding pressure on calves or thighs. The angle between the foot and the lower part of the leg should be comfortable to avoid a visible twisting strain of the infrapatellar tendon. The knees must be kept low, at or below the level of the abdomen, to avoid restricted mobility of the lower quadrant instruments by the thighs.

ANESTHESIA

For most cases, the anesthesia technique should be general endotracheal. Ventilation should be controlled because the patient must remain motionless throughout the procedure. Use of short-acting anesthetic agents will hasten recovery from anesthesia and shorten the time until the patient has gastrointestinal function and can be discharged. Our initial experience in using short-acting intravenous agents (propofol and alfentanil hydrochloride) combined with nitrous gas to avoid general inhalation agents (e.g., isoflurane) provides reason for optimism.[17] We are finding that avoiding inhalation anesthesia allows the patient to wake up promptly, oriented and comfortable, and able to move herself from the operating room table to the stretcher. These patients seem to have less minor morbidity (nausea, dizziness, malaise). A useful adjunct to general anesthesia is the posterior rectus sheath block. A long-acting local anesthetic (0.25% bupivacaine, 8 to 10 mL) is injected 5 cm cephalad and 5 cm lateral to the umbilicus just above the posterior rectus sheath, bilaterally. Needle depth is controlled by direct laparoscopic visualization. Proper placement is determined by observing a bleb just above the parietal peritoneum of the abdominal wall since the peritoneum and posterior sheath are adherent at this point. Local anesthetic markedly reduces or eliminates pain from the abdominal incisions.[18] Finally, because the insensible loss is minimal, intraoperative fluid replacement should be limited to 1 to 2 L plus blood loss replacement.

After induction of anesthesia and careful positioning and draping, it is important to intubate and empty both the stomach and the bladder. This avoids accidental penetration of the insufflating needle and trocars into these viscera or into viscera pushed into the field by these distended organs. We insert an orogastric tube, which will remain in place during the procedure, and a 14 F Foley catheter in sterile fashion after draping, which is removed before the patient leaves the recovery room.

PROCEDURE

Next, the rest of the equipment including the spring function and patency of the Veress needle is checked. The table is lowered as close to the floor as possible to gain maximal leverage at trocar insertion. The abdominal wall is elevated by grasping skin and subcutaneous tissue. Piercing towel clamps or other mechanical means of abdominal wall elevation are unnecessary and only add to the morbidity and patient discomfort. Ordinarily when the closed laparoscopy technique is used, old incisions are avoided so as not to penetrate visci or omentum. If a prior infraumbilical midline incision extends to the inferior verge of the umbilicus, the lateral or superior fold should be used for trocar placement.

CLOSED LAPAROSCOPY

To proceed with closed laparoscopy, the infraumbilical fold would usually be used. Using the correct angle to aim the insufflating needle is crucial. The needle should be aimed into the hollow of the sacrum toward the uterus to avoid aorta injury. The needle would then form a 45-degree angle to the horizontal (or 90 degrees to the elevated skin). The needle should be kept in the midline to avoid damaging the pelvic wall vessels or colon. For maximal control, the surgeon's arm should be kept at his side so that only small forearm muscles are used for placement. A twisting motion may provide better forward control.

Once the Veress needle is in place, one should set the insufflator at the lowest setting. Should visceral or vascular penetration have occurred, this will minimize the risk of CO_2 embolism. The intra-abdominal pressure reading should begin at less than 15 mm Hg and should optimally be less than 10 mm Hg. The maximal inflation pressure limit on the insufflator should be 15 mm Hg. If the initial pressure is high, the tip of the needle is most likely residing in the omentum or in the supraperitoneal space, and repositioning is required. Direct inspection with the scope should be performed after placement of the infraumbilical trocar and before insufflation.

Secondary trocar placement is done under direct visualization. These are usually placed in the right and left lower quadrants lateral to the inferior epigastric vessels and just below the level of the anterior superior iliac spines. Placement too low will restrict mobility of the instruments, whereas placement too high results in the secondary instruments hitting the scope intraperitoneally. Locating the epigastric vessels is best done by intraperitoneal inspection. They form a "V" above the symphysis with the lateral umbilical ligament and terminate at the internal inguinal ring medial to the round ligament. Transillumination of the abdominal wall is the least useful locating technique.

Maximal safety includes knowledge of the equipment and principles of electrosurgery and laser physics. When either laser or cautery is used, we always view the entire working end of the instrument (i.e., laser probe or fiber tip or cautery scissors) and view a wide enough field to avoid inadvertent bowel injury. When unipolar cautery is used, modern single-material conductive trocar sleeves should be used to avoid capacitance. Capacitance is electrical charge buildup from the electromagnetic field of the cautery instrument. Normally, charge buildup in the trocar can harmlessly ground through the surrounding skin. When the trocar is insulated from the skin, however, as when a nonconductive plastic collar is placed to reduce inadvertent dislodging of the trocar, charge stored in the trocar can discharge when the bowel is in close proximity and cause a burn (Fig 1). Additionally, the lowest unipolar current setting that is effective should be used to avoid arcing and unintended burns. Defects in instrument insulation may permit unintended current leaks and burns (Fig 2). A regular testing program to assess the integrity of reusable cautery instrument insulation is wise. The Electroshield (Electroscope, Inc., Boulder, Colo) is an electrically conductive metal tube surrounded by insulation through which up to 5-mm instruments may be inserted (Fig 3). The Electroshield is connected through the Electroshield Monitor to the return electrode (Fig 4) to harmlessly conduct stray current away from the surgical site. When current leak from defective insulation or capacitance is detected, the inhibit adaptor attached to the electrosurgical unit disables it and produces both audible and visual indications (Fig 5). The dis-

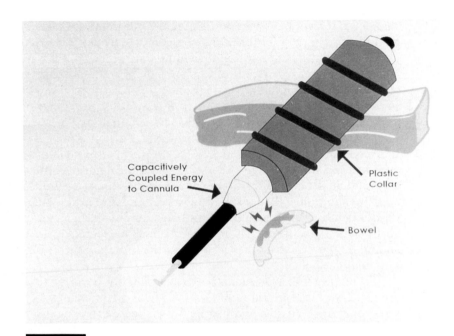

FIGURE 1.
Capacitive coupled fault condition. (Courtesy of Electroscope, Inc., Boulder, Colo.)

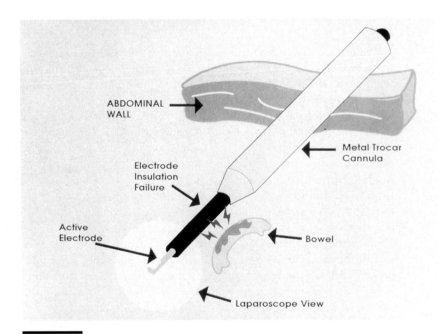

FIGURE 2.
Insulation failure. (Courtesy of Electroscope, Inc., Boulder, Colo.)

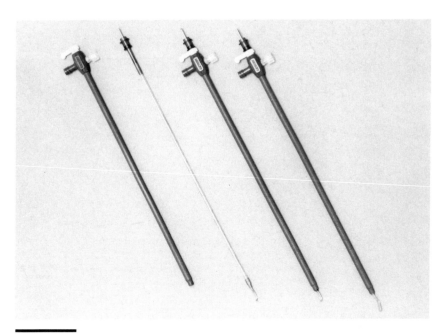

FIGURE 3.
From left to right: electroshield sheath, optional cautery probe insert, hook insert in its sheath, and spatula insert in its sheath. (Courtesy of Electroscope, Inc., Boulder, Colo.)

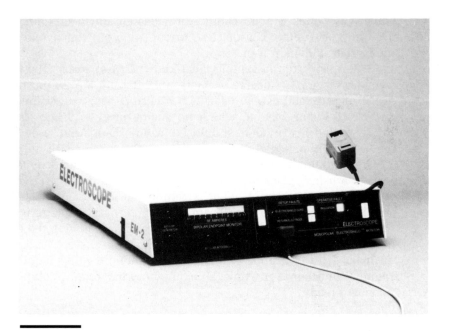

FIGURE 4.
Electroshield monitor. (Courtesy of Electroscope, Inc., Boulder, Colo.)

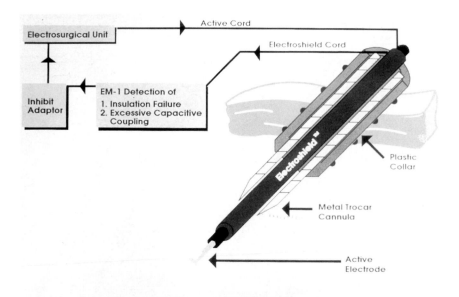

FIGURE 5.

Electroshield EM-1 monitor system. (Courtesy of Electroscope, Inc., Boulder, Colo.)

advantage to using the Electroshield is that the smallest trocar that can be used is 7 mm. Bipolar cautery provides an added measure of safety over unipolar cautery because the current cannot travel beyond the tip of the forceps, although heat can.

When using the laser, one must know its properties. The CO_2 laser provides the greatest degree of safety since irrigation fluid (normal saline or Ringer's lactate) can be used as a backstop. The extinction length in water is 0.1 mm, beyond which no energy passes. Plastic trocars and plastic-coated instruments should be avoided since the laser will melt them. Brightly polished metal trocars and instruments will reflect the laser light and produce unintended burns. Metal equipment should be burnished, brushed, blackened, or anodized to scatter or absorb the laser energy. Always be aware of what is behind the tissue being lased, which will be affected by the laser beam after target tissue penetration. A safe backstop may include irrigation fluid, the abdominal wall, the uterus, an appropriately prepared metal rod, or a glass rod. Laser waveguides are available with backstops built in. Since a complication requiring laparotomy can occur at any time, an exploratory laparotomy setup is always open and ready.

HYSTERECTOMY

Laparoscopy can be used to replace laparotomy for hysterectomy. It does not replace vaginal hysterectomy, when that is indicated, because the laparoscopic operative time is significantly longer. When the vaginal approach is contraindicated by pelvic pain, prior pelvic inflammatory disease, endometriosis, suspected cancer, adnexal pathology, a large uterus, suspected adhesions, prior major surgery, or suboptimal vaginal anatomy, the laparoscopic approach may be considered. Whether patients recover from laparoscopic hysterectomy faster and with less morbidity as compared with vaginal hysterectomy remains to be proved, although we feel that they do. A case-controlled study to evaluate this question is under way.

LAPAROSCOPY WITH HYSTERECTOMY

The combined use of laparoscopy with hysterectomy can be described by three categories. The first is "laparoscopy plus hysterectomy," which means that the patient anatomy is such that vaginal hysterectomy is technically feasible but direct visualization of the peritoneal cavity by laparoscopy is necessary to investigate and possibly treat pain or endometriosis. Other patients may have a small pelvic mass, which also could be investigated and possibly treated by laparoscopy. Once this investigation is done and it is clear that the patient could have a vaginal approach rather than an abdominal approach for hysterectomy, the vaginal approach can be performed. The benefits are shorter hospital stay and less pain than after abdominal hysterectomy and shorter operating time than is required by the other procedures.[19]

LAPAROSCOPIC-ASSISTED VAGINAL HYSTERECTOMY

The second category is "laparoscopic-assisted vaginal hysterectomy," which is generally a vaginal hysterectomy performed with the assistance of laparoscopy. This is more similar to a vaginal hysterectomy than to an abdominal hysterectomy. The majority of the hysterectomy surgery is done through the vagina by the vaginal hysterectomy technique, and the minority of the surgery is done by laparoscopy. Laparoscopy can be used to free up the ovaries and tubes, which may not be able to be reached by the vaginal approach, or to release scar tissue to make vaginal surgery safer. Laparoscopic surgical techniques may be used to control (ligate or cauterize) and transect round and infundibulopelvic ligaments. The upper cardinal ligament might be stapled and transected (Endo GIA, U.S. Surgical Corp., Norwalk, Conn) or transected after bipolar cauterization. The vaginal surgery would include control and transection of the vaginal cuff, uterosacral and cardinal ligaments, and uterine arteries. The vaginal cuff would be closed vaginally.

LAPAROSCOPIC ABDOMINAL HYSTERECTOMY

The third category is "laparoscopic hysterectomy," or "laparoscopic abdominal hysterectomy." Even though the laparoscopic approach is used, the technique is the same as the abdominal hysterectomy technique in that the direction of surgery proceeds from the superior pedicle to the vagina. All of the surgery is performed abdominally, except occasionally for cutting the vaginal mucosa. The specimen is pulled out through the vagina. It is then possible to sew the vaginal cuff together vaginally, but with the laparoscopic technique this is usually done abdominally. This is the technique we prefer. Laparoscopic hysterectomy (or laparoscopic abdominal hysterectomy) should be viewed as abdominal hysterectomy plus the reduction of morbidity by the use of laparoscopy as a secondary (modifying) procedure.

Before 1989 no case of laparoscopy and hysterectomy was reported, and the bulk of the cases were reported in 1992 (Table 2). Laparoscopic-assisted vaginal hysterectomy is being performed more commonly than laparoscopic hysterectomy. Less laparoscopic skill and operative time are required when much or most of the procedure is performed vaginally.

The choice of technique for laparoscopic hysterectomy depends on surgeon preference. Since in our hands use of the Endo GIA stapler for control of uterine vessels and the cardinal ligament did not reduce operative time, we prefer to use bipolar cautery and sharp or unipolar cautery transection. The disadvantage of the stapling technique is that it requires a larger trocar (12 mm) and is costly. Use of four cartridges for an average case (two for the infundibulopelvic ligament and two for the cardinal) increases the hospital's equipment cost by $1,000 to $1,500. For hysterectomy (with or without adnexectomy) without lymphadenectomy or removal of a large adnexal mass, we prefer to use an 11-mm infraumbilical trocar (the size will depend on the diameter of the laparoscope) and one 5-mm Hunt-Reich (Apple Medical Corp., Bolton, Mass) secondary cannula in either lower quadrant. The shafts of these self-retaining trocars are wrapped by fascia anchoring threads, so they are retained well in the abdominal wall. They are short, however, and may not be suitable for use in large patients. Uterine manipulation is performed with a Kronner Manipujector (Unimar, Wilton, Conn; Fig 6). For removal of a large mass or lymphadenectomy, a fourth (10-mm) trocar is placed in the suprapubic site. This will allow removal of larger portions of tissue and will permit use of the Endo Clip (U.S. Surgical Corp., Norwalk, Conn). Virtually all patients are discharged on postoperative day 1, and none are given intramuscular or intravenous narcotics.

TABLE 2.

Operative Laparoscopy—Hysterectomy*

Procedure[†]	Patients (n)	Age (yr)	Operative Time (min)	EBL[†] (mL)	Discharge Day	Cost ($)
L + VH[19, 20]	44	42	56	?[†]	4	2,681
L + AH[19]	4	37	93	?	5	3,133
LAVH[21–25]	61	55	160	184	3	?
LH[8, 22, 23, 26–32]	167	40	124	185	2	3,772

*Data were not available for all patients, so the results in each column may not be comparable between groups.

†L + VH = laparoscopy plus vaginal hysterectomy; L + AH = laparoscopy plus abdominal hysterectomy; LAVH = laparoscopic-assisted vaginal hysterectomy; LH = laparoscopic hysterectomy; EBL = estimated blood loss; ? = not available.

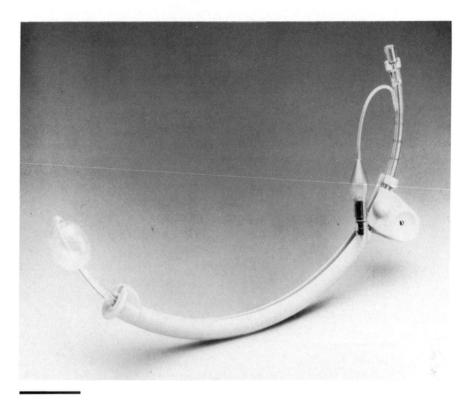

FIGURE 6.

Kronner Manipujector with a 10-mL balloon *(left)* that holds the manipulator inside the uterus. (Courtesy of Unimar, Wilmar, Conn.)

Laparoscopic hysterectomy begins with exploration of the abdominopelvic cavity (Fig 7). Pelvic cytology is performed if indicated (e.g., with endometrial cancer or a mass). The patient is placed in the 20- to 30-degree Trendelenburg position in order to keep the bowel out of the pelvis. The posterior parietal peritoneum is divided sharply, with scissors, lateral to the infundibulopelvic ligament. Dissection and identification of pelvic wall structures is carried out. After identifying the ureter, the infundibulopelvic ligament is sharply skeletonized, occluded with bipolar paddle forceps, and transected sharply. The round ligament is treated similarly (Figs 8 and 9). The course of the ureter, especially the point crossed by the uterine artery, must be carefully identified and skeletonized if needed to avoid injury by cautery or stapling. The bladder flap peritoneum is sharply incised and the bladder sharply dissected from the anterior of the cervix (Fig 10). The uterine vessels are skeletonized at the sides of the uterus. The location of the vaginal packing, previously placed at the apex, is noted visually or by palpation with a probe. Bipolar cautery is used to occlude the uterine vessels and to control the cardinal ligament 2 cm above the ureter (Fig 11). The uterosacral ligaments are cauterized and transected high on the posterior of the cervix. The cardinal ligament is taken down and the vagina circumscribed with unipolar cautery scissors (Fig 12). Should loss of pneumoperitoneum place the bowel in close proximity to the vaginal cuff, cautery should not be used for this step. To avoid unintended cautery injury, only sharp dissection should

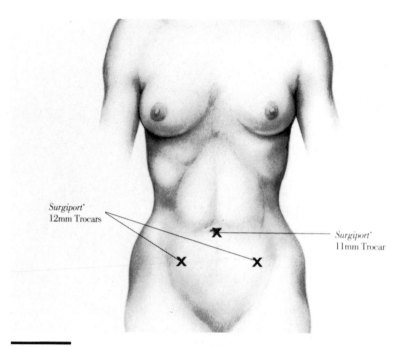

FIGURE 7.

Suggested trocar placement for hysterectomy; 12-mm lateral trocars are required for use of the Endo GIA stapler. (Courtesy of U.S. Surgical Corp., Norwalk, Conn.)

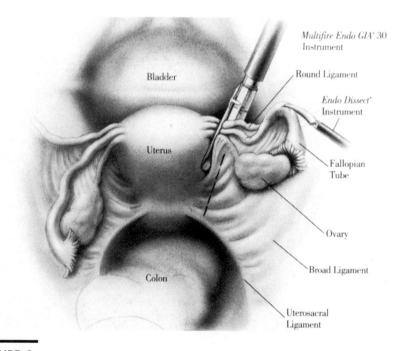

FIGURE 8.

Endo GIA stapler used for ligation of the ovarian ligament and round ligaments when salpingo-oophorectomy is not performed. (Courtesy of U.S. Surgical Corp., Norwalk, Conn.)

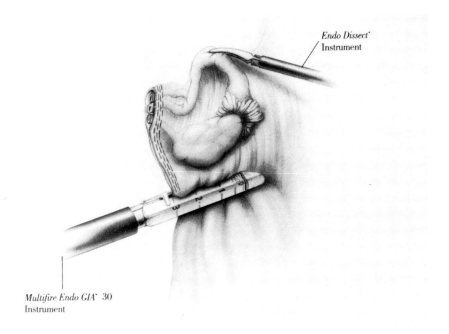

Endo Dissect
Instrument

Multifire Endo GIA 30
Instrument

FIGURE 9.

Endo GIA stapler used for ligation of the infundibulopelvic ligament and broad ligament below the ovary when salpingo-oophorectomy is performed. (Courtesy of U.S. Surgical Corp., Norwalk, Conn.)

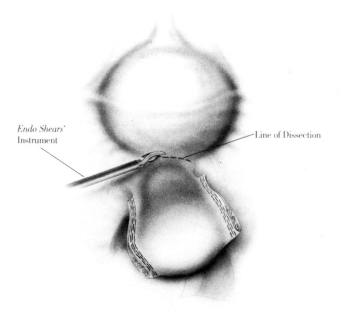

Endo Shears
Instrument

Line of Dissection

FIGURE 10.

Dissection of bladder flap peritoneum (the superior pedicles have been ligated and transected with the Endo GIA stapler). (Courtesy of U.S. Surgical Corp., Norwalk, Conn.)

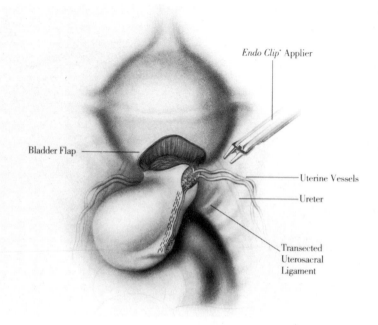

FIGURE 11.
Alternative technique to ligate uterine vessels with the Endo Clip applier. (Courtesy of U.S. Surgical Corp., Norwalk, Conn.)

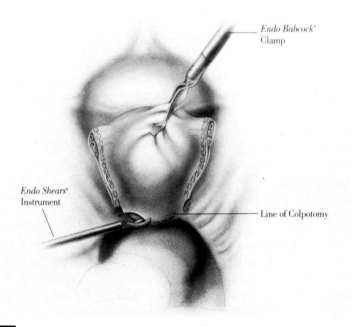

FIGURE 12.
Colpotomy performed with the unipolar electrocautery scissors. (Courtesy of U.S. Surgical Corp., Norwalk, Conn.)

be employed. Heavy hook scissors aid in transection of the tough vaginal wall. The specimen is delivered through the vagina after clamping the cervix with tenaculi. Vaginal sponges are placed to help maintain the pneumoperitoneum. Polydioxanone (Polysorb) 2-0 suture on a straight needle (Surgiwip, U.S. Surgical Corp., Norwalk, Conn) is used to sew the vaginal cuff together with the cardinal ligament and the uterosacral ligaments, if needed, in interrupted or mattress suture fashion via the 5-mm left lateral trocar (on the same side as the surgeon). The needle is brought out the same trocar, and an extracorporeal slip knot is tied[33] and pushed down with the attached knot pusher. Two additional surgeon's knots, tied intracorporeally, are placed on top of each slip knot. The pelvis is irrigated, and any secondary procedures (e.g., lymphadenectomy) are performed. The pelvis is finally inspected for bleeding with 0 to 2 mm Hg pressure. Bleeding is controlled with bipolar cautery.

The technique of laparoscopic hysterectomy is used for all cases of endometrial cancer and for all other patients with an indication for the abdominal approach to hysterectomy. This includes patients with presumed stage I ovarian cancer. Only patients with a medical contraindication to laparoscopy or with a high suspicion for or documentation of gross intraperitoneal tumor are treated by laparotomy.

LYMPHADENECTOMY

Lymphadenectomy by laparoscopy is feasible and generally practical (Table 3). The potential risk of vascular injury is high, however, as it is at laparotomy. Accordingly, this procedure should be attempted laparoscopically only by those surgeons trained, experienced, and skilled in performing lymphadenectomy by laparotomy. We perform pelvic and periaortic laparoscopic lymphadenectomy, as clinically indicated, for patients with endometrial cancer, advanced cervical cancer, and stages I and II and low–malignant potential ovarian cancers. The procedure is time consuming, however, requiring up to 1 hour of additional time for the pelvic and also for the periaortic approach.

TABLE 3.
Operative Laparoscopy—Lymph Node Surgery*

	Patients (n)		Age (yr)	Operative Time (min)	Mean No. of Nodes	Cancer Diagnosis
Procedure	All	F				
Biopsy						
Pelvic[34, 35]	13	4	63	20	NA	B, P, L
Periaortic[35]	7	3	61	?	NA	L
Removal						
Pelvic[7, 9, 20, 21, 36–40]	114	63	70	120	13	C, P, E
Periaortic[9, 20, 40]	20	18	50	?	5	C, E

*NA = not applicable; B = bladder; P = prostate; L = lymphoma; C = cervix; E = endometrium; NA = not applicable; ? = not available.

We prefer the transperitoneal approach to the nodes. The initial tro-car placement is the same as that for hysterectomy (see Fig 7); a supra-pubic trocar (10 mm) is often needed. For pelvic lymphadenectomy, the peritoneum lateral to the infundibulopelvic ligament is sharply divided in a line paralleling the ligament. Sharp, blunt, and cautery dissection are used to open the spaces. The external iliac, obturator, and common iliac nodes are sampled or completely removed as indicated. The obtura-tor nodes are most easily approached medially. Bipolar and unipolar cau-tery are used for hemostasis and lymphostasis. Drains are not employed. Medium-large or large hemoclips (Endo Clip, U.S. Surgical Corp., Nor-walk, Conn) may be used, alternatively. This instrument requires a 10-mm trocar. Because instruments and specimens are being inserted and re-moved frequently through the lateral trocars, the self-retaining Hunt-Reich Secondary Cannula, the Monoscopy brand Locking Trocar with Woodford Spike (Dexide, Inc., Fort Worth, Tex), or the Hassan SAC Stable Access Cannula with retaining balloon/cone (Marlow Surgical Technolo-gies, Inc., Willoughby, Ohio) are useful. Alternatively, trocars without re-taining devices may be sutured in place.

The periaortic nodes are approached transperitoneally by incising peritoneum along the root of the small-bowel mesentery. The key to this dissection is sufficient Trendelenburg position (30 degrees) to gravity-retract small bowel off of the aorta. We have not found it helpful to ro-tate the table to the right or left. The paracolic approach was initially at-tempted, but the required manual retraction of the colon makes this a dif-ficult approach. Unipolar and bipolar cautery are used for hemostasis and lymphostasis. Alternatively, hemoclips may be used, but placement of a 10-mm suprapubic midline trocar is often required to obtain the proper angle. Clips are used to occlude lacerations of the common iliac vein and vena cava. Reorienting the camera sideways improves surgeon orienta-tion. Additionally, when unipolar cautery is used to transect lymphatics, care must be taken to avoid grounding (i.e., coagulating) the major ves-sels. The Endo Mini-Shears or the Roticulator Endo Mini-Shears (U.S. Surgical Corp., Norwalk, Conn) are well suited to this procedure since the length of the noninsulated contact surface of the scissors is short (10 mm vs. 16 mm for Endo Shears).

Because the majority of patients with endometrial cancer will not have nodal metastases (90%), the hysterectomy is performed first. It is then sent for frozen section to analyze the grade and depth of invasion. While awaiting the frozen section result, the vaginal cuff is closed laparo-scopically, and inspection for hemostasis is carried out. Patients with 5% or less risk of pelvic node metastases[41] (grade 3 with no invasion, grade 2 with at most inner-third invasion, and grade 1 with at most middle-third invasion) are spared the additional operating time because lymph-adenectomy is not performed. Pelvic lymphadenectomy is performed for patients with a higher risk of metastases (grade 3 with inner-third inva-sion or more [9% incidence], grade 2 with middle-third invasion or more [9% incidence], and grade 1 with outer-third invasion or more [11% in-cidence]). Periaortic nodes are dissected for grades 2 or 3 with deep in-vasion only (incidence of metastases, 14% and 23%, respectively). Over-all, periaortic metastases will be found in 5% of patients.

DIAGNOSIS AND TREATMENT OF ADNEXAL MASSES

Laparoscopic diagnosis and treatment of most adnexal masses are superior to the laparotomy approach. Since most masses will be benign, most patients will be spared the morbidity of laparotomy. Even though the majority of adnexal masses are benign, thorough preoperative evaluation and malignancy risk assessment are essential. This is especially important since many of the procedures required of surgical cancer staging are beyond the scope of general gynecology practice.

Ovarian cancer affects 1 in 70 women, but a higher incidence is found in those with risk factors for the disease. One can identify women at increased risk who have normal examinations and follow them more closely for the development of cancer. For a woman with a pelvic mass, one can also determine the risk that the pelvic mass is benign or malignant and prepare the patient for surgical diagnosis and treatment or refer her to a gynecologic oncologist for specialized care, as appropriate.

Assessment of malignancy risk is based on a number of risk factors, beginning with historical factors including age, personal and familial cancer history, reproductive history, and environmental variables. As is true for most cancers, the risk of an abnormal adnexal mass being malignant increases with age. It is unusual to palpate adnexa in premenarchal patients, so all masses in this group must be considered neoplastic. In women under the age of 30 years, the chance that a pelvic mass requiring surgical intervention is malignant is 3%. Between the ages of 30 and 40 years, this risk increases to 10%. Between 40 and 50 years, it is 30%. Above the age of 50 years, the risk is relatively constant at 50%.

Reproductive and environmental risk factors are shared with cancer of the endometrium and breast. Nulliparity increases a woman's risk for contracting ovarian cancer (relative risk [RR], 2), whereas early age (<20 years) at first birth decreases it (RR, 0.2). Another risk factor is ovulatory years. This is calculated by subtracting the number of years the woman was anovulatory (pregnant, lactating, or taking birth control pills) from the time interval between menarche and menopause. A short history of ovulation (<25 years) presents a reduced risk (RR, 0.2) as compared with a long history of ovulation (>40 years). Birth control pill use decreases the risk (RR, 0.2 to 0.7) and is said to prevent 1,700 cases of ovarian cancer each year.[42] This protection seems to increase with increased duration of use.

Environmental factors also play an important role. Incidence and mortality rates for ovarian cancer are 3- to 5-fold higher in highly industrialized nations as compared with those of women in developing countries. Even within developed countries, women in rural areas have an RR of 1.2 to 1.5 in comparison to the whole population. High dietary fat consumption correlates with industrialization and confers a 2-fold increased risk.[43] Women who use talc dusting powders have a 3.3-fold increased risk.[44]

Recognition of genetic and familial tendencies is important. Inherited syndromes such as Peutz-Jeghers (familial polyposis; granulosa cell tumors in 14%), dysgenetic gonads (gonadoblastomas in 25%; secondary malignant germ cell tumors in 60% to 75% of gonadoblastomas), and benign thyroid disease (Sertoli-Leydig tumors) increase the risk.[45] A woman within a cancer family has an increased risk for ovarian, endometrial, colon, and breast adenocarcinomas of up to 50%.[46] These familial cancer syndromes occur in three patterns. The most common is the cancer family syndrome (Lynch II), including adenocarcinomas of the ovary, endometrium, colon, breast, and pancreas. The next most common is breast-ovary cancer syndrome. The least common is the site-specific familial ovarian cancer syndrome. At least 3% to 5% of ovarian cancer cases are thought to be familial. A patient with a personal history of breast or colon cancer also has a 2-fold to 4-fold increased risk.

Initial signs and symptoms may be quite mundane, so the physician must be astute in eliminating the diagnosis of ovarian cancer. Overlooking this diagnosis will result in a delay of definitive treatment and possibly decreased survival. Over half of the patients initially have abdominal pain or discomfort, and 16% have gastrointestinal symptoms (dyspepsia, early satiety, nausea). Dyspareunia, low back pain, bloating, and urinary frequency are also common.

The findings on examination may also predict risk. Physical findings include an abdominopelvic mass in 57% and ascites in 25%, generally representing extensive disease. Tumors that are larger, firmer, fixed, bilateral, or accompanied by ascites present an increased risk of being malignant. Weight loss, shortness of breath, and generalized edema are ominous but late findings. Some patients who have symptoms may not have a detectable mass on examination, especially if they are obese or unable to relax during the examination.

Risk may be assessed radiographically. Metastatic disease, ascites, or matted bowel loops on computed tomography or ultrasonography of the abdomen and pelvis are suspicious findings. Ovarian cancer is occasionally characterized by pleural effusion or, less often, parenchymal lung metastases on chest radiography. Pelvic sonography is a relatively inexpensive diagnostic test that can assess risk. Although not demonstrated to be useful for screening the general population, it can correctly predict malignant histology in 67% of ovarian masses.[47, 48] A simple cyst 8 cm or smaller in a premenopausal patient will often resolve spontaneously, thus indicating its functional nature.[49] Small simple cysts up to 5 cm in size in postmenopausal women are often neoplastic but rarely malignant. As the complexity and amount of solid material, thickness of septae, and irregularity of the capsule increases, so does the risk of malignancy.[50]

Serologic testing plays an important role in detecting ovarian cancer in high-risk groups, in confirming the probable malignant nature of the mass, and in assessing the progress of patients undergoing therapy for ovarian cancer. Many nonspecific metabolic tests may be elevated in cancer, such as liver enzymes (lactic dehydrogenase [LDH]), sedimentation rate, C-reactive protein, haptoglobin, α_1-antitrypsin, α_2-macroglobin, ferritin, amylase, white blood cell count, fibrin degradation products, complement 3b inactivator, circulating immune complex levels, serum β_2-microglobulin, protein-bound fucose, sialic acid, glycosyltransferases, glycosidases, cystine and leucine aminopeptidases, placental alkaline phosphatase, Regan isoenzyme, carcinoembryonic antigen, and human chorionic somatomammotropin. Others may be depressed, such as albumin, red blood cell count, white blood cell count, T- and B-lymphocyte counts, and immunoglobulin A. These are all nonspecific and may be abnormal in many malignant and nonmalignant conditions. α-Fetoprotein (AFP) levels are elevated in 1%, human chorionic gonadotropin (hCG) in 37%, and carcinoembryonic antigen in 38% of patients with epithelial ovarian cancer.[51, 52] AFP, hCG, and LDH are markers for some germ cell tumors.[53] More recently marketed assays for monitoring the course of breast (CA15-3), gastrointestinal (CA19-9), and gastric cancer (CA72-4) are also frequently positive in cases of ovarian cancer (55%, 56%, and 53%, respectively).

The CA-125 assay is the most specific serologic test for ovarian cancer. This immunoradiometric assay uses the monoclonal antibody OC-125 to detect the tumor-associated antigen CA-125 in patients' serum. It is positive in 85% of nonmucinous adenocarcinomas, and the level correlates with the clinical course.[54] This test may not detect the presence of mucinous epithelial tumors or germ cell or stromal tumors and may be negative in early-stage disease and with borderline tumors. An elevated CA-125 titer (>35 units/mL) and a suspicious sonogram in a postmenopausal woman have a positive predictive value for detecting cancer of almost 100%.[50] Unfortunately, in premenopausal women, the most common cause (80%) of a false positive CA-125 assay is endometriosis. Other causes of false positive test results include pregnancy, pelvic inflammatory disease, uterine leiomyomas, congestive cardiomyopathy, and nonmalignant ascites.

Indications for surgical exploration, then, are based on malignancy risk assessment. Any cystic mass in a premenopausal woman larger than 8 cm or any persistent cystic mass larger than 5 cm followed for 6 weeks, with or without birth control pill suppression, should be extirpated. The majority of functional masses, especially if 8 cm or smaller, will resolve. The majority of persistent masses will be neoplastic, although a minority will be malignant. Any complex or solid mass in a premenopausal patient should be explored. A positive CA-125 assay in this population will indicate either endometriosis or cancer once pregnancy and pelvic inflammatory disease have been ruled out. The simpler the mass appears on sonography, the lower the risk for malignancy. Patients with risk factors, however, especially those with a strong reproductive or family history of cancer, especially ovarian, should be observed with a high index of suspicion. Low–malignant potential tumors and early-grade adenocarcinomas are not infrequently manifested as simple adnexal cystic masses.

In postmenopausal patients, small (<5 cm) simple masses with a negative CA-125 result and no significant historical or physical examination risk factors may be observed with serial sonograms and CA-125 assays.[55] The risk of malignancy for these simple masses is 1% to 3%. Complex, solid, or larger masses, especially if bilateral, should be explored. Overall, 10% of masses palpable in postmenopausal women will be malignant on pelvic examination.[56] This relationship cannot be generalized to include ultrasound-diagnosed but nonpalpable masses since most of these will be small simple cysts. Once false positive causes of an elevated CA-125 have been ruled out, such as cancers in other sites, congestive heart failure, or ascites of any cause, a positive test with a pelvic mass should be assumed to indicate cancer and will require exploration. Conversely, a negative CA-125 has a high negative predictive value as long as other aspects of evaluation of the mass, such as pelvic examination and sonography, indicate low risk.

The general gynecologist would not often be performing staging for ovarian cancer, either by laparotomy or laparoscopy. Even though the gynecologic oncologist is trained to perform these procedures, preoperative planning is still important. Staging procedures such as pelvic lymphadenectomy, periaortic lymphadenectomy, and omentectomy may each require an additional hour of operating time. Additionally, trocar site placement and trocar size should be planned ahead. Additional equipment (e.g., Endo GIA or Endo Clip, U.S. Surgical Corp., Norwich, Conn) or a specialized assistant may also be required.

Numerous alternatives for laparoscopic management of adnexal masses are available. Smaller masses (2 to 4 cm) may often be removed without alteration. They can sometimes be brought out through the trocar (10 to 12 mm). A circular twisting or turning motion is helpful to reduce the width of the mass. Alternatively, small masses may often be brought directly through the abdominal wall after removal of the trocar. Small sterile endoscopy bags are available in which to place these masses. A colpotomy incision can also be made to deliver the mass.

The surgeon should be familiar with several techniques for salpingo-oophorectomy because anatomy and tumor size/location may make certain techniques inappropriate. The primary safety concern is avoiding ureteral injury. Before securing the infundibulopelvic ligament, the ureter is identified, preferably by opening the retroperitoneal space lateral to these vessels. Alternatively, the ureter may be identified transperitoneally by viewing through the parietal peritoneum medial and dorsal to these vessels. The infundibulopelvic and ovarian ligaments may be controlled with bipolar cautery followed by sharp transection. Another technique is to use the Endo GIA stapler. Two or three pre-tied Endoloops can be placed over the entire pedicle beneath the ovary. This technique is only successful if sufficient adnexal mobility is present. Otherwise, these ties may dislodge. The last technique is to make a window beneath the vessels and pass a suture laterally to medially beneath the pedicle and then back out the same trocar. If a Surgiwip suture (with the needle cut off) is used, a slip knot can be thrown and cinched down by using the attached knot pusher. Unless two or three sutures are applied, the slip knot should be secured by two intracorporeal knots. When a knot pusher is used, any suture at least 30 in. (75 cm) long with the properties of good knot security that will allow the knot to slide easily is appropriate. We prefer to use 2-0 braided nylon (Surgilon, Davis-Geck, Danbury, Conn), which ties with the facility and knot security of silk but without the intense inflammatory response induced by silk. Four half-hitch square knots can be applied one after the other. Secure tissue approximation and knotting will occur if the knot pusher is extended beyond the knot to provide countertraction while pulling the two ends of the sutures at a 180-degree angle. Both ends of the suture must be kept in tension (held in one hand) while the knot pusher is manipulated with the other hand.

Larger masses will either require a larger abdominal or colpotomy incision or will require size reduction. A large bag (Lapsac, nylon with integral polyurethane inner coating and polypropylene drawstring, 5×8 in., Cook Ob/Gyn, Bloomington, Ill) with a drawstring can be placed around the mass. The mass can then be drained or cut to reduced size so that the bag can be delivered through a trocar or colpotomy incision. Manual and automated tissue morcellators are available for this purpose. Alternatively, the neck of the bag can be brought out through the skin and the mass aspirated or cut. Laparoscopic visualization of the bag will prevent inadvertent penetration. A mass can also be drawn to and held against the colpotomy incision while aspiration per vagina is performed. When the mass diameter decreases sufficiently, it can be delivered through the vagina.

Cystic masses can be drained intra-abdominally. Rupture of an isolated ovarian malignancy raises theoretical concern over tumor spill and worsened prognosis. The bulk of the literature, however, does not demonstrate a worsened outcome.[57] Even so, to be cautious, copious irrigation is recommended after such a rupture, benign or malignant. Rupture can be controlled, avoiding detectable spill, by using a dual-lumen Topel Endoscopic Cyst Aspirator Set (Cook Ob/Gyn, Bloomington, Ill). A pretied Endoloop is first placed over the outer cannula. Suction applied to the outer 10-mm (30 cm long) cannula adheres it to the cyst wall. The central 14-gauge, 39-cm needle then pierces the cyst wall and deflates it. This is attached to separate suction. Once deflated, the 14-gauge needle is removed. Cyst wall (1 to 2 cm) can be seen to be pulled into the outer cannula. The Endoloop is then brought down to the cyst and cinched tight as the outer cannula is removed.

If ovarian cancer is found, in the absence of gross metastatic disease (>5-mm diameter) requiring cytoreduction, formal staging can be completed laparoscopically. Pelvic and periaortic lymphadenectomy are performed as described for endometrial cancer. Infracolic omentectomy is performed by bipolar cautery, stapling (Endo GIA), or pedicle tying (Endoloop or intracorporeal ties). Four-quadrant washings and biopsies can easily be performed.

APPENDICITIS

The laparoscopic approach is well suited to rule out and treat appendicitis since the organ is small (Fig 13). This procedure was first introduced by Semm[58] in 1982. The appendix is located and then mobilized by lysing any periappendiceal and pericecal adhesions (Fig 14). The mesoappendix is controlled by bipolar cautery and is transected (Figs 15 and 16). Fecal material is milked out of the appendix into the cecum. Two Endoloops are placed over the base of the appendix, and a third is placed 1 cm distal to prevent contamination of the operative field.[59, 60] Alternatively, the base of the appendix can be sealed and transected with the Endo GIA stapler[61] or occluded by a Silastic band[62] after transection (Fig 17). After transection, one or two drops of povidone-iodine solution are placed on the stump (Fig 18). Extracorporealization of the appendix, through either a secondary or the primary trocar, with appendectomy performed by traditional means, has also been reported.[63, 64]

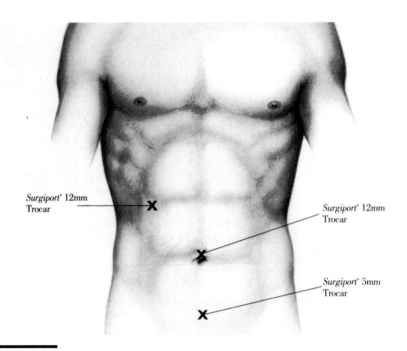

FIGURE 13.

Suggested trocar placement for appendectomy; 12-mm trocars are required for use of the Endo GIA stapler. Trocar placement as illustrated for hysterectomy is also adequate. (Courtesy of U.S. Surgical Corp., Norwalk, Conn.)

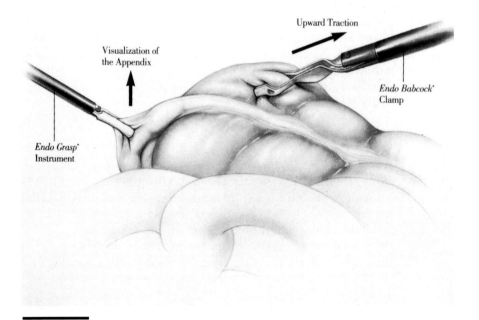

FIGURE 14.

Visualization and mobilization of the appendix. (Courtesy of U.S. Surgical Corp., Norwalk, Conn.)

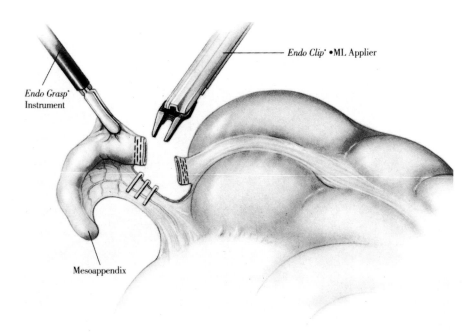

FIGURE 15.
Ligation of the mesoappendix with the Endo Clip applier after transection of the appendix with the Endo GIA stapler. (Courtesy of U.S. Surgical Corp., Norwalk, Conn.)

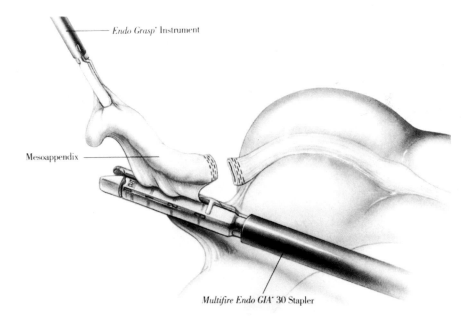

FIGURE 16.
Ligation and transection of the mesoappendix with the Endo GIA stapler. (Courtesy of U.S. Surgical Corp., Norwalk, Conn.)

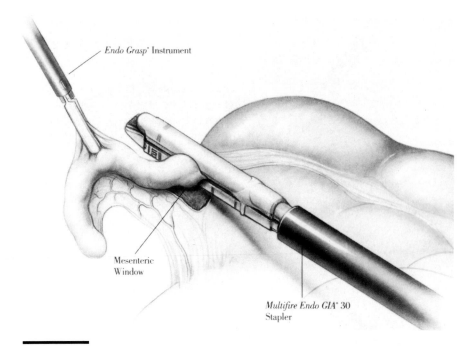

FIGURE 17.

Stapling and transection of the base of the appendix with the Endo GIA stapler after creating a mesenteric window. (Courtesy of U.S. Surgical Corp., Norwalk, Conn.)

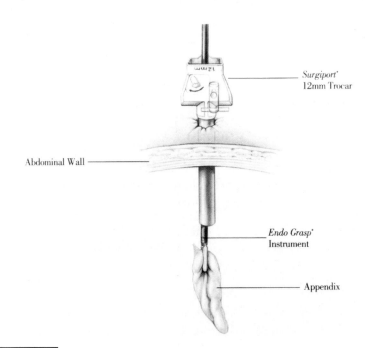

FIGURE 18.

The transected appendix may be removed via the trocar or via the skin site after removal of the trocar. (Courtesy of U.S. Surgical Corp., Norwalk, Conn.)

SECOND-LOOK LAPAROSCOPY

Operative laparoscopy is used for second-look evaluation after primary chemotherapy for ovarian cancer. This can be technically difficult secondary to adhesion formation as a result of prior cancer and surgery. Because of the high risk of bowel adhesions to the anterior abdominal wall, open laparoscopy should be performed. At times, the primary trocar site may be placed in the outer quadrants to gain entry into a clear space. If tumor is found, the procedure is completed if tumor reduction is not the goal. If no gross disease is seen, restaging and laparoscopic exploration are performed. Four-quadrant washings and biopsies are performed, and resection of residual omentum is accomplished. If lymphadenectomy was performed at the time of initial staging, repeat entry into the retroperitoneal spaces may be difficult because of fibrosis. Because laparoscopic inspection of the dorsal upper portion of the abdomen and retroperitoneum is impractical, preoperative computed tomography scanning is imperative.

FUTURE ADVANCES

Advancements in technology and our application of that technology are taking leaps and bounds. Laparoscopic equipment is improving in reliability and performance. Innovative instruments (retractors, bipolar cutting instruments, roticulators, ultrasonic aspirator) are widening the applicability of laparoscopy to surgical indications. Improvements in camera and monitor resolution will soon rival that of the human eye. Three-dimensional videography and remote operating are just over the horizon.

RADICAL HYSTERECTOMY

Radical hysterectomy is one procedure awaiting further advancement. Presently, the marked difference in patient outcome for other procedures completed by laparoscopy vs. laparotomy has not been realized for radical hysterectomy. Only three laparoscopically assisted radical vaginal hysterectomies have been reported.[9, 36] The mean operative time was 7 hours. The mean postoperative stay was 3 days.

Laparoscopic radical hysterectomy can be approached abdominally or vaginally, analogous to laparoscopic vs. laparoscopic-assisted simple hysterectomy. After exploration, the retroperitoneal spaces are opened laparoscopically. The hypogastric system is skeletonized, and the paravesical and pararectal spaces are developed. The round and infundibulopelvic ligaments (for salpingo-oophorectomy) are secured and transected (cautery, suturing, or stapling). The bladder flap is taken down sharply to 2 to 3 cm beyond the cervix. The ureter is then dissected from the cardinal ligament tunnel after coagulating or clipping the uterine artery at its origin and bringing it medially over the ureter. The uterosacral ligaments can be secured (coagulated, clipped, or stapled) at the level desired depending on the scope of the procedure.[65] The cardinal ligament parametrium can be transected after bipolar coagulation or stapling (Endo

GIA). The majority of the procedure can be completed abdominally, and the vaginal cuff margin (2 to 3 cm from the cervix) can be cut and the lower cardinal ligaments clamped and sutured from below. Alternatively, much of the procedure can be performed vaginally using the Schauta technique.[66]

In our hands a radical hysterectomy can be performed by laparotomy in 1.5 to 2.5 hours, with a mean hospital stay of 4 days. Additionally, we perform a nerve-sparing procedure with the Cavitron ultrasonic surgical aspirator (Valley Lab, Inc., Boulder, Colo). This has been shown to result in less neurogenic bladder and rectal disability.[67] We have used this technique for radical hysterectomy for the last 2 years and have noted less disability and more rapid recovery than when the standard technique of Worthheim is used.[68] This technique may be applicable to the laparoscopic approach now that the laparoscopic Cavitron adaptor (CUSALap) has been introduced. The skill level and time required for laparoscopic radical hysterectomy are high, and one should be quite adept at the procedures of laparoscopic hysterectomy, bilateral salpingo-oophorectomy, and pelvic and periaortic lymphadenectomy before it is attempted.

BOWEL RESECTION

Laparoscopic intracorporeal bowel resection and reanastomosis will also be routinely feasible in the future. Presently, most techniques rely on extracorporealization of segments to be resected and/or reanastomosed by abdominal incision, by a 3- to 4-cm trocar, or by colpotomy incision. Difficulties include the long operating time (6 to 8 hours) and the requirement to remove the large colon specimen from the abdomen. Recovery from the laparoscopic approach seems to be more rapid than with the laparotomy approach. Recovery of bowel function often occurs within 24 to 48 hours and permits hospital discharge after 2 to 3 days. This technique relies heavily on stapling.

To perform the technique entirely laparoscopically, the bowel is not exteriorized (Figs 19 to 22). After determining the segment to be resected and creating a mesenteric window (Fig 23), the colon (Fig 24) and mesentery (Fig 25) are successively stapled and transected with the Endo GIA. The correct staple size is determined by applying the Endo Gauge to the tissue first. The correct length of the staple line (30 or 60 mm) is determined by the length of tissue to be secured and by the amount of operating space in which to manipulate the instrument. A side-to-side functional end-to-end anastomosis is created by first placing the stapled ends next to each other. An endovascular clamp may be placed proximal to the anastomotic site to avoid fecal contamination. A 1-cm corner of the staple line is excised (Fig 26), and the Endo GIA 30 is inserted and fired to unite the two colonic ends and create a common lumen (Fig 27). A Multifire Endo TA 60 stapler is applied to unite and seal the two open corners (Fig 28). This same procedure is used at laparotomy to create this type of anastomosis. Defects in the mesentery may be closed by suturing or use of the Multifire Endo Hernia stapler. The abdominal cavity is then copiously irrigated, and the specimen is removed.

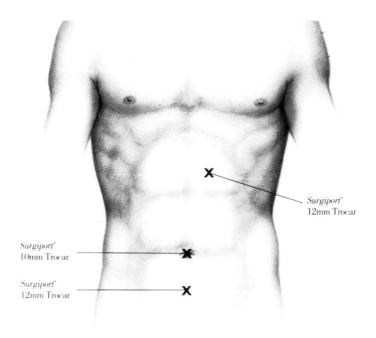

FIGURE 19.

Suggested trocar placement for hemicolectomy for a left colon lesion. (Courtesy of U.S. Surgical Corp., Norwalk, Conn.)

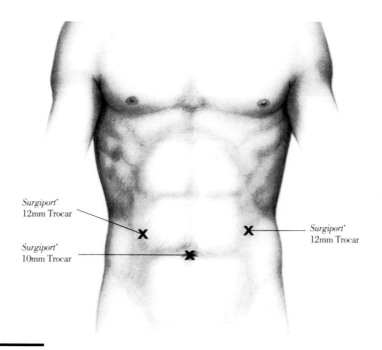

FIGURE 20.

Suggested trocar placement for resection of a transverse colon lesion. (Courtesy of U.S. Surgical Corp., Norwalk, Conn.)

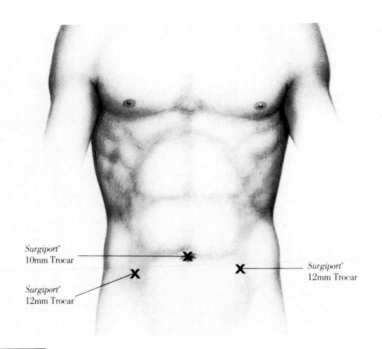

FIGURE 21.

Suggested trocar placement for resection of a rectosigmoid colon lesion. (Courtesy of U.S. Surgical Corp., Norwalk, Conn.)

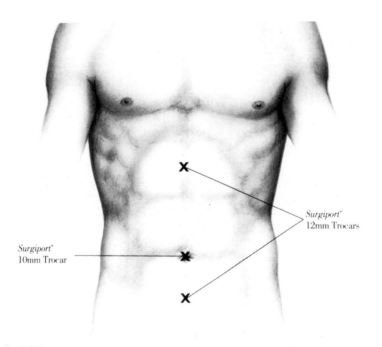

FIGURE 22.

Suggested trocar placement for resection of a right colon lesion. (Courtesy of U.S. Surgical Corp., Norwalk, Conn.)

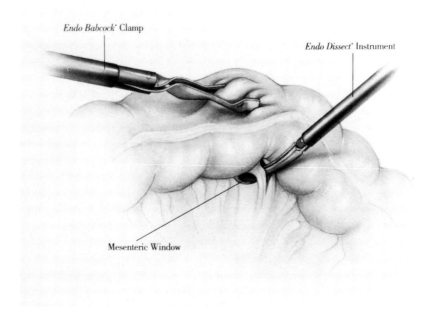

FIGURE 23.

Creation of a mesenteric window. (Courtesy of U.S. Surgical Corp., Norwalk, Conn.)

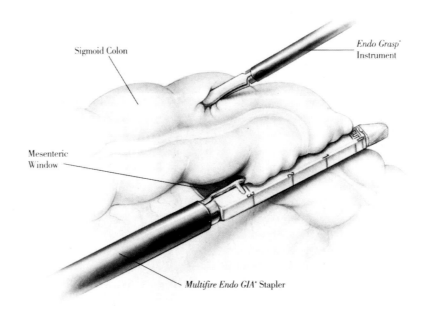

FIGURE 24.

Transection of the colon with an Endo GIA stapler. (Courtesy of U.S. Surgical Corp., Norwalk, Conn.)

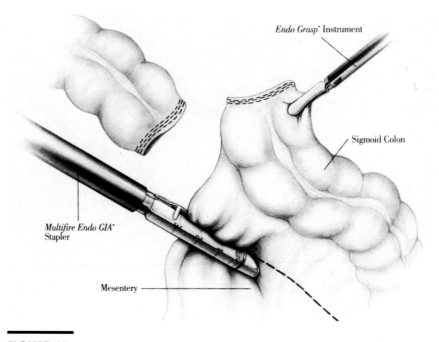

FIGURE 25.
Transection of mesentery with an Endo GIA stapler (Courtesy of U.S. Surgical Corp., Norwalk, Conn.)

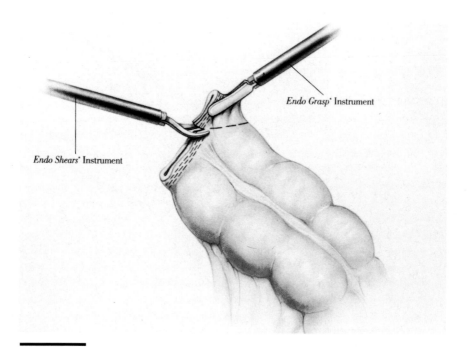

FIGURE 26.
Resection of a corner of the staple line to prepare for side-to-side, functional end-to-end anastomosis. (Courtesy of U.S. Surgical Corp., Norwalk, Conn.)

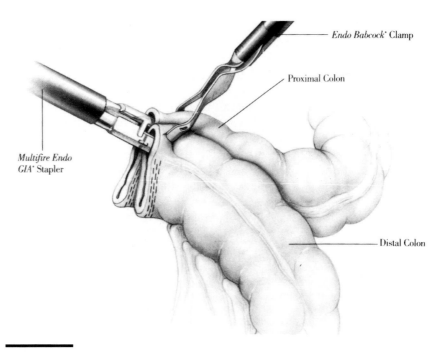

FIGURE 27.
Creation of a side-to-side anastomosis and lumen with the Endo GIA stapler.
(Courtesy of U.S. Surgical Corp., Norwalk, Conn.)

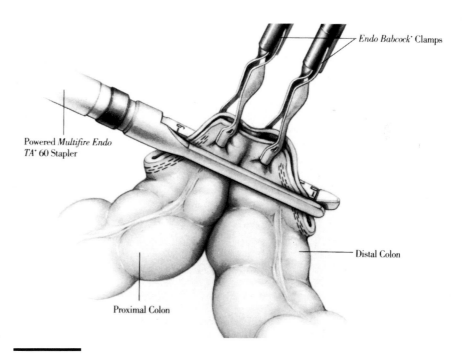

FIGURE 28.
Completion of a colocolostomy with the Endo TA stapler. (Courtesy of U.S. Surgical Corp., Norwalk, Conn.)

To perform laparoscopic-assisted resection, the segment to be resected can be removed before or after stapling transection. Removal before resection may require a larger incision. If the resection line is rectosigmoid, the EEA (end-to-end anastomotic stapler) can be used. After intracorporeal staple transection, the proximal end can be delivered through the abdominal wall (a 4-cm incision may be required). A purse-string suture is then placed and the staple line excised. The EEA anvil is placed into the proximal stump and the purse-string suture tied (Fig 29). The stump is placed back into the abdominal cavity and the abdominal incision closed. The EEA is inserted into the anus, with the white trocar point retracted, and advanced to the distal staple line. The trocar tip is advanced through the staple line and removed (Fig 30). Under direct visualization, the anvil is inserted into the stapler, locked in place, closed, and fired. After opening the stapler, it is removed from the rectum. The integrity of the anastomosis can be tested by injection of a dilute povidone-iodine solution rectally.

CYTOREDUCTION

Laparoscopic cytoreduction is presently too tedious and time-consuming to be practical. Introduction of a laparoscopic ultrasonic aspirator handpiece (CUSALap, Valley Lab, Inc., Boulder, Colo) will make this procedure more feasible, especially for a small number of implants or for small-volume implants. The CUSALap ultrasonic accessory extends

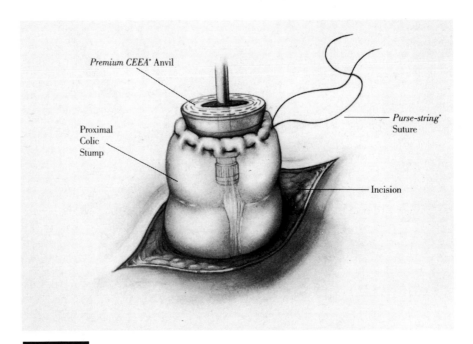

FIGURE 29.

Exteriorization of the proximal end of the colon to be anastomosed; the CEEA anvil is inserted and secured with a purse-string suture. (Courtesy of U.S. Surgical Corp., Norwalk, Conn.)

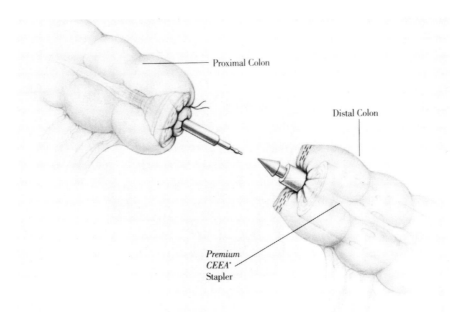

FIGURE 30.

CEEA inserted transrectally; the white trocar point will be removed before locking the anvil to the stapler. (Courtesy of U.S. Surgical Corp., Norwalk, Conn.)

the length of the CUSA System 200 handpiece to 31 cm in length. This can be used through a 10-mm trocar and provides the functions of aspiration and irrigation in addition to the electrosurgical cut and coagulation capability (with the addition of the CEM Module) available to the handpiece used at laparotomy. Use of the CUSA has already been demonstrated to improve the completeness of cytoreduction of intraperitoneal malignancy at laparotomy.[69]

SPLENECTOMY

Laparoscopic splenectomy also requires a great degree of care and skill. Splenectomy is performed by the same technique used at laparotomy (Fig 31). Great care must be taken to clamp or bipolar-cauterize all pedicles before resection since bleeding may be vigorous (Fig 32). The anterior approach begins by opening the lesser omental sac. The greater omentum is divided along the greater gastric curvature by bipolar cautery, clipping, or stapling (Fig 33). The short gastric vessels must be secured before cutting (Fig 34). The tail of the pancreas should be identified to avoid injury. The splenic artery can be identified, dissected free for 1 cm, and triply clipped (Fig 35). This will often result in reduction of the size of the spleen as it empties of blood. The gastrocolic ligament and splenic hilar vessels must then be secured with double clips or by use of the Endo GIA stapler (Fig 36). The spleen can be removed after its placement into a bag.

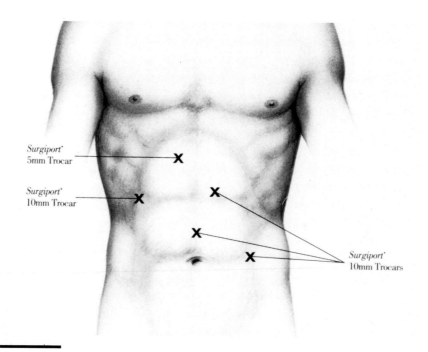

Surgiport®
5mm Trocar

Surgiport®
10mm Trocar

Surgiport®
10mm Trocars

FIGURE 31.
Suggested trocar placement for splenectomy. (Courtesy of U.S. Surgical Corp., Norwalk, Conn.)

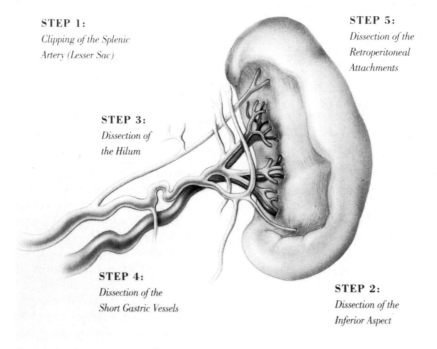

STEP 1:
*Clipping of the Splenic
Artery (Lesser Sac)*

STEP 5:
*Dissection of the
Retroperitoneal
Attachments*

STEP 3:
*Dissection of
the Hilum*

STEP 4:
*Dissection of the
Short Gastric Vessels*

STEP 2:
*Dissection of the
Inferior Aspect*

FIGURE 32.
The splenic anatomy guides the resection. (Courtesy of U.S. Surgical Corp., Norwalk, Conn.)

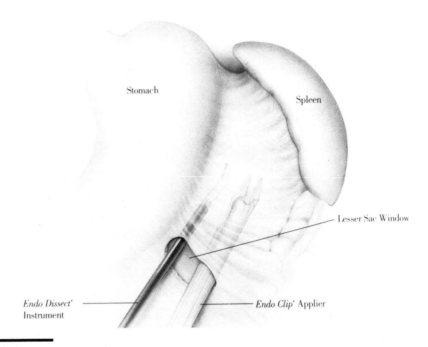

FIGURE 33.

Opening the lesser omental bursa via a window in the greater omentum. (Courtesy of U.S. Surgical Corp., Norwalk, Conn.)

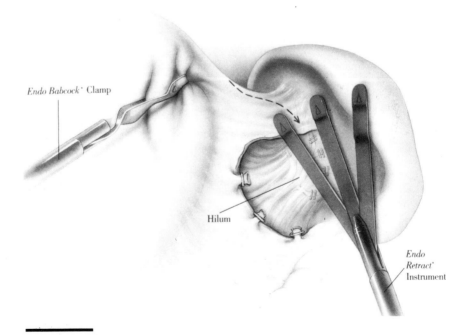

FIGURE 34.

The short gastric vessels must be secured before cutting. (Courtesy of U.S. Surgical Corp., Norwalk, Conn.)

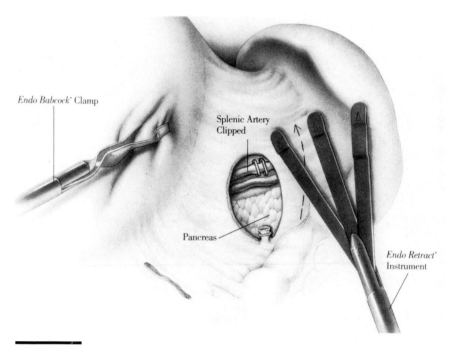

FIGURE 35.

Identification of the tail of the pancreas to avoid injury; clips on the splenic artery. (Courtesy of U.S. Surgical Corp., Norwalk, Conn.)

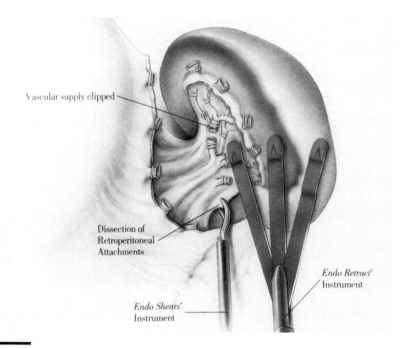

FIGURE 36.

The vascular supply to the spleen is clipped before transection. (Courtesy of U.S. Surgical Corp., Norwalk, Conn.)

SUMMARY

The future of laparoscopic surgery begins now, and rapid improvements are expected. Physician training is necessary to keep the complication rate to a minimum while maximizing the widespread use of operative video laparoscopy. Since operative laparoscopy requires a higher technical skill and a precise knowledge of anatomy, attendance at a didactic course and dry laboratory is important. Skill can then be improved by practice in the animal laboratory under the supervision and guidance of an experienced operative laparoscopist. A preceptorship for the first patient cases performed is generally recommended.

REFERENCES

1. Jacobaeus HC: Uber die moglichkeit, die zystoskopie bei untersuchung seroser hochlungen anzuwenden. *Munch Med Wochenschr* 1910; 57:2090–2092.
2. Soulas A: Television bronchologie et pneumologie. *Presse Med* 1956; 64:97–99.
3. Berci G, Kont LA: A new optical system in endoscopy with special reference to cystoscopy. *Br J Urol* 1969; 41:564–571.
4. Eisenberg J: Uber eine apparatus zur schonenden und kontrollierbaren gasfullung der bauchhohle fur die laparoskopie. *Klin Wochenschr* 1966; 44:593.
5. Semm K: Advances in pelviscopic surgery. *Curr Probl Obstet Gynecol* 1982; 5:7–42.
6. Shapiro HI, Adler DH: Excision of an ectopic pregnancy through the laparoscope. *Am J Obstet Gynecol* 1973; 117:290–291.
7. Querleu D, Leblanc E, Castelain B: Laparoscopic pelvic lymphadenectomy in the staging of early carcinoma of the cervix. *Am J Obstet Gynecol* 1991; 164:579–581.
8. Reich H, DeCaprio J, McGlynn F: Laparoscopic hysterectomy. *J Gynecol Surg* 1989; 5:213–216.
9. Nezhat CR, Burrell MO, Nezhat FR, et al: Laparoscopic radical hysterectomy with paraaortic and pelvic node dissection. *Obstet Gynecol* 1992; 166:864–865.
10. Levine R: Economic impact of pelviscopic surgery. *J Reprod Med* 1985; 30:655–659.
11. Zouves C, Urman B, Gomel V: Laparoscopic surgical treatment of tubal pregnancy. A safe, effective alternative to laparotomy. *J Reprod Med* 1992; 37:205–209.
12. Brumsted J, Kessler C, Gibson C, et al: A comparison of laparoscopy and laparotomy for the treatment of ectopic pregnancy. *Obstet Gynecol* 1988; 71:889–892.
13. Vermesh M, Silva PD, Rosen GF, et al: Management of unruptured ectopic gestation by linear salpingostomy: A prospective, randomized clinical trial of laparoscopy versus laparotomy. *Obstet Gynecol* 1989; 73:400–404.
14. Baumann R, Magos AL, Turnbull A: Prospective comparison of videopelviscopy with laparotomy for ectopic pregnancy. *Br J Obstet Gynaecol* 1991; 98:765–771.
15. Nezhat F, Nezhat C, Gordon S, et al: Laparoscopic versus abdominal hysterectomy. *J Reprod Med* 1992; 37:247–250.
16. Romanowski L, Reich H, Adelson MD, et al: Upper extremity compression neuropathies following advanced laparoscopic surgery. *Fertil Steril*, in press.

17. Raftery S, Sherry E: Total intravenous anaesthesia with propofol and alfentanil protects against postoperative nausea and vomiting. *Can J Anaesth* 1992; 39:37–40.

18. Smith BE, Suchak M, Sigins D, et al: Rectus sheath block for diagnostic laparoscopy. *Anaesthesia* 1988; 43:947–948.

19. Kovac SR, Cruikshank SH, Retto HF: Laparoscopy-assisted vaginal hysterectomy. *J Gynecol Surg* 1990; 6:185–193.

20. Childers JM, Surwit EA. Case report. Combined laparoscopic and vaginal surgery for the managemment of two cases of stage I endometrial cancer. *Gynecol Oncol* 1992; 45:46–51.

21. Photopulos GJ, Stovall TG, Summitt RL: Laparoscopic-assisted vaginal hysterectomy, bilateral salpingo-oophorectomy, and pelvic lymph node sampling for endometrial cancer. *J Gynecol Surg* 1992; 8:91–94.

22. Minelli L, Angiolillo M, Caione C, et al: Laparoscopically assisted vaginal hysterectomy. *Endoscopy* 1991; 23:64–66.

23. Nezhat C, Nezhat F, Burrell M: Brief clinical report. Laparoscopically assisted hysterectomy for the management of a borderline ovarian tumor: A case report. *J Laparoendosc Surg* 1992; 2:167–169.

24. Magos AL, Broadbent JAM, Amso NN: Laparoscopically assisted vaginal hysterectomy. *Lancet* 1991; 338:1091–1092.

25. Fernandez H, Lelaidier C, Frydman R: Laparoscopically assisted vaginal hysterectomy. *Lancet* 1992; 339:123.

26. Nezhat C, Nezhat F, Siflen SL: Laparoscopic hysterectomy and bilateral salpingo-oophorectomy using multifire GIA surgical stapler. *J Gynecol Surg* 1990; 6:287–288.

27. Maher PJ, Hill DJ: Video-assisted laparoscopic vaginal hysterectomy. *Med J Aust* 1991; 154:427.

28. Scrimgeour JB, Ng KB, Gaudoin MR: Laparoscopy in vaginal hysterectomy. *Lancet* 1991; 338:1465–1466.

29. Pelosi MA, Pelosi MA: Special report: Laparoscopic hysterectomy with bilateral salpingo-oophorectomy using a single umbilical puncture. *N J Med* 1991; 88:721–726.

30. Pelosi MA, Pelosi MA: Laparoscopic supracervical hysterectomy using a single-umbilical puncture (minilaparoscopy). *J Reprod Med* 1992; 37:777–784.

31. Padial JG, Sotolongo J, Casey MJ, et al: Laparoscopy-assisted vaginal hysterectomy: Report of seventy-five consecutive cases. *J Gynecol Surg* 1992; 8:81–85.

32. Liu CY: Laparoscopic hysterectomy. A review of 72 cases. *J Reprod Med* 1992; 37:351–354.

33. Weston PV: A new clinch knot. *Obstet Gynecol* 1991; 78:144–147.

34. Hald T, Rasmussen F: Extraperitoneal pelvioscopy: A new aid in staging of lower urinary tract tumors. A preliminary report. *J Urol* 1980; 124:245–248.

35. Salky BA, Bauer JJ, Gelernt IM, et al: The use of laparoscopy in retroperitoneal pathology. *Gastrointest Endosc* 1988; 34:227–230.

36. Canis M, Mage G, Wattiez A, et al: Vaginally assisted laparoscopic radical hysterectomy. *J Gynecol Surg* 1992; 8:103–105.

37. Schuessler WW, Vancaillie TG, Teich H, et al: Transperitoneal endosurgical lymphadenectomy in patients with localized prostate cancer. *J Urol* 1991; 145:988–991.

38. Tierney JP, Kusminsky RE, Boland JP, et al: Laparoscopic pelvic lymph node dissection. *W V Med* 1991; 87:151–152.

39. Ferzli G, Raboy A, Kleinerman D, et al: Extraperitoneal endoscopic pelvic lymph node dissection vs. laparoscopic lymph node dissection in the stag-

ing of prostatic and bladder carcinoma. *J Laparoendosc Surg* 1992; 2:219–222.

40. Childers JM, Hatch K, Surwit EA: The role of laparoscopic lymphadenectomy in the management of cervical carcinoma. *Gynecol Oncol* 1992; 47:38–43.

41. Creasman WT, Morrow CP, Bundy BN, et al: Surgical pathologic spread patterns of endometrial cancer: A Gynecologic Oncology Group study. *Cancer* 1987; 60:2035–2041.

42. Smith LH, Ol RH: Detection of malignant ovarian neoplasms: A review of the literature. I. Detection of the patient at risk: Clinical, radiological, and cytological detection. *Obstet Gynecol Surv* 1984; 39:313–328.

43. Cramer DW, Welch WR, Hutchinson GB, et al: Dietary animal fat in relation to ovarian cancer risk. *Obstet Gynecol* 1984; 63:833–838.

44. Cramer DW, Welch WR, Scully RE, et al: Ovarian cancer and talc: A case control study. *Cancer* 1982; 50:372–376.

45. Greene MH, Clark JW, Blayney DW: The epidemiology of ovarian cancer. *Semin Oncol* 1984; 11:209–226.

46. Lynch HT, Watson P, Bewtra C, et al: Hereditary ovarian cancer: Heterogeneity in age at diagnosis. *Cancer* 1991; 67:1460–1466.

47. vanNagell JR, Higgins RV, Donaldson ES, et al: Transvaginal sonography as a screening method for ovarian cancer. *Cancer* 1990; 65:573–577.

48. Ozasa H, Noda Y, Takahide M, et al: Diagnostic capability of ultrasound vs. computerized tomography for clinically suspected ovarian mass with emphasis on detection of adhesions. *Gynecol Oncol* 1986; 25:311–318.

49. Spanos WJ: Preoperative hormonal therapy of cystic adnexal masses. *Am J Obstet Gynecol* 1973; 116:551–556.

50. Finkler NJ, Benacerraf B, Lavin PT, et al: Comparison of serum CA-125, clinical impression, and ultrasound in the preoperative evaluation of ovarian masses. *Obstet Gynecol* 1988; 72:659–664.

51. Smith LH, Ol RH: Detection of malignant ovarian neoplasms: A review of the literature. II. Laboratory detection. *Obstet Gynecol Surv* 1984; 39:329–345.

52. Smith LH, Ol RH: Detection of malignant ovarian neoplasms: A review of the literature. III. Immunological detection and ovarian cancer-associated antigens. *Obstet Gynecol Surv* 1984; 39:346–360.

53. Friedman M, White RG, Nissenbaum MM, et al: Serum lactic dehydrogenase as a possible tumor marker for an ovarian dysgerminoma: A literature review and report of a case. *Obstet Gynecol Surv* 1984; 39:247–251.

54. Bast RC Jr, Klug TL, St. John E, et al: A radioimmunoassay using a monoclonal antibody to monitor the course of epithelial ovarian cancer. *N Engl J Med* 1983; 309:883–887.

55. Goldstein SR, Subramanyam B, Snyder JR, et al: The postmenopausal cystic adnexal mass: The potential role of ultrasound in conservative management. *Obstet Gynecol* 1989; 73:8–10.

56. Barber HRK, Graber EA: The PMPO syndrome (postmenopausal palpable ovary syndrome). *Obstet Gynecol* 1971; 38:921–923.

57. Adelson MD: Is rupture of a malignant ovarian cyst of prognostic importance? Submitted for publication.

58. Semm K: Endoscopic appendectomy. *Endoscopy* 1983; 15:59–64.

59. Bryson K: Laparoscopic appendectomy. *J Gynecol Surg* 1991; 7:93–95.

60. Nezhat C, Nezhat F: Incidental appendectomy during videolaseroscopy. *Am J Obstet Gynecol* 1991; 165:559–564.

61. Daniell JF, Gurley LD, Kurtz BR, et al: The use of an automatic stapling device for laparoscopic appendectomy. *Obstet Gynecol* 1991; 78:721–723.

62. Gangal HT, Gangal MH: Laparoscopic appendicectomy. *Endoscopy* 1987; 19:127–129.

63. Pelosi MA, Pelose MA: Laparoscopic appendectomy using a single umbilical puncture (minilaparoscopy). *J Reprod Med* 1992; 37:588–594.
64. Fleming JS: Laparoscopically directed appendicectomy. *Aust N Z J Obstet Gynaecol* 1985; 25:238–240.
65. Piver MS, Rutledge FN, Smith PJ: Five classes of extended hysterectomy of women with cervical cancer. *Obstet Gynecol* 1974; 44:265–270.
66. Querleu D: Hysterectomies enlargies de Schauta-Amreich et Schauta-Stoeckel assistees par coelioscopie. *J Gynecol Obstet Biol Reprod* 1991; 20:747–748.
67. Yabuki Y, Asamoto A, Hoshiba T, et al: Dissection of the cardinal ligament in radical hysterectomy for cervical cancer with emphasis on the lateral ligament. *Am J Obstet Gynecol* 1991; 164:7–14.
68. Meigs JV: Carcinoma of the cervix—the Wertheim operation. *Surg Gynecol Obstet* 1944; 78:195–198.
69. Adelson MD, Baggish MS, Seifer DB, et al: Cytoreduction of ovarian cancer with the Cavitron ultrasonic surgical aspirator. *Obstet Gynecol* 1988; 72:140–143.

Editor's Comment

Dr. Adelson has provided the clinician with an extensive review of laparoscopy including anesthesia, preoperative evaluation, a discussion of postmenopausal masses, and indications for laparoscopic excision. I am in agreement with Dr. Adelson that with increasing experience and new technology, laparoscopic surgery will continue to assume a more prominent role in the management of the gynecologic and gynecologic oncology patient. Although Dr. Adelson discusses laparoscopic hysterectomy, which requires a significant skill level and considerable operative time, he points out that surgical skills in the open abdomen have improved sufficiently to permit the procedure to be performed in 1½ to 2½ hours and to require a mean hospital stay of only 4 days. Laparoscopic node dissection with a vaginal Schauta radical hysterectomy may provide us with an alternative to the abdominal radical hysterectomy procedure. Dr. Adelson also reviews laparoscopic bowel resection and splenectomy.

Laparoscopic surgery and the equipment used continue to change at a rapid pace. For the past several decades, laparoscopy and endoscopy have been the sole purview of the obstetrician/gynecologist. During the past 5 years, our general surgery colleagues have begun to appreciate their usefulness and, unfortunately, occasionally practice these techniques without sufficient training and skills. It is incumbent upon us as clinicians to develop experience with laparoscopic techniques and to stay abreast of fast-changing technology in this field. Recognizing that acquisition of laparoscopic skill is associated with a steep learning curve, all attempts should be made to practice these procedures at a certified animal facility and perform the initial procedures under the guidance of a laparoscopic surgeon.

Ira R. Horowitz, M.D.

The Ultrasonic Surgical Aspirator in the Gynecologic Oncology Patient

THOMAS J. HERZOG, M.D.

JANET S. RADER, M.D.

T he ultrasonic surgical aspirator (USA) has become a valuable instrument in the modern-day treatment of the gynecologic oncology patient. The USA is an instrument that permits ultrasonic emulsification of tissue by using a hand-held device containing both suction and irrigating modes. The USA provides the capability to selectively and rapidly remove tissue samples that are readily available for pathologic evaluation. Intraabdominal surgical debulking and treatment of vulvar intraepithelial neoplasia represent two of the most common applications of the USA in gynecologic oncology patients. In addition to widespread use in gynecologic oncology surgery, the USA has been employed in neurosurgery, otolaryngology, urology, colorectal endoscopy, and general surgery. This chapter will discuss the historical background and physics of the USA as well as the specific applications of the USA in gynecology.

HISTORICAL BACKGROUND

The concept of ultrasonic aspiration arose from phacoemulsification, a method developed to minimize the invasiveness of ophthalmologic surgery. Clinical application of ultrasonic surgical aspiration was reported by Kelman[1] in 1969 as he removed cataracts through a 2-mm incision by fluid irrigation and aspiration coupled with emulsification through a titanium tip. The advancement of this technique was well established by 1973 when Kelman[2] reported on a series of 500 consecutive cataract emulsifications with excellent results and a complication rate not exceeding that with conventional techniques.

These results spurred the development of a larger, more powerful ultrasonic aspiration unit that found immediate application in neurosurgery. The newly designed unit featured a single multifunctional handpiece capable of fragmenting and aspirating tissue while clearing the surgical field with irrigation. Neurosurgery sought an instrument that was capable of highly selective tissue removal and yet caused only minimal bleeding and trauma to adjacent tissue. Ultrasonic surgery surpassed the performance of the conventional cutting loop, primarily by decreasing thermal trauma to surrounding tissue.

Flamm and coworkers[3] presented preliminary results of USA application in 38 neurosurgery cases in 1978. Clinically promising results were obtained in intracapsular resection of meningiomas, acoustic neuromas, and other tumors. Animal studies that compared the USA with suction-cautery established the efficacy and safety of the USA. These laboratory studies showed that the aspirating tip would penetrate neither dura nor meningioma capsule even at maximal power. Further studies by Young and colleagues[4] reported that the USA did not adversely affect either blood flow or function of spinal cord white matter beyond 1 to 2 mm from ultrasonically induced lesions in animal models. These findings combined with other clinical trial data established a firm clinical niche for surgical ultrasonic aspiration in brain and spinal cord surgery.

The advantages of ultrasonic aspiration, including selective tissue removal, a clear surgical field, and decreased blood loss and tissue trauma, prompted widened interest in the use of this modality outside neurosurgery. In 1979, Hodgson et al.[5-7] described the result of USA application in both laboratory and clinical settings. Animal studies were performed in which comparative biopsy samples were taken from the liver, spleen, stomach, small bowel, kidney, and lung by using a scalpel and the USA. The USA caused necrosis only 2 to 3 cells beyond the cut edge, which was only slightly greater than destruction observed with the scalpel. No difference in healing was noted between the USA and scalpel. Superior results were found when using the ultrasonic modality for liver and spleen surgery to selectively remove tissue, control cauterization, or preserve blood vessels. The parenchyma of the liver was removed while small vessels were cauterized and larger blood vessels were preserved and easily visualized for hemostatic clamping. Similar results were obtained for pancreatic surgery; prominent blood vessels and ducts were preserved by running the surgical aspirator parallel to the course of these structures. The USA performance was also excellent in selectively stripping the mucosa of bowel for villous adenomas, with subsequent normal mucosal regeneration. Lung and stomach dissections with the USA were not so successful; increased bleeding and increased time of dissection were reported. It should be noted that the capsule of these organs, including the liver and spleen, required cold knife incision before USA mesenchymal dissection for optimal results.

Hodgson employed the USA for precise hemostatic control to preserve normal anatomy and function in gastrointestinal surgical procedures. For example, a 59-year-old male underwent fulguration of an obstructive rectal carcinoma in lieu of a diverting colostomy. The procedure provided excellent palliation with minimal blood loss. The USA was then employed with good results in several other bowel and liver resection cases for carcinoma and was used in ten patients with head and neck tumors in which both anatomy and function were preserved better than by conventional means. An initial concern that the USA might be slower than conventional methods was dispelled by laboratory and clinical assessment. The USA actually saved time by effecting improved hemostasis.[5, 7] Hodgson identified three functional components of ultrasonic surgery: tissue aspiration, incision, and dissection. These surgical procedures can be accomplished individually or in combination by altering the amount of irrigation and temperature as well as by controlling movement of the USA handpiece.

Larger, more recent series have used the USA for hepatic resections with excellent results in patients with primary and secondary liver tumors. Little and Holland[8] reported a series of 50 consecutive liver resections, half of which were performed with the USA. Benefits found in the USA-treated group included a significant reduction in blood loss, mean hospital stay, and transfusion rate. These findings were confirmed in a series by Fasulo et al.[9] in which 34 hepatic resections were performed with the USA and compared with historical controls. Resections with the USA exhibited decreased morbidity, including decreased blood loss, without any change in mean operative time.

Adaptation of the USA to urologic surgery by Chopp et al.[10] and Addonizio et al.[11] followed in the early to mid-1980s. Contrary to Hodgson's findings, partial nephrectomy with the USA resulted in a marked reduction of blood loss relative to both electrocautery and the cold scalpel. The USA was able to fragment and aspirate parenchyma selectively while preserving higher collagen content tissue consisting of collecting system ducts and blood vessels. These findings were confirmed by laboratory and clinical trials in which the renal artery was spared. Biopsy of resection margins showed that the depth of cell damage imparted by the USA was equal to that by cold knife but less than one third that seen with electrocautery. After 3 weeks, healing in animal models was equal between those treated with the USA, electrocautery, and cold knife. The optimal power setting for partial nephrectomy was 50% fragmentation vs. 80% to 90% fragmentation used for partial hepatectomy. A dragging maneuver of the handpiece that relies on tactile feedback facilitated excellent aspiration and visualization of blood vessels 2 mm or greater in renal parenchyma. Clinical trials with partial nephrectomy validated animal studies; the average blood loss was reduced from 1,000 to 250 mL in a large series of patients.

The promising results obtained in neurologic, urologic, and general surgery prompted adaption of the USA to gynecologic surgery. Once again, the ability to selectively remove tissue while decreasing blood loss and operating time served to intensify interest in the USA. Vascular soft tissue masses in gynecologic oncology patients are often encountered in areas in which they are difficult to remove by cold knife. Resolution of this intraoperative dilemma coupled with the importance of optimal cytoreduction in certain gynecologic malignancies formed the basis for introduction of the USA into gynecologic oncology. Since its introduction, several other uses of the USA in gynecology have emerged and will be discussed later.

PHYSICS OF THE ULTRASONIC SURGICAL ASPIRATOR

In order to better understand how the USA functions, a brief discussion of the physical principles of sound wave propagation is helpful. Ultrasound waves exceed the frequency of sound detected by human hearing

(>18,000 Hz) and are longitudinal, which allows these waves to be focused. The velocity of the wave depends on the density or viscosity of the medium through which it is transmitted and can be expressed mathematically as frequency (hertz) × wavelength (λ) (Table 1). The frequency of a wave is the number of peaks or troughs that pass a particular point per unit of time. The wavelength is the distance between these peaks or troughs (Fig 1). Therefore, the velocity of a sound wave is dependent largely on the density of the transmission media. The velocity of sound in air (330 m/sec) is exceeded by that in liquid (about 1,500 m/sec), which is further exceeded by the velocity of sound in solids (2,000 to 12,000 m/sec). In discussing the function of the USA, the medium of interest is primarily liquid in both the intracellular and extracellular compartments. Thus a sound wave is actually the transmission of a pressure disturbance, and this alternating increase and decrease in pressure above and below ambient pressure causes particulates within the liquid to be displaced back and forth as the wave propagates through the liquid.

The physical properties that govern generation of sound waves can be viewed as the delivery of a sudden change of energy that results in the rapid vaporization of fluid and resultant rapid radial expansion of gases.[12] A spherically expanding wave of compressed fluid forms and exists at increased pressure, temperature, and density relative to the surrounding fluid. The sinusoidal ultrasonic wave propagates at discrete frequencies described as positive (or compressive) and negative (or tensile pressures)[12] (Fig 1). It is the generation of the negative-pressure component during rarefication that leads to the formation of bubbles in fluid. This phenomenon is known as cavitation and, in simplistic terms, can be thought of as a boiling water effect. A decrease in pressure causes an increase in the size of these submicroscopic bubbles, and an increase in pressure causes the bubbles to rapidly collapse. This collapse causes large instantaneous increases in pressure and temperature within the bubbles and results in energy transfer and tissue destruction (Fig 2). Indeed, local temperatures of 5,000 K have been measured as a result of high-intensity

---

TABLE 1.

Physics of Ultrasonic Aspiration

1.	Velocity = Frequency × Wavelength
	$V = f \times \lambda$
	Example: v = 5,000 m/sec
	f = 23,000 Hz (common USA frequency)
	$\lambda = \dfrac{5,000 \text{ m/sec}}{23 \text{ kHz}}$
	$\lambda = \dfrac{500,000 \text{ cm/sec}}{23,000 \text{ cycles/sec}}$
	λ = 21.7 cm
2.	Wave amplitude $\propto \dfrac{1}{\text{Cross-sectional area of tip}}$
3.	Intensity $\propto$ Amplitude

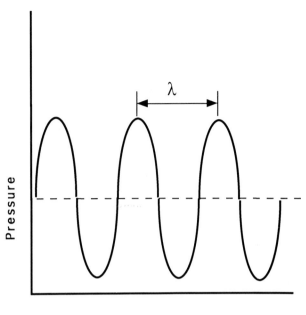

Time

FIGURE 1.

Sinusoidal ultrasonic wave. The ultrasonic wave propagates at discrete frequencies in a sinusoidal pattern. One wavelength, represented by λ, is the distance between successive peaks or troughs, and the frequency is the number of peaks or troughs that pass a particular point per second.

ultrasound-induced cavitation.[13] Violent high-energy microjets of liquid have also been associated with cavitation. The cavitation effect of ultrasound depends on the sound velocity, density, and acoustic impedance of the material that the wave strikes. Materials composed of high water content have lower densities and acoustic impedances and thus an increased susceptibility to ultrasonic cavitation and resultant tissue fragmentation.

One concern in the use of diagnostic ultrasound is the generation of waves capable of producing cavitation. Even if these pulsed waves produced only transient cavitation, free radicals might be generated that could cause biological damage by nonthermal and nonmechanical means. Free radicals have been found after diagnostic ultrasound exposure in both amniotic fluid and blood plasma; no biologically deleterious effect has ever been documented, however.[14] The threshold for transient cavitation has been found to increase with shorter pulses or higher frequencies.[15] Thus the potential for cavitation can be reduced in diagnostic ultrasound by increasing the frequency of the pulsed waves. Conversely, the ability of the USA to fragment target tissue can be enhanced by decreasing pulse frequencies. Consequently, the frequency of medical diagnostic ultrasound is in the megahertz range, whereas that of treatment ultrasound is in the kilohertz range. With maximal USA power output at 100 W with a 2-mm-diameter tip, power density is 25×10^5 mW/cm^2, and the energy output of diagnostic ultrasound is less than 10 mW/cm^2.

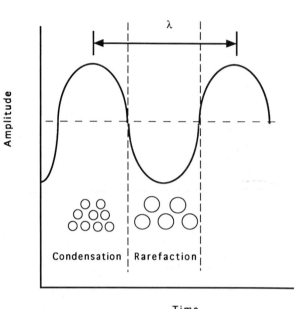

FIGURE 2.

As an ultrasonic wave propagates, a local pressure disturbance is created with pressures rising and falling relative to ambient pressures, which creates alternating areas of compression and rarefaction. This dynamic process causes submicroscopic bubbles in liquid media to expand during rarefaction and then rapidly collapse during condensation, which results in the release of energy. This energy release causes tissue destruction locally and represents the phenomenon of cavitation.

The physical properties of the USA are generated from the transducer, which converts electrical energy into mechanical motion. Ultrasonic waves can be generated from magnetostrictive transducer devices or piezoelectric crystal transducers. When the transducer is a magnetostrictive device, it is usually composed of nickel alloy laminations that increase and decrease in size when placed in an alternating magnetic field generated by electric current. The velocity of sound in the nickel alloy is 5,000 m/sec. The operating frequency of the USA operating tip is generally 23,000 Hz. Therefore, the wavelength can be calculated (velocity = frequency × wavelength) as 21.7 cm (Table 1). The mechanical vibrations generated are relayed to the operating tip and in turn to the tissue. The length from the end of the nickel alloy transducer to the end of the operational probe is one wavelength, and the unit functions as a resonant body. A piezoelectric transducer uses the vibration of crystals in an electric field to generate mechanical vibrations. The use of crystals allows for production of a lighter handpiece, which is an important feature in some USA applications. The diameter of the operating tip is also important since the amplitude of the generated wave is inversely proportional to the cross-sectional area of the tip (Table 1). Thus, the amplitude of the wave can be increased as the tip area is decreased. The standard amplitude of vibration at the end of the operating tip is 350 μm.

Considering the physical principles discussed previously, one can understand the selectivity of the USA. Biological tissues can be divided into those with high water content and those with low water (high collagen) content. Not only the parenchyma of the liver, kidney, and spleen but also many tumors have high water content. Connective tissue and blood vessel walls have low water (high collagen) content. Tissues with high water content preferentially undergo cavitation resulting in tissue destruction. All biological tissues contain water, and all tissues are susceptible to the ultrasonic-generated forces of cavitation. It is the differential water content of these tissues that imparts the selectivity and precision in tissue fragmentation witnessed in the USA applications.

THE ULTRASONIC SURGICAL ASPIRATOR UNIT

The machine consists of a console, foot pedal, and handpiece. The foot pedal allows activation of the tip vibration and irrigation modes. This pedal frees the surgeon's hands for operation of the handpiece and adds an element of safety to the unit. The console (Fig 3) essentially allows control of the handpiece. Fragmentation, irrigation, and aspiration settings can be individually varied from the console. The fragmentation mode is adjusted by controlling the amplitude of the vibrational wave by

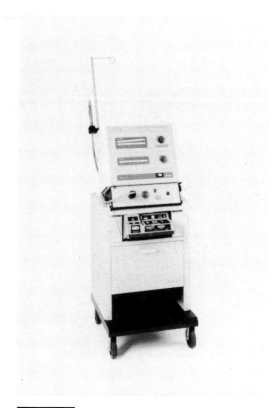

FIGURE 3.

The console is the control panel that permits modulation of the various functions of the USA handpiece. The amplitude of the ultrasonic wave can be adjusted to vary the operating tip excursion from 0 to 350 μm.

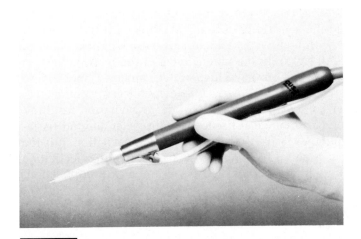

FIGURE 4.

The lightweight USA handpiece facilitates precise control. The handpiece is the operational part of the USA system that permits aspiration, irrigation, and suction.

excursion of the operational tip (from 0 to 350 μm). A 15-foot cable from the console to the handpiece carries electrical wiring and water for handpiece cooling and irrigation.

The functional portion of the USA is contained within the lightweight, gas-sterilizable, pencil-grip handpiece (Figs 4 and 5). The electrical current is carried from the outlet through the console and connecting

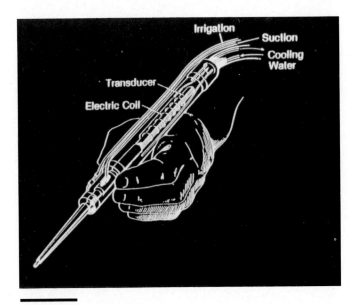

FIGURE 5.

A diagram of the components that constitute the functional handpiece is shown. The main components are the cable, transducer, coupler, and functional tip. The cable carries power and water irrigant, and the magnetostrictive helix or piezoelectric transducer converts electric energy to mechanical motion, which is then amplified by the coupler.

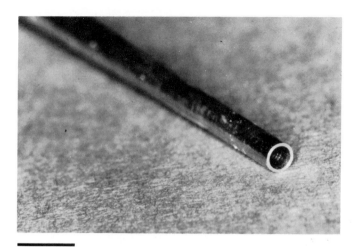

FIGURE 6.

The functional tip is composed of durable titanium and is coned to a diameter of 2 mm at the aspirating end.

cable to the piezoelectric or magnetostrictive device, which converts this energy into mechanical motion at the site of the operating tip, which oscillates along its axis at an ultrasonic frequency of 23,000 Hz. Because vibrational energy and frequency can deteriorate the probe tip, the tip is manufactured from titanium, which is relatively resistant to these forces. Housed in a protective plastic flue, the hollow tip is tapered to a diameter of 2 mm, which increases the amplitude of the vibrational wave (Fig 6). The significant heat generated at the operating tip allows cauterization of small vessels. Tissue damage and removal are limited to within a 1- to 2-mm radius of the tip. Irrigation is released around the operational tip from a separate tubing source at a rate of 3 to 10 mL/min; this irrigant facilitates both tip cooling and clearing of the surgical field. The nickel alloy composing the magnetostrictive device or the piezoelectric crystal sources is surrounded by a stainless steel, water-cooled jacket. Aspiration of the products of cavitation in the surgical field occurs through the hollow titanium probe tip. Material can be collected in a sterile trap for later histologic analysis.

The net dynamic effect of this unit, then, is that ultrasonic energy transmitted to the tissue causes cavitation and fragmentation. These particles are simultaneously aspirated, and irrigation can be employed to facilitate aspiration and control probe tip temperature. The USA is a safe, sensitive instrument capable of selective tissue removal while allowing tactile feedback to the operating surgeon.

ULTRASONIC SURGICAL ASPIRATOR IN GYNECOLOGIC ONCOLOGY

Beginning in middle to late 1980s, the USA was used on gynecologic oncology patients. The selectivity of the USA is well suited to tumors of gynecologic origin (Table 2). The tumor is readily aspirated because of its high water content, and collagen-rich blood vessels can be isolated

---

TABLE 2.

Ultrasonic Aspiration Potential in
Gynecologic Oncology

Tumor debulking from
  Diaphragm
  Small bowel
  Large bowel
  Bowel mesenteries
  Peritoneal surfaces
  Ureter
  Renal capsule
  Retroperitoneal nodes
  Spleen
  Liver
  Vagina
Vulvar intraepithelial neoplasia
Vaginal intraepithelial neoplasia
Laparoscopic lymph node removal

---

for clamping and ligation or for cauterization by using the USA tip. In addition to intra-abdominal surgery, the USA has been shown to be an effective modality in the treatment of lower genital tract lesions. These applications will be discussed individually by anatomic site.

OVARY AND FALLOPIAN TUBE

Ovarian carcinoma, which ranks highest in mortality of all gynecologic malignancies in the United States, and fallopian tube carcinoma, which accounts for fewer than 1% of all gynecologic malignancies, are both most effectively treated by surgical removal of all gross tumor.[16-18] Cancers of primary peritoneal origin with müllerian differentiation are generally grouped with epithelial ovarian tumors and are similarly treated. The therapeutic goal of optimal cytoreduction, variously defined as no residual tumor implants greater than 0.5 to 2.0 cm in diameter, is often difficult to achieve since up to 75% of patients are initially seen with advanced disease.[16] Achieving optimal cytoreduction is often limited by intimate tumor adherence to abdominal viscera such as the liver, spleen, diaphragm, and gastrointestinal tract. When optimal cytoreduction or, ideally, the removal of all gross disease can be realized, the response to chemotherapy and the 5-year disease-free and overall survival rates are increased.[16, 18]

Clearly, aggressive cytoreductive surgery is important in the treatment of patients with disseminated müllerian epithelial tumors, and any tool that optimizes tumor debulking would be valuable. The previous clinical reports that evaluated the USA in neurosurgical and general surgical applications prompted trials in tumor debulking in gynecologic oncology patients. In 1988, Adelson and associates[19] published the first report that detailed the clinical experience with the USA to obtain optimal cytoreduction in nine patients with epithelial ovarian carcinoma and one patient with fallopian tube cancer. The mean age of these patients was 65 years, and eight of ten patients had stage IIIC disease. All bulky disease in the pelvis and omentum was removed by conventional techniques (bilateral salpingo-oophorectomy, hysterectomy, and omentectomy). The USA was then employed to remove disease from the diaphragm, spleen, stomach, and small and large bowel to achieve optimal cytoreduction (all residual implants less than or equal to 0.5 cm) in nine of ten patients. It was estimated that four rectosigmoid, two abdominal colon, and two small bowel resections were prevented by the USA. Notably, the USA required an additional 49 minutes of operative time. Ten patients were excluded from this consecutive series, five because they had no gross disease and five because they had unresectable tumor (since bulky periaortic disease was deemed unresectable). No intraoperative or postoperative complications were reported in this series.

Also in 1988, Deppe and colleagues[20] reported on a second series of ovarian carcinoma patients in which the USA was used for optimal cytoreduction in 11 patients with stage III ovarian carcinoma (residual diameter not defined). Tumor that traditionally would be difficult to resect without removal of nongenital viscera was debulked with the USA. No intraoperative complications were reported, and blood loss was decreased (difference in mean blood loss volume not stated). Postoperatively, 2 patients experienced ileus, and a superficial wound infection developed in 1 patient. The USA was subjectively judged to increase resection time and was much less effective when tumor tissue was densely fibrotic.

USA application for debulking advanced ovarian carcinoma with an emphasis on diaphragmatic metastases was subsequently reported in another series by Deppe et al.[21] consisting of 12 patients in whom no complications were reported. Diaphragmatic metastases are common in ovarian cancer, and the fear of sharp dissection with possible diaphragmatic perforation is a concern when attempting to debulk implants in this area. The USA in our experience has been very useful in attaining optimal cytoreduction in patients with widespread diaphragmatic involvement. Techniques for diaphragm debulking include extension of the midline incision cephalad to the xiphoid process followed by transection of the falciform ligament and mobilization of the liver posteriorly. The ventilation rate is decreased as tolerated to limit diaphragm movement during aspiration.

Another subset of patients in whom optimal cytoreduction has been difficult to achieve is those with splenic metastases. In order to achieve optimal cytoreduction before the advent of the USA, these patients required splenectomy, which is associated with a variety of postoperative complications including thrombocytosis, clotting disorders, pancreatic pseudocysts, and an increased incidence of pneumococcal pneumonia and generalized sepsis. Adelson[22] recently reported on a series of seven patients with splenic metastases in which he achieved optimal cytoreduction with residual implants less than or equal to 5 mm while preserving the spleen. Six of the seven patients had stage IIIC ovarian cancer, and one had advanced tumor of peritoneal origin. No complications were described in Adelson's series. Splenic recurrence and survival intervals were not reported. Patsner and Rose[23] had previously reported a similar series of four patients with stage IIIC ovarian cancer metastatic to the spleen in which the USA was employed to avoid splenectomy. No complications were reported, but no survival data were presented. When using the USA for removal of tumor from the spleen, the spleen is mobilized before aspiration to expose the hilar vessels in case of uncontrolled bleeding. Mobilization is performed by transecting the gastrosplenic ligament and short gastric blood vessels. When a setting of 30% to 50% amplitude is used, little bleeding is encountered.

A definite role for the USA in obtaining optimal cytoreduction has been established by these reports and by unpublished clinical experiences of ourselves and others (Fig 7). The advantage of the USA is that not only can optimal cytoreduction be obtained but functional integrity is also preserved because splenic, bowel, hepatic, and ureteric resections can be avoided. The technique that we have found most effective in debulking a tumor includes using the USA handpiece with a dragging motion parallel to the tumor surface in the suspected course of underlying blood vessels while using an amplitude of 50%. This maneuver allows visualization of large vessels for ligation or clip application. Smaller vessels can be cauterized with built-in electrocautery units available with some USA models (Fig 8). For fibrotic tumor, electrocautery with increased cutting capability may allow resection to be performed in a more expedient manner. In addition, handpiece movement is best altered for fibrotic tumor to a thrusting motion in which the tip is moved in a plane perpendicular to the tumor surface.[22]

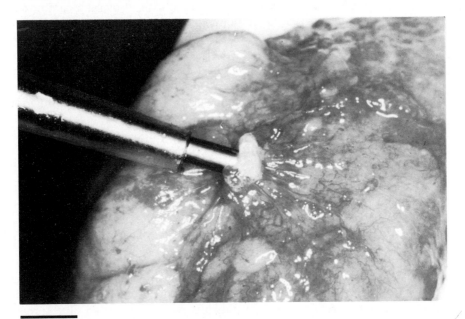

FIGURE 7.
Ultrasonic tumor aspiration by the handpiece tip permits removal of implants from bowel and mesenteric surfaces. The USA thus averts bowel resection in this patient with ovarian carcinoma while allowing optimal cytoreduction to be accomplished.

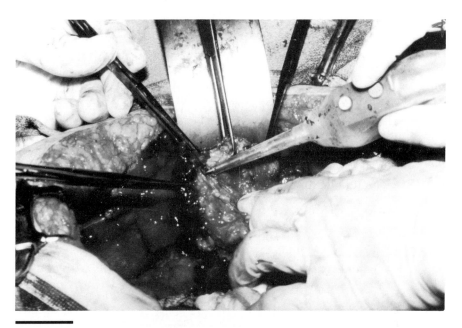

FIGURE 8.
Tumor debulking is performed in this patient with ovarian carcinoma by USA in the coagulation mode, available on some units to minimize blood loss.

UTERUS AND CERVIX

The clinical utility of the USA for treating uterine pathology has not been widely evaluated in clinical trials. Nor has any survival advantage been shown for debulking endometrial carcinoma spread beyond the pelvis. Nonetheless, the same principles of selective tissue removal relevant to ovarian debulking can be applied, especially for endometrial adenocarcinoma or sarcomas metastatic to nongenital viscera. Such selective use of the USA may obviate the need for bowel, hepatic, or splenic resection in certain cases.

The USA is generally not used for primary removal of tissue from the cervix for preinvasive or invasive disease because of the high collagen content of the cervix. The USA has been used in exenterations for centrally recurrent cervical or, occasionally, endometrial carcinomas to obtain greater margins from pelvic sidewalls or the pubic symphisis. This dissection can be accomplished hemostatically, and these additional margins can be histologically assessed for tumor involvement.

A new application of the USA in the surgical management of uterine and cervical malignancy has emerged with the recent availability of a USA laparoscopic handpiece. This handpiece can be combined with cautery and cut modes, and it is introduced through a standard 10-mm trocar port. The most obvious indications for the laparoscopic USA would be for lymph node dissections. Even in open abdominal surgery, the USA has proved effective in meticulously removing lymph-bearing tissue surrounding retroperitoneal vessels and nerves. Potentially, the USA may be employed for laparoscopic lymph node sampling in staging cervical and endometrial carcinomas. In the treatment of endometrial carcinoma, such

procedures may be combined with laparoscopic-assisted vaginal hysterectomy and bilateral salpingo-oophorectomy. A rabbit model was used
to assess the laparoscopic potential of the USA by Hurst et al.[24] The results of this analysis showed that the USA was comparable to Nd:YAG
laser and bipolar cautery with regard to pelvic sidewall adhesion formation. The USA offered a larger safety margin than did Nd:YAG and bipolar cautery, which were found to cause deeper tissue injury than desired.
The therapeutic safety and efficacy of laparoscopic ultrasonic aspiration
for lymph node dissections remain to be established in clinical trials;
nonetheless, the theoretical benefit of performing a hemostatic, thorough
lymph node dissection laparoscopically is very promising.

VULVA

The USA has been shown to be an effective modality for the treatment of
vulvar intraepithelial neoplasia (VIN) and condyloma of the vulva. Rader
and colleagues[25] reported on a series of 27 patients with noninvasive vulvar disease, 9 of whom had VIN and 18 had condylomata acuminata

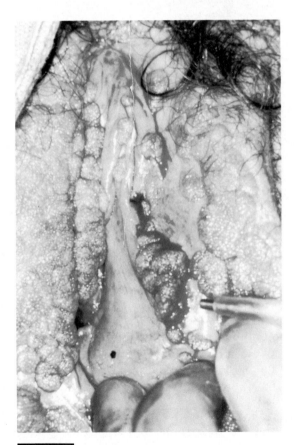

FIGURE 9.

Ultrasonic aspiration is employed to aspirate vulvar condyloma. Aspiration depth
is 2.0 to 2.5 mm for vulvar intraepithelial neoplasia and condylomas of the
vulva.[26] (From Rader J, Leake J, Dillon M, et al: *Obstet Gynecol* 1991; 77:573–
576. Used by permission.)

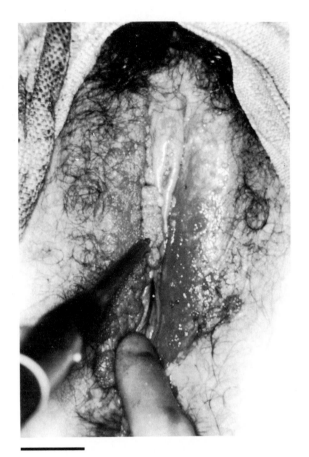

FIGURE 10.
This is the same patient as in Figure 9 with extensive condyloma of the vulva. The epithelium has been removed from the left half of the vulva by ultrasonic aspiration without charring.[26] (From Rader J, Leake J, Dillon M, et al: *Obstet Gynecol* 1991; 77:573–576. Used by permission.)

(Fig 9). Vibrating tip movement in a back-and-forth motion was performed to allow rapid epithelial removal without thermal injury to a final depth of 2 to 2.5 mm (Fig 10). An amplitude setting of 5 to 6 was employed to produce cellular fragmentation to a depth of 150 to 180 μm. Silver sulfadiazine cream was applied to the vulva following aspiration. Excellent cosmetic results with complete reepithelialization and no scarring were achieved by 5 weeks postoperatively (Fig 11). Two of the 27 patients had to be hospitalized for pain control and perineal care; no other complications of USA therapy to the vulva were reported. Recurrent disease occurred in 4 of 18 patients treated for condyloma and in 2 of the 9 cases of VIN with a mean follow-up time of 50 weeks. Importantly, the USA yielded material adequate for histopathologic diagnosis in the form of microbiopsies. All samples correlated with the clinical impression or preoperative biopsy result. The USA-generated tissue samples were also collected in a form acceptable for human papillomavirus (HPV) genotyping.

Treating intraepithelial neoplasia with the USA demonstrates the precise, hemostatic nature of this tool, and it also illustrates the potential

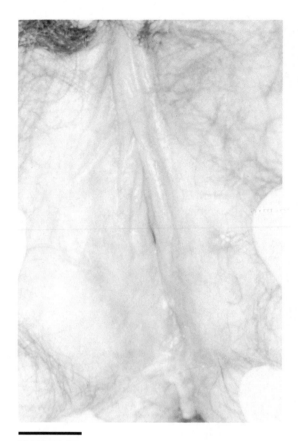

FIGURE 11.

A photograph of the patient in Figures 9 and 10 demonstrates excellent healing without scar formation 4 weeks after ultrasonic aspiration of the vulva.[26] (From Rader J, Leake J, Dillon M, et al: *Obstet Gynecol* 1991; 77:573–576. Used by permission.)

benefits of ultrasonic aspiration relative to established techniques such as laser vaporization. The main advantage of the USA in treating intraepithelial neoplasia and even condylomata is that biopsy tissue is available to possibly exclude invasive malignancy. The ability to exclude invasive disease is lost when destructive forms of therapy such as cryosurgery or chemical or laser ablation are used. An additional benefit of the USA over lasers is its greater margin of safety. Lasers in the operating room have been associated with a number of mishaps, including thermal injury to patients, to surgical drapes, and to rectal effluent. Another concern has been the production of a gas plume by lasers, which has been implicated as a possible carcinogen. These problems are largely averted with USA techniques. The potential for dispersion of tissue fragments by the USA is presently unknown; therefore, the usual operating room precautions of mask and protective eyewear should be implemented.

VAGINA

The USA can be employed for the treatment of vaginal intraepithelial neoplasia (VAIN) in a manner similar to that used for the treatment of VIN.

The specimens obtained with the USA can be assessed pathologically. Limitations of the USA in treating VAIN include those of other modalities used in treating VAIN, which consist principally of difficult access, exposure to the anterior vaginal wall, and a furrowed vaginal cuff, especially following hysterectomy. The USA can be used to remove tissue to a depth of 2 mm when no clinical, histologic, or colposcopic evidence of invasive disease is present. The USA treatment of intraepithelial neoplasia has been more completely discussed under Ultrasonic Surgical Aspirator in Gynecologic Oncology, Vulva.

Another application for the USA is palliative resection of tumors in the vagina. Deppe and coworkers[26] reported several cases of ovarian and endometrial primary tumors metastatic to the vagina that required surgical intervention to minimize bleeding and control tumor volume. The USA was successful in controlling bleeding even after packing, cautery, cryosurgery, and microfibrillar collagen had failed. These patients had also received irradiation and chemotherapy. The local control of tumor in the vagina was temporary, but no complications were reported.

WOUND HEALING

Assessment of wound healing following ultrasonic aspiration has generally been very favorable. Comparison of the USA to the carbon dioxide (CO_2) laser was performed by Rader and coworkers[27] in the laboratory on ten Hartley guinea pigs. Porcine skin histologically resembles human skin and is an established model for assessing wound healing. The back of each pig was marked with eight patches, 1 cm^2 each, that were ablated or resected alternately between laser and the USA to level of the mid-dermis. Histologic parameters of tissue damage and wound repair were assessed from 0 hours to 28 days, and peak inflammation, depth of collagen denaturation, reepithelialization, and healing at 28 days were similar in the laser- and USA-treated groups. The USA was found to be easier to control and more precise in removing tissue within the 1 cm^2 than was the laser.

Hambley and others[28] compared wound healing of skin incisions caused by a conventional scalpel, electrosurgery, CO_2 laser, and an ultrasonic knife. Porcine models were also used in this study, and scalpel-produced incisions were found to demonstrate the least injury and most rapid healing of all the modalities assessed. The ultrasonic knife–produced incisions caused less tissue damage and more rapid healing than did either electrosurgery or the CO_2 laser. Discrepancies between this study and Rader's can be explained in part by different instrumentation, wounding, and histopathologic assessment intervals. Overall, the USA appears to be at least as effective in resecting tissue as the laser and may be more precise with greater or equal healing potential without the attendant injurious risks of the laser.

PATHOLOGIC ANALYSIS OF ULTRASONIC ASPIRATES

The ability to obtain suitable specimens for pathologic analysis from the USA is a valuable asset over ablative therapy in the treatment of intraepithelial neoplasia and is often requisite for intra-abdominal surgery in cases of tissue margin resection or lymph node dissection. Original use of the USA in neurosurgery generated several reports that assessed the adequacy of specimens for histologic study. Silverman et al.[29] reported on the cytomorphologic appearance of 22 central nervous system tumors with cytology and cell block performed in each case. Three of the specimens were judged to be inadequate from both cytologic and cell block examination. All other specimens were able to be fully evaluated by light microscopy. Richmond and Hawksley[30] showed that two of two specimens obtained with the USA were adequate for histologic analysis and, in fact, were superior to standard biopsy specimens of brain tumor tissue.

The structural integrity of tissue removed by ultrasonic aspiration has been assessed from specimens of gynecologic origin as well. Paired tumor samples obtained by using the USA or a sharp knife from ten patients with epithelial ovarian cancer were examined by Thompson et al.[31] Hematoxylin-eosin–stained histologic sections from the USA showed very minimal distortion, and all samples were at least adequate for diagnosis. Flow cytometry with DNA analysis was used to confirm that both surgical methods produced matched samples. The excellent preservation of histologic architecture was also found in Rader and associates' series[25]

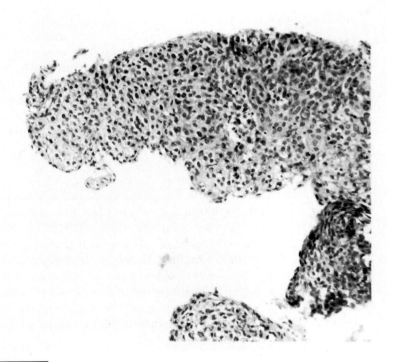

FIGURE 12.

This is a photomicrograph of a microbiopsy obtained by ultrasonic aspiration from a patient with vulvar intraepithelial neoplasia.[26] (From Rader J, Leake J, Dillon M, et al: *Obstet Gynecol* 1991; 77:573–576. Used by permission.)

in which the USA was used for VIN and condyloma; 26 of the 27 USA-obtained vulvar specimens were judged adequate. The collected tissue was in the form of microbiopsies (Fig 12).

The ability to obtain fresh sterile specimens for tissue culture purposes has become increasingly important for research, including in vitro chemosensitivity assays and viral typing. Thompson et al.[31] found no difference in initial tumor cell viability between USA- and knife-obtained specimens. Significantly, cells obtained from the USA survived and divided to a greater extent than did those obtained by knife. Both cell acquisition methods were similar with regard to the number of cell passages in culture. In a study by Oakes et al.,[32] the viability of USA-obtained specimens was further confirmed by ultrasonically aspirated human medulloblastoma cells that were successfully established in cell culture and by transplantable xenographs in immunoincompetent mice. Thus it appears that USA-obtained tissue is viable and is structurally and functionally unaltered relative to tissue obtained by conventional methods. These findings, in addition to the lack of DNA alteration on flow cytometry, suggest that tissue at resection margins left in situ is left uninjured by the USA and that the samples obtained are suitable for histopathologic analysis and tissue culture.

REFERENCES

1. Kelman CD: Phacoemulsification and aspiration. *Am J Ophthalmol* 1969; 67:464–477.
2. Kelman CD: Phacoemulsification and aspiration. A report of 500 consecutive cases. *Am J Ophthalmol* 1973; 75:764–768.
3. Flamm ES, Ransohoff J, Wuchinich D, et al: Preliminary experience with ultrasonic aspiration in neurosurgery. *Neurosurgery* 1978; 2:240–245.
4. Young W, Cohen AR, Hunt CD, et al: Acute physiologic effects of ultrasonic vibrations on nervous tissue. *Neurosurgery* 1981; 8:689–694.
5. Hodgson WJB, Poddar PK, Mencer EJ, et al: Evaluation of ultrasound powered instruments in the laboratory and in the clinical setting. *Am J Gastroenterol* 1979; 72:133–140.
6. Hodgson WJB, Sanjivani B, Harrington E, et al: General surgical evaluation of a powered device operating at ultrasonic frequencies. *Mt Sinai J Med* 1979; 46:99–103.
7. Hodgson WJB: The ultrasonic scalpel. *Buffalo N Y Acad Med* 1979; 55:908–915.
8. Little JM, Holland MJ: Impact of the CUSA and operative ultrasound on hepatic resection. *Hepatic Pancreatic Biliary Surg* 1991; 3:271–277.
9. Fasulo F, Giori A, Fissi S, et al: Cavitron ultrasonic surgical aspirator (CUSA) in liver resection. *Int Surg* 1992; 77:64–66.
10. Chopp RT, Bharat BS, Addonizio JC: Use of ultrasonic surgical aspirator in renal surgery. *Urology* 1983; 22:157–159.
11. Addonizio JC, Choudhury MS: Cavitrons in urologic surgery. *Urol Clin North Am* 1986; 13:445–454.
12. Lubock P: The physics and mechanics of lithotripters. *Dig Dis Sci* 1989; 34:999–1005.
13. Flint EB, Suslick KS: The temperature of cavitation. *Science* 1991; 253:1397–1398.
14. Crum LA, Walton AJ, Mortimer A, et al: Free radical production in amniotic

fluid and blood plasma by medical ultrasound. *J Ultrasound Med* 1987; 6:643–647.

15. Atchley AA, Frizzell LA, Apfel RE, et al: Thresholds for cavitation produced in water by pulsed ultrasound. *Ultrasonics* 1988; 26:280–285.

16. Hacker NF, Berek JS, Lagasse LD: Primary cytoreductive surgery for epithelial ovarian cancer. *Obstet Gynecol* 1983; 61:413–420.

17. Eddy GL, Copeland LJ, Gershenson DM: Fallopian tube carcinoma. *Obstet Gynecol* 1984; 64:546–552.

18. Beller U, Beckman EM, Muggia FM, et al: Surgical treatment for advanced epithelial carcinoma of the ovary. Surg Gynecol Obstet 1987; 165:279–283.

19. Adelson MD, Baggish MS, Cassell SL, et al: Cytoreduction of ovarian cancer with the cavitron ultrasonic surgical aspirator. *Obstet Gynecol* 1988; 72:140–143.

20. Deppe G, Malviya V, Malone J: Debulking surgery for ovarian cancer with the cavitron ultrasonic surgical aspirator (CUSA)—A preliminary report. *Gynecol Oncol* 1988; 31:223–226.

21. Deppe G, Malviya V, Malone J: Use of cavitron surgical aspirator for debulking of diaphragmatic metastases in patients with advanced carcinoma of the ovaries. Surg *Gynecol Obstet* 1989; 168:455–456.

22. Adelson MD: Ultrasonic surgical aspirator in cytoreduction of splenic metastases to avoid splenectomy. *J Reprod Med* 1992; 37:917–920.

23. Patsner B, Rose PG: CUSA splenorrhaphy for ovarian cytoreductive surgery. *Gynecol Oncol* 1991; 41:28–29.

24. Hurst B, Awoniyi C, Stephens J, et al: Application of the cavitron ultrasonic surgical aspirator (CUSA) for gynecologic laparoscopic surgery using the rabbit as an animal model. *Fertil Steril* 1992; 58:444–448.

25. Rader J, Leake J, Dillon M, et al: Ultrasonic surgical aspiration in the treatment of vulvar disease. *Obstet Gynecol* 1991; 77:573–576.

26. Deppe G, Malviya VK, Malone JM: Use of cavitron ultrasonic surgical aspirator for palliative resection of recurrent gynecologic malignancies involving the vagina. *Eur J Gynaecol Oncol* 1989; 10:1–3.

27. Rader J, Rest E, et al: A comparison of wound healing after epithelial resection by ultrasonic surgical aspiration and ablation by the carbon dioxide laser. *Gynecol Oncol* 1992; 46:351–356.

28. Hambley R, Hebda P, Abell E, et al: Wound healing of skin incisions produced by ultrasonically vibrating knife, scalpel, electrocautery, and carbon dioxide laser. *Dermatol Surg Oncol* 1988; 14:1213–1217.

29. Silverman J, Jones D, Unverferth M, et al: Cytopathology of neoplasms of the central nervous system in specimens obtained by the cavitron ultrasonic surgical aspirator. *Acta Cytol* 1989; 33:576–582.

30. Richmond I, Hawksley C: Evaluation of the histopathology of brain tumor tissue obtained by ultrasonic aspiration. *Neurosurgery* 1983; 13:415–419.

31. Thompson M, Adelson M, Jozefczyk M, et al: Structural and functional integrity of ovarian tumor tissue obtained by ultrasonic aspiration. *Cancer* 1991; 67:1326–1331.

32. Oakes W, Friedman H, Bigner S, et al: Successful laboratory growth and analysis of CUSA-obtained medulloblastoma samples: Technical note. *J Neurosurg* 1990; 72:821–823.

Editor's Comment

I congratulate the authors on a comprehensive review of the ultrasonic surgical aspirator in gynecologic oncology, including a section on the historical background and physics of the aspirator. I have had the opportunity to acquire experience with the ultrasonic surgical aspirator myself, and I believe it to be an essential tool in gynecologic oncology. As is discussed by Drs. Herzog and Rader, this instrumentation has resulted in a significant advance in the surgical debulking of peritoneal tumors (i.e., ovarian and fallopian tube carcinoma). Cytoreductive surgery has been maximized without increasing intraoperative and postoperative morbidity. Utilization of the ultrasonic surgical aspirator allows safe removal of tumor from the diaphragm, small bowel, colon, liver, and spleen capsule without surgically resecting these organs. The ultrasonic surgical aspirator also permits dissection of tumor in places that traditionally have required en bloc resection.

The ultrasonic surgical aspirator has proved advantageous in performing pelvic exenterations and radical hysterectomies. The surgeon can obtain greater margins adjacent to the pelvic sidewall and pubic symphisis with improved hemostasis when using the ultrasonic surgical aspirator.

Laparoscopic handpieces, devices that will improve our ability to perform laparoscopic lymph node dissections as well as second-look laparoscopy and surgical staging, are presently being introduced to the clinical setting. Dr. Rader, one of the chapter's contributing authors, has published extensively on the use of the ultrasonic surgical aspirator in vulvar disease and wound healing. This modality has proved effective in the treatment of both vulvar vaginal intraepithelial neoplasia and condyloma acuminatum. The ultrasonic surgical aspirator provides a specimen that may be evaluated histologically. Dr. Rader's review of aspirated specimens concluded that 26 of 27 specimens had excellent preservation of histologic architecture and were easily evaluated.

The ultrasonic surgical aspirator has proved to be an effective addition to the surgical instrumentation used in treating the gynecologic oncology patient. Its use will continue to be refined and redefined during the 1990s.

Ira R. Horowitz, M.D.

Molecular Biology of Gynecological Tumors

KATHLEEN R. CHO, M.D.

LORA HEDRICK, M.D.

U nderstanding the etiology and pathogenesis of human tumors has been a goal pursued by both clinical and basic science researchers for many years. Over the past decade, the application of molecular biological techniques has led to the identification of numerous genes that are thought to be important in human tumorigenesis. Furthermore, these studies have provided models that have had a major impact on our concept of how most human tumors develop. In this chapter, we will provide a general background on current concepts of the molecular basis of human tumors. The progression of colorectal tumors will be used as a model because it is one of the most thoroughly studied at the molecular level. This model provides a framework for many of the basic concepts of tumorigenesis and provides specific examples of the types of genes that are believed to play significant roles in the development of most human tumors. Within this framework we will then highlight what is known about the molecular genetics of each major gynecologic tumor type.

BACKGROUND

Epidemiologic studies have led many investigators to support the theory that the development of most if not all human tumors is a multistep process. However, the biological events underlying this process have been unclear. Recently, studies of colorectal tumorigenesis have established a model for the molecular basis of the multistep theory. Several factors make colorectal cancer particularly suitable for these types of studies. Perhaps most important, pathologists had observed that colorectal cancers arise from normal colorectal epithelium through a continuum of recognizable lesions called adenomas, which grow in size, develop increasing cytologic abnormalities, and progress finally to frankly invasive carcinomas. Therefore, researchers believed that this system might provide a good model for the progressive development of human tumors in vivo. In addition, colorectal tumors are common, and tissue from all the lesions in the progression can be obtained through either colonoscopic biopsy or surgical resection. Each lesion can therefore be studied at the molecular level. Through a series of sophisticated molecular genetic techniques investigators have identified several genes that are now believed to be at

Advances in Obstetrics and Gynecology, vol 1
© 1994, Mosby–Year Book, Inc.

least partly responsible for the development of colorectal cancer. The genes identified fall into two major categories: tumor suppressor genes and oncogenes. It is thought that alterations of these two types of genes are involved in the development of the vast majority of human tumors. Understanding the nature of these genes and the normal function of their gene products is therefore critical to unraveling the etiology and pathogenesis of cancer.

Tumor suppressor genes can be defined as genes whose gene products contribute to the neoplastic process when they are inactivated through any of several molecular mechanisms. During tumor development, it is generally thought that both gene copies must be inactivated in order for phenotypic effects to be manifested. For this reason, tumor suppressor genes are often referred to as "recessive" genes. One gene copy is often inactivated through point mutation, rearrangement, or relatively small deletional events. In many tumors, the second copy is inactivated through loss of a substantial portion of the chromosome containing the remaining wild-type allele. For this reason, losses of specific chromosomal regions in tumors, also known as allelic losses or losses of heterozygosity (LOH), are thought to target tumor suppressor genes. Consequently, analyses of various tumors for specific and frequent LOH have been used to identify tumor suppressor genes involved in the development of these specific tumor types. Because tumor suppressor genes contribute to tumorigenesis through their inactivation, it is generally accepted that the proteins they encode control cell proliferation in a negative fashion, although the mechanisms by which they control cell proliferation remain little understood. However, recent experimental evidence suggests that genes in this class may have quite diverse functions. Some appear to directly control cell proliferation through regulation of DNA synthesis, whereas others exert their effects indirectly through transcriptional regulation of other genes, which in turn influence cell growth. Other possible mechanisms for controlling cell growth are the regulation of both differentiation and cellular senescence. Terminal differentiation, which controls the number of subsequent cell divisions a cell may undertake, is a mechanism that must obviously be bypassed in tumorigenesis. Terminal differentiation and senescence may be linked in that they both control the life span of cells. However, the mechanisms by which they do so may be quite different. Therefore, it is possible that different sets of genes control the two processes and several of the involved genes could represent potential tumor suppressor genes that have yet to be identified.

Two of the most well-characterized tumor suppressor genes are p53 and Rb, which lie on chromosomes 17p and 13q, respectively. Rb was originally identified as the gene responsible for the childhood eye tumor retinoblastoma. At the genetic level, it is most commonly inactivated by interstitial deletions creating nonfunctional proteins.[1] The Rb gene encodes a nuclear protein that is thought to be involved in cell cycle control. A very recent study has also suggested a role for Rb in the control of cellular differentiation.[2] Rb mutations have been identified in several other tumor types, including osteosarcomas. The p53 gene is currently recognized as the most frequently altered gene in human tumors inasmuch as it is mutated in a wide variety of tumors. Like Rb, p53 encodes a nuclear protein that is known to bind DNA in a sequence-specific manner. Experimental evidence supports its role as a transcriptional regulator that controls cellular proliferation by regulating genes important in the cell cycle. Five other tumor suppressor genes have been identified, but little is known about the normal function of their gene products. With time, many more tumor suppressor genes will be identified. Understanding their normal functions will provide not only insights into the mechanisms of tumorigenesis but also a better understanding of normal developmental processes.

The other major class of genes altered in human tumors is oncogenes. These genes, in contrast to tumor suppressor genes, play a role in tumorigenesis when they are activated by a mutational event. Many more oncogenes have been identified than tumor suppressor genes, with a current total of approximately 50 to 60. Historically, they were identified as cellular counterparts to the transforming genes of "oncogenic" viruses. They tend to behave in a "dominant" fashion, i.e., require the activation of only one copy of the gene and leave the other in its wild-type state. The products of oncogenes are thought to be involved in controlling cell growth and proliferation in a positive manner. Thus it is understandable why the wild-type copy of the gene does not interfere with the mutant gene. The most common molecular mechanisms for activating oncogenes are gene amplification, point mutation, and rearrangement. All of these mechanisms essentially lead to the persistent "on" state of the gene product, which provides the constant proliferative stimulus necessary in tumorigenesis.

The colorectal carcinoma system is a paradigm of tumorigenesis based on the concept that tumor development involves both the inactivation of tumor suppressor genes and the activation of oncogenes. Furthermore, this model suggests that it is not the exact order in which the gene mutations occur that is critical; rather, it is the overall accumulation of these mutations that underlies the pathogenesis of neoplasia. Thus the multistep theory of tumorigenesis, recognized long before the advent of molecular oncology, translates at the molecular level into the requirement for the accumulation, in the same cell, of mutations in several tumor suppressor genes and oncogenes. It is obvious that numerous mechanisms that normally control cellular proliferation and differentiation must be overcome during the development and progression of human tumors.

GYNECOLOGIC TUMORS

In the United States alone, tumors of the female genital tract account for nearly 72,000 new cases and 24,000 cancer deaths each year.[3] The cancers that arise in the female genital tract consist of a wide variety of tumors with distinct clinical and histopathologic characteristics. It is not surprising then that there may be differences in the molecular alterations that underlie the various tumor types. However, there is reason to believe that the different tumor types may have some similarities at the molecular level. The majority of gynecologic tumors arise from epithelia lining the genital tract and covering the surface of the ovaries. These epithelia are derived embryologically from coelomic mesothelium, which gives rise to the ovarian surface epithelium and luminal epithelia of the fallopian tubes (serous), uterine corpus (endometrioid), uterine cervix (mucinous and squamous), and upper third of the vagina (squamous). Therefore, understanding the common developmental origin of these epithelia provides a unifying framework that can be used to conceptualize the histopathologic complexity of tumors arising at these sites and the molecular genetic alterations that underlie their development.

CERVICAL CANCER

In 1991, there were approximately 13,000 new cases of cervical cancer and 4,500 cervical cancer deaths in the United States. The majority of cervical cancers are squamous carcinomas and are preceded by squamous intraepithelial lesions (cervical intraepithelial neoplasia [CIN]). Widespread screening techniques involving examination of exfoliated cervical epithelium (Papanicolaou smears) have significantly reduced the incidence and death rate of cervical cancer. The identification and detection of precursor lesions and early cancers leads to therapeutic intervention in the premalignant and early (curable) stages of the disease. Consequently, the death rate from cervical cancer is relatively low in the United States. However, cervical cancer has been ranked as the predominant form of cancer in developing countries in at least one study.[4]

The sexual transmission of some factor or factors has consistently been implicated by epidemiologic studies as contributing to cervical tumorigenesis since virginity confers nearly complete protection from cervical cancer. Two DNA viruses, herpes simplex virus (HSV) and human papillomavirus (HPV), commonly infect the lower genital tract and have been extensively studied as possible etiologic agents. Early serologic and cytologic studies found a strong association between HSV-2 infection and cervical neoplasia. This association has not been supported by more recent molecular studies. In addition, at least one large prospective epidemiologic study failed to show a role for HSV-2 infection in the development of cervical cancer.[5] Thus, HSV as a causative agent has lost considerable favor.

In 1976, zur Hausen[6] proposed that certain types of HPVs were better candidates for sexually transmissible agents involved in cervical tumorigenesis. A large amount of data over the past several years accumulated from numerous immunohistochemical, molecular biological, and epidemiologic studies supports this hypothesis. Papillomaviruses are small, double-stranded DNA viruses with an 8-kilobase (kb) circular genome enclosed in a 55-nm viral capsid. Most infections by HPV cause benign cell proliferations consisting of common warts when occurring on the skin, and condylomas when occurring on the genitalia. Based on DNA sequence analyses, over 60 different types of HPVs have been identified. The different types of HPVs show host cell specificity, with approximately 20 types infecting the female genital tract. However, a single host may be infected with more than one type of HPV. The HPV types that infect the female genital tract can be broadly classified into two groups: those associated with benign or regressing lesions (primarily HPVs 6 and 11) and those strongly associated with the development of carcinoma (primarily HPVs 16, 18, and 31). These groups are based on extensive examination of the association of different types of HPV with cervical condylomas, CIN, and cervical cancers. The biological behavior of the two groups is further reflected by the fact that transfection of primary keratinocytes in vitro with cloned DNA from the high-risk but not the low risk types causes their immortalization.[7, 8] Furthermore, it has been found that in nearly all invasive cervical cancers, "oncogenic" or "high-risk" HPV types can be detected.[9] Human papillomavirus is usually maintained as a free circular molecule (episome) in condylomas and in CIN, whereas the viral DNA is integrated into the host genome in most invasive tumors and tumor cell lines.[10] The site in the host genome into which the virus integrates does not appear to be specific because several studies have failed to demonstrate a common point of integration. However, there have been at least two reports of integration of papillomavirus sequences near cellular oncogenes (specifically c-*myc* and n-*myc*) in a few cervical cancers and cancer cell lines.[11, 12] The integration of viral sequences near cellular proto-oncogenes is one mechanism that can potentially lead to oncogene overexpression/activation by interrupting the genes' normal regulatory sequences. Although the viral integration site in the host DNA may be variable, the site where the viral DNA breaks during integration is remarkably consistent. The viral genome consists of numerous overlapping open reading frames (ORFs) encoding the proteins necessary for productive viral infection. Several viral genes are expressed soon after infection and are therefore referred to as "early" genes. Their gene products are thought to be important in regulating the expression of other viral genes. In almost all cases, viral integration interrupts the early genes E1 and/or E2, which are located near the early genes E6 and E7, which remain intact. The E6 and E7 genes from "oncogenic" HPV types can immortalize primary keratinocytes in vitro in the absence of other viral sequences.[13] The E6 and E7 genes from low-risk viral types do not have this same capability. Experimental evidence suggests that the integration event may serve to release E6 and E7 from normal transcriptional regulation by E2. This deregulation of E6 and E7 expression may be critical to the biological behavior of the high-risk types, hence their association with cervical cancer.

Numerous women with histologically and colposcopically normal cervices appear to be infected with oncogenic HPV types, thus making it difficult to assign a straightforward etiologic role for HPV in cervical tumorigenesis. Infection with HPV-16 has been detected with the polymerase chain reaction (PCR) in over 70% of women, albeit at low levels.[14] Although the sensitivity of PCR introduces great potential for false positives, it is reasonable to assume that a substantial number of women with "normal" cervices are infected with high-risk HPV types. The fact that almost all cervical cancers contain HPV but cervical cancer does not develop in all cervices infected with HPV suggests that HPV may be a crucial factor in the etiology of cervical cancer but HPV alone is not sufficient. The mechanism or mechanisms of HPV contributions to cervical tumorigenesis and the additional factors necessary for cervical tumorigenesis remain little understood.

Since, as discussed above, most tumors arise through a multistep process, it is not surprising that additional cellular events are necessary for tumor formation. Given what we have learned from the colorectal model, it is likely that the additional factors include alterations in both tumor suppressor genes and oncogenes. Both epidemiologic and recent molecular studies support this hypothesis. First, only a minority of women infected with high-risk types of HPV get cervical carcinoma. Second, cervical cancer does not develop until long after (20 or more years, in most cases) the initial infection with HPV. Recent molecular studies have implicated specific genes that may be important in cervical tumorigenesis. Studies suggesting alterations of specific oncogenes in cervical tumorigenesis are summarized in Table 1. These findings are preliminary. However, they provide considerable evidence supporting the involvement of oncogene activation in the development of cervical carcinomas.

As mentioned earlier, losses of specific chromosomal regions, also known as allelic losses or LOH, are thought to target tumor suppressor genes. Studies of cervical carcinoma have described a high frequency of LOH of the short arm of chromosome 3[22] and the short arm of 17,[23] thus suggesting the possibility of suppressor genes in these regions. More extensive allelic loss studies are likely to implicate involvement of additional tumor suppressor genes.

Previous experiments have indicated that the HPV oncoproteins E6 and E7 bind to proteins encoded by tumor suppressor genes. Specifically, the products of the E6 genes of the high-risk HPV types 16 and 18 have been shown to bind the tumor suppressor protein p53.[24] There is some controversy as to whether the E6 proteins of the low-risk HPV types 6 and 11 bind to p53 at all or just with a lower affinity than that of the high-risk types. The binding of high-risk E6 to p53 promotes the degradation of p53 in vitro.[25] This degradation of p53 probably provides a functional analogue of p53 mutations in that p53 function is inactivated. Similarly, the E7 protein binds the tumor suppressor protein Rb,[26] which may also serve to inactivate the normal function of the Rb protein. From these observations, tumors harboring HPV sequences might inactivate the function of the tumor suppressor genes through these interactions. On the other hand, if p53 and Rb are important in cervical tumorigenesis, tumors lacking HPV infection are likely to have inactivating mutations in the p53 and/or Rb genes. Recent studies of Scheffner et al.[27] and Crook et al.[28] support this hypothesis. They found that HPV-infected cervical carcinoma cell lines contained wild-type copies of these genes whereas those lacking detectable HPV DNA harbored mutations in the p53 and Rb genes. A more recent evaluation of primary cervical carcinomas has yielded less straightforward results. Primary cervical tumors containing large copy numbers of oncogenic HPVs were found to lack p53 gene mutations as expected; however, HPV-negative tumors also lacked p53 gene mutations.[29, 30] These studies suggest that the development of HPV-negative tumors may involve different genetic pathways independent of p53.

The variation in the oncogenic potential between the high-risk and low-risk types of HPVs remains somewhat unclear. However, some recent studies at the molecular level have provided some early clues. Through partial mapping of functional domains in the E6 and E7 proteins, Münger et al.[31] have shown that some biochemical and biological differences between E7 proteins of HPV-6 (low risk) and HPV-16 (high

TABLE 1.
Summary of Oncogene Abnormalities in Cervical Carcinoma

Oncogene	Genetic Alteration	Summary of Results	Reference
ras Group	Overexpression of p21	Increased staining by immunohistochemistry in CIN,* invasive squamous carcinoma	Sagae et al.[15] Agnantis et al.[16]
c-HA-*ras*	Somatic deletion/codon 12 mutation	Loss of one allele in 36% of informative cases, mutations in 24% of advanced-stage carcinomas	Riou et al.[17]
c-*myc*	Overexpression	Increased staining by immunohistochemistry in 50% of invasive carcinomas, overexpression correlated with poor prognosis	Sowani et al.[18]
c-*myc*	Overexpression	Increased staining by immunohistochemistry in 2/7 high-grade CIN and in 2/4 invasive carcinomas	Di Luca et al.[19]
c-*myc*	Amplification	Amplification without structural gene rearrangement in 32% of invasive carcinomas	Baker et al.[20]
c-*myc*	Amplification or gene rearrangement	Amplification and/or gene rearrangement in nearly 90% of invasive carcinomas	Ocadiz et al.[21]

*CIN = cervical intraepithelial neoplasia.

risk) are determined by amino-terminal sequences. Specifically, the transformation properties and affinity for binding to Rb are present in the amino-terminal half of E7. Furthermore, the HPV-16 E7 protein inhibits the DNA binding properties of the Rb gene product,[32] which suggests a possible mechanism through which the interaction of E7 and Rb may contribute to tumor progression. Crook et al. have found that a C-terminal portion of the E6 protein conserved among all HPV types is important for p53 binding whereas an N-terminal domain conserved only between oncogenic HPV types promotes the degradation of p53.[33]

Several recent studies have suggested that p53 may function as an "emergency brake" in cells that have sustained DNA damage.[34, 35] Cells exposed to certain DNA damaging agents arrest in the G_1-S portion of the cell cycle. It is thought that this cell cycle arrest allows the cells to undertake DNA repair, thereby avoiding the accumulation of genetic alterations. The G_1-S arrest is temporally associated with an increase in the levels of wild-type p53. In cells containing mutant p53 genes, neither the cell cycle arrest nor the increase in p53 protein levels occurs. The interaction of p53 and HPV E6 in cells infected by papillomaviruses appears to inhibit the normal function of p53 in this important cellular response to DNA damage.[36]

Although the previous discussion has been limited to squamous carcinomas of the cervix, it is notable that many adenocarcinomas are also associated with HPV infection and that invasive adenocarcinomas contain integrated forms of the HPV genome.[37] Whether cervical adenocarcinomas and squamous carcinomas share other molecular steps in the carcinogenesis pathway has yet to be determined.

Several lines of investigation over the past several years have converged to support a critical role for the involvement of papillomaviruses in the development of cervical carcinoma. Epidemiologic studies led to the early hypothesis that HPV may play an important role in cervical tumorigenesis. More recent molecular biological and biochemical techniques have provided ample corroborating evidence for the importance of HPV infection as well as insights into the mechanisms by which oncogenic HPVs contribute to cervical neoplasia.

VULVAR CANCER

Although squamous carcinoma is the most common cancer involving the vulva, it is relatively rare, with an estimated incidence of 1 to 2 per 100,000 women.[38] Intraepithelial precursor lesions (vulvar intraepithelial neoplasia [VIN]) similar to those in the cervix have been recognized for some time. Epidemiologic studies suggest that HPV infection plays a role in the pathogenesis of at least some of these tumors. Because vulvar cancers are uncommon, thorough investigation of the role of HPV in vulvar tumorigenesis has lagged significantly behind that of the cervix. However, recent studies suggest that vulvar carcinomas may be an excellent system in which to contrast HPV-positive and -negative tumors. One study, using in situ hybridization and PCR to identify HPV-16 or -18, found HPV in nearly all cases of VIN located adjacent to invasive squamous carcinomas as well as in the associated tumors.[39] These tumors appeared to be of two specific histologic subtypes characterized as "basaloid" or "warty." In addition, several cases were observed that did not contain VIN adjacent to the invasive cancer. These cancers were usually HPV-negative and were characterized histologically as "typical" squamous carcinomas. The HPV-associated "basaloid" and "warty" carcinomas tended to occur in younger women (mean age, 55), whereas the "typical" squamous carcinomas tended to occur in older women (mean age, 77). These findings suggest the possibility that the molecular pathogenesis of vulvar cancer in these two groups may be different or may share only some steps. Recently, a cytogenetic study of six vulvar squamous carcinomas found certain consistent chromosomal abnormalities, including losses of chromosomes 3p, 8p, 22q, and the short arm of the inactive X, as well as gains of 3q and 11q. In addition, losses of 10q and 18q were found only in cases that exhibited biologically aggressive behavior.[40] Until larger studies are completed, the significance of these findings will remain unclear. In conclusion, HPV-related vulvar cancers may share several genetic alterations with cervical squamous carcinomas, whereas the molecular pathogenesis of vulvar cancer in older women may be quite different.

ENDOMETRIAL CANCER

Endometrial cancer is the most common malignancy of the female genital tract. Fortunately, the death rate from endometrial cancer is relatively low since patients are often initially seen with early-stage disease. Adenocarcinomas, characterized by glands mimicking normal proliferative endometrium (endometrioid type), are the most common type of endometrial cancer. In many cases, unopposed estrogen, either exogenous or endogenous, provides the proliferative stimulus. As in colorectal tumor development, endometrial carcinogenesis progresses along a continuum from normal to frankly malignant epithelial cells. Proliferative endometrium progresses through several stages of endometrial hyperplasia and shows increasingly severe degrees of architectural and cytologic atypia until, ultimately, an invasive cancer develops. The genetic changes accompanying this process are largely unknown.

Several studies (summarized in Table 2) have identified molecular alterations of oncogenes that may play a role in the development of endometrial adenocarcinoma. Although most of these studies are small, many of the findings have potential clinical relevance. For example, alterations of several of these genes were found to correlate with presentation at an advanced stage, high histologic grade, and/or poor prognosis. As in the colorectal tumor model, suppressor gene alterations are also likely to play a role in endometrial carcinogenesis. Imamura et al.[45] used polymorphic probes spanning all 23 chromosome pairs to evaluate 24 cases of endometrial cancer for LOH. Loss of heterozygosity was identified in 7 patients, 5 of whom lost loci on 17p. This chromosomal arm harbors the p53 tumor suppressor gene. In at least 3 of the 5 patients who had lost one copy of p53, the retained copy of p53 was mutated. Frequent LOH on chromosome 18q (containing the DCC tumor suppressor gene) has also been identified in approximately 30% of endometrial carcinomas.[46] Taken together, these findings are provocative in that they suggest that endometrial cancers may share many genetic abnormalities with colorectal tumors (specifically, K-ras, p 53, and DCC alterations). The frequent occurrence of endometrial carcinoma in patients with hereditary nonpolyposis colorectal cancer (HNPCC, or Lynch syndrome II) further supports the notion that inactivation of a common suppressor gene or genes may con-

TABLE 2.

Summary of Oncogene Abnormalities in Endometrial Carcinomas

Oncogene	Genetic Alteration	Summary of Results	Reference
ras group	Overexpression of p21	Increased staining by immuno-histochemistry in endometrial hyperplasias and invasive carcinomas	Agnantis et al.[16] Long et al.[41]
K-ras	Point mutation, K-ras codon 12	Mutant K-ras in 2/9 endometrial adenocarcinomas	Enomoto et al.[42]
fms	Overexpression of M-CSF receptor	fms Overexpression by in situ hybridization in endometrial adenocarcinomas; overexpression correlated with clinicopathologic features associated with poor prognosis	Kacinski et al.[43]
c-erbB-1 (EGF-R)	Rearrangement	Rearrangement of 5' end of erbB-1 in one case of endometrial adenocarcinoma	Zhang et al.[44]

tribute to the development of both types of tumors. Larger studies will be required to determine how often alterations of these particular oncogenes and suppressor genes are involved in endometrial cancer development. Such large studies will also allow us to determine whether these changes are restricted to certain histologic subtypes of endometrial cancer.

OVARIAN CANCER

Molecular biological studies of ovarian cancer are complicated by the histopathologic diversity of these neoplasms. The complex classification scheme for ovarian epithelial tumors reflects the ability of the ovarian surface epithelium to differentiate along several different paths resembling various epithelia of müllerian origin (serous, mucinous, endometrioid, clear cell). The distinction between subtypes is not merely semantic because tumors of different subtypes tend to exhibit different biological behaviors. To further complicate matters, each major subtype includes benign, malignant, and tumors of borderline malignancy (also known as low malignant potential [LMP] tumors). Unlike carcinomas of the colorectum, uterine cervix, and endometrium, ovarian tumor progression from adenoma to LMP tumor to frank carcinoma has not been clearly documented, further hindering efforts to study their molecular pathology. In addition, ovarian cancers are less common, and tissue is relatively difficult to obtain, especially from "early" lesions. These problems are reflected in most of the molecular studies of ovarian epithelial tumors that have been reported thus far. Although alterations of several oncogenes and suppressor genes have been described in ovarian tumors, most of these studies have evaluated relatively small numbers of cases that were of mixed histologic types. Despite these difficulties, significant progress has been made in identifying at least some of the molecular events that appear to play a role in ovarian tumorigenesis.

Oncogene activation can occur through several different mechanisms, including point mutation, amplification, and rearrangement. The result of these alterations is inappropriate or overexpression of the oncogene protein product. The recent literature contains numerous reports of oncogene activation in ovarian malignancies. Several groups have reported overexpression of erbB-2 (also known as HER-2/neu) both with and without gene amplification.[47-49] This proto-oncogene encodes a transmembrane protein with structural similarities to the epidermal growth factor receptor. The erbB-2 protein probably functions in signal transduction across the cell membrane via a tyrosine kinase domain in the intracytoplasmic portion that is activated by binding of ligand to the extracellular domain. Putative ligands for this receptor have recently been reported.[50] Using Southern blot analysis, Slamon et al.[48] found erbB-2 amplification in 26% of 120 primary ovarian malignancies studied. Overexpression of erbB-2 RNA and protein was seen in every evaluated case with gene amplification. An additional 12% of cases showed erbB-2 overexpression without evidence of gene amplification. Overexpression of erbB-2 significantly correlated with poor clinical outcome, which suggests that evaluation of expression levels of this gene may eventually become useful in predicting prognosis and determining appropriate therapy for ovarian cancer patients. Activation of the erbB-2 gene has also been identified in a substantial number of breast cancers.

The fms proto-oncogene also belongs to a family of oncogenes that transduce signals via tyrosine kinase activity. Overexpression of fms protein (M-CSF receptor) has been identified in all types of ovarian carcinomas studied (including mucinous, serous, clear cell, endometrioid, and undifferentiated). Such overexpression was not identified in either benign or LMP lesions.[51]

Unlike fms and erbB-2, which transduce signals across the cell membrane, the myc gene family encodes proteins that localize to the nucleus and affect transcription of growth-related genes by binding to specific DNA sequences. Amplification of c-myc has been reported in both hematopoietic and solid tumors and, in some neoplasms, is associated with more biologically aggressive behavior. Amplification of c-myc has been reported in 29% to 50% of ovarian cancers.[52, 53] In one of these studies, six of seven cases with c-myc amplification were of serous differentiation. None of four evaluated cases of mucinous adenocarcinoma had this change. These data support the hypothesis that different genetic alterations may be associated with or responsible for the development of different subsets of ovarian tumors. Furthermore, normal ovary, benign adenomas, and LMP tumors all failed to demonstrate c-*myc* amplification. Other oncogene abnormalities such as *ras* gene deletion, amplification, and point mutation and *fos* gene overexpression have been reported. Since these studies are limited, the biological and clinical significance of these findings remains unclear.

In keeping with the colorectal tumor model, the pathogenesis of ovarian neoplasia is also likely to involve inactivation of tumor suppressor genes. Several investigators have recently found allelic loss events at nonrandom frequencies in ovarian malignancies, but the specific genes inactivated in specific tumor subsets have yet to be identified. The results of allelic loss studies in ovarian carcinomas are summarized in Table 3. The series of Sato et al.[59] is probably the most thorough and illustrative to date. This group of investigators used a set of polymorphic DNA probes spanning all of the nonacrocentric chromosomal arms to study 37 ovarian carcinomas of mixed histologic types. Interestingly, allelic losses on 6q, 13q, and 19q were observed exclusively in serous carcinomas. Following correction for the number of informative cases, the average number of allelic losses seen in mucinous tumors was found to be significantly

TABLE 3.

Summary of Losses of Heterozygosity in Ovarian Carcinoma

Chromosomal Arms With LOH	Additional Comments	Reference
11p	Loss of one c-Ha-*ras* allele in 5/10 informative cases	Lee et al.[54]
17p (69%), 17q (77%)	12/16 cases studied were papillary serous carcinomas	Eccles et al.[55]
3p, 6q, 11p	12 cases studied	Ehlen and Dubeau[56]
6q (64%), 17p (75%), 11p (46%)	19 cases studied	Lee et al.[57]
17p (31%), 17q (77%)	19 cases studied	Russell et al.[58]
3p, 6p, 6q, 11p	30 cases studied. Losses on chromosomes 3 or 11 were not seen in low-grade lesions	Zheng et al.[47]
4p (42%), 6p (50%), 7p (43%), 8q (31%), 12p (38%), 12q (33%), 16p (33%), 16q (38%), 17p (46%), 17q (39%), 19p (34%)	37 cases studied. 6q, 13q, and 19q losses seen only in serous carcinomas. Mucinous carcinomas typically had fewer losses than other histologic subtypes	Sato et al.[59]

lower than that of other types, including serous and clear cell tumors, which tend to have a worse prognosis. Taken together, these findings suggest that alterations of several different suppressor genes are likely to play a role in ovarian cancer development and that alterations of various suppressor genes may, in part, be responsible for the variable histopathologic appearance and biologic behavior of different tumor types. The idea that certain suppressor genes may help control cellular differentiation is not unprecedented. Substantial evidence has accumulated that suggests that the DCC suppressor gene plays a critical role in both neuronal and selected epithelial differentiation.[60, 61]

The status of known tumor suppressor genes in ovarian epithelial tumors has been evaluated in a few studies. For example, homozygous deletion (loss of both copies) of the Rb gene was found in 1 of 24 ovarian carcinomas.[62] In another analysis, 36% of 34 ovarian carcinomas were found to contain p53 gene mutations, with the mutations clustered in exons 5 and 7.[63] In these tumors both copies of p53 were inactivated, either through independent mutation or, more commonly, through mutation of one allele accompanied by loss of the other. Several matched sets of primary tumor and metastasis were also evaluated, and the same mutation was identified in tumor from both sites. These findings suggest that p53 gene mutation generally precedes metastasis. Marks et al.[64] used immunohistochemical techniques to examine p53 gene expression in over 100 ovarian carcinomas. Although p53 was undetectable in several benign gynecologic tissue samples, high levels of p53 protein were detected in 50% of the cancers. As in other studies, increased levels of p53 protein were found to correlate closely with the presence of p53 gene mutation in the tumor. Thus, it appears that inactivation of the p53 gene through deletion and/or point mutation plays an important role in the development or progression of a significant number of ovarian carcinomas.

Ovarian carcinomas often involve both ovaries and/or multiple peritoneal sites at the time of initial examination. This observation has led to the suggestion that peritoneal spread, in at least some cases, may reflect multifocal tumor development in a "field" of reactive peritoneum rather than true metastasis.[65] This hypothesis is further supported by (1) occasional cases of well-documented extraovarian papillary serous neoplasia,[66, 67] (2) the occurrence of synchronous uterine endometrial carcinomas with endometrioid carcinoma of the ovary,[68] and (3) the histopathologic observation of "in situ carcinoma"–like changes in other portions of the female genital tract in patients with ovarian carcinoma. Molecular biology has provided us the tools with which to begin to address this longstanding question. Mok et al.[69] examined multifocal tumors from nine different patients. In all nine cases, the mutational pattern of the p53 gene was identical in cancer cells from different sites within the same patient. These findings suggest that these tumors were of unifocal origin and represented metastases from a single primary tumor. Using another marker of clonality (X chromosome inactivation), the same group reached a similar conclusion.[70] It is important to bear in mind, however, that studying multifocal tumors in patients with widespread disease may not be ideal in that it may introduce a bias toward patients with aggressive, widely metastatic disease. It would, perhaps, be informative to study multifocal tumors of more limited extent, e.g., bilateral ovarian disease or synchronous ovarian and endometrial tumors.

The genetic alterations described above pertain to those occurring in somatic cells during ovarian tumor development and progression. It is important to keep in mind that primary genetic factors (germ line changes) contribute to an unknown proportion of ovarian cancer cases. Hereditary predisposition to ovarian cancer has been primarily observed in three types of families: those with apparently site-specific ovarian cancer, those with frequent breast and ovarian cancer, and those with HNPCC (Lynch syndrome II). Recent epidemiologic studies have found significant heterogeneity in the age at diagnosis of ovarian cancer among patients with these different ovarian cancer–prone syndromes, thus suggesting that they may not share the same pathogenesis.[71] Linkage studies have mapped the familial breast-ovarian cancer locus to chromosome 17q12-q23, and identification and cloning of the target gene are being diligently pursued by several investigative groups. The intensive study of kindreds affected with these various syndromes is likely to pinpoint several candidate genes within the next few years. It can then be determined whether somatic alterations of these genes are playing a role in the development of sporadic ovarian cancers.

SUMMARY

The molecular pathogenesis of gynecologic tumors can now be studied by using many recently developed molecular tools. The experimental methods routinely used in molecular biology laboratories today are accessible to a large number of research laboratories. However, the importance of clinicians' and pathologists' roles in future research on gynecologic tumors cannot be overemphasized. Simply stated, the quality of the knowledge gained through an experimental approach can only be as good as the questions asked and the materials used. Clinicians offer unique insights into the biological behavior of tumors, which in turn has a large impact on the types of questions that should be asked about the individual tumor types. Pathologists can ensure that the material being studied is appropriate for the questions being asked and the techniques being employed. For example, the techniques used to analyze tumor samples for LOH rely on a comparison of normal and tumor DNA from the same patient. The ability to interpret the data depends on the analysis of relatively pure DNA samples such that tumor DNA is not heavily contaminated with normal DNA. Normal DNA contaminating tumor samples can easily conceal LOH. In addition, degraded DNA obtained from necrotic cells often leads to uninterpretable results.

The colorectal system has provided a useful model system for study of the majority of gynecologic tumors. Squamous carcinomas of the uterine cervix and adenocarcinomas of the endometrium are preceded by well-recognized intraepithelial lesions, namely, CIN and atypical endometrial hyperplasia, respectively. Cervical cancers may not progress through each degree of CIN; it is well accepted that invasive cancers generally arise from an intraepithelial precursor, however. The precursor lesions for cervical and endometrial carcinomas, like colorectal precursors, are obtainable for laboratory study at different stages along the tumor progression. In contrast, patients with ovarian cancer are usually seen with advanced-stage disease, which precludes the evaluation of possible precursor lesions and requires invasive procedures to obtain any tissue at all. Consequently, the progression of ovarian carcinoma is much more poorly understood. Despite these obstacles, molecular biological techniques have furthered our understanding of the development of these tumors.

The ultimate goal of these studies is to improve the care and management of patients with gynecologic malignancies. The identification of specific genetic alterations involved in the development of these tumors could potentially form the basis of new screening programs to detect early, curable cancers. Patients with strong family histories for specific types of cancer could be screened for inherited mutations in the relevant tumor suppressor genes. Finally, these studies may provide targeted therapeutic approaches to more effectively treat patients with advanced-stage disease.

The common gynecologic malignancies appear to develop and progress, at least in part, as a result of activation of oncogenes coupled with inactivation of tumor suppressor genes. The current goals of molecular research are to identify the specific genes involved in the different tumor types and to characterize the alterations within these genes. It is important for clinicians to stay aware of the studies emerging from the molecular approach to gynecologic malignancies. The results undoubtedly will significantly affect the diagnosis and management of cancer patients in the near future.

REFERENCES

1. Marshall C: Tumor suppressor genes. *Cell* 1991; 64:313–326.
2. Gu W, Schneider J, Conorelli G, et al: Interaction of myogenic factors and the retinoblastoma protein mediates muscle cell commitment and differentiation. *Cell* 1993; 72:309–324.
3. Boring CC, Squires TS, Tong T: Cancer statistics 1991. *CA* 1991; 41:19–36.
4. Parkin DM, Läärä E, Muir CS: Estimates of the worldwide frequency of sixteen major cancers in 1980. *Int J Cancer* 1988; 41:184–197.
5. Vonka V, Kanka J, Jelinek J, et al: Prospective study on the relationship between cervical neoplasia and herpes simplex type-2 virus. I. Epidemiological characteristics. *Int J Cancer* 1984; 33:49–60.
6. zur Hausen H: Condylomata acuminata and human genital cancer. *Cancer Res* 1976; 36:794.
7. Pirisi L, Yasumoto S, Feller M, et al: Transformation of human fibroblasts and keratinocytes with human papillomavirus type 16 DNA. *J Virol* 1987; 61:1061–1066.
8. Dürst M, Dzarlieva-Petrusevska R, Boukamp P, et al: Molecular and cytogenetic analysis of immortalized human primary keratinocytes obtained after transfection with human papillomavirus type 16 DNA. *Oncogene* 1987; 1:251–256.
9. Riou G, Favre M, Jeannel D, et al: Association between poor prognosis in early-stage invasive cervical carcinomas and non-detection of HPV DNA. *Lancet* 1990; 335:1171–1174.

10. Cullen AP, Reid R, Campion M, Lörincz AT: Analysis of the physical state of different human papillomavirus DNAs in intraepithelial and invasive cervical neoplasm. *J Virol* 1991; 65:606–612.

11. Dürst M, Croce C, Gissmann L, et al: Papillomavirus sequences integrate near cellular oncogenes in some cervical carcinomas. *Proc Natl Acad Sci U S A* 1987; 80:3812–3815.

12. Couturier J, Sastre-Garau X, Schneider-Maunoury S, et al: Integration of papillomavirus DNA near *myc* genes in genital carcinomas and its consequences for proto-oncogenes expression. *J Virol* 1991; 65:4534–4538.

13. Barbosa MS, Schlegel R: The E6 and E7 genes of HPV-18 are sufficient for inducing two-stage in vitro transformation of human keratinocytes. *Oncogene* 1989; 4:1529–1532.

14. Young L, Bevan I, Johnson M, et al: The polymerase chain reaction: A new epidemiological tool for investigating cervical human papillomavirus infection. *BMJ* 1989; 298:14–18.

15. Sagae S, Kudo R, Kuzumaki N, et al: *Ras* oncogene expression and progression in intraepithelial neoplasia of the uterine cervix. *Cancer* 1990; 66:295–301.

16. Agnantis NJ, Spandidos DA, Mahera H, et al: Immunohistochemical study of *ras* oncogene expression in endometrial and cervical human lesions. *Eur J Gynaecol Oncol* 1988; 9:360–365.

17. Riou G, Barrois M, Sheng ZM, et al: Somatic deletions and mutations of c-Ha-*ras* gene in human cervical cancers. *Oncogene* 1988; 3:329–333.

18. Sowani A, Ong G, Dische S, et al: C-*myc* oncogene expression and clinical outcome in carcinoma of the cervix. *Mol Cell Probes* 1989; 3:117–123.

19. Di Luca D, Costa S, Monini P, et al: Search for human papillomavirus, herpes simplex virus and c-*myc* oncogene in human genital tumors. *Int J Cancer* 1989; 43:570–577.

20. Baker V, Hatch K, Shingleton H: Amplification of the c-*myc* proto-oncogene in cervical carcinoma. *J Surg Oncol* 1988; 39:225–228.

21. Ocadiz R, Sauceda R, Cruz M, et al: High correlation between molecular alterations of the c-*myc* oncogene and carcinomas of the uterine cervix. *Cancer Res* 1987; 47:4173–4177.

22. Yokota J, Tsukada Y, Nakajima T, et al: Loss of heterozygosity on the short arm of chromosome 3 in carcinoma of the uterine cervix. *Cancer Res* 1989; 49:3598–3601.

23. Atkin NB, Baker MC: Chromosome 17p loss in carcinoma of the cervix uteri. *Cancer Genet Cytogenet* 1989; 37:229–233.

24. Werness B, Levine A, Howley P: Association of human papillomavirus types 16 and 18 E6 proteins with p53. *Science* 1990; 248:76–79.

25. Scheffner M, Werness BA, Huibregtse JM, et al: The E6 oncoprotein encoded by human papillomavirus types 16 and 18 promotes the degradation of p53. *Cell* 1990; 63:1129–1136.

26. Dyson N, Howley P, Munger K, et al: The human papillomavirus-16 E7 oncoprotein is able to bind to the retinoblastoma gene product. *Science* 1989; 243:934–937.

27. Scheffner M, Münger K, Byrne JC, et al: The state of the p53 and retinoblastoma genes in human cervical carcinoma cell lines. *Proc Natl Acad Sci U S A* 1991; 88:5523–5527.

28. Crook T, Wrede D, Vousden KH: p53 point mutation in HPV negative human cervical carcinoma cell lines. *Oncogene* 1991; 6:873–875.

29. Fujita M, Inoue M, Tanizawa O, et al: Alterations of the p53 gene in human primary cervical carcinoma with and without human papillomavirus infection. *Cancer Res* 1992; 52:5323–5328.

30. Kessis T, Slebos R, Han S, et al: p53 gene mutations and MDM2 amplification are uncommon in primary carcinomas of the uterine cervix. *Am J Pathol* 1993; 143:1–8.

31. Münger K, Yee CL, Phelps WC, et al: Biochemical and biological differences between E7 oncoproteins of the high- and low-risk human papillomavirus types are determined by amino-terminal sequences. *J Virol* 1991; 65:3943–3948.

32. Stirdivant S, Huber H, Patrick D, et al: Human papillomavirus type 16 E7 protein inhibits DNA binding by the retinoblastoma gene product. *Mol Cell Biol* 1992; 12:1905–1914.

33. Crook T, Tidy JA, Vousden KH: Degradation of p53 can be targeted by HPV E6 sequences distinct from those required for p53 binding and trans-activation. *Cell* 1991; 67:547–556.

34. Kastan MB, Onyekwere O, Sidransky D, et al: Participation of p53 protein in the cellular response to DNA damage. *Cancer Res* 1991; 51:6304–6311.

35. Kuerbitz S, Plunkett B, Walsh W, et al: Wild-type p53 is a cell cycle check-point determinant following irradiation. *Proc Natl Acad Sci U S A* 1992; 89:7491–7495.

36. Kessis T, Slebos R, Nelson W, et al: Human papillomavirus 16 E6 disrupts the p53 mediated cellular response to DNA damage. *Proc Natl Acad Sci U S A* 1993; 90:3988–3992.

37. Low SH, Thong TW, Ho TH, et al: Prevalence of human papillomavirus types 16 and 18 in cervical carcinomas: A study by dot and Southern blot hybridization and the polymerase chain reaction. *Jpn J Cancer Res* 1990; 81:1118–1123.

38. *Surveillance, Epidemiology, and End Results: Incidence and Mortality Data, 1973–1977.* Bethesda, Md, US Department of Health and Human Services, NIH Publication No 81-2330, 1981.

39. Toki T, Kurman RJ, Park JS, et al: Probable nonpapillomavirus etiology of squamous cell carcinoma of the vulva in older women: A clinicopathologic study using in situ hybridization and polymerase chain reaction. *Int J Gynecol Pathol* 1991; 10:107–125.

40. Worsham MJ, Van Dyke DL, Grenman SE, et al: Consistent chromosome abnormalities in squamous cell carcinoma of the vulva. *Genes Chromosomes Cancer* 1991; 3:420–432.

41. Long CA, O'Brien TJ, Sanders MM, et al: ras oncogene is expressed in adenocarcinoma of the endometrium. *Am J Obstet Gynecol* 1988; 159:1512–1516.

42. Enomoto T, Inoue M, Perantoni AO, et al: K-ras activation in neoplasms of the human female reproductive tract. *Cancer Res* 1990; 50:6139–6145.

43. Kacinski BM, Carter D, Mittal K, et al: High level expression of *fms* proto-oncogene mRNA is observed in clinically aggressive human endometrial adenocarcinomas. *Int J Radiat Oncol Biol Phys* 1988; 15:823–829.

44. Zhang X, Silva E, Gershenson D, et al: Amplification and rearrangement of c-erb B proto-oncogenes in cancer of human female genital tract. *Oncogene* 1989; 4:985–989.

45. Imamura A, Sameshima Y, Yamada Y, et al: Allelic loss on chromosome 17p and p53 mutations in human endometrial carcinoma of the uterus. *Cancer Res* 1991; 51:5632–5635.

46. Imamura T, Arima T, Kato H, et al: Chromosomal deletions and K-ras gene mutations in human endometrial carcinomas. *Int J Cancer* 1992; 51:47–52.

47. Zheng JP, Robinson WR, Ehlen T, et al: Distinction of low grade from high grade human ovarian carcinomas on the basis of losses of heterozygosity on chromosomes 3, 6, and 11 and HER-2/neu gene amplification. *Cancer Res* 1991; 51:4045–4051.

48. Slamon DJ, Godolphin W, Jones LA, et al: Studies of the HER-2/neu proto-oncogene in human breast and ovarian cancer. *Science* 1989; 244:707–712.
49. Kacinski BM, Mayer AG, King BL, et al: NEU protein overexpression in benign, borderline, and malignant ovarian neoplasms. *Gynecol Oncol* 1992; 44:245–253.
50. Peles E, Bacus SS, Koski RA, et al: Isolation of the neu/HER-2 stimulatory ligand: a 44 kd glycoprotein that induces differentiation of mammary tumor cells. *Cell* 1992; 69:205–216.
51. Kacinski BM, Carter D, Mittal K, et al: Ovarian adenocarcinomas express *fms*-complementary transcripts and *fms* antigen, often with coexpression of CSF-1. *Am J Pathol* 1990; 137:135–147.
52. Baker VV, Borst MP, Dixon D, et al: c-*myc* amplification in ovarian cancer. *Gynecol Oncol* 1990; 38:340–342.
53. Sasano H, Garrett CT, Wilkinson DS, et al: Protooncogene amplification and tumor ploidy in human ovarian neoplasms. *Hum Pathol* 1990; 21:382–391.
54. Lee JH, Kavanagh JJ, Wharton JT, et al: Allele loss at the c-Ha-*ras*1 locus in human ovarian cancer. *Cancer Res* 1989; 49:1220–1222.
55. Eccles DM, Cranston G, Steel CM, et al: Allele losses on chromosome 17 in human epithelial ovarian carcinoma. *Oncogene* 1990; 5:1599–1601.
56. Ehlen T, Dubeau L: Loss of heterozygosity on chromosomal segments 3p, 6q and 11p in human ovarian carcinomas. *Oncogene* 1990; 5:219–223.
57. Lee JH, Kavanagh JJ, Wildrick DM, et al: Frequent loss of heterozygosity on chromosomes 6q, 11, and 17 in human ovarian carcinomas. *Cancer Res* 1990; 50:2724–2728.
58. Russell SE, Hickey GI, Lowry WS, et al: Allele loss from chromosome 17 in ovarian cancer. *Oncogene* 1990; 5:1581–1583.
59. Sato T, Saito H, Morita R, et al: Allelotype of human ovarian cancer. *Cancer Res* 1991; 51:5118–5122.
60. Lawlor K, Narayanan R: Persistent expression of the tumor suppressor gene DCC is essential for neuronal differentiation. *Cell Growth Differentiation* 1992; 3:609–616.
61. Hedrick L, Cho K, Boyd J, et al: *DCC*: A tumor suppressor gene expressed on the cell surface. *Symp Quant Biol* 1992; LVII:345–351.
62. Sasano H, Comerford J, Silverberg SG, et al: An analysis of abnormalities of the retinoblastoma gene in human ovarian and endometrial carcinoma. *Cancer* 1990; 66:2150–2154.
63. Mazars R, Pujol P, Maudelonde T, et al: p53 mutations in ovarian cancer: A late event? *Oncogene* 1991; 6:1685–1690.
64. Marks J, Davidoff A, Kerns B, et al: Overexpression and mutation of p53 in epithelial ovarian cancer. *Cancer Res* 1991; 51:2979–2984.
65. Woodruff J, TeLinde R: The histology and histogenesis of ovarian neoplasia. *Cancer* 1976; 38:411–413.
66. Genadry R, Poliakoff S, Rotmensch J, et al: Primary, papillary peritoneal neoplasia. *Obstet Gynecol* 1981; 58:730–734.
67. Foyle A, Al-Jabi M, McCaughey W: Papillary peritoneal tumors in women. *Am J Surg Pathol* 1992; 5:241–249.
68. Zaino R, Unger E, Whitney C: Synchronous carcinomas of the uterine corpus and ovary. *Gynecol Oncol* 1984; 19:329–335.
69. Mok C, Tsao S, Knapp R, et al: Unifocal origin of advanced human epithelial ovarian cancers. *Cancer Res* 1992; 52:5119–5122.
70. Tsao S, Mok C, Knapp R, et al: Molecular genetic evidence of a unifocal origin for human serous ovarian carcinomas. *Gynecol Oncol* 1993; 48:5–10.
71. Lynch HT, Watson P, Bewtra C, et al: Hereditary ovarian cancer. Heterogeneity in age at diagnosis. *Cancer* 1991; 67:1460–1466.

Editor's Comment

My congratulations to Drs. Cho and Hedrick for providing a most thorough discussion of the molecular biology of gynecologic tumors. Drawing on their experience with Dr. Bert Vogelstein at the Johns Hopkins Medical Institutions, Drs. Cho and Hedrick have applied their expertise with colon carcinoma to gynecologic tumors. In addition to reporting their personal results, the authors provide an extensive review of the literature. Cervical, endometrial, and ovarian carcinomas are highlighted in this chapter. Specific attention is placed on describing various methods to activate oncogenes and to inactivate tumor suppressor genes. The authors have described mutations in specific genes that may result in gynecologic tumor formation. It is imperative that the clinician be informed about this rapidly changing technology that is making its way into the clinical setting. The coming years will increasingly emphasize gene therapy to treat the oncology patient, and the information provided in this chapter by Drs. Cho and Hedrick will be the foundation for such therapies.

Ira R. Horowitz, M.D.

Obstetrics

Substance Abuse in Pregnant Women

RAMADA S. SMITH, M.D.

SUSAN S. MARTIER, M.S.S.A.

ROBERT J. SOKOL, M.D.

Substance abuse is common in our society, and with the increased use of drugs and alcohol among younger segments of the general population, substance abuse in pregnancy occurs with relative frequency.[1] Adverse pregnancy outcomes have been variably associated with maternal consumption of alcohol and drugs. Cocaine use has become a major public health concern because of its dramatic increase over the last 10 to 15 years. Decreased costs and increased availability are responsible for the use of cocaine among all racial, ethnic, and socioeconomic groups, including the pregnant population.

Despite recognized hazards, consumption of alcohol beverages has long been an established social custom. It was only in the latter part of this century that prenatal growth deficiencies and other abnormalities were recognized in children of alcoholic mothers. Since the recognition of fetal alcohol syndrome (FAS),[2] knowledge has accumulated rapidly during the past two decades. Alcohol's potential for causing both teratogenic and fetotoxic effects has become well established, but only recently have these revelations heightened public awareness and prompted legislation to require a warning label on alcohol beverages.[3]

Human reproduction is more complicated than was once thought. Many conceptions are lost before pregnancy is even recognized.[4] Good maternal health is necessary to create a hospitable uterine environment for optimal fetal growth and development. The range of adverse effects of maternal substance abuse on pregnancy and the fetus has produced an immense and growing body of information. Needless to say, there is a considerable need for continuing medical education about chemical dependence. Pregnancy is a logical time to begin to examine the multiple aspects of substance abuse since the physician-patient relationship is frequently initiated with prenatal care.

Although drug abuse is commonly thought of as the taking of drugs prohibited by law, it has become increasingly difficult to draw a line between drug abuse and the recreational use of legal agents such as alcohol, tobacco, and caffeine. What constitutes abuse of such agents may be different for the court than for the reproductive toxicologist. "Abuse" is defined as "misuse, wrong use, or excessive use of anything."[5] For the

Advances in Obstetrics and Gynecology, vol 1
© 1994, Mosby–Year Book, Inc.

purposes of this chapter, "substance abuse" will include the abuse of the more common substances encountered in the pregnant patient, namely, alcohol, cocaine, marijuana, and opioids.

ALCOHOL

Alcohol's potential as an agent for adverse reproductive effects, although arguably observed from biblical times, has become well established in the medical sciences only during the last 2 decades. About 60% of American women drink alcoholic beverages, and about 3% can be classified as problem drinkers.[6] The proportion of women in reproductive years who drink an average of at least 14 drinks per week is about 5.5%.[7] Heavy alcohol use during pregnancy has been linked definitively to spontaneous abortion, FAS, anatomic alcohol-related birth defects (ARBDs), and more recently, neurobehavioral/developmental deficits, some of which may remain unrecognized for years after birth. Among women who are relatively heavy drinkers, the percentage of women who report at least one clinically recognized spontaneous abortion is two to three times higher than the 15% to 20% rate in the general population.[8] In fact, the alcohol-related increased risk for spontaneous abortion was seen over 2 centuries ago! Coffey et al.[9] reported an association between heavy gin drinking and pregnancy wastage during the London "Gin Epidemic" in the 1700s. Thus, alcohol use during pregnancy is considered both teratogenic and fetotoxic.

PATHOPHYSIOLOGY

A continuum of reproductive effects on the fetus is apparent with the use of alcohol. High concentrations of alcohol and its metabolite acetaldehyde appear to alter fetal development by disrupting cell differentiation and growth. Alcohol modifies maternal physiology and intermediate metabolism of carbohydrates, proteins, and fats and reduces the passage of amino acids, glucose, folic acid, zinc, and other nutrients across the placenta.[10, 11] Speculation about how these events directly or indirectly affect the fetus reflects the lack of knowledge of the actual mechanisms involved and the many effects of alcohol on the body. Some suggested mechanisms are impaired maternal nutrition, acetaldehyde toxicity, fetal hypoxia, altered placental transport, interaction with other drugs, altered prostaglandin metabolism, hormonal alterations, impaired protein synthesis, and fluidization of cell membranes in developing tissues. Animal studies have shown that some of the effects of prenatal alcohol exposure can be attenuated by maternal supplementation with high-protein diets, although supplementation of other nutrients such as folate and zinc has not successfully reversed the effects of prenatal alcohol exposure.[12]

FETAL ALCOHOL SYNDROME

Definition

In 1968, Lemoine et al.[13] in France attributed a constellation of morphologic and developmental effects in 25 children to alcoholism and alcohol abuse. Five years later, Jones and Smith in 1973[14] first applied the term "fetal alcohol syndrome" to this same pattern of effects, which they identified in 11 children in Seattle. Fetal alcohol syndrome consists of a collection of adverse effects of maternal alcohol consumption during pregnancy on the developing fetus.[15] Definitions of FAS vary with different proposed schemata, but the most commonly used is that adapted by the Research Society on Alcoholism in 1980, which specifies prenatal and postnatal growth retardation, central nervous system involvement, and cranial and/or facial abnormalities as defining characteristics. Individual anomalies are seldom all present in a given case and may not be clinically significant when considered individually. When a pattern is present, however, it can typically be related to fetal alcohol exposure. The syndrome is diagnosed only when the infant has signs in each of three categories:

1. Prenatal or postnatal growth retardation (weight, length, and/or head circumference below the 10th percentile when corrected for gestational age)
2. Central nervous system involvement
3. Characteristic facial dysmorphology with at least two of three signs: microcephaly, microphthalmos and/or short palpebral fissures or poorly developed philtrum and thin upper lip, and flattening of the maxillary area.

The median birth weight for children born with FAS is 37% lower than the normal median birth weight. Similarly, the prevalence of low birth weight, defined as less than 2,500 g, is 77% in children with FAS, much higher than the 6.8% level in children without FAS.[16] Since there may be a slightly higher incidence of preterm births for children with FAS, it is possible that differences in birth weight are due in part to differences in gestational age; however, it is probably intrauterine growth retardation that accounts for most of the decreased birth weight consistently seen in FAS. Postnatally, children with FAS have tended to remain smaller than age-matched counterparts, at least in the cohorts that have been studied to date.[17] In a more recent study, growth measures have been reported in a cohort of 359 children at 6 months, 1 year, and 5 years of age. The observed significant growth retardation was accurately predicted both by positive scores on the Michigan Alcohol Screening Test (MAST) and self-reported average daily alcohol intake during pregnancy.[18]

Prevalence
Fetal alcohol syndrome is one of the leading causes of preventable mental retardation, with an estimated Western world incidence of 33 cases per 100,000 births.[19] This incidence of 33 per 100,000 means that some 1,200 children are born each year in the United States with complete FAS. All things being equal, estimates differ among races, with a tenfold increased risk among blacks (0.3 per 1,000) when compared with whites. Establishing rates for Orientals and Native Americans has been difficult, but it is thought to be higher than for blacks and whites.[20]

ALCOHOL-RELATED BIRTH DEFECTS
Alcohol-related birth defects occur when some but not all of the criteria for FAS are expressed. These defects are also called fetal alcohol effects. In 1989, Sokol and Clarren[21] proposed a set of terminology guidelines

for use by investigators, care providers, and others that would enhance the comparability of results of clinical observations, scientific studies, and public health reporting. This would, in turn, contribute to clarifying the literature and facilitating progress in describing and understanding the mechanisms involved in producing the adverse consequences of alcohol in the offspring. Use of the term fetal alcohol effect was discouraged by Sokol and Clarren.

Alcohol-related birth defect is suggested as a term that denotes attributable observed anatomic or functional (e.g., behavioral) outcome to the impact of alcohol. It may be applied by clinical and basic scientists studying humans and animal or other biological models. In human studies, use of this term requires statistical adjustment for potential confounding factors, which increases the probability that the attribution to alcohol is correct.[21] Maternal alcohol consumption may result in a variety of fetal effects, some more serious than others. Ventricular septal defects and genitourinary anomalies such as hypospadias are most commonly found, but many others such as microphthalmos, atrial septal defects, and malformed limbs have also been noted. However, at this time no specific effect of alcohol, i.e., no effect that is attributed to alcohol use only and to no other drug or teratogen, has been isolated.

SCREENING FOR EXPOSURE

Fetal alcohol syndrome is a preventable congenital abnormality. The challenge of preventing FAS actually begins preconceptionally through effective screening programs for women during regular doctor visits. Unfortunately, the developing fetus is often exposed to alcohol before the mother realizes that she is pregnant. It has been estimated that the likelihood of some kind and degree of defect developing in the fetus because of maternal alcohol abuse during pregnancy is 2.5%. This estimate is much greater than the estimate of likelihood for similar defects in infants of women who do not drink.[8] The anatomic abnormalities detectable in the neonate are related in a clear dose-response fashion to prenatal alcohol exposure, and as would be expected embryologically, the critical period for precipitating these abnormalities is in the early first trimester. Consumption of more than 3 oz of absolute alcohol per day (i.e., six cans of beer, six glasses of wine, or six mixed drinks) greatly increases the risk of alcohol teratogenicity. The issue of "critical periods" during maturation is also evident in the findings by Clarren et al. (1990)[22] in which the direction of neurochemical changes relative to nonexposed animals was opposite for monkeys exposed to alcohol weekly throughout gestation as compared with monkeys in whom the onset of alcohol exposure was delayed until the fifth gestational week. Questions regarding "safe levels" of alcohol consumption and/or times during pregnancy when the risk is greatest or least have not been satisfactorily answered. There are multiple factors to consider when addressing the topic of exposure, including the volume of alcohol to which the fetus is exposed, the duration of such exposure, the period of pregnancy in which exposure occurs, the pattern of drinking, and last, but certainly not least, problems in ascertaining exposure.

One of the most common questions about maternal alcohol consumption is, "How much drinking is too much?" Given the amount of research on alcohol and pregnancy, the answer "it depends" seems less than adequate. Yet it does depend, for example, on the particular outcome being examined. A precise intake threshold has not been established, and even low doses of alcohol are related to an increased incidence of craniofacial anomalies.[23] Conservative estimates for risk for any clinically important adverse alcohol-related effect of one drink per day are based on averages, but this fact seems to get lost in the translation, and risk estimates are interpreted to mean one drink a day, any day. This illustrates the difficulties of dealing with estimates of risk.

In an attempt to estimate fetal alcohol exposure, one is faced with many uncertainties. Blood alcohol levels, while relatively easy to perform reliably in the laboratory, are not generally available close enough in time to exposure for accurate measures. Maternal self-report has a tendency to be unreliable, generally in the direction of underreporting, particularly in a heavy drinker. Nonetheless, there are ways to obtain the patient's drinking history that can be comfortable for both the patient and physician. Seeking evidence of alcohol tolerance seems to be a much more effective approach to obtaining an alcohol consumption history than is merely asking a patient how much she drinks. Psychological denial is a large component of alcohol dependence, and asking about tolerance appears much less likely to trigger denial than asking about volume intake. We take it as an indication of tolerance if the patient states that it takes more than two drinks to make her feel high, and this suggests to us that we need to explore her drinking behavior further. A history of being able to "hold" more than five standard drinks, e.g., a six pack of beer or a bottle of wine, certainly indicates tolerance.

Formal questionnaires have been devised to aid in identifying the woman at risk. One very reliable questionnaire has been the MAST,[24] a 25-question data collection instrument widely employed in alcohol research. Because the clinician does not have the time or office staff to administer such a test, simpler, briefer questionnaires have been devised, including the brief MAST, CAGE, and T-ACE.[25-27] The CAGE takes from 30 seconds to 1 minute to administer, is efficient, and fits well into many clinical settings (Table 1); however, it has not been used extensively with reproductive-age women. An improvement on the sensitivity of the CAGE questionnaire, known as T-ACE, has recently been developed (Table 2). Three of the CAGE questions plus a tolerance question were analyzed by multivariate statistics. A score of 2 was assigned to the tolerance ques-

TABLE 1.
"CAGE" Questions*

C	Have you ever felt that you should cut down on your drinking?
A	Have people annoyed you by criticizing your drinking?
G	Have you ever felt bad or guilty about drinking?
E	Have you ever taken a drink the first thing in the morning to steady your nerves or get rid of a hangover (eye opener)?

*From Ewing JA: *JAMA* 1984; 252:1905–1907. Used by permission.

TABLE 2.

"T-ACE" Questions*

T   How many drinks does it take to make you feel high (tolerance)?
A   Have people annoyed you by criticizing your drinking?
C   Have you felt that you ought to cut down on your drinking?
E   Have you ever had a drink the first thing in the morning to steady
    your nerves or get rid of a hangover (eye opener)?

*From Sokol RJ, Martier SS, and Ager JW: *Am J Obstet Gynecol* 1989; 160:863–870. Used by permission.

---

tion and a score of 1 to all others. When none of the answers to these questions were positive, the probability that an individual was a risk drinker was 1.5%. If the patient answered the tolerance question alone positively, the probability of risk drinking increased 8.5-fold to 11.7%. A T-ACE score of 2 or greater is considered positive for risk drinking, i.e., drinking heavy enough potentially to damage the the offspring. With all four questions answered positively, there was a 62.7% likelihood of risk drinking. When compared with other questionnaires, including the MAST, the T-ACE appears to be superior since it identifies seven out of ten risk drinkers during pregnancy.

COMMENTS

Alcohol has been clearly established as a teratogen in humans. Extensive public education efforts have alerted women to the dangers of drinking during pregnancy, and the effect, if any, of labeling alcoholic beverages is being studied. Effective prevention strategies for FAS and ARBDs probably relate to prevention of alcohol abuse in general. Identification is necessary, but refraining from moderate to heavy alcohol intake during pregnancy appears to be the best approach in preventing FAS. Unfortunately, this does not appear to be a realistic expectation. Since present interventions for FAS and ARBDs appear to be limited to encouraging abstinence, assessment of alcohol intake and subsequent fetal risk should become standard prenatal care. Most physicians lack the formal medical training necessary to recognize the risk drinkers in their practice. However, basic screening techniques can be used to identify risk drinkers. The results of these techniques may lead to secondary prevention efforts and improved pregnancy outcomes for offspring at risk for FAS and ARBDs.

COCAINE

Cocaine has become a popular recreational drug. Because of the overall increase in its use, it is logical to expect that larger numbers of women are using cocaine during pregnancy than was the case 5 to 10 years ago. Positive maternal urine tests for cocaine have been reported in 2.6% to 18% of pregnancies in various regions of the United States.[28] However, at our institution, radioimmunoassay (RIA) of the stools of 567 neonates found 20.8% to be positive for cocaine. Only 10.7% of the mothers tested admitted to drug abuse.[29] Cocaine abuse during pregnancy has attracted national attention because of concerns about possible harm to the developing embryo and fetus.

PATHOPHYSIOLOGY

Cocaine hydrochloride is a white, odorless, crystalline, water-soluble powder made from the leaves of the coca bush *Erythroxylon coca*. It is a lipophilic compound that is consumed by snorting, freebasing, or smoking "crack." It readily crosses the placenta. Its major site of action is at the nerve terminal, and its pharmacologic effects are mediated primarily through three neurotransmitter systems: norepinephrine (NE), dopamine, and serotonin.[30] Cocaine blocks the presynaptic reuptake of NE and dopamine, which allows them to accumulate at the postsynaptic receptor sites. The elevated NE levels cause vasoconstriction and an acute rise in arterial pressure, tachycardia, diaphoresis, and mild tremors. Dopaminergic effects include euphoria, sexual excitement, increased alertness, hyperactivity, and decreased appetite. After long-term use, dopamine is depleted, and the stimulant effects become overshadowed by anxiety, depression, sexual dysfunction, and exhaustion. Cocaine affects the biosynthesis of serotonin by decreasing uptake of the precursor tryptophan.

Cocaine is metabolized into water soluble metabolites, primarily benzoylecgonine and ecgonine methyl ester, by cholinesterase and other esterases in both plasma and liver and by nonenzymatic hydrolysis.[31] The elimination half-life of benzoylecgonine in adults is approximately 4.5 hours, which allows detection in urine for 24 to 48 hours after variable single intravenous doses.[32] Because cocaine is rapidly metabolized, urine drug screens can be negative even when cocaine has been ingested recently.[33] Newer technologies such as RIA of neonatal meconium and maternal hair have shown that drug histories and urine toxicologies tend to have low sensitivity but high specificity for identifying abuse of this substance.[34, 35]

MATERNAL AND FETAL COMPLICATIONS

The use of cocaine during pregnancy is associated with a variety of adverse maternal and fetal outcomes. Drug-seeking behavior has been related to a higher maternal incidence of abruptio placentae, sexually transmitted diseases, hepatitis, malnutrition, stroke, seizures, bowel ischemia, and endocarditis.[36] Many of these complications are the result of aberrant behavior such as prostitution practiced in order to support the addiction. Other complications such as infarctions are more directly due to intense vasoconstriction. Management of lethal intoxication by cocaine consists of individualized supportive measures. An antagonist like naloxone (Narcan) for opioid overdose does not exist. Fatalities are usually cardiogenic, neurologic, or respiratory in origin. The initial concern is to provide adequate maternal ventilation and perfusion.

Animal studies on the maternal lethality of cocaine have shown that susceptibility to the lethal effects of cocaine increases with repeated use. That is, a daily dose that is nonlethal during the first several days of treatment may become lethal after continued exposure.[37, 38] Since there is sensitization (rather than tolerance) to the physiologic effects of cocaine, continued cocaine use during pregnancy should increase the likelihood of morbidity and mortality in both the mother and fetus. This is in addition to the expected increased sensitivity during pregnancy related to decreased serum cholinesterase activity.

Bingol et al.[39] in 1987 were the first to report low–birth weight and small-for-gestational-age infants born to abusers of cocaine. These authors also noted an increased rate of stillbirths (related to abruptio placentae) and congenital malformations. Since this report there have been numerous publications, many of them poorly controlled studies or case reports, describing fetal complications of maternal cocaine use such as cerebral infarction, urethral obstruction, prune-belly syndrome, jejunal atresia, bowel infarction, amniotic bands, limb reduction defects, imperforate anus, horseshoe kidney, and clubfoot.[40, 41] A specific teratogenic syndrome has not been identified, but there may be an increase in major congenital malformations related to drug dose and gestational age at the time of exposure. The mechanisms by which cocaine-induced perinatal morbidity occur are uncertain but are presumed to be related to those described earlier.

According to some estimates, "crack babies" now make up more than half of the drug-associated births reported to participating clinics and children's services agencies. Recent behavioral research has identified cocaine-related dysfunctional or detrimental relationships in maternal-infant pairs.[42] Cocaine-exposed infants are reportedly poor feeders and have a low threshold for stimulation in the newborn nursery.

As thousands of drug-exposed children have now entered the classroom, teachers report that the cocaine-exposed child displays characteristics such as poor concentration, labile stimulatory overload, delayed speech, and other unique individual behaviors.[43] In addition, school systems across the country have reported a significant increase in special education referrals, thought to be due largely to the arrival of the "crack kids." A relationship to prenatal cocaine exposure is arguable and will require much further study. So far, there is little convincing evidence for such an association.

COMMENTS

A major problem in evaluating the effects of cocaine in pregnant women is that many cocaine users are also users of other drugs. As a result, it is difficult to determine whether the adverse effects seen in children born to cocaine users are related to cocaine, to the other drugs taken, or to a combination. Some studies have sought to control for many confounding variables by matching nonuser groups on age, education, race, socioeconomic status, education, other drug use, etc. These studies inherently exclude the possibility that cocaine may interact with these patient variables in unpredictable ways. With such widespread use of cocaine and so many unanswered questions, perinatal cocaine exposure has become a highly pursued area of research.

MARIJUANA

Marijuana is a crude drug preparation made from the plant *Cannabis sativa*. The principal psychoactive ingredient in marijuana is Δ-9-tetrahydrocannabinol (Δ9-THC), which is slowly released from fatty tissues; its metabolites can be detected in urine for up to 1 to 2 weeks. Marijuana is generally taken by inhalation (i.e. by smoking), and it is able to cross the placenta. Fifty-six percent of women 18 to 25 years old have reported that they have smoked marijuana.[44] Of these, 22% have used it within the past year, and 11% have used it within the past month.

Smoking marijuana may affect the fetus indirectly by elevating carbon monoxide levels in the blood. When compared with smoking of tobacco, smoking of marijuana is associated with a fivefold increase in the blood carboxyhemoglobin level, presumably because of the larger puff volumes, greater depth of inhalation, and longer breath-holding time.[45] Thus, like cigarette smoking, marijuana smoking theoretically may impair fetal oxygenation, with consequent expected impairment of growth. Fetal growth might be further impaired by the tendency of marijuana to increase the heart rate and blood pressure of the mother, thus reducing placental blood flow to the fetus. Actually, however, marijuana use during pregnancy appears to have minimal or no effects on fetal length or weight.[46-48] Transient impairment of neurobehavioral function in newborns has, however, been described in relation to maternal smoking of one or more joints per week.[45]

Studies evaluating the effects of marijuana in pregnancy, its teratogenicity, and its effect, if any, on birth weight have been hindered by inconsistent reporting of marijuana use and the inability to differentiate the effects of other substances used in conjunction with marijuana.

OPIOIDS

Opioids include agents derived from opium and synthetic compounds with similar actions. The prototypical opioid is morphine. These drugs produce euphoria, somnolence, and decreased sensitivity to pain. Heroin (diacetylmorphine) is believed to exert its effect chiefly by being metabolized to morphine. Codeine is methylated morphine and is also metabolized to the parent compound. Other opiates such as meperidine (Demerol) and methadone (Dolophine) are structurally dissimilar to morphine but share its pharmacologic properties.

The number of women who use heroin during pregnancy is difficult to ascertain since many of these women are polydrug abusers, but it is safe to say that heroin has become the forgotten drug, in part due to the wide use of cocaine. Even though the frequency of this problem seems to have decreased, its dramatic effect cannot be forgotten, especially during the acquired immunodeficiency syndrome (AIDS) crisis.

MATERNAL AND FETAL COMPLICATIONS

Women using opioids during pregnancy appear to be at high risk for premature labor, meconium-stained amniotic fluid, and intrauterine growth retardation. Near term neonatal respiratory depression can occur in addi-

tion to neonatal withdrawal consisting of tremors, irritability, hyperto-
nicity, respiratory distress, vomiting, and fever. Studies on the medical
use of opioid analgesics during pregnancy have failed to prove a teratogenic effect of these agents.[49]

Maternal withdrawal from opioids produces characteristic features
ranging from anxiety, diaphoresis, nausea, vomiting, and diarrhea to
elevated blood pressure, tachycardia, cramps, and convulsions. If the
patient is in acute withdrawal, an initial dose of Demerol of 50 to 75 mg
intravenously may be administered. The fetus does not tolerate rapid
withdrawal, and intrauterine death may occur. Abstinence from opioids
is not feasible for most users, and the possibility of occult fetal
withdrawal makes even gradual tapering problematic. Therefore, methadone maintenance is generally recommended for opiate abusers during
pregnancy. Methadone is a synthetic opioid used to "detoxify" or
maintain opioid addicts. Methadone blocks the euphoric effects of
illicitly administered opioids and prevents withdrawal symptoms. The
long half-life of methadone helps to stabilize the fetal environment, and
maternal and fetal outcomes are improved.[50] Nonetheless, methadone
maintenance is not free of complications for the newborn, and many of
these infants require prolonged hospitalization for weight loss, withdrawal symptoms, depressed suck rates, and jaundice.[51] An initial
maternal dose of 20 mg of methadone will prevent withdrawal in the
majority of patients and may be given orally or intramuscularly if the
patient is in labor or vomiting. From recent work at our institution, we
have concluded that higher maintenance dosages may improve infant
outcome with an increase in gestational duration and improved overall
growth. This could be related to less use of "street drugs" among
patients receiving "blocking" doses of methadone.

In the event of an opioid overdose, management by a physician skilled
in treating such conditions is highly recommended in caring for the gravid
victim. The obstetrician should aid in excluding entities such as eclamp-
sia, amniotic fluid embolus, and occult abruptio placenta, as well as renal and diabetic conditions, which may be confused with overdose. The
obstetrician will also be expected to supervise the assessment of fetal status and to approve agents used in maternal resuscitation. Although fetal
heart tones should be checked, stabilizing the maternal condition takes
priority over continuous fetal monitoring. Moreover, it should be recalled
that reversal of maternal hypoxia combined with maternal drug metabolism and elimination may improve an ominous fetal heart rate tracing.
Maternal withdrawal may rapidly follow successful management of an
overdose and should be recognized and controlled while remembering
that this situation poses a significant risk to the fetus.

COMMENTS

Women who inject heroin with used needles and engage in prostitution
to support their habit are at significant risk of acquiring hepatitis, subacute bacterial endocarditis, and human immunodeficiency virus and
may transmit these viruses to the fetus. These medical conditions should
be looked for along with the more direct sequelae of opioid abuse.

SUMMARY

Certain abused chemicals have well-documented, direct effects on the fetus. The problems involved in evaluating these effects in the developing fetus and infant are multiple, not the least of which are the difficulties in following these infants over a period of time. The substance abuser's environment may hamper the intensive follow-up and early intervention processes necessary to ensure maximum infant development. The substance abuser is also prone to complications in pregnancy because of factors associated with her lifestyle, thus substantially adding to the perinatal risk.

In addition to the obstetric and medical problems of alcohol and drug abuse in pregnancy, such women may have an uncooperative attitude toward medical care. There is a high rate of noncompliance in prenatal clinics, and medical advice to abstain from alcohol and drugs may be ignored. Although many believe that legislation is the best method to deal with this growing dilemma, the American College of Obstetricians and Gynecologists (ACOG) opposes legislation that would impose criminal sanctions on women who use illicit substances during pregnancy.[52] Data from our institution are consistent with the view that drug-abusing women may avoid medical care if punitive laws are in effect.[53] We support ACOG's position of opposing legislation to impose criminal sanctions. Patient cooperation may be achieved by a tactful, nonthreatening approach. One should try not to be judgmental, even though these patients can often be frustrating and difficult to manage.

Alcohol and drug-related risks to both the mother and infant persist after birth and should be considered. Infants are at increased risk for neglect, abuse, learning disabilities, and retarded growth and motor development. Maternal health may deteriorate from liver disease, AIDS, venereal disease, or a whole host of medical complications resulting from the continued abuse of various substances. A multidisciplinary approach that continues long after delivery currently appears to offer the best chance for improved maternal and infant outcome.

REFERENCES

1. American College of Obstetricians and Gynecologists: *Drug Abuse and Pregnancy*. ACOG Technical Bulletin; No 96, 1986.
2. Jones KL, Smith DW, Ulleland CN, et al: Pattern of malformations in offspring of chronic alcoholic mothers. *Lancet* 1973; 1:1267.
3. *Alcoholic Beverage Labeling*. 100th Congress Report, 1988, pp 100–596.
4. Carson SA, Simpson JL: Spontaneous abortion, in Eden R, Boehm F (eds): *Assessment and Care of the Fetus*. East Norwalk, Conn, Appleton & Lange, 1990, pp 559–574.
5. *Dorland's Illustrated Medical Dictionary*, ed 26. Philadelphia, WB Saunders, 1985, p 6.
6. Abel EL: *Marijuana, Tobacco, Alcohol and Reproduction*. Boca Raton, Fla, CRC Press, 1983.
7. Abel EL, Sokol RJ: Consequences of alcohol abuse, in Gleicher N (ed): *Principles and Practice of Medical Therapy in Pregnancy*. East Norwalk, Conn, Appleton & Lange, 1992, pp 79–85.

8. Sokol RJ, Miller FI, Reed G: Alcohol abuse during pregnancy: An epidemiologic study. *Alcohol Clin Exp Res* 1980; 4:135–145.

9. Coffey TG: Beer Street; Gin Lane: Some views of 18th Century Drinking. *Q J Stud Alcohol* 1966; 27:669.

10. Fisher SE: Selective fetal malnutrition: The fetal alcohol syndrome. *J Am Coll Nutr* 1988; 7:101–106.

11. Phillips DK, Henderson GI, Schneker S: Pathogenesis of fetal alcohol syndrome. *Alcohol Health Res World* 1989; 13:219–227.

12. Ghishan FK, Greene HL: Fetal alcohol syndrome: Failure of zinc supplementation to reverse the effect of ethanol on placental transport of zinc. *J Pediatr Res* 1983; 17:519–531.

13. Lemoine P, Harrousseau H, Borteyra J, et al: Les enfants de parents alcoholiques: Anomalies observes: A propos de 127 cas. *Quest Med* 1968; 21:476–482.

14. Jones KL, Smith DW: Recognition of the fetal alcohol syndrome in early infancy. *Lancet* 1973; 2:999–1001.

15. Schenker S, Becker HC, Randall CL, et al: Fetal alcohol syndrome: Current status of pathogenesis. *Alcohol Clin Exp Res* 1990; 14:635–647.

16. Wegman ME: Annual summary of vital statistics 1986. *Pediatrics* 1987; 80:817–827.

17. Steissguth AP: The behavioral teratology of alcohol: Performance, behavioral and intellectual deficits in prenatally exposed children, in West JR (ed): *Alcohol and Brain Development*. New York, Oxford University Press, 1986, pp 3–44.

18. Ernhart CB, Kawano T, Sokol RJ, et al: Prenatal alcohol exposure and catch up growth to age five years. *Alcoholism* 1989; 13:344.

19. Abel EL, Sokol RJ: A revised conservative estimate of the incidence of FAS and its economic impact. *Alcohol Clin Exp Res* 1991; 15:514–524.

20. Hannigan JH, Welch RA, Sokol RJ: Recognition of fetal alcohol syndrome and alcohol-related birth defects, in Mendelson JH, Mello NK (eds): *Medical Diagnosis and Treatment of Alcoholism*. New York, McGraw-Hill, 1992, pp 639–667.

21. Sokol RJ, Clarren SK: Guidelines for use of terminology describing the impact of prenatal alcohol on the offspring. *Alcohol Clin Exp Res* 1989; 13:597–598.

22. Clarren SK, Astley SJ, Bowden DM, et al: Neuroanatomical and neurochemical abnormalities in nonhuman primate infants exposed to weekly doses of ethanol during gestation. *Alcohol Clin Exp Res* 1990; 14:674–683.

23. Ernhart CB, Sokol RJ, Ager JW, et al: Alcohol related birth defects; assessing the risk. *Ann N Y Acad Sci* 1989; 562:159–172.

24. Selzer ML: The Michigan alcoholism screening test: The quest for a new diagnostic instrument. *Am J Psychiatry* 1971; 127:89.

25. Pokorny AD, Miller BA, Kapplan HB: The brief mast: A shortened version of the Michigan alcoholism screening test. *Am J Psychiatry* 1973; 129:118.

26. Mayfield D, Mcleod, Hall P: The cage questionnaire: Validation of a new alcoholism screening instrument. *Am J Psychiatry* 1975; 131:1121.

27. Sokol RJ, Martier SS, Ager J: The T-ACE questions: Practical prenatal detection of risk drinking. *Am J Obstet Gynecol* 1989; 160:863.

28. American College of Obstetricians and Gynecologists: *Cocaine in Pregnancy. Committee Opinion.* ACOG Technical Bulletin No 114, 1990.

29. Ostrea EM Jr, Brady MJ, Parks PM, et al: Drug screening of meconium in infants of drug dependent mothers: An alternative to urine testing. *J Pediatr* 1989; 115:474–477.

30. Gold MS, Washton AM, Dackis CA, et al: Cocaine abuse: Neurochemistry and Treatment. *Natl Inst Drug Abuse Res Mono Gr Ser* 1985; 61:130–150.
31. Stewart DJ, Inaba T, Lucassen M, et al: Cocaine metabolism: Cocaine and nor-cocaine hydrolysis by liver and serum esterases. *Clin Pharmacol Ther* 1979; 25:464–468.
32. Ambre J, Ruo TI, Nelson J, et al: Urinary excretion of cocaine, benzoylecgonine and ecgonine methyl ester in humans. *J Anal Toxicol* 1988; 12:301–306.
33. Mercado A, Johnson G, Calver D, et al: Cocaine, pregnancy and postpartum intracerebral hemorrhage. *Obstet Gynecol* 1989; 73:467–468.
34. Welch RA, Martier SS, Ager JW, et al: Radioimmunoassay of hair is a valid technique for determining maternal cocaine abuse. *Substance Abuse* 1990; 11:214–217.
35. Graham K, Koren G, Klein J, et al: Determination of gestational cocaine exposure by hair analysis. *JAMA* 1989; 262:3328–3330.
36. Cregler LL, Mark H: Medical complication of cocaine abuse. *N Engl J Med* 1989; 315:1495–1500.
37. Ryan L, Ehrlich S, Finnegan L: Cocaine abuse in pregnancy; effects on the fetus and newborn. *Neurotoxicol Teratol* 1987; 9:295.
38. Church MW, Dintcheff BA, Gessner PK: The interactive effects of alcohol and cocaine on maternal and fetal toxicology in the Long-Evans rat. *Neurotoxicol Teratol* 1988; 10:355.
39. Bingol N, Fuchs M, Diaz V, et al: Teratogenicity of cocaine in humans. *J Pediatr* 1987; 110:93–96.
40. MacGregor S, Keits LG, Chasnoff IJ, et al: Cocaine use during pregnancy: Adverse perinatal outcome. *Am J Obstet Gynecol* 1987; 157:686.
41. Little BB, Snell LM, Klein V, et al: Cocaine abuse during pregnancy: Maternal and fetal implications. *Obstet Gynecol* 1989; 73:157–160.
42. Horowitz FD: The psychobiology of parent-offspring relations in high risk situations. *Adv Infancy Res* 1984; 3:1.
43. Rist N: The shadow children. *Am School Board J* 2990; 177:14–24.
44. National Institute on Drug Abuse: *National Household Survey on Drug Abuse 1988 Population Estimates*. Washington, DC, US Department of Health and Human Services, 1989.
45. Wu T-C, Taskin DP, Djahed B, et al: Pulmonary hazards of smoking marijuana as compared with tobacco. *N Engl J Med* 1988; 318:347–351.
46. Fried PA, Watkinson B, Dillon RF, et al: National neurological status in a low-risk population after prenatal exposure to cigarettes, marijuana and alcohol. *J Dev Behav Pediatr* 1987; 8:318.
47. Linn S, Schoenbaum S, Monson R, et al: The association of marijuana use with outcome of pregnancy. *Am J Public Health* 1983; 73:1161.
48. Zuckerman B, Frank DA, Hingson R, et al: Effects of maternal marijuana and cocaine use on fetal growth. *N Engl J Med* 1989; 320:762.
49. Schardein JL: *Chemically Induced Birth Defects*. New York, Marcel Dekker, 1985 p 773.
50. Connaughton JF, Ruser D, Schurt J, et al: Perinatal addiction: Outcome and management. *Am J Obstet Gynecol* 1977; 129:679–686.
51. Welch RA, Dombrowski MP, Sokol RJ: Maternal chemical dependence, in Evans MI (ed): *Reproductive Risks and Prenatal Diagnosis*. East Norwalk, Conn, Appleton & Lange, 1992, pp 79–90.
52. Moore KG: Substance abuse & pregnancy: State lawmakers respond with punitive & public health measures. *COG Legis-Letter* vol 9, No 3, 1990.
53. Poland ML, Dombrowski MP, Ager JW, et al: Punishing pregnant drug users: Enhancing the flight from care. *Drug Alcohol Depend* 1993; 31:199–203.

Editor's Comment

This is a well-written chapter in which the risks of substance abuse are clearly defined. More importantly, the authors provide the clinician with clues and screening techniques to identify potential alcohol abusers. Also presented are methods that can be used to identify remote ingestion of cocaine and its related substances. Specifically, the use of maternal hair and meconium to identify remote ingestion of cocaine are methods with which all physicians should be familiar.

The authors report that the use of marijuana *may* not be as detrimental as once thought. Unfortunately, the resurgence of heroin abuse does pose immediate (overdose) and remote (withdrawal) risks of death to both the fetus and its mother. Finally, the authors stress that any form of substance abuse may be associated with other risks: bacterial endocarditis, hepatitis, and other sexually transmitted diseases including AIDS. The authors conclude with the obvious, but not often considered greatest risk that these patients pose to themselves, their fetuses, and their physicians. Specifically, these are difficult patients to manage. They are noncompliant and frequently antisocial and often have serious related psychological disorders that makes long-term prognosis for them and their fetus-infants less than ideal.

In conclusion, the information provided by the authors of this chapter is "a must." It is information that any practicing physician cannot be without in view of today's social surroundings.

Norman F. Gant, Jr., M.D.

HIV and AIDS in the Obstetrical and Gynecological Patient: A Review of the Literature With Guidelines for Care and Screening

KEVIN A. AULT, M.D.

SEBASTIAN FARO, M.D., PH.D.

B ecause the human immunodeficiency virus (HIV) is spread sexually, by blood exposure (e.g., sharing needles in intravenous drug abuse), and by perinatal exposure, obstetrician-gynecologists must be aware of the rising incidence of HIV infection and acquired immunodeficiency syndrome (AIDS) among their patients. Moreover, they must understand the pathophysiology of this spectrum of related diseases.

Human immunodeficiency virus preferentially attacks lymphocytes bearing the CD4 antigen, thus rendering the host susceptible to unusual neoplasms and opportunistic infections. Acquired immunodeficiency syndrome is a clinical entity characterized by extreme lymphocyte depletion with characteristic disease patterns. In fact, AIDS represents the end point of HIV infection and may be preceded by 8 to 10 years of asymptomatic infection,[1] during which time an individual is, however, infectious.

Women are increasingly part of the AIDS epidemic. Five percent of the newly diagnosed AIDS cases in 1987 were women, and in 1991, 14% were women.[2] This percentage will probably increase through the foreseeable future (Fig 1 and Table 1). Heterosexual transmission has become a progressively more important factor in HIV transmission.[2] Although many women are infected during sexual contact with high-risk men (known HIV-positive, bisexual, or intravenous drug users), a recent study reported that 21% of HIV-infected pregnant women had no identifiable risk factors.[3] In another study among urban adolescent pregnant women, 58% were reported to have no known risk factors.[4] Approximately 1 million Americans are now infected by the HIV virus,[5] and for every infected symptomatic individual, there are 20 to 30 asymptomatic individuals.[6]

Advances in Obstetrics and Gynecology, vol 1
© 1994, Mosby–Year Book, Inc.

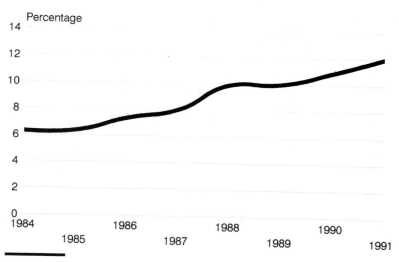

FIGURE 1.

Percentage of new AIDS patients who are women. Most women diagnosed with HIV/AIDS are in the reproductive age group. (Data from various Centers for Disease Control reports.)

Women are also involved in perinatal transmission of HIV. Neonates acquire HIV infection in utero or during the birth process by exposure to infected fluids. Approximately 6,000 neonates are exposed to HIV[7] annually, and in 25% to 50% of these infants, pediatric AIDS will develop (see later discussion). The large majority of HIV-infected women are in their reproductive years and thus are potentially at risk of delivering an infected newborn.

This chapter presents a review of the rapidly expanding knowledge base concerning women and HIV infection. Specifically, heterosexual transmission, gynecologic complications, and perinatal transmission will be reviewed. Suggested plans for caring for these women will also be presented. In June 1992, the American College of Obstetricians and Gynecologists issued a technical bulletin on HIV infections. In this bulletin, the college noted that "interaction with sexually active women . . . provide[s] a unique opportunity to educate patients about risks of infection and ways to treat them. In so doing, obstetrician-gynecologists have the chance to reduce the incidence of not only HIV disease, but also the 13 million cases of sexually transmitted diseases diagnosed annually in the United States."

TABLE 1.

Projected AIDS Cases 1992–1994*

Total	Women	Perinatal Transmission
47,000–77,000	7,000–11,000	1,050
47,000–85,000	7,000–14,000	1,100
43,000–93,000	7,000–18,000	1,200

*From Centers for Disease Control: *MMWR* 1992; 41:1–29.

HETEROSEXUAL TRANSMISSION

Approximately 30% to 50% of AIDS cases in women in the United States were acquired through heterosexual contact. Heterosexual spread of HIV is the norm throughout most of the world (as opposed to spread through homosexual contact), and case ratios of AIDS in Africa and the Caribbean are 1 to 1 male to female.[8] In the early studies reviewed by Holmes and Kriess in 1988, HIV transmission was reported to occur in both directions. Many of these studies were small, however, and the routes of infection were mixed and patients were being actively encouraged to modify their risk behavior while the studies were in progress. Transmission rates, defined as the number of HIV-positive partners per number exposed, ranged from 8% to 50% for female-to-male contact and from 0% to 45% for male-to-female contact. Risk factors identified for transmission included advanced stage of disease and heterosexual anal intercourse. Genital ulcer disease and cervicitis were found to be risk factors in several African studies. Consistent condom use was found to be protective. Another review published at the same time came to the same conclusions.[9]

A cohort study by the European Study Group on Heterosexual Transmission of HIV was recently published.[10] Index patients consisted of 159 women and 404 men and their sexual contacts. Most index cases were intravenous drug abusers. This study started in 1987, and patients were recruited when HIV was diagnosed. Seronegative partners were followed every 6 months for detection of seroconversion. Overall, 12% of male partners and 20% of female partners were infected. Risk factors for transmission included unprotected vaginal intercourse, advanced stage of disease, sex during menses, anal sex, and a history of syphilis or chlamydia. Condom usage was associated with a decrease in transmission, and use of spermicide was not found to be protective. The authors concluded that male-to-female transmission was relatively more efficient.

Use of barrier methods to prevent the heterosexual spread of HIV has received much attention in the public and scientific press. As suggested in the aforementioned study, consistent use of latex condoms has been shown to decrease transmission. Unfortunately, this method is dependent on the male partner, and the use of nonbarrier or hormonal methods such as oral contraceptives, levonorgestrel implants (Norplant), or medroxyprogesterone acetate (Depo-Provera) provides no protection against HIV infection.[11] In some African studies, increased seroconversion has been reported among women relying on oral contraceptives as their sole method of birth control.

Spermicides such as nonoxynol-9 have in vitro activity against many sexually transmitted pathogens including HIV, and a randomized trial of a spermicide-impregnated contraceptive sponge (the "Today Sponge") has been reported.[12] In this study, 116 Nairobi, Kenya, prostitutes were randomized to use a sponge or placebo. They were instructed to also continue the same method of contraception that was used before enrollment. No protection against seroconversion was conferred by use of the nonoxynol-9–impregnated sponge. During the approximately 1-year follow-up, 27 of 60 (45%) of the subjects and 20 of 56 (36%) of the controls underwent seroconversion (no statistical difference). Subjects using the sponge did, however, have a 60% reduced risk for gonococcal cervicitis.

The most remarkable finding in this study was that subjects had an increased risk of vaginitis and genital ulcers. These inflammatory processes with subsequent breakdown of the vaginal epithelium may have overcome any potential antiviral effect of the spermicide. In their accompanying editorial, Stone and Peterson[13] stated that enthusiasm for currently available spermicides as a protection against heterosexual transmission of HIV may be premature and that latex condoms remain the method of choice in sexually active women wishing to reduce their exposure to sexually transmitted disease including HIV.

GYNECOLOGIC DISEASES AND HIV INFECTION

Women with HIV have a predilection for two specific gynecologic diseases: vaginitis and cervical neoplasia. The tendency toward chronic vaginal candidiasis was recognized early in the AIDS epidemic. In a small cohort of women followed at Walter Reed Army Hospital between 1983 and 1986, 7 of 29 HIV-infected women, or 24%, had chronic vaginitis.[14] The mean CD4 count among these women was 90 (the usual normal or uninfected range is 600 to 1,000), and clinically evident AIDS developed in 6 of the 7 within the 30-month follow-up period. In all cases, vaginal infection preceded the development of oral thrush or more invasive *Candida* disease.

The hierarchical pattern of infection with *Candida* in infected women was confirmed in a recent report.[15] In this study, 66 HIV-positive women were followed for 3 years. Thirty-three of these women had *Candida* vaginitis as the initial sign of immune dysfunction, and 17 gave a history of increased frequency of vaginitis before their diagnosis of HIV infection. Oral thrush developed in 21 women during the study period, and esophageal candidiasis developed in 9. Location of the *Candida* infections was related to CD4 counts. Mean CD4 counts were as follows: no *Candida* infection, 741; vaginal, 506; oral, 320; and esophageal, 30. The authors noted a high cure rate for vaginitis with relatively normal CD4 counts; however, prolonged courses of oral antifungal medications were often necessary to relieve vaginitis as immune function deteriorated. In a subsequent letter to the editor by the same authors, it was suggested that the occurrence of *Candida* vaginitis should prompt an investigation of risk factors for HIV infection. In our opinion, testing should be offered to women with recurrent or unusual manifestations of vaginitis as well as to women with risk factors.

As mentioned previously, cervical neoplasia has been associated with HIV infection. It is well known that other women with immunosuppression are at increased risk of cervical neoplasia, so this finding is not unexpected. The issue is complicated, however, by the frequent coinfection with human papilloma virus (HPV). The results of serial screening with semiannual Papanicolaou smears have been reported in a recent multicenter study.[16] One hundred thirty-five women were enrolled at three different urban sites, and abnormal Papanicolaou smears were reported in 23% to 48% of these women. This was much higher than the baseline abnormal Papanicolaou smear rate at each institution. Only 6 women had smears suggestive of high-grade intraepithelial neoplasia. The rate of abnormal Papanicolaou smears was related to the degree of immunosuppression as measured by the CD4 count.

The relationship of neoplasia, HPV, and HIV was reported in a recent Italian study of 75 infected women.[17] At the initial visit, patients underwent colposcopy and cytologic screening with directed biopsies if abnormalities were found. A commercial kit was used to detect HPV DNA. Twenty-five patients underwent biopsies, and cervical intraepithelial neoplasia (CIN) was found in 22. All but 1 of the high-grade lesions contained HPV. Vulvar or perianal condylomas were detected in 14 women. Women with moderate or severe CIN had significantly lower mean CD4 counts. All patients with CIN completed at least 1 year of follow-up. One woman with high-grade lesions had a recurrence, but no women with mild dysplasia had recurrences. Invasive cervical cancer in HIV-infected women has been reported in two recent studies. In Kenya,[18] 200 consecutive women with invasive cervical cancer were tested for antibodies to HIV. Three women were seropositive (1.5%), a percentage similar to the 2% rate reported among blood donors in Kenya. In striking contrast with the results of the Kenya study were results reported from Brooklyn, New York.[19] Twenty percent of AIDS cases in this area of the United States occur in women. Thirty-seven women under the age of 50 were tested for HIV. Seven women (19%) tested positive, including a 16-year-old with stage IIIB cervical cancer. No HIV-positive women had early disease when compared with HIV-negative controls. The HIV-positive and HIV-negative groups were similar in age, parity, smoking, age at first coitus, and number of sexual partners. Persistent or recurrent disease developed in all HIV-positive women. Four died of cervical cancer. The median time to death from cervical cancer was 10 months in HIV-positive women as compared with 23 months in the HIV-negative group.

The effect of HIV infection on cervical histology was reported in another study from the same facility.[20] Under this protocol, 32 known HIV-positive women underwent cervical cytology and routine colposcopy. Liberal colposcopically directed biopsies were taken in abnormal areas; if no lesions were found, a random biopsy was taken from the transition zone. Evidence of CIN was seen on one Papanicolaou smear, whereas 25 of 32 (78%) had normal cytologic findings. On biopsy, however, 13 of 32 (41%) had CIN, and 6 patients had either moderate or severe dysplasia. Most of the remaining women had evidence of cervicitis. Thus, 12 of 31 women with CIN on biopsy had no evidence of dysplasia on Papanicolaou smear. Two other potential cofactors in the neoplastic process were investigated. Mean CD4 counts were lower in women with CIN. Biopsy specimens were analysed for HPV DNA with polymerase chain reaction. Seven of 12 women with CIN had evidence of HPV infection, but none of 17 with normal biopsy findings had HPV DNA in their specimen.

Does dysplasia follow a more aggressive course in HIV-positive women? This question was specifically addressed in one study.[21] Women were referred for colposcopic evaluation if squamous intraepithelial neoplasia (SIN) was found on Papanicolaou smear. The referral population was derived from a clinic dedicated to women at high risk for HIV infection; therefore, both seropositive and seronegative women had similar behavioral and socioeconomic risks for CIN. Of the 38 women who underwent colposcopy for abnormal cytology, 13 were seronegative (34%), 18 had symptomatic HIV infection, and 7 were seropositive without symptoms. In contrast to the previously cited study, overall agreement was observed between cytology and histologic findings. Only 2 women had biopsy results showing more advanced disease than was shown by cytology. No invasive cancers were found. Therapy was not altered based on HIV status, and follow-up was available on 27 of the 38 enrollees. All 3 of the treated seronegative women had normal follow-up cytologic findings, and 5 of 10 seropositive women had normal follow-up. Three had persistent disease without progression, and 2 had progression of vulvar or vaginal condyloma. Although these numbers are small, rapid progression of CIN was not seen, and seropositive patients responded well to conventional therapy.

When discussing the interrelationship of HIV and dysplasia, several methodology problems are obvious. Cervical dysplasia, like HIV, is a sexually transmitted disease with a significant transmission contribution from several behavioral factors. Epidemiologic risk factors such as age at first coitus, number of sexual partners, nonbarrier or no contraception, and coinfection with other sexually transmitted diseases (STDs), especially HPV, are well-established risk factors for cervical dysplasia and invasive cancer. It is easy to see that these are also risk factors for acquisition of HIV infection. Thus, studies of the natural history of dysplasia in HIV-positive women should include some meaningful comparison groups. In a recent review of the relevant literative on this subject, Mandelblatt et al.[22] found that 5 of 21 studies included control groups and that the relative risk of dysplasia was five times greater in seropositive patients.

What difference does this information make in the practice of clinical gynecology? Although it is difficult to find agreement in published studies concerning gynecologic care of HIV-positive women, it seems prudent to pursue more frequent cytologic sampling of these patients on a semiannual or three-times-a-year schedule. Any Papanicolaou smear abnormality should be investigated promptly and subjected to colposcopy. It is difficult at this time to recommend routine colposcopy with a normal cytology. Given the findings of Maiman et al.,[20] however, some experts recommend "baseline" colposcopic examinations. Do women with dysplasia need to undergo screening for HIV? Again, when caring for women with CIN, a discussion of the behavioral risks associated with this disease should take place, and such a discussion can serve as an evaluation for risks for HIV. Since HIV may affect the course of treatment of dysplasia and cervical cancer, women with recurrent dysplasia or young women with cervical cancer probably should be screened for HIV. In recognition of the aforementioned data, the Centers for Disease Control (CDC) in 1993 added invasive cervical cancer as an AIDS-defining illness in HIV-positive women.

Two other gynecologic complications of HIV deserve mention. An unusually aggressive vulvar squamous cell carcinoma has been reported in a 27-year-old woman.[23] This patient had a long history of vulvar condyloma, and a rapidly growing carcinoma was discovered on biopsy. The patient underwent radical vulvectomy and a single positive left inguinal lymph node was found. The patient had a recurrent lesion within 2 months of surgery, and this mass responded poorly to high-dose radiation therapy. The patient died of unspecified causes 9 months later.

Another aspect of gynecology and HIV disease that must be considered is the transmission of HIV through donor insemination. Specifically, the American Fertility Society[24] suggests that males with certain HIV risk factors should be precluded from semen donation programs. These risk factors include homosexual contact, intravenous drug use, sexual contact with a known HIV-positive woman, and evidence of exposure to or history of past STDs. All donors should undergo screening for HIV before sample collection and every 6 months while they continue to donate.

INTERACTION OF HIV AND OTHER SEXUALLY TRANSMITTED DISEASES

There are several aspects of HIV infection that relate to other STDs. The first and most obvious is the presence of one of the more traditional STDs—syphilis, gonorrhea, or chlamydia—any one of which should serve as a marker for behavioral risks for HIV. The results of a national screening program at STD clinics around the United States have been reported.[25]

Anonymous sera samples were analyzed from attendees, and selected demographic and behavioral variables were analyzed. Seroprevalence rates from 37 clinics in 27 metropolitan areas were calculated. Two of the traditional risk groups predictably had a high prevalence of HIV infection. Men who had sex with men without a history of intravenous drug use had a seroprevalence of 14.3% to 64.2%, and heterosexual drug abusers had a range of seroprevalence from 0% to 4.1%. Heterosexuals who did not abuse drugs but who exhibited other high-risk behavior were seropositive at a rate of 0% to 14.1%. Heterosexuals with no identifiable risk factors were seropositive at a rate of 0% to 10.7%. There were large geographic differences in the clinics studied.

A seroprevalence study involving a single age group within a single state[26] has been reported, and heterosexual contact was felt to be the primary mode of transmission. The overall rate of HIV seroprevalence was 4 per 1,000 adolescents attending STD clinics in Mississippi. This rate did not vary with gender, race, or geographic location. Rates were not analyzed by the underlying STD. The authors concluded that the incidence of HIV infection among teenagers does not vary by gender or by urban location as was suggested in several previous studies. They entitled this a "rural epidemic" in a state with a high level of STDs.

A uniquely female complication of two of the most common STDs, gonorrhea and chlamydia, is pelvic inflammatory disease (PID), an upper genital tract infection. This diagnosis provides an opportunity to study the interaction of STDs and HIV in a strictly female population. Sera of 333 women hospitalized with PID over the years 1985 to 1988 was retrospectively analyzed for HIV antibodies in a San Francisco–based study.[27] From a chart review, the authors identified a significant relationship between intravenous drug abuse and seropositive HIV status. Other risk factors analyzed included serum chlamydia antibody status, race, VDRL status, history of genital HPV infection, positive culture for gonorrhea or chlamydia, or active infection with *Trichomonas vaginalis*. None of these factors was significantly related to seroprevalence. The overall seroprevalence was 4.2% with increasing prevalence throughout the study. A rate of 6.7% was reported for the last year.

In a similar prospective study in New York, Hoegsberg and colleagues[28] reported an incidence of 13.6% for HIV-seropositive status in 110 women hospitalized for PID. Seropositive women were more likely to have normal white blood cell counts and also more likely to need surgery. No differences were found among rates of STDs studied. The authors stated that there appeared to be a tendency for PID to be more aggressive in HIV-positive women and that hospital management was preferred.

Another interaction between HIV and other STDs is that diseases causing genital ulceration such as herpes, syphilis, and chancroid provide a route for HIV transmission by mucosal breakdown and facilitated access to the bloodstream. These ulcers are characterized by lymphocytic infiltration. That HIV can be expressed by infected lymphocytes or acquired more easily by uninfected cells has been confirmed by epidemiologic studies of both homosexual and heterosexual transmission. In one study,[29] homosexual men with STDs or seeking testing for HIV were tested for specific treponemal antibodies (syphilis) and herpes simplex virus 2 (HSV-2) antibodies. Significant differences by logistic regression were found between seropositive and seronegative men in syphilis serology, HSV antibody titer, and clinical history of syphilis or herpes. These differences persisted when controlling for the number of sexual partners. Moreover, serologic and clinical evidence of recent primary herpes was associated with an increased rate of seroconversion for HIV. In another study of heterosexual men in Africa,[30] HIV prevalence was shown to be associated with a history of genital ulcer disease, especially chancroid. There is reason to believe that such synergy could take place in urban settings in the United States. Record increases in syphilis[31] and chancroid[32] have occurred in recent years. Epidemics of these two ulcerative diseases have occurred mainly among heterosexuals.

Also noteworthy are the special complications of syphilis that occur in HIV-positive individuals. Unusual symptoms, poor response to therapy, and rapid advancement of disease have been reported.[33] For these reasons, HIV coinfection must be considered and excluded when syphilis is diagnosed. In one study of 120 women with reactive syphilis screening during pregnancy, 7 (5.8%) were found to be HIV-positive. In another study, the relationship between HIV, syphilis, and cocaine was explored.[34] In this study, 1,206 women giving birth had urine tested for the presence of cocaine, and sera used for syphilis serology was also tested for HIV antibodies. Of the study subjects, 12.9% had urine toxicology positive for cocaine. Cocaine-positive women were six times more likely to be HIV-seropositive and ten times more likely to be positive for specific syphilis serology.

In summary, there appears to be a growing body of evidence linking STDs in heterosexuals to HIV risk. The presence of STDs may be the only identifier that a woman may have been exposed to HIV. The use of barrier contraception will decrease the acquisition of HIV as well as other STDs. For these reasons, women with STDs should undergo testing for HIV. This is especially true for syphilis and possibly for PID; the presence of HIV may alter the natural history of these STDs.

PREGNANCY AND HIV INFECTION

Many aspects of HIV infection have a direct impact on pregnancy. Maternal infection is directly responsible for pediatric AIDS through vertical transmission of HIV. Pregnancy and HIV have the potential for interaction during the course of gestation. As HIV infection in reproductive-age women becomes more common, clinicians must be familiar with methods of care for HIV-infected women.

There is much to be learned about the perinatal transmission of HIV. Generally, the most commonly cited rates of maternal-fetal transmission are 25% to 35%. Maternally acquired antibodies may persist in the newborn for up to 15 months and give a positive result on the enzyme-linked immunoassay commonly used to test for HIV antibodies. The timing of HIV transmission is variable; some fetuses are infected in utero and others in late gestation or during the peripartum period. In several placental cell lines, the CD4 receptor has been demonstrated. Human immunodeficiency virus core antigen has been localized in term placentas, and evidence of HIV infection in the products of conception have been found even in the first trimester.[35]

The perinatal transmission of HIV has been discussed in three review articles[36-38] published in 1992. The most consistently cited risk factor for perinatal transmission is the viral load in the mother. Maternal viremia in HIV is greatest at the time of initial infection and in the late stages of the disease. It is believed that there is a long quiescent period where virus is only found in the lymph nodes between these two periods. The clinical correlate to HIV load is the CD4 count, and decreased CD4 counts have been shown to be a risk factor. The presence of maternal antibodies to certain HIV epitopes has been reported to be protective; however, these data are conflicting. This fact may lead to a potential step for intervention by maternal immunization to certain HIV glycoproteins. Other factors may include placentitis and preterm delivery.

In a recent large study, the rate of maternal-fetal transmission has been shown to be lower than has been previously reported.[39] This study included 600 children born to HIV-positive mothers in ten European centers. Of children with adequate follow-up, 12.9% were infected. Of these infected children, 83% showed laboratory or clinical features of HIV infection by 6 months of age. By 12 months, 26% had pediatric AIDS, and 17% had died of HIV-related diseases. Clinical features of the pregnancy and neonatal course did not distinguish infected from uninfected children.

There is no reliable serologic test in newborns that will predict which ones will become infected.[40] Failed methodologies that have been tried include anti-HIV IgM, IgA, and IgG production from cultured lymphocytes. One study included both IgM and IgA antibody tests; IgA was found to be the most promising.[41] All infected children were positive for IgA antibodies by 12 months of age. Infected children were positive for IgA at twice the rate of IgM at the same age. Attempts to identify virus or viral DNA have also been made. Unfortunately, the HIV virus is difficult to culture, and few laboratories are equipped for the extensive precautions that are necessary. All of these tests have the distinct disadvantage of being inadequate to identify neonates infected late in gestation or perinatally.

One simplified technique was recently reported to identify HIV infection in neonates.[42] In this assay, HIV antigen-antibody complexes from neonatal sera were dissociated and subjected to testing with a commercially available test for the p24 HIV antigen. Five of eight HIV-infected neonates had p24 antigen detected in their cord blood, and two who were initially negative at birth had positive tests at 12 and 18 days. The remaining infant was lost to follow-up. There were no "false positive" results in uninfected infants.

Approximately 6,000 newborns are exposed to HIV annually—a national rate of 1.5 per 1,000[43] (Table 2). This study was done by testing anonymous heelstick samples from 38 states. The method used detected maternally derived IgG. Large regional differences were found. These data were obtained during 1989, and these figures will increase as the number of HIV-infected women continues to increase.

What effect does pregnancy have on disease progression in the HIV-infected woman? Most investigators attempting to answer this question have been limited by short observation periods and lack of a control group. The most comprehensive study yet reported, of 128 women followed for an average of 16 months, showed little effect on HIV progres-

TABLE 2.

Prevalence of HIV Infection in Childbearing Women in Selected States*

State	Prevalence per Thousand†
New York	5.8
District of Columbia	5.5
Florida	4.5
National average	**1.5**
North Carolina	1.2
Texas	1
Illinois	0.9
California	0.7
Washington	0.2

*From Gwinn M, Pappaioanou M, George J, et al: *JAMA* 1991; 265:1704–1708. Used by permission.

†Data obtained by anonymous heelstick 1988–1989.

sion.[44] No significant differences were shown between third-trimester women and nonpregnant controls. One study[45] involved 203 women enrolled in a methadone maintenance program who agreed to participate in a longitudinal study of HIV infection. During the approximately 2 years of follow-up, 24% of seropositive and 22% of seronegative women become pregnant. There were no significant differences between the two groups. Anemia and bacterial pneumonia both were more common in the seropositive group. Neonatal measures such as gestational age, birth weight, and Apgar score were similar in each group. Many of these same conclusions were reported by a comparable study[46] in which the control group was composed of women enrolled from the same prenatal clinic.

It would seem logical that HIV-infected women are at increased risk for infections during pregnancy. In one study of 56 seropositive women with controls,[47] none of the subjects had serious infectious complications if their absolute CD4 count was greater than 300. In the subset of patients with lower CD4 counts, there were 2 cases of *Pneumocytis* infection, 1 case of bacterial pneumonia, 1 case of central nervous system toxoplasmosis, and 1 case of postcesarean abscess.

Who should be tested for HIV status during pregnancy? Early in the HIV epidemic, risk could be assessed by the traditional factors of intravenous drug abuse or sexual contact with a man who was such an abuser, contact with a bisexual male, or a transfusion before the routine test of blood donors. This strategy, however, was found to be lacking in one recent analysis.[48] Testing only those women with risk factors would have identified only 57% of infected pregnant women. Voluntary testing raised this percentage considerably. Remarkably similar percentages were found in a variety of clinical settings (Table 3). Among pregnant women in rural Florida[3] and adolescents[4] and women receiving inadequate prenatal care in metropolitan Atlanta,[49] approximately 50% had no identifiable risk factors for HIV seroconversion. For these reasons, we recommend routine voluntary HIV screening of pregnant women in the United States. An eloquent editorial in *The New England Journal of Medicine* by Heagarty and Abrams[50] stated, "Surely we have reached the time when widespread testing of women and newborn infants is both warranted and justifiable. Any such program must be developed with careful attention to protection of confidentiality, but we cannot care for women and children with HIV infection without knowing who they are."

It has been our experience that a policy of routine voluntary screening will uncover many asymptomatic HIV-positive women during their prenatal care. The obstetrician-gynecologist will then be in a position to make informed management decisions about the health care of these women. Suggestions for workup (Table 4) do not differ radically from standard prenatal examination.[51] Hepatitis B surface antigen is included for testing because some women may also be intravenous drug abusers, and women with continued risk for hepatitis should be immunized. The natural history of tuberculosis is altered in HIV-positive individuals, and purified protein derivative (PPD) status should be established and appropriate follow-up undertaken. Toxoplasmosis and cytomegalovirus (CMV) are included because these diseases also have an altered course in HIV-infected women and both may cause congenital infection. Intrapartum

TABLE 3.
Selected Seroprevalence Studies in Pregnant Women

Setting*	Seroprevalence	Epidemiologic Risk Factors	Percentage Seropositive Without Risk Factors
Atlanta: 1987–1991, adolescents[4]	4.7/1,000	"Crack" cocaine	58
Atlanta: 1987–1988[49]	Receiving prenatal care 3.5/1,000 Inadequate prenatal care 14.3/1,000	Intravenous drug abuse	25–50
Baltimore: 1987–1990[48]	29/1,000	—	43
Rural Florida[3]	58/1,000	"Crack" cocaine, multiple partners, syphilis	21
United States: 38 states using anonymous neonatal heelstick[7] (see Table 2)	1.5/1,000	—	—

*See the cited references.

care should be modified to avoid the use of fetal scalp electrodes if possible in order to keep intact the potential defenses of the uninfected neonate. The route of delivery does not affect the rate of neonatal disease because many infections occur in utero. Therefore, routine cesarean delivery is not recommended. Postpartum seroconversion of infants has been thought to occur by ingestion of infected breast milk, and breast-feeding should be discouraged.[52]

TABLE 4.
Initial Workup for Women Found To Be HIV-Positive

Baseline differential CD4 lymphocyte count
PPD skin test with controls
Endocervical cultures for gonorrhea and chlamydia
Serology for syphilis—VDRL or rapid plasma reagin
Serology for cytomegalovirus and toxoplasmosis
Hepatitis surface antigen
Baseline Papanicolaou smear

The mainstay of care for HIV-infected women is periodic determination of immune depletion as measured by CD4 counts. In pregnant women with an initial count above 500 cells/mm^2, CD4 counts should be monitored every trimester. No dramatic deterioration of immune function would be expected in these patients. Women with CD4 counts less than 500 should be managed in consultation with a practitioner familiar with the care of HIV-infected women. The initial data on the use of the anti-retroviral drug zidovudine during pregnancy shows no undue risk, and use of this drug should be dictated by the clinical situation. A report concerning the use of this drug from the National Institute of Health's AIDS Clinical Trials Units was recently published.[53] In this case series of 43 pregnant women taking zidovudine, no consistent pattern of neonatal complications or toxicity was found. The most serious complications were 2 maternal toxicities of anemia and gastrointestinal disturbances that responded to dose reductions. Serious neonatal complications included 1 case each of granulocytopenia, ureteropelvic junction obstruction, congenital CMV (in a first twin), oligohydramnios, and *Mycoplasma* pneumonia. There were no congenital abnormalities in newborns with first-trimester exposure to zidovudine.

Women with CD4 counts of less than 200 should also receive prophylaxis against *Pneumocystis* pneumonia with orally administered trimethoprim-sulfamethoxazole.[54] It is possible that the zidovudine may decrease the maternal viral load and therefore decrease perinatal transmission. A National Institutes of Health–sponsored clinical trial of this hypothesis is currently in progress.

SUMMARY

A review of the current literature with recommendations for care of the HIV-infected women has been presented here. The most prominent gynecologic conditions involve vaginitis and cervical neoplasia, whereas obstetric issues involve neonatal transmission. Our suggestions for screening have appeared throughout the paper and are reviewed in Table 5. Determining whom to screen is perhaps the most difficult issue facing the clinician. During pregnancy, both neonatal transmission and partner testing must be considered. It is conceivable that when an obstetrician-gynecologist uncovers an asymptomatic HIV infection in a pregnant

TABLE 5.
Suggestions for HIV Testing

High-risk sexual contact—bisexual partner or drug-abusing partner
Intravenous drug abuse
Pregnancy
Syphilis, herpes, and other STDs
Unusual or recurrent *Candida* vaginitis
Young women with recurrent dysplasia or cervical cancer

woman, both the patient's fetus and her partner may also have the disease.

Screening for HIV must include informed consent and a frank discussion of the patient's risk and sexual behavior. The most rational and comprehensive policy in the literature was proposed by a mixed group of public health officials, obstetricians, and other professionals with a background in ethics.[55] According to this group, all pregnant women and new mothers should be told of the availability of HIV testing both in person and in writing. Testing should be voluntary, and local health departments should be involved in counseling patients and establishing laboratory standards. Existing laws regarding medical confidentiality and discrimination must be obeyed.

It is difficult to project the future of this disease. It appears likely that the obstetrician-gynecologist will be increasingly involved in the epidemic and will be at the forefront of efforts to prevent the disease and to care for the infected woman.

REFERENCES

1. Anderson R, May R: Epidemiological parameters of HIV transmission. *Nature* 1988; 333:514–519.
2. Centers for Disease Control and Preventin (CDC): Projections of the number of persons diagnosed with AIDS and the number of immunosuppressed HIV infected persons—United States 1992–1994. *MMWR* 1992; 41:1–29.
3. Ellerbrock T, Lieb S, Harrington P, et al: Heterosexually transmitted human immunodeficiency virus infection among pregnant women in rural Florida community. *N Engl J Med* 1992; 327:1704–1709.
4. Lindsay M, Johnson N, Peterson H, et al: Human immunodeficiency virus infection among inner city adolescent parturients undergoing routine voluntary screening—July 1987 to March 1991. *Am J Obstet Gynecol* 1992; 167:1096–1099.
5. Centers for Disease Control: HIV prevalence estimates and AIDS case projections for the United States: Report based upon a workshop. *MMWR* 1990; 39:1–18.
6. Padian N: Heterosexual transmission of AIDS: Epidemiology and significance for the obstetrician and gynecologist. *Am J Obstet Gynecol* 1986; 155:235–239.
7. Gwinn M, Pappaioanou M, George J, et al: Prevalence of HIV infection in childbearing women in the United States: Surveillance using newborn blood samples. *JAMA* 1991; 265:1704–1709.
8. Holmes K, Kreiss J: Heterosexual transmission of human immunodeficiency virus: Overview of a neglected aspect of the AIDS epidemic. *J Acquir Immune Defic Syndr* 1988; 1:602–610.
9. Haverkos H, Edelman R: The epidemiology of acquired immunodeficiency syndrome among heterosexuals. *JAMA* 1988; 260:1922–1929.
10. European Study Group on Heterosexual Transmission of HIV: Comparison of female to male and male to female to male transmission of HIV in 563 stable couples. *BMJ* 1992; 304:809–813.
11. Minkoff H, Dehovitz J: Care of women infected with the human immunodeficiency virus. *JAMA* 1991; 266:2253–2258.
12. Kreiss J, Ngugi E, Holmes K, et al: Efficacy of Nonoxynol 9 contraceptive sponge in preventing heterosexual acquisition of HIV in Nairobi prostitutes. *JAMA* 1992; 268:477–482.
13. Stone K, Peterson H: Spermicides, HIV and the vaginal sponge. *JAMA* 1992; 268:521–523.

14. Rhoads J, Wright D, Redfield R, et al: Chronic vaginal candidiasis in women with human immunodeficiency virus infection. *JAMA* 1987; 257:3105–3107.

15. Imam N, Carpenter C, Mayer K, et al: Hierarchical pattern of mucosal *Candida* infections in HIV seropositive women. *Am J Med* 1990; 89:142–146.

16. Marte C, Kelly P, Cohen M, et al: Papanicolaou smear abnormalities in ambulatory sites for women infected with the human immunodeficiency virus. *Am J Obstet Gynecol* 1992; 166:1232–1237.

17. Spinillo A, Tenti P, Zappatore R, et al: Prevalence, diagnosis and treatment of lower genital neoplasia in women with human immunodeficiency virus infection. *Eur J Obstet Gynecol* 1992; 43:235–241.

18. Rogo K, Linge K: Human immunodeficiency virus seroprevalence among cervical cancer patients. *Gynecol Oncol* 1991; 37:87–92.

19. Maiman M, Fruchter R, Serur E, et al: Human immunodeficiency virus infection and cervical neoplasia. *Gynecol Oncol* 1990; 38:377–382.

20. Maiman M, Tarricone N, Vieira J, et al: Colposcopic evaluation of human immunodeficiency virus–seropositive women. *Obstet Gynecol* 1991; 78: 84–88.

21. Adachi A, Fleming I, Burk R, et al: Women with human immunodeficiency virus infection and abnormal Papanicolaou smears: A prospective study of colposcopy and clinical outcome. *Obstet Gynecol* 1993; 81:372–377.

22. Mandelblatt J, Fahs M, Baribaldi K, et al: Association between HIV infection and cervical neoplasia: Implications for clinical care of women at risk for both conditions. *AIDS* 1992; 6:173–178.

23. Giorda G, Vaccher E, Volpe R, et al: An unusual presentation of vulvar carcinoma in a HIV patient. *Gynecol Oncol* 1992; 44:191–194.

24. American Ferility Society: New guidelines for the use of semen donor insemination: 1990. *Fertil Steril* 1990; 53(suppl):1–13.

25. McCray E, Onorato I: Sentinel surveillance of human immunodeficiency virus infection in sexually transmitted disease clinics in the United States. *Sex Transm Dis* 1992; 19:235–241.

26. Young R, Feldman S, Brackin B, et al: Seroprevalence of human immunodeficiency virus among adolescent attendees of Mississippi sexually transmitted disease clinics: A rural epidemic. *South Med J* 1992; 85:469–471.

27. Safrin S, Dattell B, Hauer L, et al: Seroprevalence and epidemiological correlates of human immunodeficiency virus infection in women with acute pelvic inflammatory disease. *Obstet Gynecol* 1990; 75:666–670.

28. Hoegsberg B, Abulafia O, Sedlis A, et al: Sexually transmitted diseases and human immunodeficiency virus infection among women with pelvic inflammatory disease. *Am J Obstet Gynecol* 1990; 163:1135–1139.

29. Stamm W, Handsfield H, Rompalo A, et al: The association between genital ulcer disease and acquisition of HIV infection in homosexual men. *JAMA* 1988; 260:1429–1433.

30. Greenblatt R, Lukehart S, Plummer F, et al: Genital ulceration as a risk factor for human immunodeficiency virus infection. *AiDS* 1988; 2:47–50.

31. Hutchison C, Hook E: Syphilis in adults. *Med Clin North Am* 1990; 74:1389–1416.

32. Schimd G, Sanders L, Blount J, et al: Chancroid in the United States. *JAMA* 1987; 258:3265–3268.

33. Hook E: Syphilis and HIV infection. *J Infect Dis* 1989; 160:530–534.

34. Sperling R, Joyner M, Hassett J, et al: HIV-1 seroprevalence in pregnant women testing positive on serological screening for syphilis. *Mt Sinai J Med* 1992; 59:67–68.

35. Mattern C, Murray K, Jensen A, et al: Localization of human immunodeficiency virus core antigen in term human placentas. *Pediatrics* 1992; 89:207–209.

36. Douglas G, King B. Maternal-fetal transmission of human immunodeficiency virus: A review of possible routes and cellular mechanism of infection. *Clin Infect Dis* 1992; 15:678–691.

37. Borkowsky W, Krasinski K: Perinatal human immunodeficiency virus infection: Ruminations on mechanism of transmission and methods of intervention. *Pediatrics* 1992; 90:133–136.

38. Ukwu H, Graham B, Lambert J, et al: Perinatal transmission of human immunodeficiency virus-1 infection and maternal immunization strategies for prevention. *Obstet Gynecol* 1992; 80:458–468.

39. European Collaborative Study: Children born to women with HIV-1 infection: Natural history and risk of transmission. *Lancet* 1991; 337:253–260.

40. Sison A, Campos J: Laboratory methods for early detection of human immunodeficiency virus type 1 in newborns and infants. *Clin Microbiol Rev* 1992; 5:238–247.

41. Weiblen B, Lee F, Cooper E, et al: Early diagnosis of HIV infection in infants by detection of IgA HIV antibodies. *Lancet* 1990; 335:988–990.

42. Miles S, Balden E, Magpantay L, et al: Rapid serological testing with immune-complex–dissociated HIV p24 antigen for early detection of HIV infection in neonates. *N Engl J Med* 1993; 328:297–302.

43. Gwinn M, Pappaioanou M, George J, et al: Prevalence of HIV infection in childbearing women in the United States. *JAMA* 1991; 265:1704–1708.

44. Berrebi A, Kobuch W, Puel J, et al: Influence of pregnancy on human immunodeficiency virus disease. *Eur J Obstet Gynecol Reprod Biol* 1990; 37:211–217.

45. Selwyn P, Schoenbaum E, Davenny K, et al: Prospective study of human immunodeficiency virus infection and pregnancy outcomes in intravenous drug users. *JAMA* 1989; 261:1289–1294.

46. Minkoff H, Henderson C, Mendez H, et al: Pregnancy outcomes among mothers infected with human immunodeficiency virus and uninfected control subjects. *Am J Obstet Gynecol* 1990; 163:1598–1604.

47. Minkoff H, Willoughby A, Mendez H, et al: Serious infections during pregnancy among women with advanced human immunodeficiency virus infection. *Am J Obstet Gynecol* 1990; 162:30–34.

48. Barbacci M, Repke J, Chaisson R: Routine prenatal screening for HIV infection. *Lancet* 1991; 337:709–711.

49. Lindsay M, Leng T, Peterson H, et al: Routine human immunodeficiency virus infection screening unregistered and registered inner-city parturients. *Obstet Gynecol* 1991; 77:599–603.

50. Heagarty M, Abrams E: Caring for HIV-infected women and children. *N Engl J Med* 1992; 326:887–888.

51. Nanda D, Minkoff H: Pregnancy and women at risk for HIV infection. *Primary Care* 1992; 19:157–169.

52. Van de Perre P, Simonon A, Msellati P, et al: Postnatal transmission of human immunodeficiency virus type 1 from mother to infant. *N Engl J Med* 1991; 325:593–598.

53. Sperling R, Stratton P, O'Sullivan J, et al: A survey of zidovudine use in pregnant women with human immunodeficiency virus infection. *N Engl J Med* 1992; 326:857–861.

54. Stratton P, Mofenson L, Willoughby A: Human immunodeficiency virus infection in pregnant women under care at AIDS Clinical Trials Centers in the United States. *Obstet Gynecol* 1992; 79:364–368.

55. Working Group on HIV Testing of Pregnant Women and Newborns. HIV infection, pregnant women and newborns: A policy proposal for information and testing. *JAMA* 1990; 264:2416–2420.

Editor's Comment

The title of this chapter is accurate and descriptive. Moreover, Drs. Ault and Faro present the necessary information in a concise and easily readable format with appropriate tables, figure, and references. This chapter should be required reading for all obstetricians and gynecologists.

The methods of HIV transmission are presented and followed logically by the consequences in gynecologic and then obstetric patients. The authors stress the association of HIV infection with other sexually transmitted diseases and with an association to vaginal and other sites of *Candida* infection. Finally, the association of cervical and vulvar neoplasia and its apparent increased incidence in HIV-positive women are presented.

The consequences of HIV infection on both the pregnant woman and her fetus/infant are summarized as well as an estimate of the rate of maternal-fetal transmission. The authors make recommendations concerning screening both *before* and *during* pregnancy, and they present data that screening by using standard risk assessments is inadequate medicine. They present convincing evidence that all women should be screened for HIV infection during pregnancy but acknowledge that the usual questions regarding problems with drugs for HIV do exist. As a minimum of treatment during pregnancy, the authors suggest the possible advantages of therapy with zidovudine during pregnancy and present a discussion of the minor side effects associated with its use to date.

A discussion of the newest criteria used to make the diagnosis of AIDS was not included with this chapter. This is unfortunate but should not detract from the overall usefulness of this informative review.

Norman F. Gant, Jr., M.D.

Fetal Surgical and Medical Interventions

MARK I. EVANS, M.D.

MICHAEL R. HARRISON, M.D.

N. SCOTT ADZICK, M.D.

AVIHAI REICHLER, M.D.

MARK P. JOHNSON, M.D.

T he United States recently passed the 20th anniversary of Roe vs. Wade. The first decade after the 1973 decision saw an expansion of availability of abortion services and prenatal diagnostic procedures. The second decade, however, witnessed considerable legal retrenchment of women's choices, but a continued geometric expansion of diagnostic techniques and utilization. This second decade also witnessed the first real attempts to correct birth defects before birth, as well as fetal surgical and medical interventions. These first forays into fetal treatment began the substance of the counterargument to those who argued that prenatal diagnosis was merely a "search-and-destroy" mission.

Our experiences, as well as those of other groups, clearly show that such is not the case. Not every fetus with an abnormality is aborted. In fact, for both chromosomal and structural malformations, there is a direct correlation between the severity of the defect and the likelihood that the couple will choose termination.[1, 2] Our experiences also show that when there is the possibility of either neonatal or prenatal correction, considerable parental weight is given to that option and that there is a much lower rate of abortion of these fetuses than in situations in which there is no likely treatment.

A simple fact for us as physicians is that *one cannot treat anything before it is diagnosed.* An increasing number of disorders can now be treated in utero. When a potentially correctable fetal anomaly is diagnosed, several issues must be addressed[3]:

1. What is the natural history of this anomaly if repair procedures are delayed until after birth? Will additional or irreversible damage be caused to the fetus?
2. Can the anomaly or its consequences be corrected in utero? Will the procedure change the natural outcome?
3. What is the risk to the mother and the fetus?

Advances in Obstetrics and Gynecology, vol 1
© 1994, Mosby–Year Book, Inc.

As fetal surgical and medical interventions have developed over the past decade, approaches have generally been categorized by fetal disease or by modality of treatment. We have found the latter to be more useful and divide fetal interventive therapies into percutaneous in utero surgical procedures, open fetal surgical procedures, and noninvasive medical therapies.

PERCUTANEOUS FETAL SURGERY

The first attempts at fetal surgery were transfusions for hemolytic anemias by Liley in the early 1960s.[4] With the increasing sophistication of ultrasound, the development of intravascular transfusions, and the prevention of Rh disease with $Rh_o(O)$ immune globulin (RhoGAM), severe complications or fetal death from fetal anemia are much less common than a generation ago.[5]

FETAL VENTRICULOMEGALY

In the early 1980s, considerable interest in the potential treatment of obstructive ventriculomegaly[6] (Fig 1) emerged from (1) the relative ease of diagnosis by ultrasound and (2) the success rates of a simple shunting procedure performed in the neonate. The hope for interventive surgical therapy in the fetus, as developed in animal models, was that early shunting of ventriculomegaly in utero might prevent the irreversible damage caused by prolonged increased intracranial pressure.

Human clinical experience, however, proved to be very disappointing for ventriculoamniotic shunts. As of March 1993, 45 cases of fetal ventriculomegaly treated in utero by chorionic ventriculoamniotic shunts have been reported to the International Fetal Registry, all of them before 1986.[7] In the majority of cases, the shunting was performed on fetuses presumed to have ventriculomegaly-hydrocephalus secondary to aqueductal stenosis. Of 41 fetuses with hydrocephalus treated by ventricular amniotic shunting, 34 have survived (83%). Of the 7 deaths that occurred, 4 could be directly attributed to trauma at the time of placement of the shunt or to premature labor and delivery occurring within 48 hours of shunt placement. Of 34 surviving children, 14 (33.5%), all with aqueductal stenosis, are reported as normal at follow-up evaluation. Twenty of 34 survivors have all exhibited varying degrees of neurologic handicap; the majority of these children (18 of 34 survivors; 53%) are classified as having severe handicaps. These infants all exhibited gross delay in reaching developmental milestones, and the tested developmental quotient was always less than 60. Five of these infants have cortical blindness, 3 have seizure disorders, and 2 have spastic diplegia. Outcome among survivors was related principally to the primary etiology of obstructive hydrocephalus. Aqueductal stenosis of uncertain etiology was the most common etiologic factor for obstructive hydrocephalus (28 of 41 cases; 68%), and the only intact survivors were found in this group.

Because the results of these ventriculoamniotic shunting cases for fetal ventriculomegaly were so disappointing,[8] most investigators have observed a de facto moratorium since the early 1980s. The rationale of intervention was that fetuses that otherwise would be severely impaired by

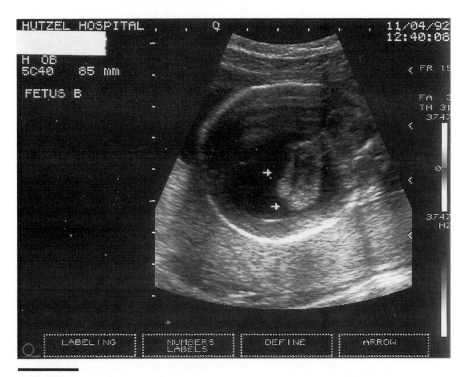

FIGURE 1.

Ventriculomegaly with a choroid plexus cyst (*arrows*) in a fetus at 24 weeks by dates and femurs, but biparietal diameter compatible with 35 weeks.

ventriculomegaly could avoid irreversible damage by undergoing intrauterine surgical treatment. These happy results were not attained, however, and surgical treatment in a few instances contributed to the survival of severely affected infants who otherwise would have died.

Despite the poor outcomes in treated fetuses, the investigation of in utero shunting for ventriculomegaly should possibly be reinstituted for several reasons.[3] Analysis of the reported cases in the registry of ventriculoamniotic shunt placement performed in the 1980s shows that selection criteria were not always employed appropriately and that fetuses with ventriculomegaly associated with other severe anomalies (i.e., holoprosencephaly or autosomal trisomies) were also given the "benefit" of intrauterine treatment despite the fact that even with therapy the prognosis was extremely poor.

Recent reports are suggestive that the natural history of fetal ventriculomegaly is dismal[7] (Table 1). The major prognostic determinants are the association with other intracranial or extracranial malformations. Additional malformations are found in 70% to 85% of fetuses with ventriculomegaly, and all such cases suffer high perinatal mortality or severe morbidity. Even if a diligent search for additional malformations is performed by combining a detailed ultrasound study of the fetus, amniocentesis for karyotype, and amniotic fluid α-fetoprotein and acetylcholinesterase determinations, about 20% of abnormalities are not detected, even by experienced personnel. It is clear, from reevaluation of old data, that the prin-

TABLE 1.

Groups and Outcomes

Category	Treatment	Outcome
Ventriculomegaly with other anomalies	No	90%–100% Severe*
Ventriculomegaly with other anomalies	Yes	70%–90% Moderate-severe*
Isolated ventriculomegaly, nonprogressive	No	80% Normal
Isolated ventriculomegaly, progressive	Yes	50%–80% Moderate-severe*

*Neurologic sequelae.

cipal mistake was poor selection of shunt candidates. With our current understanding of pathophysiology, it should be possible to limit selection to instances in which there is a greater likelihood of success.

The "likely" potential candidates for in utero ventricular shunting are the fetuses with *isolated* progressive ventriculomegaly. These are limited in number by the high rate of associated anomalies and by the relative failure to exclude additional malformations prenatally. When the only two midtrimester options are termination of pregnancy or inactive observation of progressive dilatation of the ventricles, placement of a ventriculoamniotic shunt should be a welcome third option in selected isolated cases. Given the small number of good candidates and the need to develop a new shunt catheter (none is currently available), a future study should be performed in one of the centers experienced in the technical aspects of ventriculoamniotic shunt placement. Such a study might resolve the questions of efficacy and usefulness of a fetal shunt procedure for the prevention of long-term sequelae in obstructive ventriculomegaly-hydrocephaly.

OBSTRUCTIVE UROPATHY IN THE FETUS

The development of high-resolution ultrasound has allowed detection of numerous parenchymal and collecting system abnormalities of the fetal urogenital system[9] (Fig 2). Many reports have documented the poor prognosis of fetuses with persistent urinary obstruction, particularly those with oligohydramnios and resultant pulmonary hypoplasia.[9, 10] The timing of onset and the degree of obstruction are crucial determinants in the development of irreversible renal and pulmonary damage. The onset of these abnormalities before 22 weeks' gestation is associated with a poorer outcome if intervention is not attempted.[11–14] As documented in animal studies, chronic obstructive hydronephrosis predisposes to dysplastic degeneration within the renal parenchyma.[12] The severe oligohydramnios associated with urinary tract outlet obstruction results in pressure deformities of the face and climbs and in pulmonary hypoplasia. Paradoxically, neonatal death is caused by respiratory insufficiency rather than renal

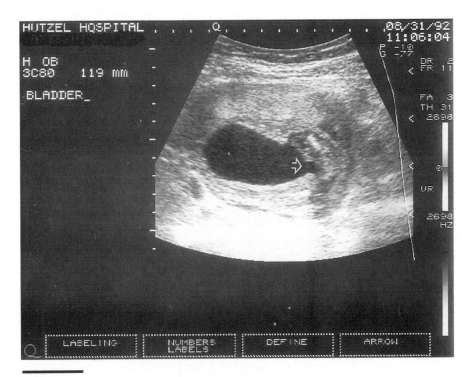

FIGURE 2.

Megalocystis: enlargement of the bladder with the keyhole sign (*arrow*) and oligohydramnios secondary to the obstruction.

failure. Our concepts of fetal renal pathophysiology have evolved considerably over the past several years. Initial simplistic models of obstruction, destruction, and possible rescue of tissue have been replaced by a more sophisticated understanding of what happens to the genitourinary architecture under increased pressure and the sequelae of attempting to bypass the obstruction.

We are presently investigating the histologic changes that occur throughout the course of the fetal urinary tract as a consequence to chronic obstruction. In fetuses with classic outlet obstructions secondary to urethral atresia or posterior urethral valves, we have observed a remarkable hypertrophic and hyperplastic response of the smooth muscle component from the origin of the obstruction ascending through the entire urinary tract to include the renal pelves.[15] These changes have been found as early as 16 weeks and are progressive through gestation with chronic obstruction. By the late second trimester, the fetus is left with markedly thickened, less compliant walls within the bladder and ureters and marked distortion of the critical ureterovesical angles (Fig 3). Neonatal response to interventive postnatal therapy such as vesicostomy, in the rare infant who survives the devastating effects of classic obstruction on pulmonary and renal development and function, is extremely poor, and these changes are only partially reversible. Such histologic evidence of progressive developmental derangements serves to underscore the importance of early diagnosis, detailed evaluation, and early in utero surgical intervention.

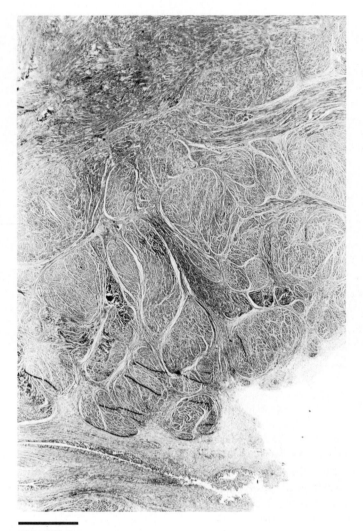

FIGURE 3.
Photomicrograph demonstrating the tremendous smooth muscle hyperplasia and
hypertrophy that occur in cases of true anatomic obstructive uropathy.

Several parameters have been used prenatally in the evaluation of renal function in fetuses with obstructive uropathy, including amniotic
fluid volume, ultrasound appearance of the kidneys, and biochemical
composition of fetal urine. The critical issue is that the fetus must be
"worked up" as carefully as any other surgical candidate before intervention.

Visualization

In the antepartum evaluation of obstructive uropathy, sonographic evaluation of the urinary tract as well as a complete fetal survey to rule out
associated anomalies is an essential component. The presence of other
anomalies would make one suspect an underlying chromosomal or genetic syndrome etiology. In such cases, intervention would not be expected to alter or improve the long-term prognosis of the fetus. One of
the greatest challenges of sonographic evaluation of the fetus is that vi-

sualization is limited secondary to the severe oligohydramnios, which is generally present. Because of this, we routinely precede our detailed fetal surveys with an amnioinfusion procedure. With warm 5% dextrose in lactated Ringer's solution (D_5LR), we restore amniotic fluid volume to low-normal levels over a 10- to 15-minute period. This restores the fluid-fetal interface and markedly enhances fetal examination.

After other anomalies have been ruled out, we carefully evaluate the entire urinary tract. The finding of a thick-walled megalocystis with a typical "keyhole" sign (Fig 3) indicates a bladder outlet obstruction at the level of the proximal aspect of the urethra. (As noted earlier, the greater the wall thickening, the less compliant and elastic the bladder is, and the poorer the prognosis for return to normal function following neonatal correction.) The ureterovesical junctions are examined next, together with both ureters. Massively distended, serpiginous hydroureters with open ureterovesical angles secondary to gross reflux are associated with a poorer prognosis.

Renal findings characteristically show dilated renal pelves, calyces, and lower collecting systems with a narrow rim of echo-dense renal parenchyma. The more compressed or narrowed the rim of parenchyma, the poorer the prognosis, particularly if this rim is brightly echo dense on ultrasound. Fibrotic and dysplastic changes in the parenchyma are progressive and reflected in the size and echo density of these tissues. In early obstructive hydronephrosis, the kidneys are enlarged and not significantly increased in echo density. With increasing fibrosis and damage, the kidneys become more echo dense and smaller, and the rim of cortical parenchyma narrows. Careful examination of the renal parenchyma for the presence of cortical microcystic or macrocystic changes is vital. Such changes are associated with advanced, irreversible dysplasia within the cortical parenchyma, and no degree of intervention will improve the prognosis.

Findings in fetuses that would be good candidates for in utero surgical intervention include a mild to moderately thickened megalocystis with the "keyhole" sign, absence of intact ureterovesical angles without gross reflux, mildly dilated hydroureters, and moderate hydronephrosis with retained, mildly echo-dense parenchyma without cortical cysts. Cases undergoing evaluation and workup for possible in utero intervention should always have documented decreasing amniotic fluid volumes and oligohydramnios before proceding with amnioinfusion. Cases of obstructive uropathy in a setting of normal or increased amniotic fluid volume most likely represent transient, partial, or intermittent obstruction and, unless the amniotic fluid volume begins to fall significantly, should not be considered for in utero surgical intervention. In our experience, underlying renal compromise is absent or minimal, and the risks of invasive intervention are not warranted.

Karyotyping

Intrauterine treatment should therefore be reserved for cases with bladder outlet obstruction and bilateral upper urinary tract dilation, demonstrated reasonable renal function, decreased amniotic fluid volume, and no associated life-threatening anomalies.[14] *Cytogenetic anomalies* and congenital malformations of other systems are diagnosed in about 15% of cases of fetal obstructive uropathy. The evaluation should include a karyotype (by amniocentesis, transabdominal chorionic villus sampling, or cordocentesis), echocardiography, and a detailed ultrasound examination to assess renal size and parenchymal thickness as noted previously, to evaluate fetal bladder filling, and to exclude additional malformations.[14] Different types of chromosomal abnormalities seem to be related to different patterns of renal defects. In mild hydronephrosis, the most common chromosome abnormality is trisomy 21, whereas in moderate/severe hydronephrosis, multicystic kidneys, or renal agenesis, the most common abnormalities are trisomies 18 and 13. If fetal visualization is hampered by severe oligohydramnios, amnioinfusion will improve sonographic visibility and fetal assessment. The observation of fetal behavior (drinking, filling of the stomach and bladder) makes the study of fetal anatomy more accurate.

Urine Biochemistry

A few groups, including Mueller[16] and Dumez[17] and their colleagues, have evaluated multiple urinary parameters and found sodium, β_2-microglobulin, NH_3, and creatinine to be good predictors of renal function and long-term outcome[16, 17] (Table 2). Our data from Detroit suggest that a single fetal urine sample may be insufficient to declare irreversible damage.[14, 18] Following ultrasound-guided bladder drainage, improvement in urine biochemistry or its lack thereof as shown by serial measurements may be more representative of underlying renal function and more predictive of ultimate outcome. Drainage by either percutaneous needle aspiration or in utero shunting is warranted in carefully selected cases and can save fetuses that would otherwise very likely be doomed. Overall, the best ultrasonic indicator of the severe progression of this disease appears to be a decrease in amniotic fluid volume. As noted previously, when severe oligohydramnios develops in a fetus before the 20th week of gestation, the prognosis is usually dismal.

We feel that serial urine aspirations for biochemical profile are an essential part of the workup of obstructive uropathies. The initial urine ob-

TABLE 2.

Fetal Urine Biochemistry*

	Dead	Alive	Good Function	Poor Function
Na, mmol/L	112	53	46	57
Ca, mg/dL	1.99	0.93	0.67	1.27
PO$_4$, mg/24 hr	1.40	0.28	0.08	0.51
Glu, mg/dL	2.89	0.38	0.19	0.65
NH$_3$, mg/L	192	654	767	493
Cr,† mg/dL	5.61	8.65	9.20	8.00
TP,† mg/dL	1.18	0.04	0.02	0.06
β2M,† mg/dL	16.0	3.16	1.02	5.7

*Adapted from Mueller F, Dumez Y: *Genetics* 1991; 49(suppl 4):175.
†Cr = creatinine; TP = total protein; β2M = β_2-microglobulin.

tained by percutaneous bladder aspiration represents "old" urine that has been present in the bladder over a period of time. Because of this, its osmotic and electrolyte configuration may have changed according to the laws of passive diffusion and/or active transport and may therefore not reflect present renal status. From serial aspirations at 48- to 72-hour intervals, one can observe continued deterioration of renal function parameters, a steady state, or in some cases a progressive improvement in electrolyte profiles consistent with underlying renal reserve. It is the latter cases that most often benefit from shunting. Evidence has been reported that if the system is allowed to drain, the underlying pathologic process may stabilize and further progression may be prevented.

SHUNT PROCEDURES

Most procedures of vesicoamniotic shunt placement have been performed percutaneously with ultrasonographic guidance.[14, 19] A double-coiled nylon catheter has been used in most cases with good results. One-way valve catheters are not necessary because the pressure in the obstructed bladder usually exceeds that in the amniotic fluid and there is no apparent harm in amniotic fluid entering the fetal bladder.

The function of these shunts, however, may be impaired by occlusion or displacement and necessitate close observation and replacement of the nonfunctioning shunt. When weeks to months of continuous drainage are required, some favor open surgical decompression by bladder marsupialization or bilateral ureterostomies. However, this would involve an increased risk to both the mother and fetus.

The Fetal Surgery Registry, coordinated by Dr. Frank Manning of the University of Manitoba, lists 98 cases as of March 1993 treated by indwelling shunts (personal communication). The longest follow-up is over 11 years, and the overall survival rate has been 40.8%. Particularly at the beginning of the series, a number of patients were inappropriately chosen for surgery, which would serve to considerably lower the survival statistics. For example, several fetuses were shunted before the elucidation of a chromosome abnormality. When appropriately stratified by etiology, survival rates reach as much as 70% for a male fetus with a posterior urethral valve.

Attempts to develop more accurate assessments of the degree and reversibility of renal compromise, specific etiologies, and the likelihood for successful prenatal or postnatal treatment have been thwarted by a poor understanding of normal fetal urine biochemistry. Such confusion has been further compounded by conflicting inferences about the significance of different biochemical parameters in compromised situations. Originally, Rodeck et al. (personal communication) proposed that a sodium concentration of greater than 100 mg/dL indicated irreversible renal damage. Mueller and Dumez[16] and Dumez et al.[17] have recently proposed that β_2-microglobulin might be a more sensitive indicator and have further demonstrated gestational age variations for several fetal urine parameters. Data from our center in Detroit have recently demonstrated that evaluation of proteinuria in combination with sodium and osmolality provides the best predictive combination of good potential long-term prognosis.[18] However, no parameter or combination is presently believed to offer satisfactory evidence of long-term renal competence or compromise, and the search to find more specific markers of long-term outcome continues.[16]

We believe that the earlier in pregnancy that diagnosis and potential therapy take place, the more likely it is that progressive damage can be prevented in selected patients. Furthermore, we have become concerned that the "accepted" parameters for fetal urine biochemistry obtained on a single initial sampling must be inherently inaccurate since initial aspiration of obstructed urine from the bladder must by definition be "old" and not reflective of "current" fetal renal function. Autopsies of some fetuses with "classic" lower obstruction on ultrasound evaluation and urine profiling have failed to document the presence of any obstructing anatomic abnormality as the cause of the apparent megalocystis. In addition, we have seen several cases in which megalocystis failed to redevelop following initial bladder drainage. We therefore propose that in certain cases, relief of the intravesicular pressure might subsequently relieve a possible "physiologic" obstruction by allowing a functional valve or spasm in the bladder neck or upper part of the urethra to "fall open." In those instances in which "suboptimal" fetal urine biochemistry failed to improve despite decompression and the relief of obstruction, our prediction of poor prognosis was confirmed on neonatal follow-up or postmortem examination by the documentation of poor renal function or histologically by extensive renal fibrosis and dysplasia.

Percutaneous transabdominal intrauterine vesicoamniotic shunting has been accomplished under ultrasound guidance with a Rodeck shunt apparatus (Rocket of London). The shunt loader has an outer 16-gauge metal tube with a sharp central trocar and a side channel for specimen aspiration. After a directional approach has been chosen under ultrasound guidance, the maternal skin is anesthetized with 1% lidocaine, and a scalpel blade is used to nick the skin. Under continuous real-time ultrasound guidance, the shunt loader is inserted into the uterine cavity and suprapubically into the fetal bladder. After a urine sample is obtained, the central trocar is removed. A plastic, double pig-tailed catheter with a central wire stylet is inserted down the entire length of the shunt loader. The wire stylet is then removed. A short plunger is used to push the distal half of the catheter into the fetal bladder. A long plunger is inserted down the shaft to touch the proximal end of the catheter. The outer component of the shunt loader is then pulled back while holding the plunger steady, with the result that the proximal half of the catheter is extruded into the amniotic cavity (Fig 4).

The many patients who have undergone successful shunting procedures are a testimonial to the potential benefits of early, aggressive evaluation of fetal renal function and fetal treatment in selected cases of obstructive uropathies. Our own data also suggest that placement of a suprapubic vesicoamniotic shunt need not be considered *the rule* in primary treatment of obstructive uropathies. One must consider alternatives while keeping in mind the long-term problems associated with an indwelling catheter (obstruction, displacement, anatomic damage, and iatrogenic ventral wall defects) before committing a fetus to such therapy.

At the current stage of development, it is still unclear as to the exact benefits and risks of decompression. It is certain that correlation of oligo-

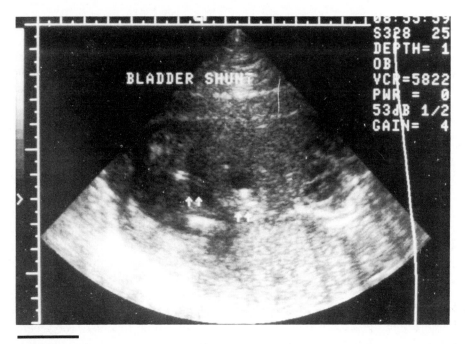

FIGURE 4.
Bladder shunt catheter in the fetal bladder *(right set of arrows)* and leading out into the amniotic cavity *(left arrows).*

hydramnios is critical to pulmonary development and likely prevents phenotypic deformations. Without a "reasonable" amniotic fluid volume, one can expect pulmonary hypoplasia and no subsequent chance for survival.

Whether decompression prevents, reverses, or merely forestalls renal damage cannot yet be concluded. We believe that serial evaluation is better than a single measurement, particularly if initial values are "abnormal." It seems reasonable that the relief of obstruction would allow a rapidly developing fetal organ to either regenerate or at least not suffer further damage.

With increasing ultrasound and biochemical sophistication, it is obvious that most of the initial early attempts at fetal urinary diversion were performed on poorly chosen patients. Given our more advanced understanding of the processes and our abilities to diagnose, we now need to start afresh in creating a database to evaluate the natural history, pathophysiology, and possibilities for intervention.

No one center is likely to have enough cases to develop criteria that are universally applicable; therefore, a flexible approach based on each center's data and experience will be required over the next several years. Our data and those from other centers suggest an approach to the management of obstructive uropathy. Some points follow directly from the data, but others must still be considered speculative. All studies to date, including our own, are to varying degrees uncontrolled, and therefore all points have to be considered somewhat tentative. Clearly a randomized trial of intervention would be the most scientifically rigorous approach to the problem, but this would require significant multicenter cooperation. Such a study has been proposed by the International Fetal Medicine and Surgery Society but is not yet active.

From the major investigators in the field, an approach to the evaluation of fetuses with obstructive uropathies is beginning to emerge. Key points in the management of fetal obstructive uropathies can be summarized as follows[14]:

1. Urinary tract decompression has a place in the management of isolated distal obstruction in fetuses who do not have underlying irreversible renal pathology.

2. Decompression with restoration of amniotic fluid volume should improve pulmonary status, but it is presently unclear as to the "reversibility" of damaged renal paraenchyma following decompression.

3. Early, aggressive identification of potential candidates for shunting is appropriate in obstructive uropathies. The mere drainage of urine may be enough to open up a urethral or bladder outlet obstruction and should be the first attempt at interventive therapy.

4. Our experience with fetuses of very early gestational age in both needle decompression and bladder shunting is encouraging and suggests that the earlier a pathology can be reversed, the greater the potential for return to normal function.

5. A single evaluation of fetal urine may not correctly reflect current or long-term renal function. The relief of obstruction may often bring about improved parameters from which we can speculate about the resiliency of fetal renal tissues.

6. It is not yet possible to distinguish factors concerning the amelioration of lung pathology for those fetuses that show improved renal function and are therefore candidates for vesicoamniotic shunting, but improvement of amniotic fluid volume following decompression or shunting will likely prove to be an important element in fetal lung development and maturation.

7. Iatrogenic abdominal wall defects may become a recognized complication of urinary shunts secondary to active or passive fetal displacement of the indwelling catheters.

8. Fetuses with persistent megalocystis but whose biochemical parameters demonstrate incremental improvement (sodium, <100; osmolality, <200) following initial decompression as documented by successive aspirations probably represent the group most likely to require and benefit from invasive interventive fetal therapy.

Thoracoamniotic Shunting

Intrauterine intrathoracic and mediastinal compression by conditions such as cystic adenomatoid malformation and pleural effusions can lead to the development of hydrops and polyhydramnios, which are associated with a high risk of premature delivery and intrauterine or neonatal death.

Isolated pleural and pericardial effusions or pulmonary cysts in the fetus may resolve spontaneously, or they can be treated effectively after birth. Nevertheless, in some cases where onset is early in gestation or progression is rapid, severe and chronic compression of the fetal lungs can result in pulmonary hypoplasia and subsequent neonatal death. In others, mediastinal compression may lead to the development of hydrops and polyhydramnios, which are associated with a high risk of premature delivery and perinatal death.

The data from fetuses with isolated idiopathic pleural or pericardial effusions suggest that short-term decompression by thoracocenteses or temporary drainage may in some cases disrupt the underlying pathology. However, in the majority of cases the fluid reaccumulates within 24 hours and requires repeated procedures, which are likely to be more traumatic than thoracoamniotic shunting.

Thoracoamniotic shunting is also an effective and apparently safe method of treatment for chronic drainage of fetal pleural effusions or pulmonary cysts. It can reverse idiopathic nonimmune fetal hydrops, resolve polyhydramnios and thereby reduce the risk of preterm delivery, and may also prevent pulmonary hypoplasia. Nevertheless, in a high proportion of nonimmune hydropic fetuses (50% in our series), thoracoamniotic shunting did not prevent their ultimate death from the underlying disease processes responsible for the hydrops.

OPEN FETAL SURGERY

Although the percutaneous approach under ultrasonographic guidance seems to be the preferred method for placing a shunt in a hollow enlarged viscus, correction of more extensive fetal anomalies requires more extensive and more invasive surgery on both the mother and the fetus.[20] The feasibility of open fetal surgery was first tested in the 1960s when an open technique was used for intrauterine exchange transfusions in erythroblastosis fetalis. However, preterm labor and abortion made this initial experience so discouraging that direct extrauterine exposure of the fetus was abandoned for over a decade. In the late 1970s and early 1980s, interest in open fetal surgery was revived by two factors. Several simple, anatomic defects (e.g., fetal pulmonary hypoplasia secondary to urinary tract obstruction or diaphragmatic hernia) were being diagnosed prenatally more easily and earlier. At the same time, neonatologists and pediatric surgeons were coming to grips with the futility of attempting to salvage these babies after birth. It became increasingly apparent that the only way to salvage fetuses with these lesions was by open extrauterine fetal surgery.

In the early 1980s, a group at the University of California, San Francisco, studied the pathophysiology of diaphragmatic hernia and hydronephrosis in animal models, defined the natural history and outcome of diaphragmatic hernia and obstructive uropathy in human fetuses, and developed the anesthetic, pharmacologic, and surgical techniques in the nonhuman primate necessary to make open fetal surgery safe for both the mother and fetus.[21]

Throughout the 1980s and early 1990s, the San Francisco group performed over two dozen open fetal surgeries for obstructive uropathies, congenital diaphragmatic hernias (CDHs), and congenital cystic adenomatoid malformations of the lung. Creating vesicostomies for obstructive uropathy and lobectomies for cystic adenomatoid malformations associated with hydrops fetalis have been quite successful in salvage of most of these severely affected fetuses.[22] Repair of CDH, however, has proved difficult. Despite extensive work in animal models, the first attempts failed because of unforeseen technical problems, the most serious of which was the unexpected finding of significant amounts of liver as well as bowel in the chest cavity.[20] The bowel could be reduced without difficulty. However, when attempts were made to reposition the liver into its normal intra-abdominal position, the umbilical vein would kink and vascular collapse would occur. Eventually, the presence of a significant proportion of the liver in the chest became an exclusion criteria. The seventh patient proved to be the first successful delivery of a viable infant following this revolutionary new surgery.[19] Since then, in patients who meet the new criteria, the survival rate has been about 50%.

There is considerable controversy as to the efficacy of open fetal surgery for CDH. Survival rates by concurrent therapy, i.e., postnatal extracorporeal membrane oxygenation (ECMO) and surgery, vary from 5% to 50%. It is clear that the only way to resolve the question of the role of prenatal surgery in CDH will be to perform a randomized, controlled study of fetal surgery vs. postnatal treatment. Such a study is now under way as a National Institutes of Health (NIH) trial.

A major side benefit of the fetal surgery program has been the discovery that fetal wounds seem to heal without a scar.[23] Extensive work now suggests that the mechanism by which the fetus heals is fundamentally different from that of an adult in the organization of collagen deposition and the composition of the extracellular matrix, especially hyaluronic acid.[23]

There are several potential uses for the knowledge gained from the study of fetal scar formation or the lack thereof.[24] Scarless healing would allow plastic surgeons to do less obtrusive reconstructive and plastic repairs. Craniofacial malformations and some types of cleft lip and palate may in the future be corrected early in utero in order to take advantage of rapid scar-free healing and the prevention of secondary disruption sequences in these disorders.[25–27] The recent enthusiasm for endoscopic surgical approaches has also engendered a shift in the possible direction of fetal surgery. Given the newly developed fiber optics and instruments, many more manipulations are now possible without opening the uterus. As more sophisticated facilities and experience are generated, it is reasonable to expect that many procedures now requiring open surgery might be done either completely transcutaneously or trans utero with a maternal incision. Likely possibilities include excision of amniotic bands, marsupialization of anterior fetal bladder obstruction, and excision of prematurely fused cranial sutures or other joints.

MEDICAL FETAL THERAPY

The spectrum of pharmacologic interventions includes (1) attempts to correct documented reversals of pathophysiology, (2) prevention of structural anomalies, and (3) biochemical alterations of questionable clinical significance. With evolving sophistication of diagnostic techniques and increasing confidence in our abilities to transfer agents into the fetus, the debate now focuses on determining whom to treat, when to treat, and the best way to treat the fetus, i.e., either indirectly through the mother and placenta or directly into the fetus by injection or via cordocentesis.

Although surgical experiments, particularly the first successes of open fetal surgery,[19] have gained more notoriety than have medical therapies, some of the most significant advances in fetal therapy have been pharmacologic. Medical fetal therapy has been effective in two main areas: the prevention of external genital masculinization in female fetuses affected with 21-hydroxylase deficiency (congenital adrenal hyperplasia [CAH]) and the correction of fetal cardiac arrhythmias that can lead to nonimmune fetal hydrops and fetal death. The pharmacology of the fetus can be altered in other ways, but the effectiveness of such alterations has not been established. Correction of fetal cardiac arrhythmias has been accomplished in hundreds of cases.

FETAL CARDIAC THERAPY

The treatment of fetal cardiac anomalies is an extensive topic far beyond the space available here. However, just as cardioversion is accomplished neonatally with pharmacologic agents targeted to the specific arrhythmia, the same approach is applicable to the fetus. The major difference, of course, is the indirect route to the fetus through the mother, which exposes the pharmacologic agent to degradation by the maternal liver before reaching the fetus.

Fetal Rhythm and Rate

Early in gestation, the fetal heart rate averages 140 beats per minute (bpm). As the fetus approaches 40 weeks' gestation, the mean heart rate is more in the range of 120 bpm. Although early in gestation there is very little variability in heart rate, beat-to-beat variability develops in the fetus as it matures concomitant with the development of parasympathetic innervation to the sinus node. Sinus arrhythmia may occur in the latter stages of pregnancy. As a general rule, fetal tachycardia is defined as heart rates greater than 180 bpm, and bradycardia is defined as rates less than 100 bpm.

Benign arrhythmias are common and do not require any intervention. Sinus bradycardia is the most common of these rhythms[28] and occurs commonly early in pregnancy. It is also noted frequently during abdominal ultrasonography since the umbilical cord may be compressed or placental blood flow compromised by the gravid uterus compressing the maternal vena cava and aorta when the pregnant woman is lying flat on her back during examination. This type of intermittent sinus bradycardia is benign. It must be distinguished from an apparently slow heart rate caused by blocked premature atrial contractions. A fetal echocardiogram is helpful in distinguishing the two. Sinus bradycardia that is not intermittent is unusual but can be associated with severe fetal compromise and may represent a preterminal event. There is no treatment per se for persistent sinus bradycardia, although the mother and the fetus should be observed carefully for the development of untoward events.

Atrial and ventricular ectopic beats are generally benign. Atrial ectopy is much more common than ventricular ectopy and is more likely to occur in the latter third of pregnancy. These rhythms are not uncommon during labor and are generally not associated with physiologic or anatomic abnormalities. As mentioned previously, ectopic beats should be distinguished from sinus bradycardia. Although it has been reported that fetal atrial ectopy can lead to supraventricular tachycardia, this is not generally accepted.

More significant fetal arrhythmias may lead to hydrops fetalis.[29] Approximately 30% of nonimmune hydrops is related to a cardiac disorder, and half of these may be related to fetal arrhythmias. It is generally felt that intermittent arrhythmias alone do not result in hydrops. Hydrops fetalis, however, is a true fetal emergency, and efforts to diagnose a particular arrhythmia and institute treatment are extremely important.

Specific arrhythmias appropriate for treatment include complete atrioventricular block and atrial and ventricular tachycardias. Agents for treatment have evolved over time in a manner parallel to the development of cardiac agents for adults. A major debate presently exists as to whether newer, longer-acting drugs should be introduced into the fetus by direct injection or by cordocentesis to obviate the need for transplacental transfusion in those cases in which incomplete passage of the drug is established fact. Direct injection would reduce the risk of maternal toxicity, which is a major factor when considering in utero treatment. As noted earlier, a significant percentage of maternally administered drug can be lost in the first and subsequent passages through the maternal liver. Newly developed approaches may allow for continuous vascular access to the fetus.[30]

Congenital Adrenal Hyperplasia

The fetal adrenal gland can be pharmacologically suppressed by maternal replacement doses of dexamethasone.[31, 32] In CAH caused by 21-hydroxylase deficiency, impaired metabolism in the pathway between cholesterol and cortisol creates excess 17-OH progesterone, which is shunted via other pathways into the production of androstenedione and androgens. Consequently, genetically normal females are exposed to excess androgens and can be masculinized. The subsequent abnormal sexual differentiation can vary from clitoral hypertrophy to complete formation of a phallus and apparent scrotum.

In an attempt to prevent this birth defect, Evans et al.[31] first administered dexamethasone, a fluorinated steroid, to an at-risk mother beginning the tenth week of gestation. Maternal estriol and cortisol values indicated rapid and sustained fetal and maternal adrenal gland suppression. This fetus ultimately turned out to be a carrier for 21-hydroxylase deficiency. Following this initial observation, Forrest and David[32] used the same protocol of 0.25 mg of dexamethasone four times daily beginning at 9 weeks to treat several fetuses and demonstrated that fetuses known to be clinically affected with the severe form of 21-hydroxylase deficiency CAH were protected from external congenital masculinization. To date, several infants with classic CAH, who clearly would have been masculinized, have been born with normal genitalia. In a few cases, some masculinization has still been observed following this regimen beginning at 9 weeks. Our current protocol, therefore, is to begin therapy at 7 weeks, although there have been too few cases to assess this modification.[33, 34] These events represent the first prevention of a birth defect and may serve as a model for other attempts at pharmacologic fetal therapy. In all of these cases, therapy had to begin long before a diagnosis was possible. With the autosomal recessive genetics of CAH, only one of eight pregnancies would be expected to benefit (females with CAH). With the present availability of a molecular probe for the CAH gene,[35] a nearly definitive diagnosis may be possible by DNA analysis of chorionic villi in the first trimester. Although diagnosis of CAH still comes several weeks after steroid therapy must be initiated to be effective, this earlier diagnosis of CAH certainly represents progress.

The fundamental principles addressed in such attempts to prevent feminine masculinization are logically extended to other medical fetal therapies. The concepts of a thorough, informed consent procedure, thorough documentation of progress, and high-risk obstetric management have generally been followed by investigators in this field.

NEURAL TUBE DEFECTS

Despite maternal serum α-fetoprotein screening, each year 2,500 infants are born in the United States with neural tube defects (NTDs), and an additional unknown number of affected fetuses is aborted.[36] Anencephaly is incompatible with life beyond early infancy, and the majority of severe cases of spina bifida have some degree of paralysis and loss of bowel and urinary control. The estimated annual medical cost for all persons with spina bifida exceeds $200 million. Except for some success in identifying a small number of cases that are part of other genetic syndromes, most cases remain unexplained. This fact points to the possibility of identifying from trend epidemiologic data a nongenetic etiology that can be modified or corrected to reduce the risk of NTDs.

Epidemiologic studies have demonstrated a very wide variation in prevalence between different countries, between different social and ethnic groups, and from decade to decade in the same population.[37] In many parts of the world, the birth prevalence of NTDs has been declining since 1950. In the United States, two birth defect surveillance systems, the Nationwide Birth Defect Monitoring Program and the Metropolitan Atlanta Congenital Defects Program, have found a decrease in rate from 1.3 per 1,000 live births in 1970 to 0.6 per 1,000 births in 1989.[38] The recurrence rate is 2% to 3%. This decline strongly suggests the importance of an environmental etiology. The commonly proposed explanation for the decline includes population changes in the pool of genes, improved and more widespread prenatal diagnostic facilities, and of particular interest, better nutritional intake by mothers. Dietary deficiencies associated with an increased rate of NTDs were noted when food was scarce in Germany after World War II and in Holland following the famine of 1944–1945. In England, the same association was found for the lower social classes in which diet was poor.

The possibility that folic acid might be involved was raised in 1964, when folic acid deficiency combined with aminopterin (folate antagonist) in animal experiments produced neural tube and other defects. Blood concentrations of vitamins such as folic acid and vitamin C and B_{12} were found to be lower on average among women who later gave birth to infants with NTDs, and the quality of diet was found to be poorer. However, this evidence is nonspecific because deficiency of one nutrient is correlated with deficiency of other nutrients as well as nonnutritional factors. In vitro studies with various nutrients found that only inositol was associated with NTDs. Therefore, no clear animal or in vitro evidence exists that vitamin supplementation protects against isolated NTDs.

Human observational data have been accumulating for the last decade and have shown that vitamins, including folic acid supplementation in the periconceptional period, can reduce the incidence of NTDs.[39–44] Published data are available from randomized and nonrandomized intervention trials and from observational studies. Early studies were conducted only in high-risk groups because of the rarity of the disease, and the majority of data have been derived from England, where the background risk is significantly higher than in the United States. Most of the studies have been retrospective and inconclusive.

In 1980–1981, the results of two interventional studies were published in which vitamin supplementation around the time of conception was given to women who had had a pregnancy with an NTD.[39] The South Wales study was a small, randomized trial of folic acid supplementation alone. The study yielded inconclusive results when it was analyzed according to randomly allocated groups but yielded a significantly lower recurrence rate in the supplemented group when analyzed by ignoring randomization. In the second nonrandomized study,[39] women were given a mixture of eight vitamins including folic acid (0.36 mg/day) in comparison to a control group of already pregnant women who declined to take the vitamins. The study showed a sevenfold ratio in risk between supplemented and unsupplemented women. This finding, while impressive, has been criticized because of self-selection of the women, overrepresentation of the high-risk area in the unsupplemented group, and association between high social class and the supplemented group. Patient selection apparently did introduce some bias to this multicenter study; however, it is impossible to assess whether bias explains all the results. There may also have been a direct preventive effect, and it was not known whether the responsible component was folic acid or one of the other vitamins.

A large, randomized, double-blind intervention trial was launched in July 1983 by the British Medical Research Council (MRC)[43] that involved 33 centers. The study was halted in 1991 by the ethical committee after abundant information and clear results were obtained on this issue so that all women at risk could receive the potential benefits of the supplementation. The population tested was a high-risk group of women who had had a previous pregnancy with an NTD. These women were randomly assigned to one of four supplementation groups: group A received 4.0 mg of folic acid; group B, a multivitamin preparation also containing 4.0 mg of folic acid; group C, neither multivitmains nor folic acid; and group D, multivitamins without folic acid. To test the effect of folic acid, investigators compared the outcomes of groups A and B with those of groups C and D. To test the effect of multivitamins, they compared the outcomes in groups B and D with those of groups A and C. The early results of the MRC study showed that high doses of folic acid reduced the risk of having a subsequent NTD-affected pregnancy by 70%, which is a threefold ratio. The study also demonstrated that folic acid alone is an effective agent; thus the need to use a mixture of vitamins and concern over possible toxicity of other vitamins are avoided.

Some questions remain. A very large trial is needed to estimate the relative efficacy of different doses and to determine the minimal effective dose of folic acid. Also, the MRC-sponsored study had insufficient power to answer the question of the safety of using high doses of folic acid for public health purposes. The fact that 95% of the cases of NTD occurred in the low-risk general population raises the last and most important question: are the results of this study restricted to the high-risk group, which has ten times the general risk? It is extremely unlikely that a method of preventing the second occurrence of NTD will not also tend to prevent the first, although the quantitative effect may be different. A 1993 study now suggests a 0.4 relative risk of primary NTD occurrence in women taking folic acid.[44]

To determine whether periconceptional vitamin supplementation can reduce the incidence of a first occurrence of NTD, four other observational studies and one recent nonrandomized interventional Cuban experience were published. All but one showed a lower risk for first-occurrence NTD in the general population for women who consumed 0.4 to 0.8 mg/day of folic acid from multivitamin supplementation, but all may have suffered from selection and memory bias. Recently the results of a Hungarian carefully designed, randomized controlled trial of multivitamin/mineral periconceptional supplementation (including 0.8 mg/day of folic acid) involving almost 5,000 women who had not had a previous NTD-affected pregnancy were reported.[45] This study was also stopped when the evidence of an NTD-protective effect became apparent. However, we cannot be sure that the preventive effect was due to folic acid alone or in combination with other components of the supplementation. Supplemental folic acid did not prevent all cases of NTD, possibly because these disorders may be heterogeneous in etiology, and further research will be needed to identify the causes of NTDs that are not averted by folic acid supplementation.

In summary, from a synthesis of information from several studies, it can be inferred that folic acid alone at levels of 0.4 mg/day will reduce the risk of NTDs. A reasonable estimate of the expected reduction in the United States is 50%.

From the aforementioned evidence, the U.S. Public Health Service has recommended that all women of childbearing age in the United States who are capable of becoming pregnant should consume 0.4 mg/day of folic acid to reduce their risk of having a pregnancy affected by spina bifida or other NTD.[46] Women who have had an affected pregnancy should consume 0.4 mg of folic acid per day, unless they are planning a pregnancy. In that case they should follow the August 1991 guideline[47] and consult their physician about the desirability of using 4.0 mg of folic acid per day, according to the data from the most rigorous study directed at the high-risk group.

The possibility of reducing NTDs through daily consumption of folic acid presents an important opportunity in public health, and an effort must be made to decide which is the best approach to deliver folic acid to the general population. The authors of this paper, however, have concerns about the possible medicolegal effects of such broad and easy-to-misunderstand expectations.

SUMMARY

The field of fetal therapy, both medical and surgical, has expanded at a geometric rate. The sophistication of questions now being asked is dumbfounding by comparison with the fundamental issues being addressed only a few years ago. Just as the space race of the 1960s produced profound changes in related areas such as computer technologies, so did the surgical principles that emerged from the work on CDH lead to a better understanding of wound healing, fetal physiology, premature labor, and placental blood flow. Changing technology and our growing depth of understanding will continue to spur investigations into treatment of fetal disease. Gene therapy, the direction of the future, will be discussed in the next chapter. What is not discussed are the social, medical, ethical, and legal implications of these new technologies. The topic has been discussed at length elsewhere[48] and will not be touched upon here except to caution that enthusiasm should be tempered by a thorough understanding of all the issues involved. That something can be done does not necessarily require that it should be done.

REFERENCES

1. Drugan A, Krause B, Canady A, et al: The natural history of prenatally diagnosed ventriculomegaly. *JAMA* 1989; 261:1785–1789.
2. Pryde PG, Odgers AE, Isada NB, et al: Determinants of parental decision to abort (DTA) or continue for non-aneuploid ultrasound detected abnormalities. *Obstet Gynecol* 1992; 80:52–56.
3. Evans MI, Drugan A, Manning FA, et al: Fetal surgery in the 1990's. *Am J Dis Child* 1989; 143:1431–1436.
4. Liley AW: Intrauterine transfusion of foetus in haemolytic disease. *BMJ* 1963; 2:1107–1109.
5. Berkowitz RL, Chitkara U, Goldberg JD, et al: Intrauterine transfusion in utero: The percutaneous approach. *Am J Obstet Gynecol* 1986; 154:622–627.
6. Clewell WH, Johnson ML, Meier PR: A surgical approach to the treatment of hydrocephalus. *N Engl J Med* 1982; 306:1320.
7. Manning FA, Harrison MR, Rodeck C, et al: Special report: Catheter shunts for fetal hydronephrosis and hydrocephalus. Report of the International Fetal Medicine and Surgery Society Registry. *N Engl J Med* 1986; 315:336–340.
8. Berkowitz RL, Tertora M, Hobbins JC, et al: The management of fetal hydrocephalus. *Am J Obstet Gynecol* 1985; 151:993.
9. Callan NA, Blakemore K, Park J, et al: Fetal genitourinary tract anomalies: Evaluation, operative correction, and follow-up. *Obstet Gynecol* 1990; 75:67–74.
10. Helin I, Persson PH: Prenatal diagnosis of urinary tract abnormalities by ultrasound. *Pediatrics* 1986; 78:879–883.
11. Smith D, Egginton JA, Brookfield DSK: Detection of abnormality of fetal urinary tract as a predictor of renal tract disease. *BMJ* 1987; 294:27–28.
12. Adzick NS, Harrison MR, Glick PL, et al: Fetal urinary tract obstruction: Experimental pathophysiology. *Semin Perinatol* 1985; 9:79.

13. Weiner C, Williamson R, Monsib MS, et al: In utero bladder diversion problems with patients selection. *Fetal Ther* 1986; 1:196.

14. Evans MI, Sacks AJ, Johnson MP, et al: Sequential invasive assessment of fetal renal function and the intrauterine treatment of fetal obstructive uropathies. *Obstet Gynecol* 1991; 77:545–550.

15. Chamberlain C, Qureshi F, Jacques SM, et al: Why vesicoamniotic shunts need to be placed early: Histologic comparison of urinary tracts with fetopsy-proven anatomical obstructions and with no anatomic obstruction in fetal obstructive uropathy. Presented at the annual meeting of the Society of Perinatal Obstetricians, San Francisco, February 1993.

16. Mueller F, Dumez Y: Contribution of biochemistry to prenatal diagnosis of obstructive uropathies. Proceedings of 8th International Congress of Human Genetics. 1991; 49(suppl 4):175.

17. Dumez Y, Revillon Y, Dommergues M, et al: Long-term predictive value of fetal renal function. Presented at the Fifth Meeting of the International Fetal Medicine and Surgery Society, Bonn, Germany, June 1988.

18. Johnson MP, Bukowski TP, Kithier K, et al: Fetal urine albumin/globulin ratio in the in utero evaluation of obstructive uropathies. Presented at the 42nd Annual Meeting of the American Society of Human Genetics, San Francisco, CA (abstract 1022). *Am J Hum Genet* 1992; 51:259.

19. Harrison MR, Adzick NS, Longaker MT, et al: Successful repair in utero of a fetal diaphragmatic hernia after removal of herniated viscera from the left thorax. *N Engl J Med* 1990; 322:1582–1584.

20. Jennings RW, Adzick NS, Harrison MR: The fetus as a surgical patient, in Evans MI (ed): *Reproductive Risks and Prenatal Diagnosis.* East Norwalk, Conn, Appleton & Lange, 1992.

21. Jennings RW, Adzick NS, Longaker MT, et al: New techniques in fetal surgery. *J Pediatr Surg* 1992; 27:1329–1333.

22. Adzick NS, Harrison MR, Flake AW, et al: Fetal surgery for cystic adenomatoid malformation of the lung. *J Pediatr Surg* 1993; 28:806–812.

23. Adzick NS, Longaker MT (eds): *Fetal Wound Healing.* New York, Elsevier Science Publishers, 1992.

24. Adzick NS, Longaker MT: Scarless fetal healing: Therapeutic implications. *Ann Surg* 1992; 215:3–6.

25. Sullivan WG: In utero cleft lip repair in the mouse without an incision. *Plast Reconstr Surg* 1989; 84:723–730.

26. Estes JM, Whitby DJ, Lorenz HP, et al: Endoscopic creation and repair of fetal cleft lip. *Plast Reconstr Surg* 1992; 90:743–746.

27. Estes JM, MacGillivray TE, Hedrick MH, et al: Fetoscopic surgery for treatment of congenital anomalies. *J Pediatr Surg* 1992; 27:950–954.

28. Allen LD: Fetal arrhythmias, in Long WA (ed): *Fetal and Neonatal Cardiology.* Philadelphia, WB Saunders, 1990, p 170.

29. Allen LD, Crawford DG, Sheridan R, et al: Etiology of non-immune hydrops: The value of echocardiography. *Br J Obstet Gynaecol* 1986; 93:223.

30. Hedrick MH, Jennings RW, MacGillivray TE, et al: Endoscopic catheterization of placental vessels for chronic fetal vascular access. *Surg Forum* 1992; 43:504–505.

31. Evans MI, Chrousos GP, Mann DL, et al: Pharmacologic suppression of the fetal adrenal gland: Attempted prevention of 21-hydroxylase deficiency congenital adrenal hyperplasia in utero. *JAMA* 1985; 253:1015.

32. Forrest M, David M: Prenatal treatment of congenital adrenal hyperplasia due to 21-hydroxylase deficiency (abstract 911). Presented at the Seventh International Congress of Endocrinology, Quebec, Canada, 1984.

33. Shulman DI, Mueller OT, Gallardo LA, et al: Treatment of congenital adrenal hyperplasia in utero. *Pediatr Res* 1989; 25:2.

34. Pang S, Pollack MS, Marshall RN, et al: Prenatal treatment of congenital adrenal hyperplasia due to 21-hydroxylase deficiency. *N Engl J Med* 1990; 22:111–115.

35. Phillips JA III, Burr IM, Orlando P, et al: DNA analysis of human steroid 21-hydroxylase genes on congenital hyperplasia (abstract). *Am J Hum Genet* 1985; 37:171.

36. Evans MI, Dvorin E, O'Brien JE, et al: Alpha-fetoprotein and biochemical screening, in Evans MI (ed): *Reproductive Risks and Prenatal Diagnosis*. East Norwalk, Conn, Appleton & Lange, 1992, p 223.

37. Hunt GM: Open spina bifida; outcome for a complete cohort treated unselectively and followed into adulthood. *Dev Med Child Neurol* 1990; 32:108.

38. Yen IH, Khoury MJ, Erickson JD, et al: The changing epidemiology of neural tube defects, U.S. 1986–1989. *Am J Dis Child* 1992; 146:857–861.

39. Smithells RW, Sheppard S, Schorah CJ, et al: Vitamin supplementation and neural tube defects. *Lancet* 1981; 1:425.

40. Milunsky A, Jick H, Jick SS, et al: Multivitamin/folic acid supplementation in early pregnancy reduced the prevalence of neural tube defects. *JAMA* 1989; 262:2847.

41. Mills JL, Rhoads GG, Simpson JL, et al: The absence of a relation between the periconceptional use of vitamins and neural tube defects. *N Engl J Med* 1989; 321:430.

42. Mulinare J, Cordero JF, Erickson JD, et al: Periconceptional use of multivitamins and the occurrence of neural tube defects. *JAMA* 1988; 260:3141.

43. MRC Vitamin Study Research Group: Prevention of neural tube defects: Results of the Medical Research Council Vitamin Study. *Lancet* 1991; 337:131.

44. ACOG Committee Opinion. Folic acid for the prevention of recurrent neural tube defects. American College of Obstetricians and Gynecologists, No 120, Washington, D.C., March 1993.

45. Czeizel AE, Dudas I: Prevention of the first occurrence of neural tube defects by periconceptional vitamin supplementation. *N Engl J Med* 1992; 327:1832–1835.

46. Centers for Disease Control: Recommendations for the use of folic acid to reduce the number of cases of spina bifida and other neural tube defects. *MMWR* 1992; 41:1–7.

47. Centers for Disease Control: Use of folic acid for prevention of spina bifida and other neural tube defects. *MMWR* 1993; 40:513–516.

48. Evans MI, Fletcher JC, Dixler AO, et al (eds): *Fetal Diagnosis and Therapy: Science, Ethics, and the Law*. Philadelphia, JB Lippincott, 1989.

Fetal Gene Therapy

MARK PAUL JOHNSON, M.D.

MICHAEL R. HARRISON, M.D.

N. SCOTT ADZICK, M.D.

AVIHAI REICHLER, M.D.

MARK I. EVANS, M.D.

In the past decade, advances in molecular genetics and recombinant DNA technology have been quite dramatic and have led to the development of sensitive diagnostic techniques for a continuously increasing number of single-gene disorders. Cutting DNA with restriction endonucleases and analyzing restriction fragment length polymorphisms (RFLPs), sequence-specific DNA isolation techniques, and cloning of single-stranded DNA have allowed the formation of highly specific gene probes. These have increased not only the accuracy of diagnosis of abnormal conditions but also our basic understanding of normal gene function and regulation, with specific emphasis on understanding the development of the mechanisms of cancer and its treatment.[1, 2] The next natural step in this evolving technology is the development of techniques to introduce purified or cloned gene sequences into cultured cells and living animals to correct single-gene defects. Attention can then be directed to their application to the treatment and care of single-gene disorders in the human.

APPROACHES TO GENE THERAPY

Approaches to gene therapy can be broadly divided into three categories: modification of existing material, removal of material, and addition of material.

MODIFICATION

Modification has been used with initial success in hemoglobinopathies. Ley and colleagues[3] have demonstrated that 5-azacytidine and other demethylating agents can induce the expression of fetal hemoglobin in baboons and humans with β-thalassemia and sickle cell anemia. The genes for hemoglobin F and A are adjacent on chromosome 11. 5-Azacytidine removes the methyl group attached to cytosine (C) and some CG sequences. The methyl group normally acts as an inhibitor of transcription. Demethylation results in increased production of hemoglobin F, and some clinical improvement has been documented. Unfortunately, the effects have been short-lived, and currently available drugs are quite toxic.

Advances in Obstetrics and Gynecology, vol 1
© 1994, Mosby–Year Book, Inc.

A technique known as "site-directed homologous recombination" has been used to modify the expression of a specific gene in a mouse model.[4] The process involves construction of a "targeting gene" that carries homologous sequences at each of its ends with an intervening nonfunctional or marker gene region to assess integration into the host genome. Once introduced into the target nucleus, this gene aligns itself with the homologous regions of the target gene. When somatic recombination, which is analogous to meiotic crossing over, occurs, insertion into or replacement of the target gene by the incoming DNA segment results. This technique can be used to disrupt a normal gene or to replace it with a mutant copy. Alternatively, it can be used to replace a mutant gene with a normal copy (i.e., gene therapy). Subsequent assay of successful integration can be easily accomplished by RFLP or polymerase chain reaction (PCR) to probe for the original gene or an inserted segment. In gene therapy applications, the return of a function absent before therapy would be a sign of successful integration. This approach may someday prove useful for the modification of specific genetic disorders and could in principle be done not only in somatic cells (e.g., erythroid, lymphoid, or liver) but even at a preimplantation embryonic level.

REMOVAL

Removal of genetic material is theoretically possible in conjunction with in vitro fertilization. Multiple phenotypic abnormalities such as those seen with Down's syndrome are caused by the extra copy of chromosome 21. If it were possible to remove or destroy the expression of the extra material, development should occur normally. By birth, the baby will have only 5% of adult body weight, but 90% of the total cell number, and the additional chromosome will appear in all of them. Attempt at any removal would have to be applied extremely early in pregnancy— probably at the single-cell stage. Although irrelevant for most couples, for those at extremely high risk (e.g., balanced translocation carriers), in vitro fertilization with immediate karyotype analysis and potential ablation or removal of extra material may someday be feasible, although it is far beyond existing technology.

ADDITION

Addition of material is the most promising approach for stable correction of defects. Anderson defined three potential levels of genetic engineering and therapy[5, 6]:

1. Somatic cell gene therapy: insertion of a gene into the body cells of an affected individual to correct a genetic disorder in this individual only.
2. Germ line gene therapy: insertion of a gene into the germ cells of an affected individual to correct a disorder in the patient and his or her future offspring.
3. Enhancement genetic engineering: insertion of a gene into a normal individual to enhance a desirable known characteristic.

Active workers in the field now agree that human gene therapy will be feasible and should be applied to at least some serious genetic disorders.[7] It is also generally held that human gene therapy should not be applied at this time to germ cells, but only to somatic cells which cannot transmit the altered genetic material to subsequent generations.[8] The first target for human gene therapy would therefore be the somatic cell.

SOMATIC CELL GENE THERAPY

Gene products are required for normal growth and development, homeostasis and metabolism, complex organ function, immunity, and reproduction. Abnormal gene function causes diseases such as the hemoglobinopathies, inborn errors of metabolism, coagulopathies, or endocrine disorders. Somatic gene therapy for such diseases would involve the introduction of a normal recombinant gene into the body cells of an individual to reconstitute specific gene products and their functions.[9] From this definition for somatic cell gene therapy there evolve a few requirements about those disorders likely to be attempted:

1. The disorder should be severe and crippling enough to justify offering experimental treatment.
2. The symptoms of the disorder should be reversible with gene therapy treatment.
3. The disease should be correctable by gene insertion into bone marrow cells, which is the only tissue that can be extracted, treated in vitro, and successfully returned at this time.
4. The defect should be a single-gene alteration with simple regulation, most probably an enzymatic defect that can be corrected by relatively low expression of the inserted gene.
5. The deficiency must be caused by a known, identified, and cloned gene.
6. A safe and effective method of introducing the cloned gene into the treated cells must be available.

Three diseases are among the most likely to be first treated by gene therapy: Lesch-Nyhan syndrome, an X-linked disorder caused by hypoxanthine-guanine phosphoribosyltransferase (HGPRT) deficiency; severe combined immunodeficiency syndrome (SCID), caused by adenosine deaminase (ADA) deficiency; and immunodeficiency resulting from purine nucleoside phosphorylase (PNP) abnormalities.[10] These diseases meet most of the criteria. Moreover, heterologous bone marrow transplantation has been found to be beneficial for some of these patients.[11] Diseases correctable by bone marrow transplantation[12] are the natural candidates for human somatic cell gene therapy. The problems associated with allogeneic bone marrow transplantation (availability of histocompatible bone marrow donors, graft-vs.-host disease, and the need for complete lymphoid and hematopoietic ablation in the recipient before transplant) would be avoided by the use of autologous bone marrow treated by gene insertion.

TECHNIQUES FOR GENE INSERTION

The several techniques of gene insertion into mammalian cells have been summarized recently.[8-10, 13] The most common method, transfection, uses calcium phosphate precipitation to facilitate the uptake and stable integration of microprecipitates of exogenous DNA. The advantages of this procedure include technical simplicity and the ability to manipulate highly purified gene sequences.[8] It is, however, relatively inefficient and unstable, and even in the best recipient cell lines, overall efficiency is minimal.[10] Other physical methods of gene insertion include cell fusion, electroporation, and microinjection. This last method seems to be ideal in terms of efficiency, but only a few cells may be injected with soluble DNA at a time, and many of these subsequently die. Consequently, microinjection has limited value in somatic cell gene therapy but is the ideal method of treatment for germ cell therapy—injecting the purified DNA in solution into the pronucleated embryo. The incorporated genetic material would subsequently appear in all cells derived from multiplication of the injected one-cell embryo, including the germ cells.

A still more efficient way of inserting exogenous DNA into cells is the use of biological vectors—DNA and RNA viruses. Several DNA viruses have been used, such as the simian virus 40 (SV40), bovine papillomavirus, and adenovirus.[10] Experiments with SV40 were limited by the amount of foreign DNA that the virus could carry, and the bovine papillomavirus was not successful in integrating the DNA into chromosomes of replicating cells. Adenoviruses may be of the greatest use because they infect a wide range of host cells; however, the systems for their use are still poorly defined and the potential risk of neoplastic transformation of the infected cells exists.[8, 14]

RNA viruses of the retrovirus type are presently the center of most interest as biological vectors for gene insertion in animal models. These are simple viruses with small and well-defined viral genomes. For purposes of expression and replication, they insert a reverse transcript of their viral RNA into host DNA that is integrated as a single copy at a single site. If portions of the viral genome are replaced by exogenous sequences, the virus will often lose its ability to replicate. However, if the recombinant retroviral genome containing the gene of interest is transfected into cells previously infected with a wild virus, complementation of functions can occur and give rise to new retroviral particles that contain the defective recombinant genome and are infectious to suitable target cells.[10] By using this method, a large number of proliferating cells can be effectively infected and the recombinant DNA introduced into their genome. As long as target cells are proliferating, retroviruses demonstrate little tissue specificity and only minimal species specificity.[9]

Several problems and potential dangers are associated with the use of retroviral delivery systems. The site of integration of the retrovirus is random, which leads to potential problems of stability and expression of the inserted gene. It may occasionally integrate into the middle of an otherwise normal gene and create new mutations by insertional mutagenesis.[15] The strong promoter usually encoded in the viral long terminal repeat (LTR) could accidentally activate proto-oncogenes adjacent to the insertion site, thus leading to damage of the cell (and the organism).[16]

Excision and mobilization to a new location in the genome may further increase the risk for loss of function and mutagenesis.[10]

Retroviruses have been used in animal studies to introduce human intact genes that were subsequently expressed in vitro by the cultured cells. Mouse primary hepatocytes, NIH 3T3, and hepatoma cells were infected successfully with human phenylalanine hydroxylase (PAH) genes.[17, 18] Human β-globin genes have been introduced into mouse erythroleukemia cells.[19] Although they were inserted in foreign positions, the gene maintained normal regulation. Expression was roughly comparable to that of endogenous mouse β-globin genes. Canine hematopoietic progenitor cells in culture were infected by retrovirus packaging cell lines, and the genes inserted conferred resistance to antibiotics and methotrexate.[20]

In human cells cultured in vitro, the retrovirus delivery system has been used for infection and integration of glucocerebrosidase into type 2 Gaucher fibroblasts.[21] Secretion of fully active factor IX has also been demonstrated in human skin fibroblasts.[22] The introduction of the ADA gene into ADA-deficient skin fibroblasts[23] and correction of ADA deficiency[24] have been achieved in cultured human T and B cells by retrovirus insertion of the ADA gene. Retrovirus-mediated transfer and expression of drug-resistant genes were achieved in human hematopoietic progenitor cells,[25] and thioguanine-resistant human leukemia cells were sensitized by retroviral insertion of the human HGPRT gene.[26] Efficient introduction of plasmid DNA into human hematopoietic cells has also been demonstrated for DNA viruses.[27]

Another important principle for gene transfer is selectivity. To increase the number of cells taking up and expressing the gene, that gene must convey some advantage during cell proliferation. Cellular transformation by drug-resistant genes and cell growth in media containing the antiproliferative drug will favor the proliferation of genetically transformed cells. The combination of methotrexate and methotrexate-resistant genes was the first such selective system used in gene transfer in vivo and is still the most practical for clinical use.[8, 28] Other systems include selection by resistance to antibiotics (aminoglycoside G-418) and 6-thioguanine.[29] One must choose a selection system carefully because conferred resistance to some drugs will eliminate the potential therapeutic use of that agent to treat disease in that organism.

CURRENT STATUS

Although progress has been great in gene transfer into cultured cells, studies extending this technology into live animals are still in preliminary stages. It is possible to infect the whole animal with viral vectors to produce transformation of cells with the recombinant gene product in vivo, although the loss of target specificity may entail greater risks.[19] A safer approach would involve introduction of the recombinant gene in vitro and then transplanting the transformed cells into live animals. This method is applicable only to tissues that are able to proliferate in vitro, such as bone marrow, skin fibroblasts, or liver cells. Bone marrow infected with recombinant retroviruses containing the bacterial neomycin resistance gene and transplanted into live mice will express the product of the recombinant gene in vivo.[19, 30] Recombinant mouse fibroblast clones transplanted into the peritoneal cavity of nude mice express human α_1-antitrypsin gene in vivo, with enzymatic activity in both sera and the epithelial surface of the lungs.[31] An advantage in proliferation of recombinant bone marrow cells is conveyed by total-body irradiation with ablation of endogenous bone marrow cells. However, more limited skeletal irradiation (300 rad to the femur) appears to allow engraftment.[32]

Hematopoietic stem cell (HS-cell) transplantation offers another approach. Fetal-derived early HS-cells can be isolated from fetal liver preparations. These stem cells would possess the potential to differentiate into any of the hematologic cell lines and could carry their genetic information for gene product synthesis with them. The impact of this on such disorders as β-thalassemia, ADA deficiency, or SCID is obvious. Of fetal origin, HS-cells would also be devoid of antigenic cell surface markers and could be transplanted early into fetuses by intra-abdominal or umbilical artery injection, where they would colonize the fetal marrow and produce a chimera. If transplanted early, tolerance may occur to any cell-specific surface antigenic markers that might develop on these cells later in the fetus or neonate and thereby circumvent the problems of graft rejection or graft-vs.-host disease.

A recently developed technique for creating transgenic animals uses embryonic stem cells (ES-cells) as carriers of genetic information. Embryonic stem cells are derived from the inner cell mass component of the early blastocyst. These cells are pluripotential and give rise to the endodermal, ectodermal, and mesodermal compartments.[33] This stage of development is therefore the ideal time for introduction of genetically manipulated material.

Embryonic stem cells have been shown to remain in undifferentiated form in vitro if maintained on embryonic fibroblast feeder layers. If placed into cell suspension culture, they will begin differentiation and eventually form embryoid bodies with elements of glandular cells, heart and skeletal smooth muscle, nerve cells, keratin-producing cells, and even melanocytes.[34]

Embryonic stem cells can be modified "in vitro" by any of the aforementioned techniques and then microinjected back into the blastocyst cavity of a developing embryo, where they integrate into the inner cell mass to form a chimera. The earlier in development this procedure is done, the higher the percentage of chimera cells and the greater the chance of incorporation into germ cell lines and subsequent transmission to future generations of offspring.

Gossler and colleagues[35] used the transfection technique to introduce a circular plasmid containing the neomycin-resistant gene into mouse ES-cells. The successfully transfected cells were injected back into mouse blastocysts, where they incorporated into the developing inner cell mass and resulted in chimeric animals.

Other approaches to gene introduction have included injection of retroviruses carrying a specific gene sequence into ES-cell nuclei or into pre-implantation embryos, with nonspecific genome integration of these genes.[36] Culturing ES-cells on embryonic fibroblast feeder layers that have been transfected with retrovirus carrying an inserted gene sequence has resulted in successful transfection and incorporation of that sequence into these cells. The nonspecific integration into the host genome, the inability to select or screen before implantation, and the additional possibility of insertional mutagenesis are the major drawbacks of these methods.

Embryonic stem cell transplants offer a unique system to introduce modified genetic information into early pluripotential embryonic cells with successful integration and expression of this information in the resulting chimeric animal. Very early transplants carry the possibility of integration of this new material into germ cell lines and transmission onto subsequent generations. This system further allows the selection and screening of pretransplanted cells to ensure the appropriate gene number and orientation before introduction back into the embryo. We have recently attempted stem cell transplantation for β-thalassemia diagnosed by chorionic villus sampling in the first trimester. Unfortunately, the fetus was miscarried before information about engraftment could be obtained. Approximately ten such transplants have been attempted with one certain success in a fetus with bare lymphocyte syndrome.[37] In the other instances, either the patients miscarried or engraftment could not be confirmed because of induced abortion or low-level activities. Much further work remains to be done, but the results, we believe, will be very promising.

GERM LINE GENE THERAPY

Insertion of genetic material can be accomplished via micromanipulation of a pronucleus in a single-cell embryo. The resultant incorporated material would be duplicated in every cell of the organism, including germ cells for future generations. Two methods—microinjection of purified DNA into one of the two pronuclei[38, 39] and nuclear transplantation[40]—have proved successful in animal studies and produced transgenic mice, rabbits, sheep, and pigs. Following appropriate gene insertion into the pronucleus, murine hereditary dwarfism[41] and thalassemic mice[42] have been cured. The HGPRT gene has been introduced in mouse embryos and expressed in the central nervous system of such transgenic mice.[43] Since the possibility of diagnosing HGPRT deficiency in the preimplantation mouse embryo has been reported recently,[44] a putative scenario can be developed on this model. Women at risk for having children with Lesch-Nyhan syndrome would be referred to a center for in vitro fertilization and preimplantation diagnosis. Maternal eggs would be obtained after adequate hormonal stimulation and fertilized in vitro. Male and female embryos would be differentiated by means of a Y-DNA probe. Female embryos would be returned to the uterus by the usual methods of embryo transfer either in the treatment cycle or in a natural cycle after cryopreservation. In male fetuses HGPRT deficiency tests would be employed. In those found to be deficient, HGPRT gene microinjection could be used and gene expression assessed in culture as an index of the success of treatment. About one in five cells could be expected to be permanently transfected by microinjection.[6] Embryos for which treatment was successful could then be cryopreserved and transferred in a later cycle.

The arguments in favor of germ line gene therapy include efficiency and expression of the gene in all organs, including some that are not accessible to somatic cell gene therapy (e.g., the brain). Disadvantages of the germ line modality are the yet undefined risks of embryonic and fetal death, tumors and malformation that may occur, the absence of control over the site of insertion of the injected DNA in the recipient genome (with implications in terms of tissue specificity and expression of the inserted gene and insertional mutagenesis), and the current high failure rate of the procedure. The available data suggest that 10% to 20% of transgenic mice may carry recessive mutations of essential genes.[45] In animal studies involving microinjection of an immunoglobulin gene into mouse eggs, only 64% of the injected eggs were considered to be healthy enough to be transferred to surrogate mothers. Only 3.7% proceeded to live birth, and only 2% carried the injected gene. In a cumulative study from in vitro fertilization centers in the United States, a 12.6% clinically confirmed pregnancy rate (per egg retrieval) was reported, about half of them resulting in live births.[46] In view of current data and the potential problems, the arguments for germ line therapy are not as compelling as those for somatic cell experiments, and therefore clinical trials need to await further basic advancement. Accumulation of data and experience from basic biological research and animal studies may render human germ line therapy feasible in the future.

ENHANCEMENT OF GENETIC ENGINEERING

Genetic engineering (or eugenics) is considerably different from the previously discussed approaches. Here the goal is not to try to correct a genetic abnormality but to insert additional genetic material into a normal individual in order to change or enhance a specific characteristic such as linear growth.

The body exists in a very complex and delicate homeostasis, on the cellular as well as the whole organism level. The intricate pathways of interaction are as yet only poorly defined. Insertion of additional genetic information can alter this delicate balance, with consequences that cannot be appreciated at our present state of knowledge. These consequences are probably justifiable if a normal gene is inserted to replace a faulty one. As emphasized by Anderson, we know too little about the human body to attempt to insert a gene designed for "improvement" into a normal individual.

Fletcher[47] has underlined a moral distinction between the use of human gene therapy in cases where it may relieve severe morbidity or mortality and in cases where the intent is to alter characteristics that have nothing to do with disease. In the first situation, accepting some risks, even if poorly defined, is in the best interest of the affected individual. In the latter cases, the benefit obtained may be very slight, if any, and the potential wrong done to the individual may be severe. It should also be remembered that although the technical possibility exists today to insert a gene into a cell population, we do not have methods yet to extract or inactivate a specific gene once it is inserted. Therefore a gene, once inserted, even if it is later found to be harmful, will continue to act until the death of the cell or the individual.

The principles of justice are also violated by applying gene therapy to normal individuals. When resources are scarce, they should be used to alleviate suffering and early death and should not be used to promote special interests of normal persons. Moreover, enhancement genetic experiments would probably be more susceptible to control by interested societies and governments.[47]

Changing traits such as appearance, intelligence, and character are not possible in the foreseeable future. These traits are influenced by interactions between numerous genes, in pathways not presently clear. Environmental factors also have an effect on these traits. In time, however, the genes and their interactions may be discovered, and the technical availability of enhancement genetic engineering may become a reality. The scientific community and the public should cooperate in evaluating the medical, ethical, and philosophical aspects of this issue. Such debate and resolution should be accomplished well before these procedures are technically possible.

ETHICAL ISSUES

From animal studies we have learned that most problems associated with somatic cell gene therapy (definition of target disorders, mode of delivery for the gene, expression, and safety) can be overcome and that human somatic gene therapy is at our doorstep. As with every experimental procedure, before transferring it from the laboratory to clinical treatment in humans, the ethical implications should be considered. Some of the main questions involve "risk assessment"[48] of morbidity and mortality rates associated with the disease, existing therapy and its effectiveness, and the possibility of therapy to stop or reverse clinical deterioration. The safety of the protocol for gene insertion and the effectiveness of gene expression in the treated cells should be judged on the basis of well-controlled animal studies. As with other "first of their kind" experiments such as artificial organ and xenograft transplantations, human studies must be scupulously fair in patient selection and conscientious in obtaining informed consent.[49] Questions of privacy and confidentiality may also arise.

The Working Group on Human Gene Therapy, an interdisciplinary subgroup of the National Institutes of Health Recombinant DNA Advisory Committee, has published a guiding document representing a framework for review in each specific case of the most important areas of concern affected by human gene therapy.[50] The following are the major topics discussed in this document:

1. Objectives and rationale of proposed research
2. Research design, anticipated risks and benefits
3. Selection of patient
4. Informed consent
5. Privacy and confidentiality

In addition to the professional review suggested by these guidelines, a special public review mechanism has been established to evaluate proposals to perform gene therapy in humans. In early experiments, however, the information given to the patients and family for informed consent or for review would be based only on animal studies. Thus long-term consequences and safety can only be speculative.

SUMMARY

Genetic therapy has the potential to offer a cure to individuals affected by serious disorders that are the cause of severe disability and early death. Somatic cell gene therapy is technically possible and ethically permissible; human treatment in these aspects is ready to be applied. The first attempts to treat ADA deficiency have been made in children at the National Institutes of Health. Problems of control of the insertion site and regulation of gene expression in specific tissues still need to be solved when specific genes are being transplanted. Hematologic stem cell and embryonic stem cell transplant therapy are technically possible and in use with animal models, and first attempts in humans are occurring. Isolation and propagation of cell lines for human transplantation are problems presently being addressed. The long-term immunologic consequences of stem cell transplants remain the major concern. Germ line gene therapy is technically possible, but the high loss rate of the procedure and the possibility of inducing malformation and tumors in the offspring cause this procedure to be unacceptable at this time. Once these technical problems are solved, this procedure will be potentially applicable. Enhancement genetic engineering may, in the future, be technically possible, but it remains ethically unacceptable because the consequences of inserting additional genetic material into a normal, genetically balanced individual may be severe, and the scientific basis for such engineering does not at present exist.

REFERENCES

1. Miller WL: Recombinant DNA and the pediatrician. *J Pediatr* 1981; 99:1.
2. Antonarakis SE, Phillips JA, Kazazian HH: Genetic disease: Diagnosis by restriction endonuclease analysis. *J Pediatr* 1982; 100:845.
3. Ley TJ, DeSimone J, Anagnou NP, et al: 5-Azacytidine selectively increases gamma-globulin synthesis in a patient with beta-thalassemia. *N Engl J Med* 1982; 307:1469.
4. Doetschman T, Maeda N, Smithies O: Targeted mutation of the Hprt gene in mouse embryonic stem cells. *Proc Natl Acad Sci U S A* 1988; 85:8583.
5. Anderson WF: Human gene therapy—scientific and ethical considerations. *J Med Philos* 1985; 10:275.
6. Anderson WF: Prospects for human gene therapy in the born and unborn patient. *Clin Obstet Gynecol* 1986; 29:586.
7. Human Genetic Engineering, Hearings Before the Subcommittee on Investigations and Oversight of the Committee on Science and Technology (US House of Representatives 97th Congress No 170). Washington, DC, US Government Printing Office, 1983.
8. Cline MJ: Gene therapy: Current status. *Am J Med* 1987; 83:291.
9. Ledley FD: Somatic gene therapy for human disease: Background and prospects. *J Pediatr* 1987; 110:1.
10. Shapiro LJ, Comings DE, Jones OW, et al: New frontiers in genetic medicine. *Ann Intern Med* 1986; 104:527.

11. Markert ML, Hershfield MS, Schiff RI, et al: Adenosine deaminase and purine nucleoside phosphorylase deficiencies: Evaluation of therapeutic intervention in eight patients. *J Clin Immunol* 1987; 7:389.

12. Milewski EA: Discussions on human gene therapy. *Recomb DNA Tech Bull* 1986; 9:88.

13. Griffin JA: Recombinant DNA—Potential for gene therapy. *Am J Med Sci* 1985; 289:98.

14. Lacey M, Alpert S, Hanahan D: Bovine papillomavirus genome elicits skin tumours in transgenic mice. *Nature* 1986; 322:609.

15. Ling W, Patel MD, Lobel LI, et al: Insertion mutagenesis of embryonal carcinoma cells by retroviruses. *Science* 1985; 228:554.

16. Hayward WS, Neel BG, Astrin SM: Activation of a cellular oncogene by promoter insertion in ALV induced lymphoid leukosis. *Nature* 1981; 290:475.

17. Ledley FD, Grenett HE, McGinnis Shelnott M, et al: Retroviral mediated gene transfer of human phenylalanine hydroxylase into NIH 3T3 and hepatoma cells. *Proc Natl Acad Sci U S A* 1986; 83:409.

18. Ledley FD, Darlington GJ, Hahn T, et al: Retroviral gene transfer into primary hepatocytes: Implications for genetic therapy of liver-specific functions. *Proc Natl Acad Sci U S A* 1987; 84:5335.

19. Rund D, Dobkin C, Bank A: Regulated expression of amplified β globin genes. *Blood* 1987; 70:733.

20. Kwok WW, Schuening F, Stead RB, et al: Retroviral transfer of genes into canine hemopoietic progenitor cells in culture: A model for human gene therapy. *Proc Natl Acad Sci U S A* 1986; 83:4552.

21. Choudary PV, Tsuji S, Martin BM, et al: The molecular biology of Gaucher disease and the potential for gene therapy. *Cold Spring Harbor Symp Quant Biol* 1987; 51:1047.

22. Anson DS, Hock RA, Austen D: Towards gene therapy for hemophilia B. *Mol Biol Med* 1987; 4:11.

23. Palmer TD, Hock RA, Osborne WRA, et al: Efficient retrovirus mediated transfer and expression of a human adenosine deaminase gene in diploid skin fibroblasts from an adenosine deaminase deficient human. *Proc Natl Acad Sci U S A* 1987; 84:1055.

24. Kantoff PW, Kohn DB, Mitsuya D, et al: Correction of adenosine deaminase deficiency in cultured human T and B cells by retrovirus-mediated gene transfer. *Proc Natl Acad Sci U S A* 1986; 83:6563.

25. Hock RA, Miller AD: Retrovirus-mediated transfer and expression of drug resistant genes in human haemotopoietic progenitor cells. *Nature* 1986; 320:275.

26. Howell SB, Murphy MP, Johnson J, et al: Gene therapy for thioguanine-resistant human leukemia. *Mol Biol Med* 1987; 4:157.

27. Oppenheim A, Peleg A, Fibach E, et al: Efficient introduction of plasmid DNA into human hemopoietic cells by encapsidation in simian virus 40 pseudovirions. *Proc Natl Acad Sci U S A* 1986; 83:6925.

28. Robertson M: Gene therapy—desperate appliances. *Nature* 1986; 320:213.

29. Woo SLC, DiLella AG, Marvit J, et al: Molecular basis of phenylketonuria and potential somatic gene therapy. *Cold Spring Harbor Symp Quant Biol* 1986; 51:395.

30. Dick JE, Magli MC, Haszar D, et al: Introduction of a selectable gene into primitive stem cells capable of long term reconstitution of the hematopoietic system in W/WV mice. *Cell* 1985; 42:71.

31. Garver RI, Chytil A, Courtney M, et al: Clonal gene therapy: Transplanted mouse fibroblast clones express human alpha-1 antitrypsin gene in vivo. *Science* 1985; 237:762.

32. Cline MK: Perspectives for gene therapy. Inserting new genetic information

into mammalian cells by physical technique and viral vectors. *Pharmacol Ther* 1985; 29:69.

33. Doetschman TRC, Eistetter H, Katz M, et al: The in vitro development of blastocyst-derived embryonic stem cell lines: Formation of visceral yolk sac, blood islands and myocardium. *J Embryol Exp Morphol* 1985; 87:27.

34. Doestschman T, Williams P, Meada N: Establishment of hamster blastocyst-derived embryonic stem (ES) cells. *Dev Biol* 1988; 127:224.

35. Gossler A, Doetschman T, Korn R, et al: Transgenesis by means of blastocyst-derived embryonic stem cell lines. *Proc Natl Acad Sci U S A* 1986; 83:9065.

36. Rubenstein JLR, Nicolas JF, Jacob F: Introduction of genes into preimplantation mouse embryos by use of a defective recombinant retrovirus. *Proc Natl Acad Sci U S A* 1986; 83:366.

37. Touraine JL, Raudrant D, Royo C, et al: In-utero transplantation of stem cells in bare lymphocyte syndrome. *Lancet* 1989; 1:1382.

38. Gordon JW, Ruddle FH: Gene transfer into mouse embryos: Production of transgenic mice by pronuclear injection. *Methods Enzymol* 1983; 101:411.

39. Hammer RE, Pursel VG, Rexroad CE, et al: Production of transgenic rabbits, sheep and pig by microinjection. *Nature* 1985; 315:680.

40. Willadsen SM: Nuclear transplantation in sheep embryos. *Nature* 1986; 320:63.

41. Hammer RE, Palmiter RD, Brinster RL: Partial correction of murine hereditary growth disorder by germ line incorporation of a new gene. *Nature* 1984; 311:65.

42. Costantini F, Chada K, Magraw J: Correction of murine beta thalassemia by gene transfer into the germ line. *Science* 1986; 233:1192.

43. Stout JT, Chen HY, Brennand J, et al: Expression of human HPRT in the central nervous system of transgenic mice. *Nature* 1985; 317:250.

44. Monk M, Hardy K, Handyside A, et al: Preimplantation diagnosis of deficiency of hypoxanthine phosphoribosyl transferase in a mouse model for Lesh-Nyhan syndrome. *Lancet* 1987; 2:423.

45. Muller H: Human gene therapy: Possibilities and limitations. *Experientia* 1987; 43:375.

46. Seibel MM: A new era in reproductive technology. *N Engl J Med* 1988; 318:828.

47. Fletcher JC: Ethical issues in and beyond prospective clinical trials of human gene therapy. *J Med Philos* 1985; 10:293.

48. Walters L: The ethics of human gene therapy. *Nature* 1986; 320:225.

49. Drugan A, Evans WJ, Evans MI: Fetal organ and xenograft transplantation. *Am J Obstet Gynecol* 1989; 160:288.

50. National Institutes of Health/Recombinant DNA Advisory Committee: Points to consider in the design and submission of human somatic-cell gene therapy protocols. *Recomb DNA Tech Bull* 1985; 8:116.

Editor's Comment

What fun! What a joy to read these two chapters! Anyone who enjoys medical practice and appreciated "Star Wars" will read these chapters non-stop. Drs. Evans and Johnson and their colleagues take us on a medical trip to the future. This trip begins from what is today simple fetal surgery via a percutaneous needle (drainage of various fetal cavities such as ventricles and bladders) and goes through fetal medical therapy for cardiac arrhythmias and congenital adrenal hyperplasia, to fetal gene therapy. The only criticism this editor has is that he didn't want the trip to end!

Norman F. Gant, Jr., M.D.

Index

A

Abdominal hysterectomy, total, for pelvic
    inflammatory disease, 95
Abdominal pregnancy, 76
Abdominal sacrocolpopexy, 151, 153
Abscess, tubo-ovarian, diagnosis of, 92
Acquired immunodeficiency syndrome
    (AIDS)
  heterosexual transmission of, 385–386
  in obstetrical/gynecological patient,
      383–396
  in women, incidence of, 383–384
Adnexal mass, laparoscopy in diagnosis
    and treatment of, 301–305
Adnexectomy, unilateral, for pelvic
    inflammatory disease, 95
Adrenal hyperplasia, congenital, fetal
    therapy for, 416–417
Alcohol use in pregnancy, 370–374
  birth defects related to, 371–372
  fetal alcohol syndrome from, 370–371
  pathophysiology of, 370
  screening for, 372–374
α-Adrenergic agents in urinary
    incontinence management, 126
Anabolic steroids for osteoporosis, 172
Analgesia, endoscopic complications
    related to, 20
Androgens
  in menopause management, 160–161
  for osteoporosis, 172
Anesthesia, endoscopic complications
    related to, 18
Antibiotics for pelvic inflammatory
    disease, 94–95
Antidepressants, tricyclic, in urinary
    incontinence management, 126
Antiestrogens for osteoporosis, 172
Antrum, 213
Appendicitis laparoscopic management of,
    305–308
Arrhythmias, cardiac
  complicating pneumoperitoneum, 19
  fetal, medical therapy for, 415–416
Arteries supplying urethra, 107

Ascites, urinary, complicating endoscopy,
    22

B

Bacteria, endogenous, in microbial
    etiology of PID, 86–87
Bacterial vaginosis (BV) microorganisms in
    microbial etiology of PID, 86–87
Bacteriodes sp. in microbial etiology of
    PID, 86
Behavioral training in urinary
    incontinence management,
    124–125
Bethesda system for Papanicolaou smear
    interpretation, 265–269
  merits of, 266–267
  problems with, 267–268
    resolution of, 268–269
Biofeedback in urinary incontinence
    management, 125
Biology, molecular, of gynecological
    tumors, 347–361 (see also
    Molecular biology)
Biopsy
  blastocyst, in preimplantation diagnosis,
    240–241
  cone, for cervical intraepithelial
    neoplasia, 271
  embryo, in preimplantation diagnosis,
    239–240
  endometrial, in pelvic inflammatory
    disease diagnosis, 91
Biphosphonates for osteoporosis,
    171–172
Birth defects, alcohol-related, 371–372
Bladder
  anatomic support of, stress incontinence
    and, 114–116
  dysfunction of, intrinsic, stress
    incontinence and, 116–117
  mobilization of, for total laparoscopic
    hysterectomy, 43–44
Blastocyst, biopsy of, in preimplantation
    diagnosis, 240–241
Bleeding complicating endoscopy, 22

Blood count in ectopic pregnancy
diagnosis, 61
Blood supply to urethra, 107
Bone density, gonadotropin-releasing
hormone agonists and, 186
Bovie electrocautery for cervical
intraepithelial neoplasia, 272
Bowel injuries complicating endoscopy, 21
Bowel resection, laparoscopic, 310–316
Bradyarrhythmias complicating
pneumoperitoneum, 19
Breast
cancer of
estrogen use and, 163–164
GnRH agonists in, 200
disease of, fibrocystic, GnRH agonists in,
199

C

CA-125 assay for ovarian cancer, 303
CAGE questions in FAS screening, 373
Calcitonin for osteoporosis, 170–171
Calcium channel blockers in urinary
incontinence management, 126
Calcium for osteoporosis, 167–168
CA-125 levels in endometriosis, GnRH
and, 191
Cancer
breast
estrogen use and, 163–164
GnRH agonists in, 200
cervical
molecular biology of, 350–354
ultrasonic aspiration for, 337–338
endometrial
estrogen use and, 164–165
GnRH agonists in, 200
molecular biology of, 355–356
fallopian tube, ultrasonic aspiration for,
334–337
ovarian (see Ovary(ies), cancer of)
uterine, ultrasonic aspiration for,
337–338
vaginal, ultrasonic aspiration for,
340–341
vulvar
molecular biology of, 354–355
ultrasonic aspiration for, 338–340
Candidiasis, vaginal, HIV infection and,
386
Carbon dioxide gas for hysteroscopy, 8–9
Carbon dioxide laser therapy for cervical
intraepithelial neoplasia,
273–274

Carbon dioxide pneumoperitoneum,
complications of, 19–20
Cardiac arrhythmias complicating
pneumoperitoneum, 1919
Cardiovascular system, effects of estrogens
on, 162–163
Cefoxitin for pelvic inflammatory disease,
94
Central nervous system (CNS), side effect
of gonadotropin-releasing
hormone agonists affecting,
186–187
Cervical intraepithelial neoplasia (CIN),
261–278
Bovie electrocautery for, 272
carbon dioxide laser therapy for,
273–274
cone biopsy for, 271
cryotherapy for, 272–273
electrocoagulation diathermy for, 272
endocervical curettage for, 270–271
epidemiology of, 261–264
HIV infection and, 386–388
loop excision procedures for, 274–276
management of, 269–270
screening for, 261–264
treatment of
excisional vs. destructive methods in,
270–274
selection of technique for, 276–278
Cervical neoplasia, HIV infection and,
386–388
Cervical pregnancy, 75
Cervix, cancer of
molecular biology of, 350–354
ultrasonic aspiration for, 337–338
Chlamydia trachomatis in microbial
etiology of PID, 86
Circumferential culdotomy in total
laparoscopic hysterectomy, 44
Citrovorum factor in ectopic pregnancy
management, 73
Clindamycin for pelvic inflammatory
disease, 94–95
Cocaine use in pregnancy, 374–376
Coculture of embryos, 248–249
Colposcopy for "atypical" Papanicolaou
smear patient, 269–270
Condyloma of vulva, ultrasonic aspiration
for, 338–340
Cone biopsy for cervical intraepithelial
neoplasia, 271
Congenital adrenal hyperplasia, fetal
therapy for, 416–417

Continence, neurologic control of, 113–114

"Crack babies," 376

Cryopreservation, embryo, in augmenting pregnancy, 243–246

Cryotherapy for cervical intraepithelial neoplasia, 272–273

Cul-de-sac of Douglas, closure of, during hysterectomy, 144–148, 149

Culdocentesis in ectopic pregnancy diagnosis, 66–67

Culdoplasty, McCall, suspension with, in total laparoscopic hysterectomy, 44–45

Culdotomy, circumferential, in total laparoscopic hysterectomy, 44

Curettage
  dilation and, endometrial sampling by, in ectopic pregnancy diagnosis, 67–68
  endocervical, for cervical intraepithelial neoplasia, 270–271

Cystocele, stress incontinence and, 116

Cystometry in urinary incontinence evaluation, 121–123

Cytoreduction, laparoscopic, 316–317

D

Danazol for endometriosis, GnRH versus, 190

Detrusor hyperreflexia, definition of, 117

Detrusor instability, idiopathic, definition of, 117

Dextran 70 for hysteroscopy, 9

Dextrose 5

for hysteroscopy, 9–10

Diathermy, electrocoagulation, for cervical intraepithelial neoplasia, 272

Dilation and curettage, endometrial sampling by, in ectopic pregnancy diagnosis, 67–68

Ditropan in urinary incontinence management, 126

Donor insemination, HIV transmission through, 389

Doxycycline for pelvic inflammatory disease, 94

E

Ectopic pregnancy, 55–77
  abdominal, 76
  cervical, 75
  diagnosis of, 55–69
    abdominal tenderness in, 60
    blood count in, 61
    culdocentesis in, 66–67
    endometrial sampling by dilation and curettage in, 67–68
    estradiol in, 63
    human chorionic gonadotropin assays in, 61–62
    invasive testing in, 66–68
    laboratory evaluation in, 60–64
    laparoscopy in, 68
    laparotomy in, 68
    nonsurgical, algorithms for, 68–69, 70
    pelvic examination in, 60
    physical examination in, 58–60
    relaxin in, 63–64
    renin in, 64
    serum progesterone in, 62–63
    sonography in, 64–66
    vital signs in, 59
  epidemiology of, 55, 56
  history of, 57–58
  management of, 69–76
    fimbrial expression in, 72
    methotrexate in, 72–75
    nonsurgical, 72–75
    for persistent ectopic gestation, 72
    for ruptured vs. unruptured gestation, 69–71
    salpingectomy in, 72
    salpingostomy in, 71–72
    surgical approaches in, 71–72
  nontubal, 75–76
  ovarian, 76
  risk factors for, 57
  symptoms of, common, 57–58

Electrical stimulation in urinary incontinence management, 125–126

Electrocautery, Bovie, for cervical intraepithelial neoplasia, 272

Electrocoagulation diathermy for cervical intraepithelial neoplasia, 272

Embolism, carbon dioxide, complicating pneumoperitoneum, 19–20

Embryo(s)
  coculture of, 248–249
  cryopreservation of, in augmenting pregnancy, 243–246
  micromanipulation of, 238–243
  in assisted reproduction, 238–243

Embryo transfer, GnRH agonists in, 192–194

Endocervical curettage (ECC) for cervical intraepithelial neoplasia, 270–271

Endocrinology, reproductive, 157–258
  menopause and, 159–173 (see also
      Menopause)
Endometrial biopsy in pelvic inflammatory
      disease diagnosis, 91
Endometrial receptivity, effects of GnRH
      agonists on, 194
Endometriomas, gonadotropin-releasing
      hormone agonists for, 191
Endometriosis
  CA-125 levels in, GnRH and, 191
  danazol for, GnRH versus, 190
  gonadotropin-releasing hormone
      agonists for, 189–191
  stage IV, laparoscopic hysterectomy in,
      47–50
Endometrium
  ablation of
      GnRH agonists before, 199
      hysteroscopy in, 10
  cancer of
      estrogen use and, 164–165
      GnRH agonists in, 200
      molecular biology of, 355–356
  sampling of, by dilation and curettage in
      ectopic pregnancy diagnosis,
      67–68
Endoscopy, complications of, 13–24
  analgesic, 20
  anesthesia-related, 18
  bowel injuries as, 21
  in descriptive and cohort studies, 16–18
  incisional, 20–21
  infectious, 20–21
  pneumoperitoneum-related, 19–20
  surveys of, 13–16
  from trocar insertion, 22–23
  urologic injuries as, 21–22
  vascular, 22
  from Veress needle insertion, 22–23
Enterocele, preventing, 144–148
Estradiol in ectopic pregnancy diagnosis,
      63
Estrogens
  cardiovascular effects of, 162–163
  exogenous, in urinary incontinence
      management, 126–127
  in menopause management, 161–165
  for osteoporosis, 168–169
  replacement therapy with, GnRH
      agonists and, 197–198
  risks from use of, 163–165
Ethical issues in fetal gene therapy,
      431–432

Exercise(s)
  for osteoporosis, 167
  pelvic muscle, in urinary incontinence
      management, 125

F
Fallopian tube carcinoma, ultrasonic
      aspiration for, 334–337
Fertilization, in vitro (see In vitro
      fertilization (IVF))
Fetal alcohol syndrome (FAS), 370–371
  screening for, 372–374
Fetus
  gene therapy for, 423–432 (see also
      Gene therapy, fetal)
  medical therapy for, 414–420
      for cardiac anomalies, 415–417
      for congenital adrenal hyperplasia,
          416–417
      for fetal heart rhythm and rate
          abnormalities, 415–416
      for neural tube defects, 417–420
  obstructive uropathy in, in utero
      intervention for, 404–413
      karyotyping in, 407–408
      shunt procedures in, 409–413
      urine biochemistry for, 408–409
      visualization for, 406–407
  surgery on
      open, 413–414
      percutaneous, 402–413
  surgical/medical interventions in,
      401–420
  ventriculomegaly in, shunting for,
      402–404
Fibrocystic breast disease, GnRH agonists
      in, 199
Fibroids, uterine, gonadotropin-releasing
      hormone agonists for, 187–189
Fimbrial expression for ectopic pregnancy,
      72
Fitz-Hugh-Curtis syndrome (FHCS), 87–88
Fluoride for osteoporosis, 169–170
Folic acid in neural tube defect
      prevention, 417–420
Follicle compartment, structure of,
      213–214
Follicle stimulating hormone (FSH) in
      graafian follicle development,
      214–215
Folliculogenesis, 212–213
  growth factor concept of, 215–216
  two-gonadotropin/two-cell concept of,
      214–215

Forceps, Kleppinger bipolar, for
    laparoscopic hysterectomy, 34

G

Gamete intrafallopian transfer (GIFT),
    249–251
Gametes, micromanipulation of, 238–243
Gene insertion techniques, 426–427
Gene therapy, fetal, 423–432
    by addition of genetic material,
        424–425
    approaches to, 423–425
    ethical issues in, 431–432
    germ line, 429–430
    by modification of existing material,
        423–424
    by removal of genetic material, 424
    somatic cell, 425–429
Genetic engineering, enhancement of,
    430–431
Genital ulcer disease, HIV and, 390
Gentamicin for pelvic inflammatory
    disease, 95
Germ line gene therapy, 429–430
Gonadotropin-releasing hormone (GnRH)
    agonists of, 179–201
        activity of, 179–180
        bioavailability of, 182–183
        biochemistry of, 179–187
        bone density and, 186
        in breast cancer, 200
        central nervous system side effects of,
            186–187
        delivery systems for, 182–183
        emerging applications with, 198–200
        before endometrial ablation, 199
        in endometrial cancer, 200
        endometrial receptivity and, 194
        for endometriomas, 191
        for endometriosis, 189–191
        estrogen replacement therapy and,
            197–198
        in fibrocystic breast disease and
            mastalgia, 199
        granulosa cell function and, 194
        for hirsutism, 198–199
        in intrauterine insemination cycles,
            195
        in in vitro fertilization-embryo
            transfer, 192–194
        lipoprotein profiles and, 185–186
        mechanism of action of, 180–181
        menopausal symptoms from, 184–185
        oocyte quality and, 194

in ovarian cancer, 200
for ovulation induction, 191–196
pituitary function and, 187
in pregnancy, inadvertent use of, 187
for premenstrual syndrome, 198
progestin replacement therapy and,
    196
response to, in in vitro
    fertilization-embryo transfer
    cycles, prognostic value of, 194,
    195
side effects of, 184–187
structure of, 179–180
therapy with, initiation and
    monitoring of, 183–184
for triggering ovulation, 195–196
for uterine leiomyomas, 187–189
analogues of (GnRHa), in ovarian
    hyperstimulation for in vitro
    fertilization, 233, 235–237
pulsatile, in ovulation induction,
    221–222
Gonadotropins
human chorionic, assays of, in ectopic
    pregnancy diagnosis, 61–62
human menopausal
    in ovarian hyperstimulation for in
        vitro fertilization, 231–235
    in ovulation induction, 219
        with growth hormone cotreatment,
            220–221
Graafian follicle
development of, two-gonadotropin/
    two-cell concept of, 214–215
insulin-like growth factor system in,
    217–219
structure of, 213–214
Granulosa cells, 213
function of, effect of GnRH agonists on,
    194
Growth factor concept of folliculogenesis,
    215–216
Growth hormone, human menopausal
    gonadotropin cotreatment with, in
    ovulation induction, 220–221
Gynecological tumors, molecular biology
    of, 347–361 (see also Molecular
    biology)
Gynecologic diseases, HIV infection and,
    386–389

H

Habit training in urinary incontinence
    management, 125

Haemophilus influenzae in microbial etiology of PID, 86
Halban cul-de-sac closure, 145, 147–148
Heroin use in pregnancy, 377–378
Hirsutism, gonadotropin-releasing hormone agonists for, 198–199
Human chorionic gonadotropin (hCG), assays of, in ectopic pregnancy diagnosis, 61–62
Human immunodeficiency virus (HIV) infection
  gynecologic diseases and, 386–389
  heterosexual transmission of, 385–386
  interaction of, with other sexually transmitted diseases, 389–391
  in obstetrical/gynecological patient, 383–396
  perinatal transmission of, 391
  pregnancy and, 391–395
  in women, incidence of, 383–384
Human menopausal gonadotropins (hMG)
  in ovarian hyperstimulation for in vitro fertilization, 231–235
  in ovulation induction, 219
    with growth hormone cotreatment, 220–221
Human papillomavirus (HPV), cervical cancer and, 350–354
Hysterectomy
  adjunct support to vaginal cuff during, 148–153
  classical abdominal Semm, 30–31
  laparoscopic, 292–299
    procedure for, 295–299
    radical, 309–310
    supracervical, 30–31
  laparoscopy in, 29–52 (*see also* Laparoscopic hysterectomy (LH))
  preventing enterocele following, 144–148, 149
  preventing vaginal prolapse at time of, 142–144
  total abdominal, for pelvic inflammatory disease, 95
  vaginal
    diagnostic laparoscopy with, 30
    laparoscopic-assisted, 30, 293
Hysteroscopy, 3–10
  complications of, 6
  contraindications for, 5–6
  historical perspective on, 3
  indications for, 3–5
  media for, 8–10
  technique for, 6–8
  therapeutic considerations on, 10

I

Incontinence, urinary, 103–132 (*see also* Urinary incontinence)
Infectious complications of endoscopy, 20–21
Infertility
  in endometriosis patients, GnRH and, 190–191
  male, gamete micromanipulation in therapy of, 242–243
Insemination, donor, HIV transmission through, 389
Insulin-like growth factor (IGF) system in graafian follicle, 217–219
Intrauterine insemination cycles, GnRH agonists in, 195
In vitro fertilization (IVF)
  donor oocyte, 246–248
  GnRH agonists in, 192–194
  ovarian hyperstimulation, controlled, for, 231–238
    luteal phase in, 238
    progesterone monitoring in, 237–238
    treatment schedules for, 231–237

K

Kegel exercises in urinary incontinence management, 125
Kleppinger bipolar forceps for laparoscopic hysterectomy, 34

L

Laparoscopic-assisted vaginal hysterectomy, 30
Laparoscopic hysterectomy (LH), 29–52
  complications of, 45–46
  contraindications to, 32–33
  definition of, 30
  equipment for, 33–34
  goal of, 29
  indications for, 31–32
  with laparoscopic rectocele repair, 50
  with laparoscopic uterosacral-vaginal suspension, 50
  patient positioning for, 34–35
  postoperative considerations in, 45
  preoperative preparation for, 34–35
  scoring system for, 50–52
  special problems related to, 46–50
  in stage IV endometriosis, 47–50
  total, 30
    bladder mobilization for, 43–44

circumferential culdotomy in, 44
exploration for, 43
incisions for, 35–42
laparoscopic vaginal vault closure in, 44–45
suspension with McCall culdoplasty in, 44–45
technique for, 35–45
underwater examination in, 45
upper uterine blood supply in, 44
ureteral dissection for, 43
uterine vessel ligation in, 44
vaginal preparation for, 43
with very large fibroid uterus, 46–47
Laparoscopic pelvic reconstruction (LPR), 31
Laparoscopic supracervical hysterectomy (LSH), 30–31
Laparoscopy
diagnostic, with vaginal hysterectomy, 30
in ectopic pregnancy diagnosis, 68
in gynecologic oncology management, 283–321
in hysterectomy, 29–52 (see also Laparoscopic hysterectomy (LH))
operative video, 283
in adnexal mass diagnosis and treatment, 301–305
advantages of, 284–285
anesthesia for, 288
for appendicitis, 305–308
closed, 288–292
disadvantages of, 285
future advances in, 309–320
bowel resection as, 310–316
cytoreduction as, 316–317
radical hysterectomy as, 309–310
for hysterectomy, 292–299
procedure for, 295–299
for lymphadenectomy, 299–300
positioning for, 286–287
preoperative preparation for, 285–286
procedure for, 288
second-look, 309
splenectomy as, 317–320
in pelvic inflammatory disease diagnosis, 91–92
vaginal hysterectomy assisted by, 293
Laparotomy in ectopic pregnancy diagnosis, 68
Laser, carbon dioxide, for cervical intraepithelial neoplasia, 273–274

Leiomyomas, uterine, gonadotropin-releasing hormone agonists for, 187–189
Lipoprotein profiles, gonadotropin-releasing hormone agonists and, 185–186
Loop excision procedures for cervical intraepithelial neoplasia, 274–276
Luteal phase in ovarian hyperstimulation for in vitro fertilization, 238
Luteinizing hormone (LH) in graafian follicle development, 214
Lymphadenectomy by laparoscopy, 299–300
Lymphatics of urethra, 107

M

Male infertility, gamete micromanipulation in therapy of, 242–243
Marijuana use in pregnancy, 377
Marshall-Marchetti-Krantz (MMK) procedure for urinary incontinence, 127, 128, 129–132
Mastalgia, GnRH agonists in, 199
McCall cul-de-plasty, modified, 143, 144
McCall culdoplasty, suspension with, in total laparoscopic hysterectomy, 44–45
Menopause, 159–173
osteoporosis and, 165–172 (see also Osteoporosis)
replacement therapy for, 160–165
androgens in, 160–161
estrogens in, 161–165
progestins in, 161–165
symptoms of, from gonadotropin-releasing hormone agonists, 184–185
Methadone maintenance in pregnancy, 378
Methotrexate in ectopic pregnancy management, 72–75
Micromanipulation
of embryos
in assisted hatching, 243
and gametes, 238–243
for preimplantation diagnosis, 239–242
of gametes in male infertility therapy, 242–243
Molecular biology
of cervical cancer, 350–354

Molecular biology *(cont.)*
  of endometrial cancer, 355–356
  of gynecological tumors, 347–361
    background of, 347–349
  of ovarian cancer, 356–360
  of vulvar cancer, 354–355
Moschcowitz procedure for deep
        cul-de-sac closure, 145–146, 148,
        149
Muscles of urethra, 107–110
Mycoplasma hominis in microbial etiology
        of PID, 86

N

Needle urethropexy for urinary
        incontinence, 127, 128–129
Neisseria gonorrhoeae in microbial
        etiology of PID, 86
Nerves supplying urethra, 107, 110–111
Neural tube defects (NTDs), fetal therapy
        for, 417–420
Neurologic examination in urinary
        incontinence evaluation, 120

O

Obstetrics, 367–434
  fetal surgical/medical interventions in,
        401–420 (*see also under* Fetus)
  HIV/AIDS in, 383–396 (*see also*
        Acquired immunodeficiency
        syndrome (AIDS); Human
        immunodeficiency virus (HIV))
  substance abuse in pregnancy and,
        369–379 (*see also* Substance
        abuse in pregnancy)
Obstructive uropathy in fetus, in utero
        intervention for, 404–413
  karyotyping in, 407–408
  shunt procedure in, 409–413
  urine biochemistry for, 408–409
  visualization for, 406–407
Oncology, gynecologic
  laparoscopy in management of, 283–321
        (*see also* Laparoscopy, operative
        video)
  ultrasonic surgical aspirator in, 325–343
        (*see also* Ultrasonic surgical
        aspiratory (USA))
Oocyte(s)
  donor, in vitro fertilization with, 246–248
  quality of, effect of GnRH agonists on,
        194
Operative video laparoscopy, 283
Opioid use in pregnancy, 377–378

Osteoporosis, 165–172
  anabolic steroids for, 172
  androgens for, 172
  antiestrogens for, 172
  biphosphonates for, 171–172
  calcitonin for, 170–171
  calcium for, 167–168
  estrogen for, 168–169
  exercise for, 167
  fluoride for, 169–170
  laboratory workup for, 166–167
  progestins for, 172
  therapeutic intervention for, 167–172
  thiazides for, 172
  vitamin D for, 167–168
Ovarian pregnancy, 76
Ovary(ies)
  ablation of, in polycystic ovary disease,
        ovulation induction after, 223
  cancer of
    GnRH agonists in, 200
    molecular biology of, 356–360
    risk factors for, 301–302
    serologic testing for, 302–303
    signs and symptoms of, 302
    ultrasonic aspiration for, 334–337
  hyperstimulation of, controlled, for in
        vitro fertilization, 231–238
    luteal phase in, 238
    progesterone monitoring in, 237–238
    treatment schedules for, 231–237
  polycystic, ovulation induction in
        patient with, GnRH agonist
        therapy for, 191–192
Ovulation
  induction of
    basic advances in, 211–219
    clinical advances in, 219–223
    following ovarian ablation in
        polycystic ovary disease, 223
    gonadotropin-releasing hormone
        agonist therapy for, 191–196
    human menopausal gonadotropin
        cotreatment with growth hormone
        in, 220–221
    human menopausal gonadotropins in,
        219
    in premature ovarian failure, 222–223
    pulsatile gonadotropin-releasing
        hormone in, 221–222
    superovulation and, 219–220
  triggering, GnRH agonist for, 195–196
Oxybutynin in urinary incontinence
        management, 126

P

Papanicolaou smear
  "atypical", management of, 269–270
  in cervical intraepithelial neoplasia
        screening, 262–264
  interpretation of, Bethesda system for,
        265–269
  specimen collection for, improvements
        in, 264–265
Papillomaviruses, human, cervical cancer
        and, 350–354
Pelvic examination in ectopic pregnancy
        diagnosis, 60
Pelvic inflammatory disease (PID), 85–98
  atypical, 88
  diagnosis of, 88–92
     criteria for, 88–91
     endometrial biopsy in, 91
     laparoscopy in, 91–92
     ultrasound in, 91
  epidemiology of, 85
  Fitz-Hugh-Curtis syndrome and, 87–88
  HIV and, 389–390
  microbiology of, 85–87
  pathogenesis of, 85–87
  prevention of, 96–97
  sequelae of, long-term, 96
  treatment of, 92–96
     medical, 93–95
     surgical, 96
Pelvic muscle exercises in urinary
        incontinence management, 125
Pelvic reconstruction, laparoscopic, 31
Penicillins for pelvic inflammatory
        disease, 95
Peptostreptococcus sp. in microbial
        etiology of PID, 86
Percutaneous fetal surgery, 402–413
Percutaneous transabdominal intrauterine
        vesicoamniotic shunting for
        obstructive uropathy in fetus, 410,
        411
Pharmacologic therapy of urinary
        incontinence, 126
Phenylpropanolamine (PPA) in urinary
        incontinence management, 126
Physiotherapy in urinary incontinence
        management, 125–126
Pituitary function, gonadotropin-releasing
        hormone agonists and, 187
Pneumoperitoneum, complications of,
        19–20
Polar body analysis in preimplantation
        diagnosis, 241–242

Polycystic ovaries, ovulation induction in
        patient with, GnRH agonist
        therapy for, 191–192
Polycystic ovary disease, ovarian ablation
        in, ovulation induction after, 223
Pregnancy
  alcohol use in, 370–374 (*see also*
        Alcohol use in pregnancy)
  ectopic, 55–77 (*see also* Ectopic
        pregnancy)
  HIV infection and, 391–395
  inadvertent use of
        gonadotropin-releasing hormone
        agonists during, 187
  substance abuse in, 369–379 (*see also*
        Substance abuse in pregnancy)
Premature ovarian failure (POF), 222–223
Premenstrual syndrome (PMS),
        gonadotropin-releasing hormone
        agonists for, 198
Progesterone
  monitoring of, in ovarian
        hyperstimulation for in vitro
        fertilization, 237–238
  serum, in ectopic pregnancy diagnosis,
        62–63
Progestins
  in menopause management, 161–165
  for osteoporosis, 172
  replacement therapy with, GnRH
        agonists and, 196
Propantheline in urinary incontinence
        management, 126
Pulsatile gonadotropin-releasing hormone
        in ovulation induction, 221–222

Q

Q-tip testing in urinary incontinence
        evaluation, 121
Quinolones for pelvic inflammatory
        disease, 95

R

Rectocele repair, laparoscopic,
        laparoscopic hysterectomy with, 50
Relaxin in ectopic pregnancy diagnosis,
        63–64
Renin in ectopic pregnancy diagnosis, 64
Reproductive endocrinology, 157–258 (see
        also Endocrinology, reproductive)
Reproductive technology, assisted,
        231–252
  coculture of embryos in, 248–249
  cryopreservation in, 243–246

Reproductive technology (cont.)
  micromanipulation of embryos and
      gametes in, 238–243
  ovarian hyperstimulation for in vitro
      fertilization in, 231–238 (see also
      Ovary(ies), hyperstimulation of,
      controlled, for in vitro
      fertilization)
  tubal transfer procedures in, 249–251
  in vitro fertilization as, donor oocyte,
      246–248
Respiratory pathogens in microbial
    etiology of PID, 86
Retropubic urethropexy for urinary
    incontinence, 127, 128, 129–132

S

Sacrocolpopexy, abdominal, 151, 153
Sacrospinous ligament fixation for vaginal
    support, 150–151, 152
Salpingectomy
  bilateral, for pelvic inflammatory
      disease, 95
  for ectopic pregnancy, 72
Salpingitis, atypical, 88
Salpingo-oophorectomy, bilateral, for
    pelvic inflammatory disease, 95
Salpingostomy for ectopic pregnancy,
    71–72
Semm hysterectomy, classical abdominal,
    30–31
Serologic testing for ovarian cancer,
    302–303
Sexually transmitted diseases (STDs),
    interaction of HIV with, 389–391
Sexually transmitted pathogens in
    microbial etiology of PID, 85–86
Shoulder-hand syndrome complicating
    pneumoperitoneum, 20
Shunting for fetal ventriculomegaly,
    402–404
Sling procedures for urinary incontinence,
    129
Somatic cell gene therapy, 425–429
Sonography in ectopic pregnancy
    diagnosis, 64–66
Sphincter, artificial, for urinary
    incontinence, 129
Splenectomy, laparoscopic, 317–320
Steroids, anabolic, for osteoporosis, 172
Streptococcus pneumoniae in microbial
    etiology of PID, 86
Streptococcus pyogenes in microbial
    etiology of PID, 86

Stress incontinence, definition of, 117
Substance abuse in pregnancy
  with alcohol, 370–374
  with cocaine, 374–376
  with marijuana, 377
  with opioids, 377–378
Superovulation, 219–220
Supracervical hysterectomy, laparoscopic,
    30–31
Syphilis, HIV and, 390

T

T-ACE questions in FAS screening,
    373–374
Theca externa, 213–214
Thiazides for osteoporosis, 172
Thoracoamniotic shunting for obstructive
    uropathy in fetus, 412–413
Transabdominal sonography in ectopic
    pregnancy diagnosis, 64–65
Transvaginal sonography in ectopic
    pregnancy diagnosis, 65–66
Tricyclic antidepressants in urinary
    incontinence management, 126
Trocar insertion, endoscopic
    complications involving, 22–23
Trocar sleeves for laparoscopic
    hysterectomy, 33–34
Tubal transfer procedures, 249–251
Tubo-ovarian abscess (TOA), diagnosis of,
    92
Tumors, gynecological, molecular biology
    of, 347–361 (see also Molecular
    biology)
Tumor suppressor genes, 348–349
Two-gonadotropin/two-cell concept,
    214–215

U

Ulcers, genital, HIV and, 390
Ultrasonic surgical aspirator (USA)
  for cervical malignancy, 337–338
  for fallopian tube carcinoma, 334–337
  in gynecologic oncology, 333–341
  historical background of, 325–327
  for ovarian carcinoma, 334–337
  pathologic analysis of aspirates from,
      341–343
  physics of, 327–331
  unit for, 331–333
  for uterine malignancy, 337–338
  for vaginal malignancy, 340–341
  wound healing following, 341
Ultrasound in pelvic inflammatory disease
    diagnosis, 91

Ureter
    dissection of, in total laparoscopic
        hysterectomy, 43
    injuries to, complicating endoscopy,
        22
Urethra
    anatomy of, 107–111
    "sphincter" mechanism of
        external, 113
        internal, 112–113
Urethral pressure profilometry in urinary
        incontinence evaluation, 123–124
Urethrocystometry in urinary incontinence
        evaluation, 123
Urethropexy
    needle, for urinary incontinence, 127,
        128–129
    retropubic, for urinary incontinence,
        127, 128, 129–132
Urge incontinence, 118–119
Urinary incontinence, 103–132
    anatomy and, 106–107
    contemporary concepts of, 107–111
    evaluation of, 117–124
        cystometry in, 121–123
        history in, 118–120
        laboratory tests in, 121
        neurologic examination in, 120
        physical examination in, 120
        Q-tip testing in, 121
        urethral pressure profilometry in,
            123–124
        urethrocystometry in, 123
        uroflowmetry in, 124
    management of
        nonsurgical, 124–127
        surgical, 127–132
    overflow, definition of, 117
    pathophysiology of, 111–117
    scope of problem of, 103–106
    stress, definition of, 117
    urge, 118–119
Uroflowmetry in urinary incontinence
        evaluation, 124
Urologic injuries complicating endoscopy,
        21–22
Uropathy, obstructive, in fetus, in utero
        intervention for, 404–413
    karyotyping in, 407–408
    shunt procedures in, 409–413
    urine biochemistry for, 408–409
    visualization for, 406–407
Uterine vessel ligation in total
        laparoscopic hysterectomy, 44

Uterosacral-vaginal suspension,
        laparoscopic, laparoscopic
        hysterectomy with, 60
Uterovaginal prolapse, 149, 150, 151
Uterus
    carcinoma of, ultrasonic aspiration for,
        337–338
    fibroid, very large, laparoscopic
        hysterectomy with, 46–47
    leiomyomas of, gonadotropin-releasing
        hormone agonists for, 187–189
    perforation of, complicating endoscopy,
        23
    upper, blood supply of, in total
        laparoscopic hysterectomy, 44

V

Vagina, cancer of, ultrasonic aspiration
        for, 340–341
Vaginal cuff, adjunct support to, during
        hysterectomy, 148–153
Vaginal hysterectomy
    diagnostic laparoscopy with, 30
    laparoscopic-assisted, 30, 293
Vaginal intraepithelial neoplasia (VAIN),
        ultrasonic aspiration for,
        340–341
Vaginal vault closure, laparoscopic, in
        total laparoscopic hysterectomy,
        44–45
Vaginal vault prolapse, 141–155
    anatomy related to, 141
    management of, 153–155
    prevention of
        adjunct support to vaginal cuff in,
            148–153
        enterocele prevention and, 144–148
        at time of hysterectomy, 142–144
Vaginal vesicourethropexy for urinary
        incontinence, 127, 128
Vaginitis, HIV infection and, 386
Valtchev uterine mobilizer for
        laparoscopic hysterectomy, 33
Vascular injuries complicating endoscopy,
        22
Venous drainage of urethra, 107
Ventriculomegaly, fetal, shunting for,
        402–404
Veress needle insertion, endoscopic
        complications involving, 22–23
Vesicourethropexy, vaginal, for urinary
        incontinence, 127, 128
Vitamin D for osteoporosis, 167–168

Voiding, prompted, in urinary
    incontinence management, 125
Vulva, cancer of
  molecular biology of, 354–355
  ultrasonic aspiration for, 338–340
Vulvar intraepithelial neoplasia (VIN)
  ultrasonic aspiration for, 338–340
  vulvar cancer and, 354

W

Wound healing after ultrasonic aspiration,
    341

Z

Zygote intrafallopian transfer (ZIFT), 249,
    250, 251